Bone Marrow Disorders
THE BIOLOGICAL BASIS
OF TREATMENT

Bone Marrow Disorders
THE BIOLOGICAL BASIS OF TREATMENT

A.J. BARRETT MD, FRCPath
Department of Haematology, Royal Postgraduate Medical School
Hammersmith Hospital, London

M.Y. GORDON DSc, FRCPath
Leukaemia Research Fund Centre, Institute of Cancer Research
Chester Beatty Laboratories, London

FOREWORD BY
M.F. GREAVES PhD, MRCPath, Hon MRCP
Professor of Cell Biology and Director
Leukaemia Research Fund Centre, Institute of Cancer Research
Chester Beatty Laboratories, London

OXFORD
BLACKWELL SCIENTIFIC PUBLICATIONS
LONDON EDINBURGH BOSTON
MELBOURNE PARIS BERLIN VIENNA

© 1985, 1993 by
Blackwell Scientific Publications
Editorial Offices:
Osney Mead, Oxford OX2 0EL
25 John Street, London WC1N 2BL
23 Ainslie Place, Edinburgh EH3 6AJ
238 Main Street, Cambridge
   Massachusetts 02142, USA
54 University Street, Carlton
   Victoria 3053, Australia

Other Editorial Offices:
Librairie Arnette SA
2 rue Casimir-Delavigne
75006 Paris
France

Blackwell Wissenschafts-Verlag
Meinekestrasse 4
D-1000 Berlin 15
Germany

Blackwell MZV
Feldgasse 13
A-1238 Wien
Austria

All rights reserved. No part of this
publication may be reproduced, stored
in a retrieval system, or transmitted,
in any form or by any means,
electronic, mechanical, photocopying,
recording or otherwise without the
prior permission of the copyright
owner.

First published 1985
Second edition 1993

Set by
Excel Typesetters Company, Hong Kong
Printed and bound in Great Britain
by Hartnolls Ltd, Bodmin, Cornwall

DISTRIBUTORS

Marston Book Services Ltd
PO Box 87
Oxford OX2 0DT
(*Orders*: Tel: 0865 791155
         Fax: 0865 791927
         Telex: 837515)

USA
Blackwell Scientific Publications, Inc.
238 Main Street
Cambridge, MA 02142
(*Orders*: Tel: 800 759-6102
         617 876-7000)

Canada
Times Mirror Professional Publishing
Ltd
130 Flaska Drive
Markham, Ontario L6G 1B8
(*Orders*: Tel: 800 268-4178
         416 470-6739)

Australia
Blackwell Scientific Publications Pty
Ltd
54 University Street
Carlton, Victoria 3053
(*Orders*: Tel: 03 347-5552)

A catalogue record for this title is
available from the British Library

ISBN 0-632-03353-3

Library of Congress
Cataloging in Publication Data

Barrett, A.J. (Austin John)
   Bone marrow disorders:
   the biological basis of treatment /
   A.J. Barrett, M.Y. Gordon.
      p.   cm.
   Gordon's name appears first
   on the earlier edition.
   Includes bibliographical references
   and index.
   ISBN 0-632-03353-3
   1. Bone marrow – Diseases.
   2. Hematopoietic stem cells.
   I. Gordon, M.Y. (Myrtle Y.)
   II. Title.
      [DNLM: 1. Bone Marrow Diseases.
   WH 380 B274b]
   RC645.7.B37   1993
   616.4'1 – dc20

Contents

FOREWORD, viii

PREFACE TO THE SECOND EDITION, ix

PREFACE TO THE FIRST EDITION, xi

1 ADVANCES IN EXPERIMENTAL HAEMATOLOGY, 1
   Introduction, 1
   Measurement of haemopoietic stem cells, 4
     Blast colony-forming assay, 5
     The long-term bone marrow culture system, 6
     Colony formation on stromal layers, 7
     Proliferation in multiwells, 8
     Transplantation in immune-deprived mice, 9
   Molecular biology of growth factors and their receptors, 10
     Molecular cloning of the HGFs and interleukins, 12
     Structure–function relationships, 18
     Molecular cloning of the HGF receptors, 21
     Kinetics of growth factor binding to receptors, 28
     Cell surface expression of growth factor receptors, 30
     Receptor characterization, 35
     Receptor regulation, 36
     Chromosomal localization of growth factor and receptor genes, 37
     Signal transduction, 40
   Biological effects of growth factor–target cell interactions, 43
     Human HGFs and their targets, 44
     The influence of serum-free culture conditions, 50
     Enriched progenitor cell populations and the influence of accessory cells, 51
     Physiology of the growth factor response, 53
   References, 60

2 TREATMENT STRATEGIES IN BONE MARROW DISORDERS, 73
   Haematological malignancies, 73
     Introduction, 73
     Relevance of malignant cell biology to treatment, 74
     Treatment implications, 80
     Treatment planning, 84
     Treatment strategies in individual haematological malignancies, 93
   Congenital bone marrow disorders, 112
     Introduction, 112
     Bone marrow transplantation, 114
     Cytokines, growth factors and other agents, 115
     Gene therapy, 117
   Aplastic anaemia and drug-induced cytopenias, 122
     Pathophysiology of aplastic anaemia, 122
     Treatment, 125
     Drug-induced cytopenias, 127
   References, 133

3 MOLECULAR PATHOLOGY OF HAEMATOLOGICAL DISORDERS, 141
  Introduction, 141
  Methods, 143
    Morphology and cytochemistry, 143
    Phenotype, 144
    Karyotype, 144
    Southern analysis, 145
    Northern analysis, 146
    Restriction fragment length polymorphisms, 147
    The polymerase chain reaction, 147
    Altered protein products, 149
    Progenitor assays, 150
    Tracking and localizing cells *in vivo*, 150
  Genes and proteins of special interest, 152
  Applications to haematological disease, 156
    Chronic myeloid leukaemia, 156
    Myeloproliferative disorders, 162
    Acute myeloid leukaemia, 163
    Myelodysplasia, 167
    Bone marrow transplantation, 168
    Lymphoid neoplasia, 172
    Aplastic anaemia, 178
    Haemoglobinopathies, 179
    Other inherited deficiencies, 180
    Overview, 181
  References, 181

4 BONE MARROW TRANSPLANTATION, 190
  Historical introduction, 190
  Current results of BMT, 194
  Animal models of BMT, 195
  Stem cells and engraftment, 200
  Recovery of haemopoiesis after BMT, 204
  Immune recovery, 208
  Tissue typing and matching, 211
  Clinical outcome and it relationship to the source of stem cells used for transplantation, 224
  Cure of leukaemia by allogeneic BMT, 225
  Cure of haematological malignancies by ABMT, 233
  Cure of non-malignant disorders by BMT, 238
  GVHD, 242
  Pathophysiology of acute GVHD, 245
  Prevention and treatment of GVHD, 248
  Graft failure, 253
  Infections after BMT, 258
  Non-haematological complications after BMT, 266
  References, 271

5 CLINICAL APPLICATION OF HAEMOPOIETIC GROWTH FACTORS, 281
  Introduction, 281
    General features of HGF responses *in vivo*, 282

Experimental background, 288
  Preclinical models of growth factor therapy, 288
  Effects of high-level, continuous exposure to HGFs *in vivo*, 289
Principles and practice of HGF therapy, 292
  Administration, 292
  Toxicity, 293
  Contraindications, 294
Clinical HGF therapy, 296
  Treatment of aplastic anaemia with HGFs, 297
  Treatment of neutropenia with HGFs, 299
  Treatment of thrombocytopenia with HGFs, 301
  Treatment of anaemia with HGFs, 302
  Effects of HGF treatment on neoplastic cell growth, 304
  Treatment of myelodysplasia with HGFs, 305
  Treatment of acute myeloid leukaemia with HGFs, 307
  Treatment of non-myeloid leukaemias with HGFs, 308
  Treatment of infections with HGFs, 308
  The value of HGFs in chemotherapy, 309
  The value of HGFs in bone marrow transplantation, 311
Overview, 314
References, 316

6 IMMUNOTHERAPY, 324
Historical introduction, 324
Tumour immunobiology, 326
  Relationship between the immune system and haematological malignancies, 326
  Experimental methods for the study of immune interactions with haematological malignancies, 329
  Tumour cells as targets for immune attack, 336
  Immune responses against haematological malignancies, 348
  NK and LAK cells, 349
  Lymphocytes expressing the $\alpha\beta$ receptor, 353
  $\gamma\delta$ T cells, 354
  Other cells, 354
Immunotherapy, 355
  Cytokines and interleukins, 355
  Interferons, 358
  Clinical applications of interferons, 361
  IL-2, 367
  TNF, 379
  IL-4, 382
  IL-6, 382
  M-CSF, 382
  Tumour-specific immune cells, 383
  Antibodies, 387
  Future developments, 393
References, 395

INDEX, 405

Foreword

If a week is a long time in politics, then 7 years in the field of bone marrow biology and pathology is almost a geological time span, given the remarkable pace of recent developments. It is therefore both inevitable and desirable that Drs Barrett and Gordon should provide us with a completely new edition of their successful book. As previously, the attraction of the publication is in its impressive breadth of coverage and the complementary interests and knowledge which a laboratory based scientist and clinical researcher have skillfully interwoven. This provides for a more cohesive set of chapters than is usually possible in multi-authored books.

In this edition, the newer molecular data takes a prominent position particularly with respect to growth factors, their receptors and oncogenes. The biology presented is of very considerable interest in its own right but the spirit and the special appeal of the book lies in the application of fundamental laboratory based investigations to the management of patients with bone marrow disorders. The timing could hardly be more appropriate as we are now in the exciting early phases of these clinical applications. Barrett and Gordon are to be congratulated on providing such a comprehensive, lucid and altogether excellent new book.

Mel F. Greaves

Preface to the Second Edition

We live in exciting times. The past decade has witnessed major advances in our understanding of the function of the bone marrow and the cytokines and growth factors which regulate haemopoiesis and immune function. The technological advances that have enabled us to probe into normal and malignant cells and their cytokine products, and characterize events at a molecular level have also facilitated the development of new treatments for malignant and non-malignant bone marrow diseases. Investigation and treatment are closely linked as never before and the interval between the identification, for example, of a new growth factor, its molecular characterization, synthesis and clinical application, has diminished remarkably. The shrinking interval between scientific discovery and clinical application is well illustrated by the time elapsed between the description of the first granulocyte-monocyte colony-stimulating factor in the mouse by Bradley and Metcalf in 1967, its identification in man by Pike and Robinson in 1970, its subsequent molecular and genetic characterization in the 1980s and its first use in clinical trials in man, about 20 years later. This 20 year story contrasts markedly with the brief interval elapsing between the first description of the stem cell growth factor (SCF) in 1987 and the first production of SCF for clinical trials in 1991 – an interval of only 4 years. The consequence of these technological advances has been the availability for clinical use of a large variety of growth factors and cytokines. Almost inevitably they have been applied empirically because the pace of advance has outstripped detailed understanding of the physiology of these factors. Clinicians need to know as much as possible about the underlying biology of the potent therapeutic weapons they now wield, while scientific researchers need to perceive the potential clinical applications of the biologically potent agents that they can so readily produce.

In this book, we attempt to bring together the advances that have occurred in the basic biology of bone marrow stem cells, the immune system and cytokines and growth factors relevant to the clinical advances that are occurring in the treatment of malignant and non-malignant bone marrow disorders. We have concentrated on reviewing the new advances in the biology of stem cells, haemopoietic growth factors, cytokines and their receptors, attempting to show how this knowledge is used both in the characterization and detection of disease states and in treatment strategies. In subsequent chapters we describe the principles in biology of bone marrow transplantation, the application of haemopoietic growth factors and the rational basis for the use of immunotherapeutic approaches in the treatment of haematological malignancies. We hope that this book will find a place on the shelves of clinicians and research scientists who have the common goal of improving the lot of patients with life-threatening bone marrow diseases.

ACKNOWLEDGEMENTS

We wish to acknowledge the help of our many colleagues who have borne with us while we struggled over our word processors. In particular Ed Kanfer for his enormous patience and help in reviewing the manuscript and to Sue Robson who typed much of it.

John Barrett and Myrtle Gordon

Preface to the First Edition

It is nearly 20 years since Bradley and Metcalf in Australia and Pluznik and Sachs independently in Israel first showed that it was possible to identify haemopoietic progenitor cells from mice by *in vitro* cloning techniques. The later application of the technique to studies on human bone marrow cells brought about a revolution in our understanding of the nature of haemopoiesis and the abnormalities found in bone marrow disorders. Advances in the treatment and support of patients have followed this broader understanding. With the advent of molecular biology, we are on the threshold of using *in vitro* cell culture methods for even more fundamental investigations, and of applying advanced experimental techniques directly to treating haematological disease.

It is, therefore, appropriate to review the achievements that have established the biological basis for clinical problems in haematology. This book is intended to provide for the clinician the experimental background to the diseases that he treats and, for the experimentalist, an outline of the practical problems encountered in the management of bone marrow disorders.

We have largely restricted our review to work done with human bone marrow cells, rather than relying on more extensive but less germane studies in animals. We have also restricted ourselves to blood disorders where culture work has provided important insight into the pathogenesis of disease or has contributed directly to patient management.

We would like to thank Dr Ted Gordon-Smith for writing the foreword to this volume and Drs John Goldman, Donald McCarthy, Jill Hibbin and Alastair Munro for their helpful criticism and advice. We would also like to thank Drs Inês Nolasco, Jill Hibbin, Donald McCarthy, Sally Pittman and Lyndal Kearney for some of the illustrations and Jan Brayley for typing the manuscript.

Myrtle Gordon and John Barrett

Chapter 1
Advances in Experimental Haematology

Introduction, 1
Measurement of haemopoietic stem cells, 4
  Blast colony-forming assay, 5
  The long-term bone marrow culture system, 6
  Colony formation on stromal layers, 7
  Proliferation in multiwells, 8
  Transplantation in immune-deprived mice, 9
Molecular biology of growth factors and their receptors, 10
  Molecular cloning of the HGFs and interleukins, 12
  Structure–function relationships, 18
  Molecular cloning of the HGF receptors, 21
  Kinetics of growth factor binding to receptors, 28
Cell surface expression of growth factor receptors, 30
Receptor characterization, 35
Receptor regulation, 36
Chromosomal localization of growth factor and receptor genes, 37
Signal transduction, 40
Biological effects of growth factor–target cell interactions, 43
Human HGFs and their targets, 44
The influence of serum-free culture conditions, 50
Enriched progenitor cell populations and the influence of accessory cells, 51
Physiology of the growth factor response, 53
References, 60

INTRODUCTION

The last 5 years have witnessed major advances in our understanding of the haemopoietic system and molecular biology has given us a new perspective on haemopoietic growth factors and their receptors. The haemopoietic system produces all of the myeloid and lymphoid cells that circulate in the blood and populate the bone marrow and lymphoid organs. These mature cells are produced by a series of proliferative and maturational changes that ultimately derive from a common pool of pluripotent, self-renewing stem cells. It has become customary to display the intermediate stages as a series of discrete but concatenated stem and progenitor cell compartments. This view comes from the development of clonogenic assays for haemopoietic progenitor cells in the 1960s, initially for murine myeloid cells and subsequently for murine and human progenitor cells of all lineages of haemopoietic cell differentiation (Fig. 1.1).

Haemopoietic progenitor cells respond to haemopoietic growth factors (HGFs) and other cytokines that are listed in Table 1.1. Cytokines that influence the functions of more mature cells are also included in the table. The information that originally led to the associations between HGFs and their target cells has been summarized in an earlier review (Gordon and Barrett, 1985). More recently, work in this area has been concerned with the precise definition of growth

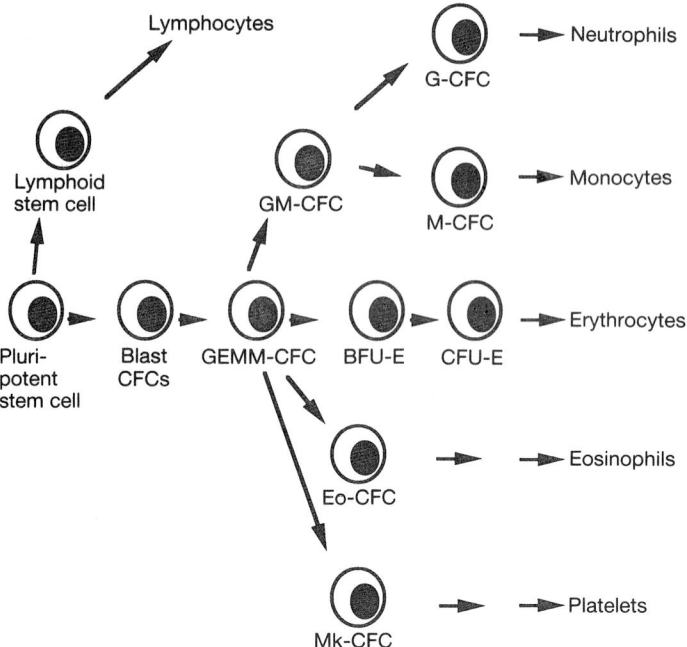

Fig. 1.1 Haemopoietic progenitor cell compartments.

factor–target cell relationships using recombinant HGFs and cytokines and highly enriched progenitor cell populations. Also, rapid progress in the cloning of growth factors and their receptors has made possible a spectrum of biological, biochemical, molecular and clinical studies. The growth factors listed in Table 1.1 will be considered later. A new stem cell factor, which is homologous to the product of the Steel locus in mice and is the ligand for c-kit (the product of the murine W locus) has recently been cloned (Martin et al., 1990). Leukaemia inhibitory factor (LIF), the interferons and transforming growth factor β (TGFβ) are included because they have been shown to influence haemopoietic cell proliferation and differentiation. The original operational definition of the HGFs granulocyte-macrophage colony-stimulating factor (GM-CSF), granulocyte (G-CSF) and macrophage colony-stimulating factor (M-CSF) was partially superseded when the term 'interleukin' was introduced in 1979. Newly discovered growth factors and cytokines are now named according to their biological activity and assigned an interleukin number once they have been cloned.

Recombinant technology has helped to clarify relationships between biologically defined growth factors, and some molecules responsible for a variety of activities are now known to be identical. For example, the activity described as haemopoietin-1 is now known to be molec-

Table 1.1 Growth factors in haemopoiesis with their alternative names

Multi-CSF	IL-3; pluripoietin
GM-CSF	Burst-promoting activity (BPA)
M-CSF	CSF-1
G-CSF	
BPA	GM-CSF
Erythropoietin	
Eo-CSF	
IL-1	Haemopoietin-1; lymphocyte-activating factor; osteoclast-activating factor
IL-2	T cell growth factor
IL-3	Multi-CSF; pluripoietin
IL-4	B cell stimulatory factor-1; hybridoma growth factor; β_2-interferon; B cell-stimulating factor-2; hepatocyte-stimulating factor
IL-5	
IL-6	
IL-7	
IL-8	Neutrophil activating protein (NAP-1)
IL-9	
IL-10	Cytokine synthesis inhibitory factor (CSIF)
IL-11	
Interferon (IFN) α/γ	
TGFβ	
TNFα/β	
Steel factor	c-*kit* ligand; stem cell factor; mast cell growth factor
LIF	Leukaemia inhibitory factor; human interleukin for DA cells (HILDA); differentiation inhibiting activity (DIA)

ularly identical to interleukin 1α (IL-1α); GM-CSF and erythroid burst-promoting activity (BPA) are also one and the same gene product. Other advances have been made in detection systems and radio-immunoassay (RIA) and enzyme-linked immunosorbent assays (ELISA) are becoming more widely available. However, the antigenicity required for these systems does not necessarily correspond structurally to the requirements for biological activity.

In vivo, haemopoiesis is restricted to the haemopoietic organs and, in adults, occurs exclusively in specific parts of the skeleton. It is now generally accepted that this localization of haemopoietic activity reflects a requirement for stromal cells and other factors constituting the haemopoietic microenvironment. This concept is based on a large volume of information derived from clinical and experimental bone marrow transplantation, experiments using Dexter's long-term bone marrow culture system (Dexter *et al.*, 1977) and many other *in vivo* and *in vitro* studies.

The soluble factors that stimulate haemopoietic colony formation *in vitro* probably represent a mechanism for inducing the rapid production of cells in times of physiological emergency, such as infection or bleeding, whilst an association between haemopoietic cells and stromal cells is responsible for the homeostatic maintenance of blood cell production under normal conditions. The cellular and molecular biology of haemopoietic cell regulation is considered in detail in the rest of this chapter.

MEASUREMENT OF HAEMOPOIETIC STEM CELLS

Figure 1.1 emphasizes the rather distal position in the haemopoietic hierarchy held by *in vitro* colony-forming cells. Although colony assays have provided valuable information about haemopoiesis in a variety of diseases and about the effects of therapy on the haemopoietic system, they do not provide a satisfactory measure of the pluripotent stem cell population. In recent years, therefore, efforts have been made to develop assays for human haemopoietic stem cells. The expression of the antigen CD34 by stem and progenitor cells (Katz *et al.*, 1985) and the availability of monoclonal antibodies have played a part in our ability to enrich stem cells for experimental purposes.

Differentiation of haemopoietic stem cells along the different lineages must be accompanied by changes in transcription and expression of tissue-specific genes (see Gordon *et al.*, 1990) and the isolation of normal multipotent progenitors is important for studies on the molecular regulation of haemopoietic cell development. Aspects that have been studied include the factors determining the accessibility of lineage-specific genes for transcription using DNAse I hypersensitivity as a marker. This property indicates that particular genes are in an uncoiled conformation allowing access of certain DNA-binding proteins and RNA polymerase enzymes. The amount of DNA methylation also influences the availability of genes for transcription. The expression of transcription factors implicated in the control of haemopoietic cell differentiation is under intensive investigation.

The 'homeobox' genes are now thought to be involved in haemopoiesis. This group of transcription-regulating genes have certain structural features in common and encode sequence-specific DNA-binding proteins (see Chapter 3). Expression of the Hox family of homeobox genes has been investigated in haemopoietic cells and activity of the Hox 2 gene has been demonstrated in erythroid cell lines but not in myeloid cell lines (Magli *et al.*, 1991). Furthermore, expression of two homeobox genes in CD34-positive cells from human bone marrow was reduced by treating the cells with haemopoietic growth factors, indicating that expression is related to the stage of cellular maturation (Deguchi and Kehri, 1991). In the lymphoid system, the Hox 2.3 gene has been associated with cellular activation since it is expressed in activated, but not in resting, T and B cells (Deguchi *et al.*, 1991).

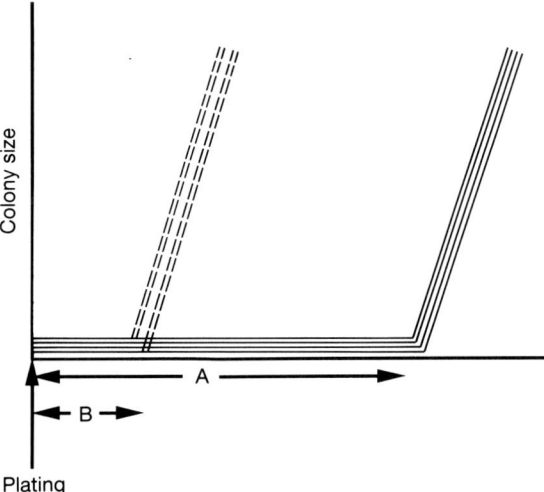

Fig. 1.2 Influence of growth factors on the onset of colony formation in Ogawa's blast colony assay. (A) Time for G_0 blast progenitors to enter cell cycle in absence of inducing factors; (B) time for G_0 blast progenitors to enter cell cycle in presence of inducing factors.

Blast colony-forming assay

The assay for blast colony-forming cells described by Ogawa (see Ogawa, 1989) is an extension of semisolid culture technology. Due to the primitive nature of these blast colony-forming cells, the formation of the blast colonies is delayed relative to the formation of granulocyte-macrophage colonies and erythroid bursts, but their appearance can be hastened by adding certain growth factors (IL-6 + IL-3; IL-1 + IL-3) to the culture system. This reduction in the time required for the onset of blast colony formation has been used to identify growth factors that induce resting (G_0) blast colony-forming cells to enter the cell cycle and to show that the subsequent rate of colony development is not altered by the addition of these factors (Fig. 1.2). In this way, G-CSF, IL-6, IL-11, stem cell factor and LIF have been identified as factors acting on primitive G_0 cells (Ogawa, 1991).

Almost all of the blast colony-forming cells are out of cycle in the marrow and the colonies produced by them contain further blast colony-forming cells, produced by self-renewal, which can be detected by replating the cells from the colony in a secondary culture. Similarly, lineage-restricted progenitor cells can be detected in replating experiments. Thus, this blast colony-forming cell possesses the characteristics of an early haemopoietic stem cell.

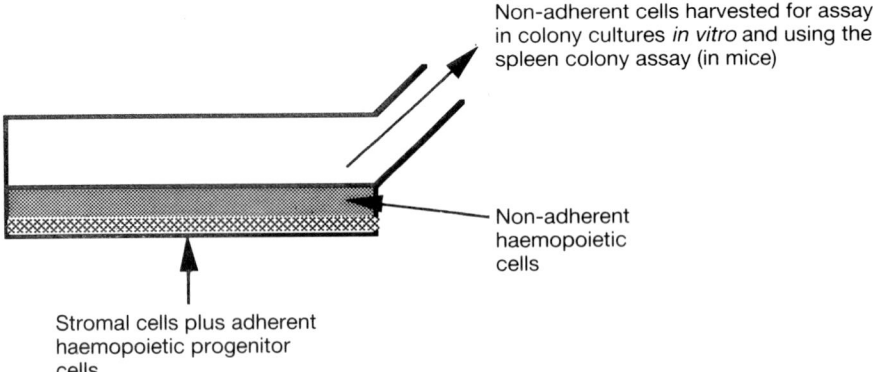

Fig. 1.3 Elements of the long-term bone marrow culture (LTBMC) system.

The long-term bone marrow culture system

Long-term bone marrow culture was originally used to study murine haemopoiesis (Dexter *et al.*, 1977). In outline, a bone marrow cell suspension is introduced into culture flasks and a stromal layer is produced by some of the cells that settle on the plastic surface. These cells can support the proliferation of stem cells in the cultures and haemopoietic activity is measured by the output of progenitor cells into the culture supernatant (Fig. 1.3). These include stem cells that form colonies on the spleens of irradiated, transplanted mice (spleen colony-forming cells – CFU-S) and *in vitro* colony-forming cells.

Adaptation of the system for human bone marrow culture led to the development of a two-stage method where one bone marrow cell suspension is used to produce the stromal layer. Once the stroma is established, a second marrow suspension containing the stem cells for assay is added and the output of colony-forming cells into the supernatant is measured. By digesting the stromal layer with collagenase, Coulombel *et al.* (1983) demonstrated that progenitor cells could also be detected amongst the stromal cells. Further studies indicated that these cells are more primitive than those released into the supernatant medium (Cashman *et al.*, 1985).

In an attempt to define the cells responsible for haemopoiesis in long-term cultures, Andrews and colleagues (1990) have obtained highly purified populations of CD34+, CD33− marrow cells which lack T cell, B cell and myeloid cell-associated antigens and do not produce colonies in semisolid culture systems. These cells are capable of haemopoietic activity when cultured on preformed marrow-derived stromal layers and a single cell can produce several myeloid colony-forming progeny. Similar studies by Sutherland *et al.* (1989a) identified cells, by flow cytometry, with low light-scattering properties, low HLA-DR expression, high CD34 expression and the potential to initiate haemopoiesis in long-term bone marrow cultures. These cells also express the CD45 isoform known as 'RO' (Lansdorp et al., 1990).

A low level of staining with the fluorescent dye rhodamine 123, which accumulates preferentially in the mitochondrial membranes of live cells, provides a further selective characteristic of primitive progenitors assayed in long-term cultures (Udomsakdi et al., 1991). This property has generally been thought to reflect a lack of mitochondrial activity in early cells but recent studies indicate that it may be the result of expression of the multidrug-resistance gene MDR1, which encodes a transmembrane efflux pump for a group of lipophilic compounds (Chaudhary and Roninson, 1991). This finding suggests that haemopoietic stem cells, like a variety of malignant cell types that express MDR1 (see Chapter 3), might be resistant to cancer chemotherapy.

The stromal layer produced in the long-term cultures is heterogeneous and consists of fibroblasts, endothelial cells, adipocytes and macrophages. Despite some study, it is still not certain which of these cell types is essential for haemopoiesis in this system. No growth factors are added to the long-term cultures and it is assumed that all of the necessary stimuli are supplied by the stromal layer. Production of a number of growth factors has been demonstrated by Northern analysis of messenger RNA (mRNA) in stromal cells (Gimble et al., 1989) but it is uncertain which of them is necessary for prolonged haemopoietic activity. Recently, platelet-derived growth factor (PDGF), IL-1 and TGFβ have been implicated in the direct or indirect regulation of haemopoiesis in long-term cultures of human marrow (Cashman et al., 1990).

There is no evidence that lymphopoiesis occurs in standard long-term marrow cultures. In 1982, Whitlock and Witte adapted the system for the proliferation of murine B cells (see Kincade et al., 1989, for review). A number of cloned stromal cell lines that influence B lymphopoiesis in vitro have been derived from murine stromal cultures and there is now evidence that cells of both the B lymphoid and myeloid lineages can be grown from a single stem cell in vitro (Ohara et al., 1991). Recently, McGinnes and colleagues (1991) reported that human marrow-derived stromal cells support human B cell development in vitro.

Colony formation on stromal layers

Following up an observation made by Cohen et al. (1980) that colonies of adherent haemopoietic cells (cobblestone areas) were produced

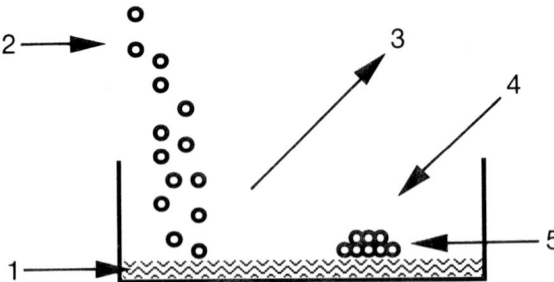

Fig. 1.4 Procedure for culturing stroma-adherent blast colony-forming cells: (1) grow stroma; (2) add cells; (3) wash; (4) add agar; (5) count colonies.

when murine marrow was added to preformed stromal layers, Gordon et al. (1985) added human marrow mononuclear cells to stroma, using the procedure shown in Figure 1.4, and obtained the growth of similar adherent colonies (Plate 1.1, facing p. 148). The properties of these colony-forming cells are consistent with them occupying an early position in the haemopoietic hierarchy. Also, Verfaillie et al. (1990) have shown that the cells responsible for sustained haemopoiesis in long-term cultures adhere to cultured stroma, as do progenitors of granulocyte-macrophage colony-forming cells (Dowding and Gordon, 1991). This information indicates that adherence to stroma is a property shared by a spectrum of early haemopoietic progenitor cells.

Very similar colonies can be grown by adding mouse bone marrow to stromal layers. Ploemacher et al. (1989) have equated these murine colony-forming cells with the population that repopulates the marrow of irradiated transplanted mice, suggesting that they are very primitive stem cells. Their potential for lymphoid repopulation is unknown.

Proliferation in multiwells

The need to study purified progenitors at the single cell level and the availability of recombinant growth factors has led to the use of very small-volume liquid cultures. Terstappen et al. (1991) sorted CD34+ CD38− cells singly into 72-well plates, supplied them with IL-3, IL-6, GM-CSF, G-CSF and erythropoietin and incubated them for 28–34 days. The contents of the wells were then subcultured several times. In this way, single CD34+ CD38− progenitor cells were shown to be capable of producing up to five generations of colony-forming cells with signs of morphologically detectable differentiation occurring in the fourth generation.

Transplantation in immune-deprived mice

Immunodeficient (bg/nu/xid) mice have reduced numbers of natural killer (NK) and lymphokine-activated killer (LAK) cells and can be used as recipients for infusions of human bone marrow (Kamel-Reid and Dick, 1988). The human cells repopulate the murine haemopoietic system with macrophage progenitor cells that persist for more than 5 weeks. This system has been proposed as a human stem cell assay. Similarly, mice with severe combined immunodeficiency (SCID) have been used as hosts for human T and B lymphocyte development (McCune et al., 1988; Mosier et al., 1988). However, lymphoid engraftment was transient and it will be necessary to have a better understanding of the mechanisms involved in xenografting human cells before this approach can be taken further. Nevertheless, these approaches have already been explored as experimental models of leukaemia, solid tumours, infectious diseases and autoimmunity and may contribute to the development of antibodies against agents that cannot be used to immunize humans (see Dick, 1991).

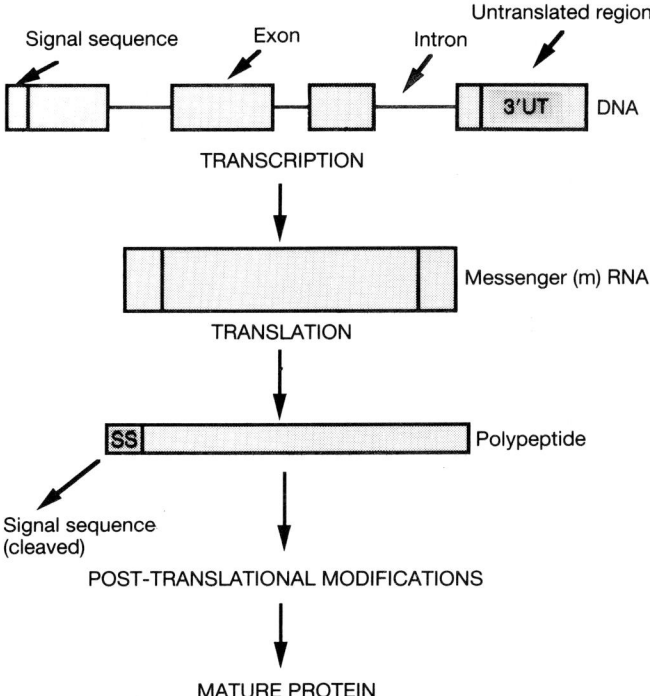

Fig. 1.5 Generalized structure of growth factor genes and their products.

MOLECULAR BIOLOGY OF GROWTH FACTORS AND THEIR RECEPTORS

In general, the haemopoietic growth factors and the lymphokines are proteins or glycoproteins encoded by genes that are present as a single copy per cell. Interferon α (IFNα) is an exception: there are more than 20 genes for IFNα although there is only one IFNβ and one IFNγ gene. Like most eukaryotic genes, the growth factor genes consist of exons separated by introns. When the genes are transcribed to produce mRNA, the regions complementary to the exons are retained and those complementary to the introns are spliced out to produce the mature message (Fig. 1.5). Most of the genes in question here are composed of four or five exons and three or four introns and are flanked by 5' signal sequences and 3' untranslated regions (Table 1.2). The signal sequences are important for the secretion of soluble growth factors.

The cloning of the human colony-stimulating factor and lymphokine genes has been reviewed by Sieff (1988) and Hamblin (1988). Essentially, two approaches have been used to isolate the complementary (c) DNA corresponding to growth factor genes from cDNA libraries. The first requires knowledge of at least part of the amino acid sequence of the growth factor protein so that oligonucleotides can be synthesized and used to probe a cDNA library derived from cells producing the factor of interest. The second approach bypasses the

Table 1.2 Molecular features of some human growth factor genes and proteins

Growth factor	Exons	Introns	Gene size (kb)	Protein length (aa)	Cysteine residues	Leader (aa)	Potential N-gly sites	Potential O-gly sites
GM-CSF	4	3	2.5	144	4	25	2	
G-CSF	5	4	2.2	207	5	30	0	yes
M-CSF	10	9	21.0	224	6	32	2	yes
IL-3	5	4	2.5	152	2	19	2	
Erythropoietin	5	4	5.4	166	4	27	3	
IL-1α	7	6		271		no		
IL-1β	7	6		269	no	no	no	
IL-2	4	3		153	3	20		1
IL-4	4	3	9.0	153	6	22	2	
IL-5	4	3	1.9	134	2	19	2	
IL-6	5	4	4.7	212	4	28	2	
IL-7				177	6	25	3	
IL-9	5	4		144			4	
TNFα	4	3		233		76		
TNFβ	4	3		205	yes	34		
IFNα/β		0		166	4/3	16–23	0/1	
IFNγ	4	3		146	2	23	2	
TGFβ				391	7–9		0	0

For abbreviations see Table 1.1.

need for protein purification by isolating mRNA from a suitable cell type to provide a template for making cDNA. Since the expression of growth factor genes is often induced by stimulating the cells, rather than being constitutive, it is possible to narrow the search for the relevant mRNA by comparing mRNA species from stimulated and unstimulated cells. The RNA message is translated either in a cell-free system or, more commonly, in *Xenopus* oocytes, yeast, bacteria or mammalian cells. The translation product is identified using bioassays or immunoassays and the sequence can then be used to identify a cDNA clone containing a full-length cDNA insert.

The production of growth factors in response to inducing signals is controlled at the level of gene transcription and the common regulatory sequences found in the 5' flanking regions of, for example, GM-CSF, IL-2, IL-3 and IFNγ may account for the fact that these genes are often coordinately expressed in stimulated cells.

The sequences of the cloned cDNAs predict the amino acid sequence of the mature protein product and provide clues about its structure. Most of the cDNAs for haemopoietic growth factors have a 5' hydrophobic signal sequence (Table 1.2) which is necessary for the extracellular secretion of the protein. The positions of cysteine residues indicate the potential for disulphide bond formation that is important for protein folding. Also, identification of potential glycosylation sites indicates some of the post-translational modifications that can be made to the molecule inside the cell.

The large-scale production required for growth factors to be clinically useful has led to developments in the manufacturing processes and strategies used to obtain high yields, purity and quality control. The options available have been reviewed by Thatcher (1990) and include the possibility of modifying the natural protein structure to improve the efficacy of the product.

Studies on HGF receptors have provided information about their cellular distribution, variables influencing growth factor binding (e.g. glycosylation), numbers and affinities. These aspects of growth factor–receptor interactions are important in the context of biotherapy and have implications for the industrial production of the factors for clinical use. The results of receptor ligand studies have also been applied to the development of sensitive radioreceptor-binding assays for the measurement of growth factors in solution.

Most of the HGF receptors are expressed in very low numbers on progenitor cells and cell lines have been used for many studies because they are more accessible and provide larger amounts of material. Also, large amounts of purified ligand are needed for receptor research and these were not available until the cognate growth factors were cloned.

Molecular cloning of the HGFs and interleukins

The basic structural features of the HGF and interleukin genes, together with features of the deduced amino acid sequences encoded by them, are summarized in Table 1.2.

GM-CSF

Human cDNA clones for GM-CSF have been isolated by screening cDNA or genomic libraries (see Gasson, 1991). Comparison of amino acid sequences and the effects of neutralizing antibodies in *in vitro* marrow culture systems have shown that GM-CSF and erythroid BPA are one and the same gene product (Kohama *et al.*, 1988). Moreover, the biologically active protein produced by the expression of the cloned gene in monkey Cos cells stimulates the formation of myeloid and erythroid colonies *in vitro*.

The recombinant protein expressed in Cos cells has an M_r of 20–23 kDa (Kaushansky *et al.*, 1986) whilst unglycosylated protein produced in *Escherichia coli* has an M_r of 14.7 kDa (Schrimsher *et al.*, 1987). Expression of GM-CSF in yeast results in variably glycosylated protein products (Miyajima *et al.*, 1986). Similarly, the GM-CSF protein purified from the Mo cell line exhibits a range of sizes (M_r 14–35 kDa) as a result of variable glycosylation.

G-CSF

The human G-CSF gene was isolated from the human bladder carcinoma cell line, 5637 (Souza *et al.*, 1986), from a human squamous carcinoma cell line (Nagata *et al.*, 1986a) and from a human genomic library (Nagata *et al.*, 1986b). The cDNA sequence encodes a protein of 18.6 kDa with no predicted N-linked glycosylation (there are no asparagine residues) and there is no N-linked glycosylation in the natural protein, only O-linked glycosylation (Welte *et al.*, 1985). As a result, the recombinant protein is less heterogeneous in size than recombinant GM-CSF or recombinant IL-3 (Souza *et al.*, 1986).

M-CSF

Transcripts of the M-CSF gene undergo differential splicing to generate multiple mRNA species. The cDNAs corresponding to biologically active forms of human M-CSF have been cloned from pancreatic carcinoma or trophoblastic cell lines. Precursor proteins of 256 and 554 amino acids are predicted from the cDNA sequence and each

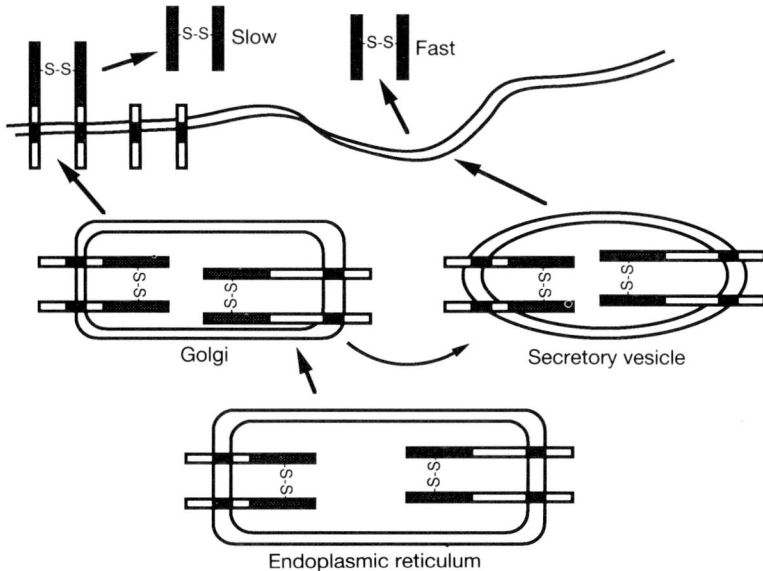

Fig. 1.6 Processing of M-CSF precursor molecules showing soluble and membrane-bound forms.

consists of a signal sequence, 'spacer' region, growth factor sequence, hydrophobic region and carboxyterminal tail. Processing of the various precursor proteins results in secreted growth factor and a small dimeric form that retains its membrane-binding properties and is stably expressed at the cell surface (Rettenmier and Sherr, 1989; Fig. 1.6). This occurs because the 554 amino acid form has a recognition site for an intracellular protease which releases it from the membrane whilst the 256 form does not, and this results in the expression of the membrane-bound form.

IL-3

A cDNA encoding the multilineage growth factor IL-3 was isolated from the gibbon T cell line MLA-144 to obtain the homologous sequence (90%) from a human genomic library (Yang *et al.*, 1986). In a separate study, Dorssers *et al.* (1987) exploited a non-coding murine sequence that is highly conserved to obtain a human cDNA clone by hybridization with murine IL-3 cDNA. This strategy was successful despite the fact that the predicted amino acid sequence of human IL-3 is only 29% homologous with that of murine IL-3. More recently, cDNA clones encoding IL-3 have been isolated from a human T cell library (Otsuka *et al.*, 1988). Translation of the mRNA gives a protein of 15–25 kDa.

Erythropoietin

Erythropoietin was first described by Carnot and Deflandre in 1906. Human erythropoietin has been purified from the urine of patients with aplastic anaemia and is a 35 kDa glycoprotein (Miyake *et al.*, 1977). Subsequent cloning and expression of the gene in Chinese hamster ovary (CHO) cells produced a protein that was biologically active *in vivo* and *in vitro* (Jacobs *et al.*, 1985; Lin *et al.*, 1985). This does not support the hypothesis that erythropoietin is released as a biologically inactive prohormone that requires processing for full biological activity (see Gordon and Barrett, 1985, for references).

Steel factor/stem cell factor

Genomic clones of human stem cell factor (SCF) have been isolated using probes based on rat cDNA sequence (Martin *et al.*, 1990). SCF exists in a soluble form consisting of 164/5 amino acids or as a cell surface molecule of 248 amino acids. This corresponds to the expression of exon 6 which encodes a proteolytic cleavage site and thereby determines whether or not the protein is removed from the cell surface. The cell surface molecule has the potential to act as a cell adhesion molecule by binding to its receptor on target cells (Flanagan *et al.*, 1991).

IL-1

In spite of almost identical biological activities and binding to a common receptor, IL-1α and IL-1β are quite dissimilar in their amino acid sequences (26% homology). They are encoded by two distinct, but distantly related, genes (Auron *et al.*, 1984; March *et al.*, 1985) with homologous structural organization (Clark *et al.*, 1986; Furutani *et al.*, 1986). It is now known that IL-1α is identical to the factor previously known as haemopoietin-1 (Mochizuki *et al.*, 1987).

Both IL-1α and IL-1β are first synthesized as intracellular prohormones that are subsequently processed for secretion. Macrophages release more IL-1β than IL-1α, which possibly reflects the greater efficiency of the β gene promoter compared with the α promoter (March *et al.*, 1985).

IL-2

The human T cell line Jurkat III can be induced with concanavalin A to produce 1000 U/ml of IL-2 and was used to obtain IL-2 cDNA (see

Taniguchi et al., 1986). Human IL-2 consists of 133 amino acids, including three cysteine residues. Two of them form a disulphide bridge that is essential for the biological activity of IL-2. Some heterogeneity in the size of the IL-2 molecule is associated with variations in O-linked glycosylation.

IL-4

Human IL-4 clones have been isolated from activated T cell-derived libraries and the complete nucleotide sequence of the human IL-4 gene has been determined (see Yokota et al., 1988). The recombinant protein of 153 amino acids includes a signal sequence of 22 amino acids. There are two potential N-linked glycosylation sites and six cysteine residues and the deduced molecular weight is 15 kDa (see Paul, 1991, for references).

IL-5

The IL-5 gene has been cloned from cDNA or genomic libraries and expressed in monkey Cos cells or *Xenopus* oocytes (Azuma et al., 1986; Campbell et al., 1987). Gel electrophoresis under non-reducing conditions suggests that IL-5 normally exists as a dimer (see Takatsu et al., 1988; Yokota et al., 1988) of approximately 45 kDa. The intron–exon organization of the IL-5 gene suggests some phylogenetic relationship with the genes for GM-CSF, IL-2, IL-4 and IFNγ but there is negligible sequence homology between IL-5 and the other haemopoietic growth factors and lymphokines (Campbell et al., 1987; Tanabe et al., 1987).

IL-6

Complementary DNA clones for IL-6 have been isolated from cDNA libraries derived from induced human fibroblasts and lymphocytes. Human and murine genomic IL-6 genes share highly homologous regions upstream of the cap site (i.e. where RNA transcription is initiated). Several potential transcriptional control elements have been identified in the conserved region and are implicated in the regulation of IL-6 gene expression (see Hirano et al., 1990). The molecular weight of human IL-6 is 22–29 kDa.

IL-7

The finding that long-term stromal cultures can support the growth of B cell precursors in murine marrow (Whitlock and Witte, 1982) led the way to cloning the cDNA for murine IL-7. Murine cDNA from a stromal cell-derived library was used to isolate the human homologue from a human hepatoma cDNA library. Expression of the gene in Cos cells yielded a recombinant IL-7 protein that stimulated human and murine pre-B cell proliferation (Goodwin et al., 1990). The cDNA for human IL-7 encodes a protein of 177 amino acids with three potential N-glycosylation sites and a predicted molecular weight of 17.4 kDa.

IL-8

The neutrophil activating factor IL-8 is released from human monocytes and has been purified from monocyte supernatants. It belongs to a group of 10 or more cytokines that are involved in inflammatory responses (Holmes et al., 1991). The complete 72 amino acid sequence was used to synthesize and clone a gene that was then expressed in E. coli. The molecular weight of IL-8 is approximately 10 kDa. Tests of the recombinant product on neutrophil activation showed that it was functionally equivalent to the natural protein (Lindley et al., 1988).

IL-9

The cDNA encoding human IL-9 has been isolated by expression cloning based on its ability to stimulate proliferation by a human megakaryocytic cell line (Yang et al., 1989). The gene consists of five exons and four introns. The protein consists of 144 amino acids with a calculated molecular weight of 16 kDa and has four potential sites for N-linked glycosylation. It is the homologue of the murine T cell growth factor, p40.

IL-10

The human equivalent of murine cytokine synthesis inhibitory factor (CSIF; IL-10) has been cloned using a tetanus toxin-specific human T cell clone. It has extensive sequence homology with an open reading frame in the Epstein–Barr virus (EBV) genome and the protein (predicted M_r 18.7 kDa) inhibits cytokine synthesis by activated human peripheral blood mononuclear cells (Moore et al., 1990; Vieira et al., 1991).

IL-11

Interleukin 11 was cloned from an immortalized primate bone marrow-derived stromal cell line by Paul and colleagues (1990). The cDNA contains a single long open reading frame of 597 nucleotides encoding a predicted 199 amino acid polypeptide with a hydrophobic signal sequence and lacking cysteine residues, potential sites for N-linked glycosylation and an apparent M_r of about 23 kDa.

LIF

The cDNA for human LIF has been cloned (Gough et al., 1988; Moreau et al., 1988) and mRNA has been detected in bone marrow-derived fibroblast cell lines (Libbert et al., 1989). The cDNA sequence predicts a mature protein of 170 amino acids.

Interferons

The interferons are a heterogeneous group of proteins and, in different organisms, varying numbers of unique genes encode the IFNs α and β (type I/viral interferon) and IFNγ (type II/immune interferon). In humans, there are more than 20 IFNα genes, one IFNβ gene and one IFNγ gene. The IFNs α are a closely related multigene family and evolutionarily related to IFNβ; all of the genes in this family lack introns. Interferon $β_2$ is now known as IL-6.

Interferon γ has little, if any, homology to IFNs α and β (see Hamblin, 1988; Langer and Petska, 1988; Hauser, 1990). It is produced by stimulated lymphocytes whereas IFNs α and β are produced by fibroblasts. The molecular weight of natural IFNγ is 35–70 kDa and it appears to consist of two glycosylated species that normally aggregate (see Trinchieri et al., 1987).

TGFβ

The TGFβ family comprises a number of dimeric proteins which are particularly homologous in seven to nine conserved cysteine residues in the C-terminal region. They can form homodimers ($TGFβ_1$ and $TGFβ_2$) or heterodimers ($TGFβ_{1.2}$ and $TGFβ_{1.3}$). Human cDNA clones encoding TGFβ were isolated by Derynck and colleagues (1985) using protein purified from platelets. The mature protein of 112 amino acids (M_r 24 kDa) is derived from a 391 amino acid precursor that is cleaved slowly, removing a sequence containing three potential glycosylation sites, by an elastase-like enzyme (Pandiella and Massague, 1991).

Tumour necrosis factor (TNF)

Complementary DNA derived from HL60 cells was used to clone TNFα. The molecular weights of native and recombinant TNFα are the same (17 kDa) due to the complete absence of glycosylation. Lymphotoxin (TNFβ) is closely related to TNFα but is glycosylated and lacks the disulphide bond found in TNFα. Native TNFβ is a glycosylated trimer with a molecular weight of 60–70 kDa that dissociates to 20 kDa under reducing conditions (see Hamblin, 1988; Balkwill, 1989).

Structure–function relationships

The HGFs and interleukins are multifunctional molecules and it is likely that different structural domains correspond to their different activities. This line of research has been pursued actively to gain insight into the biology of growth factor–target cell interactions and has raised the possibility that selectively active cytokine fragments could be used in therapy. For example, analysis of the structure and function of the IL-1β molecule has shown that a peptide in position 190–202 has hyperalgesic effects in rats (Ferreira et al., 1988) whilst a pentapeptide loop (165–169) appears sufficient for its immunostimulatory effects (Boraschi et al., 1990). In addition, substitution of the N-terminal amino acids of G-CSF can produce a two to four fold increase in its activity in vivo and in vitro and this could be valuable in treatment (Okabe et al., 1990). Likewise, fusion of the coding region of human GM-CSF and IL-3 resulted in a protein with enhanced haemopoietic activity (Curtis et al., 1991).

Glycosylation

Many of the natural growth factors are extensively glycosylated but the recombinant growth factors are either not glycosylated (if produced in bacteria) or may be inappropriately glycosylated (if produced in yeast or mammalian cells). However, comparisons of glycosylated and non-glycosylated GM-CSF and studies of the effect of mutating potential glycosylation sites indicate that the carbohydrate component of the molecule is not necessary for its biosynthesis, secretion or biological activity. In fact, deglycosylation of recombinant GM-CSF produced in yeast increased its biological activity (Moonen et al., 1987). Also, deglycosylation of IL-4 does not affect its biological activity (see Paul, 1991). There are two potential N-glycosylation sites in human, but not in murine, IL-6, which suggests that glycosylation may not be required for the activity of this cytokine either (Chiu et al., 1988). In contrast, glycosylation is essential for erythropoietin activity in vivo, though not in vitro, and is thought to protect the molecule from degradation or elimination (Goldwasser et al., 1990). A specific requirement for N-linked oligosaccharides has recently been demonstrated for erythropoietin (Wasley et al., 1991).

Disulphide bridges

A requirement for the integrity of disulphide bridges joining cysteine residues has been demonstrated for GM-CSF, IL-3, erythropoietin and IL-7 (Clark-Lewis and Schrader, 1982; Kaushansky et al., 1987; Namen et al., 1988; Wingfield et al., 1988; Goldwasser et al., 1990). These bonds are important for maintaining the secondary and tertiary structure and often are required for biological function. For example, there are two possible disulphide bridges in the IL-3 molecule, although only one of them is needed for biological activity. There are six cysteine residues in IL-7 and at least some of them are functionally important since IL-7 can be inactivated by treatment with β-mercaptoethanol. Similarly, the activity of IL-4 is completely destroyed by reduction and alkylation (see Paul, 1991).

Protein folding

The tertiary conformation of the HGFs and cytokines is becoming better understood and it is now clear that these proteins, which have

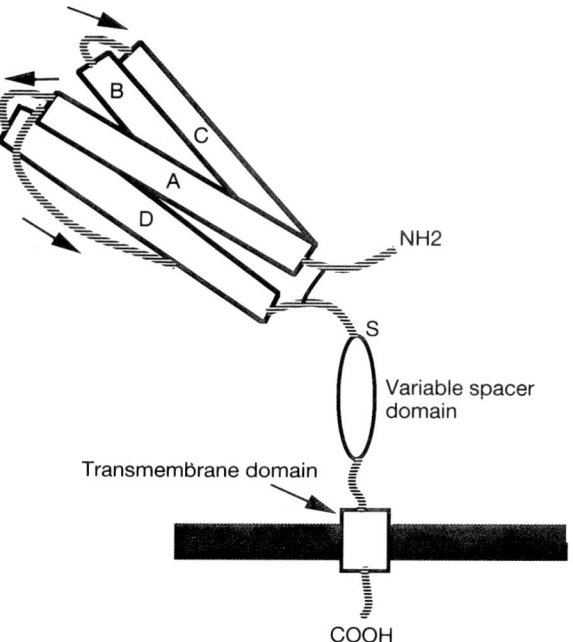

Fig. 1.7 Simplified diagram of the common tertiary structures of SCF and M-CSF proposed by Bazan (see text for details).

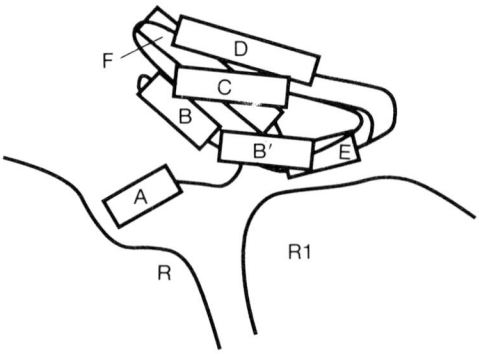

Fig. 1.8 Model of the three dimensional structure of interleukin-2 showing protein domains A–F and binding to the two IL-2 receptor chains, R and R' (after Brandhuber et al., 1987).

very little amino acid sequence similarity, can be grouped into families that are rich in α-helices (GM-CSF, G-CSF, erythropoietin, IL-2, IL-5, IL-6 and IFNα), families with extensive β structure (IL-1β) and those like IL-3 with features of both groups (Parry et al., 1988; Bazan, 1990a,b,c). Recently, Bazan (1991) has drawn attention to the similarities between SCF and M-CSF in the α-helical structure of their extracellular domains and has proposed that there is an evolutionary relationship between the two growth factors. The conservation of structural features, in particular the occurrence of four α-helical bundles, suggests that they are important for biological activity (Fig. 1.7).

Residues 14–25 of the GM-CSF molecule are predicted to form the first α-helix and are essential for its function whilst residues 14–121 are sufficient for complete biological activity (Clark-Lewis et al., 1988). Likewise, the conserved part of the G-CSF molecule is important for bioactivity but the divergent N-terminal sequence is not necessary (Kuga et al., 1989; Okabe et al., 1990). Part of the α-helical structure of GM-CSF is predicted to be involved in binding to the cognate receptor and is clearly essential (Kaushansky et al., 1989). Studies with monoclonal antibodies to IL-2 peptides indicate that portions of the A and B' helices and the peptide joining them are candidate receptor-binding regions (Fig. 1.8) and other studies demonstrate the importance of helical structure for protein folding and biological function (Brandhuber et al., 1987; Ciardelli et al., 1988). Alpha helices may also be involved in binding growth factors to proteoglycans in the extracellular matrix (see Gordon, 1991).

Receptor binding

Bazan (1990a) has suggested that the conformation of the α-helical cytokines is crucial for their binding to their receptors. Some of the supporting evidence is summarized in the previous paragraph. D'Andrea *et al.* (1990) have produced four monoclonal antibodies that bind to erythropoietin, two of which inhibit erythropoietin binding to its receptor. These and similar antibodies (Goto *et al.*, 1989; Wognum *et al.*, 1990b) will be valuable in further investigating the structural basis of erythropoietin-receptor recognition.

A series of anti-GM-CSF monoclonal antibodies has been used to identify regions of the molecule involved in receptor binding and to map non-functional epitopes. The latter reagents can be predicted to be useful for labelling GM-CSF without interfering with its biological activity (Kanakura *et al.*, 1991).

Molecular cloning of the HGF receptors

The molecular characterization of the growth factor receptors has revealed that they, like their cognate ligands, can be grouped into families. The IL-1 and M-CSF receptors are members of the immunoglobulin superfamily, based on similarities in the extracellular portion that binds the ligand. Recently, a large new receptor superfamily, designated the 'haematopoietin receptor superfamily', has been identified (Cosman *et al.*, 1990). It was discovered during studies on the IL-4 receptor by Idzerda *et al.* (1990) who found DNA sequences that are homologous with sequences in the DNA encoding the human IL-6 receptor, the human IL-2 receptor β chain and the erythropoietin receptor. Other studies demonstrated homologies with the IL-7 receptor (Goodwin *et al.*, 1990).

The members of the haematopoietin receptor superfamily now include receptors for interleukins 2, 3, 4, 6 and 7, GM-CSF and erythropoietin (Fig. 1.9). The major region of homology resides in a stretch of 210 amino acids in the extracellular ligand-binding domain which, in all members, contains four cysteine residues (CCCC) and a sequence of five amino acids (WSXWS) just outside the membrane-spanning region. This segment is duplicated in the IL-3 receptor (Fig. 1.9). The IL-6 and G-CSF receptors overlap the two families having an N-terminal immunoglobulin domain as well as the 210 amino acid sequence characteristic of the haematopoietin receptor superfamily. These different types of receptor probably correspond to the different structural groupings of their ligands (see Bazan, 1990a and above).

Immunoglobulin-like receptors

M-CSF/CSF-1 receptor. The M-CSF receptor is encoded by the c-*fms* proto-oncogene and exhibits ligand-induced protein tyrosine kinase activity. The human M-CSF receptor is an integral transmembrane

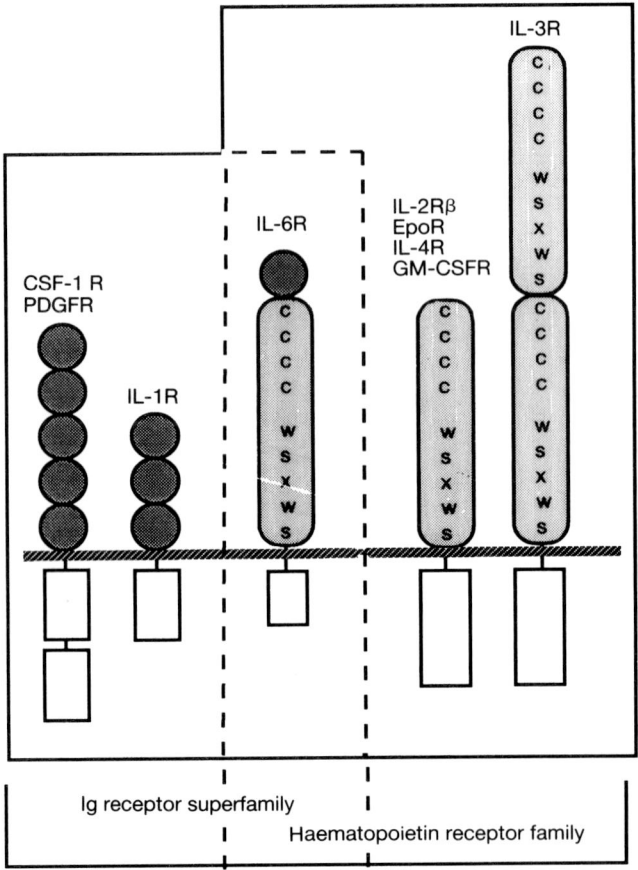

Fig. 1.9 The immunoglobulin-like and haematopoietin receptor families.

glycoprotein of 972 amino acids and has a molecular mass of 165 kDa. The extracellular domain consists of five disulphide-bonded, extensively glycosylated immunoglobulin-like loops and the intracellular domain has the sequences necessary for tyrosine kinase activity (Fig. 1.10; Sherr, 1990).

IL-1 receptor. An IL-1-specific binding protein (80 kDa) has been cloned and identified as a member of the immunoglobulin superfamily. The cytoplasmic sequence of this protein does not resemble the protein tyrosine kinases, although there is a potential protein kinase C phosphorylation site. Other IL-1-binding proteins have been identified by cross-linking experiments, ranging in size from 26 to 220 kDa, and one or more of them may combine with the 80 kDa protein to form a functional, signal-transducing IL-1 receptor (see Dinarello *et al.*, 1989).

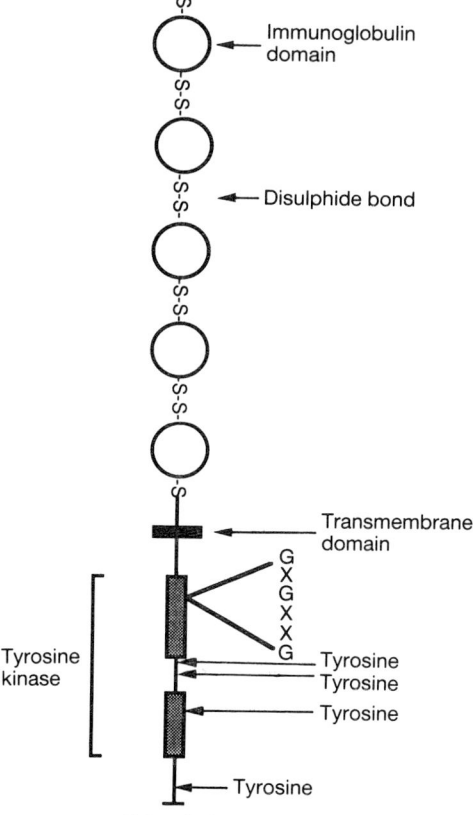

Fig. 1.10 Predicted structure of the receptor for M-CSF (after Sherr, 1990).

c-kit. The c-*kit* proto-oncogene encodes a transmembrane receptor that is structurally related to the M-CSF receptor. It is expressed as a 145 kDa cell surface molecule with tyrosine-specific autophosphorylation activity. The sequence of 953 amino acids includes six cysteine residues and nine potential N-glycosylation sites (Yarden et al., 1987).

The haematopoietin receptor superfamily

GM-CSF receptor. The GM-CSF receptor consists of at least two components (α and β subunits) which together form the high-affinity receptor. Gearing et al. (1989) isolated two cDNA clones encoding human GM-CSF-binding protein (α subunit) of 80 kDa from a placental cDNA library which binds GM-CSF with low affinity when transfected into Cos cells. The cDNA for the β subunit was isolated initially as the human homologue of the murine low-affinity IL-3 receptor but high-affinity binding of GM-CSF was obtained when it was coexpressed with the GM-CSF receptor α chain (Kitamura et al., 1991a). In chemical cross-linking studies, both the α and β subunits bind to GM-CSF, showing that both components of the high-affinity receptor bind to the growth factor (Hayashida et al., 1990). Interestingly, the β chain of the GM-CSF receptor is shared with the IL-3 and IL-5 receptors (Kitamura et al., 1991b; Tavernier et al., 1991).

IL-3 receptor. An IL-3-binding component of the murine IL-3 receptor has been cloned and is a member of the haematopoietin receptor superfamily with duplication of the characteristic extracellular domain (Itoh et al., 1990). The protein expressed in Cos cells or fibroblasts showed specific low-affinity binding of IL-3 with no ligand-dependent receptor internalization and no tyrosine phosphorylation in IL-3-stimulated transfected cells. The cytoplasmic domain lacks a consensus sequence for tyrosine kinase and this finding, plus the low binding affinity of IL-3, suggests that additional components are necessary for the functional high-affinity IL-3 receptor. These β components appear to be shared between the GM-CSF and IL-3 receptors in human cells whereas murine cells possess two distinct β subunits (Kitamura et al., 1991a,b), although the murine GM-CSF β chain is also a component of the murine IL-5 receptor (Takaki et al., 1990; Devos et al., 1991).

Erythropoietin receptor. The gene for the human erythropoietin receptor has recently been cloned (Jones et al., 1990; Winkelman et al., 1990). The derived amino acid sequence of 508 amino acids is 83% homologous to the murine erythropoietin receptor and there are no major differences between the species. Sequence comparison between the erythropoietin receptor and the IL-2 receptor β chain shows significant homology and justifies inclusion of the erythropoietin receptor in the haematopoietin receptor superfamily (D'Andrea et al., 1989).

IL-2 receptor. Interleukin 2 binds to two distinct receptor molecules, IL-Rα (p55) and IL-2Rβ (p75). The α chain has a low affinity for IL-2 and is recognizable as the Tac antigen whilst the β chain has an intermediate binding affinity and belongs to the haematopoietin receptor superfamily. The combination of the α and β chains produces the high-affinity IL-2 receptor (Fig. 1.11; Hatakeyama et al., 1989).

The p55 component (α chain) lacks a significant cytoplasmic domain and is not functional in the absence of p75. In contrast, p75 binds IL-2 and functions in signal transmission on its own. It consists of an extracellular domain and a transmembrane region and has a large cytoplasmic domain that probably is responsible for IL-2-mediated signal transduction. However, transfection of p75 cDNA into non-

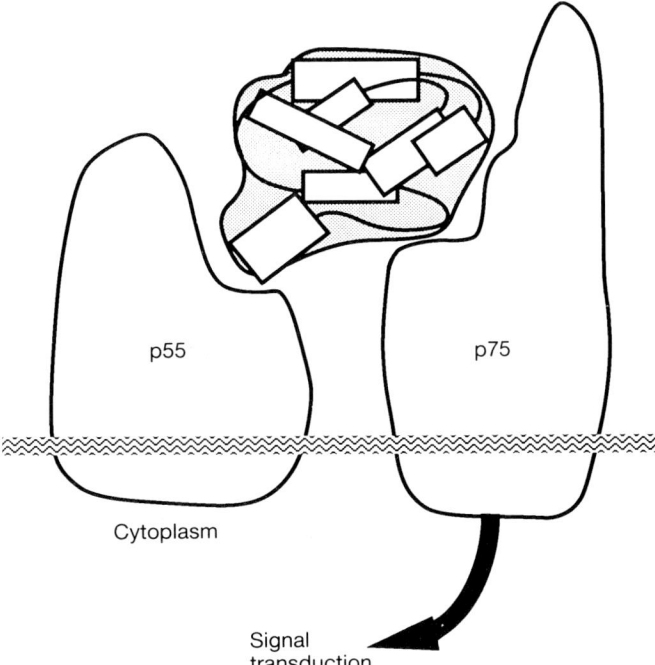

Fig. 1.11 Stylized diagram of the interaction between interleukin 2 and its receptor.

lymphoid cells resulted in expression of p75 that did not bind IL-2. Evidence from murine studies suggests that this could be explained by a requirement for an additional subunit, p40, for a functional high-affinity IL-2 receptor (Saragovi and Malek, 1990).

IL-4 receptor. The cDNA for the human high-affinity IL-4 receptor encodes a single transmembrane protein of 140 kDa (Idzerda *et al.*, 1990). The cytoplasmic domain of the IL-4 receptor has no consensus sequences for tyrosine kinase activity but it does have potential phosphorylation sites for protein kinase C. In murine cells, there is an alternatively spliced mRNA that is translated to produce a secreted form of the IL-4 receptor (Moseley *et al.*, 1989) but an analogous human cDNA has not been isolated. However, recent evidence suggests that a second, low-affinity, IL-4 receptor exists on human cells (see Callard, 1991).

IL-5 receptor. The IL-5 receptor α chain has been identified as a member of the haematopoietin receptor superfamily and the β chain of the high-affinity receptor is shared with GM-CSF (Tavernier *et al.*, 1991) which in turn shares its β chain with IL-3 (Kitamura *et al.*, 1991b). Thus, this group of three receptors have β chains in common.

IL-7 receptor. Goodwin *et al.* (1990) isolated cDNAs encoding three species of IL-7-binding protein. One of them encoded a protein of 459 amino acids, including a signal sequence of 20 amino acids, with a transmembrane hydrophobic region and a calculated molecular weight of 49.5 kDa. There are six potential N-linked glycosylation sites and candidate sites for O-linked glycosylation. The cytoplasmic domain does not contain sequences typical of protein tyrosine kinases. Another cDNA is suggested to result from alternative splicing and encodes a protein with an abbreviated cytoplasmic domain whilst the third lacks sequences for the transmembrane-spanning region and would be predicted to encode for a soluble form of the IL-7 receptor. This hypothesis was confirmed by demonstrating that supernatant medium from Cos cells expressing the soluble IL-7 receptor inhibited IL-7 binding to its cell surface receptor target cells.

Interferon receptors. The receptors for IFNα and β (type I) and IFNγ (type II) have been cloned (Aguet *et al.*, 1988; Uze *et al.*, 1990). There is evidence that they are evolutionarily related and qualify for membership of the haematopoietin receptor superfamily (Bazan, 1990b,c).

Hybrid receptors

These receptors have features that are characteristic of both the immunoglobulin superfamily and the haematopoietin receptor superfamily.

G-CSF receptor. The murine G-CSF receptor has been cloned and is a 90 kDa polypeptide of 812 amino acids. Its similarity to the rat prolactin receptor places it in the haematopoietin receptor superfamily (Fukunaga *et al.*, 1990). Human G-CSF receptor cDNA has been isolated from a placental library (Larsen *et al.*, 1990). Two cDNAs were cloned and encoded high-affinity transmembrane G-CSF receptors of 759 and 812 amino acids respectively. The two proteins differ in their carboxy-termini as a result of alternative splicing. The extracellular portion of the receptor contains an immunoglobulin-like domain and a type III fibronectin-like domain which suggests it may have originated in an ancestral molecule resembling N-CAM, the neuronal cell adhesion molecule.

IL-6 receptor. The cDNA encoding the human IL-6 receptor has been cloned (Yamasaki *et al.*, 1988). The receptor consists of 28 amino acids and is a transmembrane glycoprotein of M_r 80 kDa (Hirata *et al.*, 1989). The cytoplasmic domain does not contain tyrosine kinase sequences and recent work (Hirano *et al.*, 1990) suggests that the

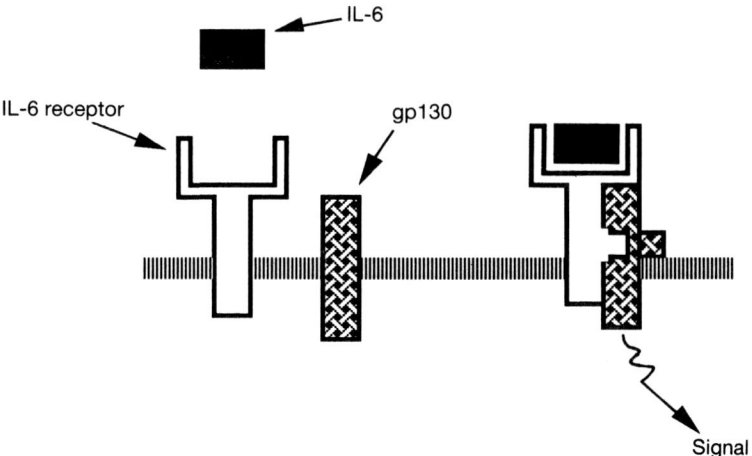

Fig. 1.12 Proposed mechanism of IL-6 induced cell stimulation.

complex of IL-6 and its receptor binds to a cell surface molecule that is involved in signal transduction. This latter component (gp130) does not associate with the IL-6 receptor unless IL-6 is complexed with it and it is found also on cells that do not express the IL-6 receptor. It is suggested that the association of the extracellular region of the IL-6 receptor with gp130 causes an allosteric change in the receptor and leads to transduction of a signal across the cell membrane (Fig. 1.12).

The nerve growth factor receptor superfamily

The members of this family are characterized by three or four cysteine-rich motifs of about 40 amino acids in the extracellular part of the sequence (Mallett and Barclay, 1991).

The TNF receptor. Various cells express low levels of two distinct receptors (55 and 75 kDa) for TNF. Both forms of the human TNF receptors have been cloned and they show a high degree of sequence homology with the extracellular domain of the nerve growth factor (NGF) receptor (Loetscher et al., 1990; Schall et al., 1990; Smith et al., 1990). A soluble TNF-binding protein is derived from the cell surface by proteolysis.

Other receptors

Some growth factor receptor structures do not appear to fit into the haematopoietin, NGF or immunoglobulin families, although they may belong to other receptor superfamilies such as the G protein-linked receptors (e.g. IL-8).

IL-5 receptor. The murine IL-5 receptor has been cloned and consists of an αβ heterodimer of molecular weights 60 and 130/140 kDa respectively (Mita *et al.*, 1991). The human IL-5 receptor α chain has also been cloned (Tavernier *et al.*, 1991) and it interacts with a β chain (shared with the GM-CSF and IL-3 receptors) to form the high-affinity IL-5 receptor (Kitamura *et al.*, 1991b).

IL-8 receptor. The IL-8 receptor belongs to the superfamily of G protein-linked receptors characterized by seven hydrophobic domains that are presumed to span the cell membrane and N-linked glycosylation sites near the amino-terminus. The cDNA encodes a protein of 350 amino acids and the smaller molecular size of the translated receptor (40 kDa) compared with that of the neutrophil receptor identified by cross-linking studies (67 kDa) may be accounted for by differences in glycosylation (Holmes *et al.*, 1991; Murphy and Tiffany, 1991).

The TGFβ receptor. Three structurally distinct TGFβ receptors have been identified by affinity cross-linking studies. The type I band has a molecular weight of 65 kDa, type II 85–95 kDa and type III 280–330 kDa (Massague and Like, 1985; Cheifetz *et al.*, 1987). Recent work has identified the high molecular weight (type III) TGFβ receptor as a proteoglycan with glycosaminoglycan side chains of heparan sulphate and chondroitin sulphate (Cheifetz *et al.*, 1988; Segarini and Seyedin, 1988).

Kinetics of growth factor binding to receptors

This area of receptor research is concerned with the kinetics of binding interactions between growth factors and their cell surface receptors. The methods used to investigate the receptors in this context have been reviewed in detail by Park *et al.* (1990) and will only be summarized in this text. The second part of this section describes the information that has been obtained about the numbers, distribution and affinities of growth factor receptors on the surface of haemopoietic cells.

Methods used in receptor research

The fundamental requirements for these studies are preparations of the receptors, purified growth factor, systems for measuring the interaction between the growth factor and its receptor and a means of separating bound from unbound ligand. The growth factor receptors are expressed in very low numbers on haemopoietic progenitor cells and the cells themselves are not usually sufficiently accessible for studies to be performed using them. The exception to this restriction is the use of erythroid colony-forming cells (E-CFC) which have been purified and used in studies of the erythropoietin receptor (Krantz et al., 1990). Otherwise, receptors have been studied using cell lines, mature cell populations such as neutrophils or lymphocytes, or leukaemic blast cells, all of which can be obtained as large homogeneous populations.

In studies of receptor binding, the ligand is usually labelled with a radioisotope so that the interaction can be measured quantitatively. The availability of recombinant growth factors has made it possible to label the purified ligands to high specific activity. In most cases, the growth factors have been labelled by covalently attaching iodine-125 to lysine (Bolton Hunter method) or tyrosine (chloramine T or lactoperoxidase reactions), the success of which depends on the amounts and accessibility of these residues in the target molecule.

It is necessary to optimize the incubation conditions used for the interaction between the receptor and its ligand. These need to be established for each individual receptor–ligand pair and include the time required to reach equilibrium and the temperature of the reaction. As a rule, haemopoietic growth factor binding reaches equilibrium more rapidly at 37°C than at 4°C but at the higher temperature it is necessary to include 0.2% sodium azide in the incubation mixture to prevent the complex of receptor and bound growth factor from being transferred from the cell surface to the cytoplasm (internalized) and degraded.

To determine the amount of specific binding, as opposed to the amount of non-specific binding, the amount of radiolabelled growth factor bound in the absence (for total binding) and in the presence (for non-specific binding) of a large excess amount of unlabelled factor is measured (Fig. 1.13). The amount of specific binding can then be determined by subtraction of the non-specific binding from the total. Linear transformation of the binding data is most often done using the Scatchard method which provides information about the affinity of the interaction and the receptor density from the slope of the line and its intercept on the x-axis respectively (Fig. 1.13).

The receptors can be further characterized by treating the receptor–ligand complex with a bifunctional cross-linking agent such as dithiobis(succinimidylpropionate) to stabilize it. The ligand plus receptor can then be extracted, by solubilizing the cell in detergent, and analysed by SDS-polyacrylamide gel electrophoresis (SDS-PAGE)

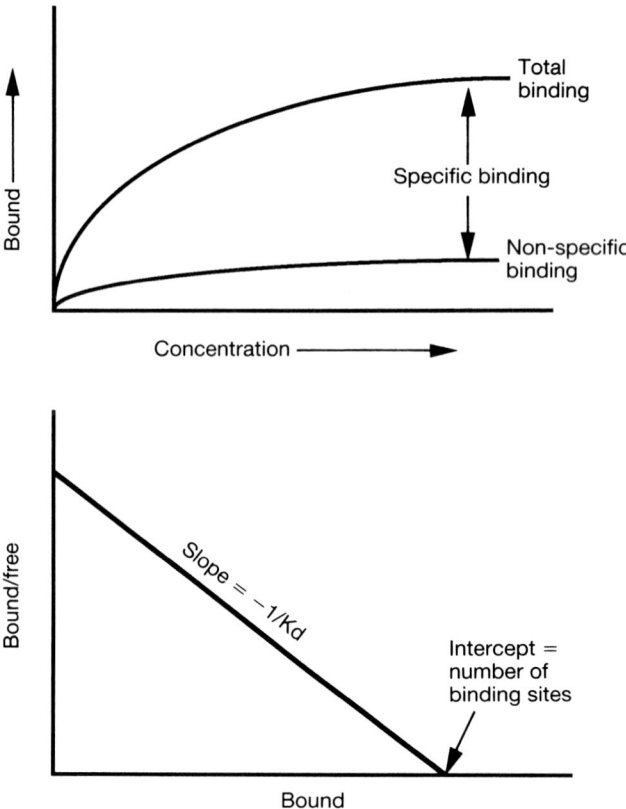

Fig. 1.13 Measurements used in Scatchard analysis of ligand binding affinities and receptor numbers.

and autoradiography. This allows the molecular weight of the receptor to be determined by subtracting the M_r of the unbound factor from that of the receptor–ligand complex. In these studies, it is very important to inhibit cellular proteases during the procedure so that the receptor is not degraded and its molecular weight is not underestimated.

Monoclonal antibodies can be used to characterize growth factor receptors by immunoprecipitation. Highly abundant receptors may be present in sufficient quantity for purification and amino acid sequencing. As we have seen, molecular cloning of the receptors leads to predictions about their structure and can reveal relationships with other members of gene families.

Cell surface expression of growth factor receptors

Cellular distribution

Haemopoietic growth factor receptors have been detected on a variety of malignant and non-malignant haemopoietic and non-haemopoietic cell types. The information regarding their distribution is summarized in Table 1.3 and gives an impression of the potential target cell range of each factor.

Table 1.3 Cell surface expression of haemopoietic growth factor receptors

Growth factor	Target cells	
GM-CSF	Progenitor cells Eosinophils Myeloid leukaemic blasts	Neutrophils Monocytes
G-CSF	Progenitor cells Myeloid leukaemic blasts Human placenta Small cell lung cancer	Neutrophils Trophoblasts
M-CSF	Progenitor cells Macrophages Choriocarcinoma	Monocytes Trophoblasts
IL-3	Progenitor cells Eosinophils Myeloid leukaemic blasts	Monocytes Pre B/B cell lines
Erythropoietin	Progenitor cells (CFU-E) Erythroblasts	
IL-1	Progenitor cells Fibroblasts Mesangial cells	T and B cells Keratinocytes Glial cells
IL-2	T cells NK cells	Activated B cells Monocytes
IL-4	B and T cells Burkitt's lymphoma Epithelial and endothelial cell lines Fibroblasts	Monocytes
IL-5	Eosinophils	
IL-6	Progenitor cells T and B cells Hepatocytes Nerve cells	Megakaryocytes Plasmacytoma/myeloma Mesangial cells Keratinocytes
IL-7	Pre-B cells	T cells
IL-8	Neutrophils	
IL-9	Megakaryocytes Erythroid progenitors	
IL-10	Monocytes	Mast cells
IL-11	(Megakaryocytes – indirectly) B cells/plasmacytoma	
TGFβ	Most cell types	

For abbreviations see Table 1.1.

Receptor numbers and affinities

GM-CSF receptor. The most mature normal cells express the greatest number of GM-CSF receptors. Neutrophils, eosinophils and monocytes express up to 2000 high-affinity sites per cell with K_d values falling between 40 and 600 pM (Park *et al.*, 1986; Budel *et al.*, 1989a; Lopez *et al.*, 1989; Chiba *et al.*, 1990; DiPersio *et al.*, 1990). In addition, monocytes express as many as 10 000 low-affinity (K_d 1–2 nM) GM-CSF receptors per cell (Chiba *et al.*, 1990). The concentration of GM-CSF required to occupy 50% of the receptors is two to three orders of magnitude higher than the concentration needed for a biological response, which indicates that GM-CSF can exert an effect by binding to only a few receptors.

Human recombinant GM-CSFs expressed in different cells vary in their receptor-binding affinities. For example, the affinity of GM-CSF expressed in *E. coli* is higher (K_d 20 pM) than that of the CHO-derived protein (K_d 500 pM–1 nM) (Kelleher *et al.*, 1988). The higher affinity of the *E. coli*-derived GM-CSF was shown also by Chiba *et al.* (1990) who found that a 50–100 molar excess of CHO-derived GM-CSF was needed to compete with the bacterial factor for binding to the receptor.

Several studies have examined the expression of GM-CSF receptors by fresh leukaemic blast cells and a consistent theme of interpatient variability has emerged with receptor numbers ranging from undetectable to 1300 per cell and affinities between 3 and 400 pM (K_d). There is no straightforward relationship between receptor expression and a proliferative response to GM-CSF. There is, however, some correlation with French-American-British (FAB) classification with receptor numbers being somewhat lower in the M1 and M2 categories and higher in M4 and M5 (Kelleher *et al.*, 1988; Budel *et al.*, 1989b; Park *et al.*, 1989; Onetto-Pothier *et al.*, 1990).

G-CSF receptor. Specific G-CSF receptors are expressed by normal neutrophils and acute myeloid leukaemia (AML) blasts. In one study, neutrophils expressed a single class of 700–1300 receptors per cell with a K_d of 405–648 pM (Budel *et al.*, 1989a); in another, they expressed, on average, 190 receptors per cell with a K_d of 77 pM (Avalos *et al.*, 1990), and in a third study chronic myeloid leukaemia (CML) neutrophils expressed 1400 receptors with a K_d value of 245 pM (Hanazono *et al.*, 1991).

M-CSF/CSF-1 receptor. Receptors for M-CSF are found on placental trophoblasts and on choriocarcinoma cell lines as well as on monocytes, macrophages and their precursor cells (see Sherr, 1990, for review). At least in the mouse, there are very large numbers (>50 000 per cell) of high-affinity receptors on monocytes. In normal humans, receptor expression is restricted to cells of the mononuclear phagocyte lineage (Ashmun et al., 1989).

IL-3 receptor. The binding of IL-3 to its cell surface receptor has been studied using human eosinophils, neutrophils, monocytes and leukaemic blast cells. It binds to human eosinophils via a single class of high-affinity (K_d 470 pM) receptors but not to human neutrophils (Lopez et al., 1989). Monocytes express low numbers (168 per cell) of high-affinity binding sites (Urdal and Park, 1988; Elliot et al., 1989). High- and low-affinity receptors have been demonstrated on primary AML blast cells but not on acute lymphoblastic leukaemia (ALL) blast cells. In common with the expression of other receptors, this did not correlate with proliferation *in vitro* (Urdal and Park, 1988; Budel et al., 1989b; Park et al., 1989).

A degree of competition for binding between IL-3 and GM-CSF has been demonstrated and can probably be explained by interaction between distinct receptors for the two factors on cells where both receptors are expressed (Elliot et al., 1989; Gesner et al., 1989) and competition for the shared receptor β chain.

Erythropoietin receptor. Studies of the binding of erythropoietin to its receptor on relatively early progenitor cells have been possible using purified erythroid colony-forming cells (CFU-E) which express 200 high-affinity (K_d 0.1 nM) and 850 low-affinity (K_d 0.57 nM) receptors per cell (Krantz et al., 1990).

Steel factor/SCF receptor. The receptor for SCF is the c-*kit* proto-oncogene product which is expressed on 4% of normal low-density marrow mononuclear cells. These cells belong to progenitor cell and colony-forming cell populations and to maturing mast cell populations (Ashman et al., 1991). Flanagan and Leder (1990) expressed SCF as a cell surface protein on 3T3 fibroblasts and found that it bound the kit protein (receptor) with a K_d of 30 nM.

IL-1 receptor. Information about the IL-1 receptor which binds IL-1α and IL-1β has been reviewed recently by Dinarello et al. (1989). Interleukin 1 binds to IL-1-responsive T cell lines which express 238 receptors per cell with an affinity of 3.6 nM and to fibroblast cell lines expressing 5×10^3 receptors per cell with an affinity of 2.6 nM (Dower et al., 1986).

IL-2 receptor. Interleukin 2 binds to two distinct receptor molecules (Rα, p55 and Rβ, p75) on activated T cells. The β chain has the higher affinity of the two (K_d 0.82 nM) and accounts for 10% of the 500–5000 IL-2 receptors. The K_d value for the α chain is 18 nM and when the two chains combine to form a high-affinity receptor the K_d is 18 pM (Robb et al., 1987).

IL-4 receptor. Human IL-4 binds specifically to high-affinity (K_d 70 pM) receptors on a Burkitt's lymphoma cell line which expresses 1200 binding sites per cell; lower-affinity sites have also been described (see Yokota et al., 1988). Most T and B cell lines express a few hundred receptors per cell and binding sites have also been detected on epithelial and endothelial cells and on fibroblasts. The soluble form of the IL-4 receptor has the same binding kinetics and affinity as the membrane-bound form (Jacobs et al., 1991).

IL-5 receptor. Interleukin 5 binds rapidly and specifically to its receptor on an IL-5-responsive cell line which expresses 200 high-affinity (K_d 400 pM) and 1000 low-affinity (K_d 1.1 nM) binding sites per cell (Takatsu et al., 1988).

IL-6 receptor. Epstein–Barr virus-transformed B cells express a single class (K_d 370 pM) of 2700 binding sites per cell but none are found on Burkitt's lymphoma cell lines. Normal B cells express receptors only after activation (600 per cell; K_d 420 pM) but expression by T cells is constitutive (300 per cell; K_d 140 pM; Taga et al., 1987).

IL-8 receptor. The IL-8 receptor is expressed exclusively on neutrophils and binds IL-8 with an apparent affinity of 1.2 nM (Thomas et al., 1991).

Interferon receptors. A wide variety of cell types express different numbers (200–10 000) of high-affinity receptors for IFNα. The curvilinear Scatchard plot suggests that there may also be a fairly high number of low-affinity receptors. Interferon β binds to the same receptor as IFNα and has similar binding properties. The IFNγ receptor is separate but has a similar affinity to the α/β receptor (K_d 1 nM–10 pM) and is expressed in similar numbers (see Langer and Petska, 1988).

TGFβ receptor. Virtually all cells have high-affinity (K_d 1–60 pM) receptors for TGFβ$_1$ which are of three types (M_r 280, 85 and 65 kDa) and most cells express all of them at the cell surface (Cheifetz et al., 1987). An inverse relationship between the receptor affinity and the numbers expressed per cell is such that different cell types bind the same number of molecules at physiological concentrations (Wakefield et al., 1987).

TNF receptor. The tumour necrosis factors TNFα and TNFβ (formerly known as lymphotoxin) share a common receptor. Binding studies using monocyte membrane preparations revealed the presence of 230 high-affinity (K_d 26 pM) and 3800 low-affinity sites per cell (Imamura et al., 1987).

Receptor characterization

Chemical cross-linking of radiolabelled ligand to receptor is a sensitive way of determining the molecular weight of growth factors and the published results are summarized in Table 1.4 and by Park et al. (1990). In some cases, binding proteins of different sizes have been detected. This may be because more than one binding protein is required to constitute a functional high-affinity receptor (e.g. the IL-2 receptor), because of differences in glycosylation between one cell type and another or because of proteolytic degradation during preparation of the sample. Hanazona et al. (1991) interpret their finding of two G-CSF binding proteins on normal and CML neutrophils as indicative of alternate splicing of message from a single gene. The size of the erythropoietin receptor obtained by cross-linking iodinated

Table 1.4 Molecular mass (M_r) of some human haemopoietic growth factor/interleukin receptors determined by chemical cross-linking

Receptor	M_r (kDa)	Reference
GM-CSF	84	DiPersio et al. (1990)
	150, 115, 95	Chiba et al. (1990)
	93	Gesner et al. (1989)
G-CSF	150, 120	Uzumaki et al. (1989)
	160, 110	Hanazono et al. (1991)
IL-3	69	Gesner et al. (1989)
	170, 130, 70	Tamura et al. (1990)
Erythropoietin	66, 100	Jones et al. (1990)
		Winkelman et al. (1990)
IL-1	80	Dinarello et al. (1989)
	26–220	Dinarello et al. (1989)
IL-2	α-55; β-75	
IL-4	70, 140	Yokota et al. (1988)
IL-7	68, 75, 153	Goodwin et al. (1990)
IFNγ	90, 50–55	see Langer and Petska (1988)
TGFβ	280, 65, 85	Cheifetz et al. (1987)

For abbreviations see Table 1.1.

erythropoietin does not agree with the molecular weight predicted by its cDNA sequence. Recently, studies with biotinylated erythropoietin and using a ligand-blotting technique demonstrated that the native erythropoietin receptor exists as a single protein of 60–65 kDa (Wognum et al., 1990a; Atkins et al., 1991).

Use of reducing versus non-reducing conditions for electrophoresis can show whether or not a receptor molecule is likely to exist as a dimer. For example, the two G-CSF-binding proteins in placenta were not disulphide-linked components of a single receptor complex since their M_r values were the same under reducing and non-reducing conditions. They could be the same protein differently glycosylated or the 120 kDa protein could result from degradation of the 150 kDa species (Uzumaki et al., 1989).

Antibodies to a number of receptors are available and can be used for protein characterization by immunoprecipitation. Some antibodies that block receptor binding to its ligand can be used to analyse the structure of the ligand-binding site. Highly abundant receptors may be available in sufficient quantity for purification and protein sequencing. As we have seen, molecular cloning of the receptors leads to predictions about their structure and can reveal relationships with other members of gene families.

Receptor regulation

It is now realized that studies of growth factor binding to receptors under equilibrium conditions give an unrealistic picture of their potential to interact because cells can regulate the numbers and affinities of the receptors they express. In common with most other growth factor–receptor interactions, occupation of an HGF receptor by its ligand results in internalization of the complex and degradation inside the cell (Nicola et al., 1988; Cannistra et al., 1990). This sequence can be referred to as 'homologous down-modulation' (see Nicola, 1991). A more complex pattern of heterologous receptor down-modulation, known as 'trans down-modulation', has been described in studies on mouse bone marrow cells by Walker et al. (1985). This involves occupation of a receptor by its ligand and a reduction in the capacity of other receptors to bind their respective ligands. A hierarchical sequence was discerned which showed that IL-3 down-regulated receptors for GM-, G- and M-CSFs; GM-CSF down-regulated G- and M-CSF receptors, and G- and M-CSF only influenced the expression of other receptors when they were present at very high concentrations. An example of cross-modulation is provided by the apparent interaction between IL-3 and GM-CSF receptors which occurs equally in both directions and involves only the high-affinity class of receptors (Cannistra et al., 1990; DiPersio et al., 1990; Nicola, 1991).

The HGFs can also be down-modulated by exposure to bacterial lipopolysaccharide, phorbol ester, IFNγ, TNF and the chemotactic peptide f-met-leu-phe (fMLP). Receptor expression can be up-regulated as well as induced as shown by the effect of IFNγ on the TNFα/β receptor and the treatment of HL60 cells with dimethyl sulphoxide (Aggarwal et al., 1985; Tsujimoto et al., 1986; Nicola, 1987).

Changes in receptor affinity are another way of regulating receptor function. All of the HGFs can exist in high- and low-affinity forms (K_d 1–100 pM and 1–10 nM). This suggests either that there are separate high- and low-affinity receptors or that the one form can be converted into the other. Nicola (1991) proposed that the latter explanation is correct and has presented a molecular model to account for the conversion. It is already clear that the high-affinity receptors for IL-2 and IL-6 consist of ligand-binding and non-binding components (see above) and Nicola (1991) suggests that similar associations are involved in regulating HGF receptor affinities.

Thus, the low-affinity HGF receptors share and compete for common subunits which convert them into high-affinity receptors (Fig. 1.14a). In fulfilment of this hypothesis, the α chains for the human IL-3, GM-CSF and IL-5 receptors have now been cloned and shown to associate with a common β chain (Fig. 1.14b) when they form high-affinity receptors (Gearing et al., 1989; Kitamura et al., 1991a,b; Tavernier et al., 1991). It should not be forgotten that receptors can be up-regulated by exposure to some growth factors as well as down-regulated. Thus, growth factors acting early in cell development can induce expression of receptors for growth factors required later in cell development.

Chromosomal localization of growth factor and receptor genes

The availability of cloned cDNA probes for genes encoding the HGFs has led to their karyotypic localization using in situ hybridization or hybridization with chromosomes isolated by high-resolution sorting methods. The information obtained from these studies has been relevant to our understanding of the evolutionary relationships between growth factor genes and ways in which abnormalities in growth factor production might be implicated in haematological disease. For example, as shown in Table 1.5, the genes for GM-CSF, IL-3, M-CSF, IL-5 and IL-9 are found very close together on chromosome 5. The genes for GM-CSF and IL-3 are arranged in tandem on chromosome 5 and separated by 9 kb, suggesting that they may have evolved from the same ancestral gene (Yang et al., 1988). The two IL-1 genes are located

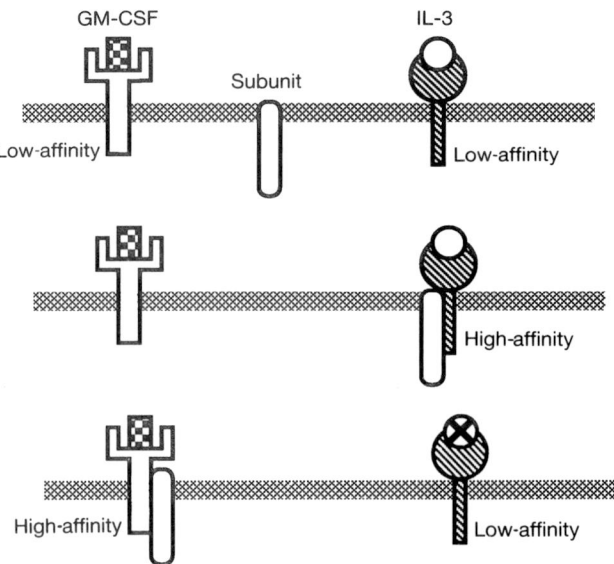

Fig. 1.14a Nicola's hypothesis for the interaction between low-affinity receptors and common subunits in the formation of high-affinity growth factor receptors.

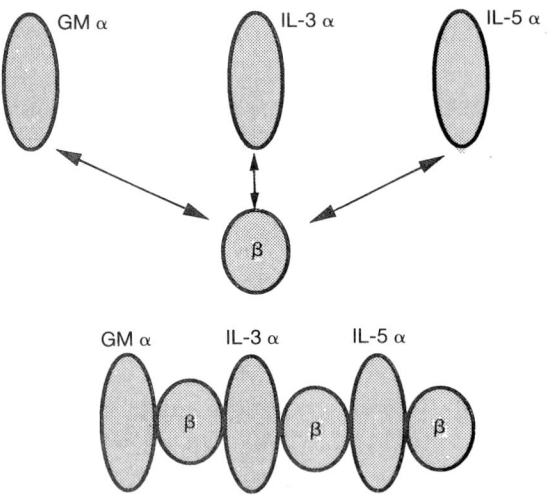

Fig. 1.14b Kitamura's model for the formation of high-affinity receptors: α = individual α chains for the IL-3, IL-5 and CSF receptors; β = common β chain receptors for IL-3, IL-5 and GM-CSF.

in the same chromosomal region on chromosome 2. This finding, together with the apparent structural relationship between the two genes and the close similarity or identity of their receptors, suggests that they may have arisen by duplication of a single gene.

Table 1.5 Chromosomal localization of haemopoietic growth factor genes

Growth factor	Chromosome	Band	Reference
GM-CSF	5q	23–32	Yang et al. (1988)
IL-3	5q	23–32	Yang et al. (1988)
G-CSF	17		Simmers et al. (1987)
M-CSF	5q	33.1	Pettenati et al. (1987)
Erythropoietin	7		Powell et al. (1986)
IL-1α	2q	13	Lafage et al. (1989)
IL-1β	2q		Webb et al. (1986)
IL-2	4q		Seigel et al. (1984)
IL-4	5q	23–31	Le Beau et al. (1989)
IL-5	5q	23.3–32	Sutherland et al. (1988)
IL-6	7		Sehgal et al. (1986)
IL-7	8q	12–13	Sutherland et al. (1989a)
IL-9	5q	31–32	Kelleher et al. (1991)
IFNα/β	9q	22	Trinchieri et al. (1987); Pitha (1990)
IFNγ	12		Trinchieri et al. (1987)
TGFβ	19q		Derynck et al. (1985)
TNFα/β	6		Hamblin (1988)
LIF	22q	12	Sutherland et al. (1989b)

For abbreviations see Table 1.1.

Haemopoietic growth factor genes may be altered in association with several haematological diseases. Genes found in the q23–32 region of chromosome 5 are deleted in the 5q– syndrome (Pettenati et al., 1987; Sutherland et al., 1988, LeBeau et al., 1989). Similarly, rearrangement or loss of IFNα and β genes may occur when chromosome 9p is altered in lymphoid leukaemias. This region has been identified as a putative location for a tumour suppressor gene which may be the IFN gene itself or some other closely related gene (see Pitha, 1990). Growth factor genes may also be involved in translocations: the G-CSF gene is close to the breakpoint on chromosome 17 that is involved in the t(15;17) characteristic of promyelocytic leukaemia (Simmers et al., 1987).

Similar considerations apply to the chromosomal localization of growth factor receptor genes. Recently, the GM-CSF receptor gene has been found to be located in the pseudoautosomal regions of the X and Y chromosomes, which are so called because alleles in this region can be exchanged between male and female sex chromosomes and escape X inactivation. This means that they can be inherited as if they are truly autosomal. The finding that GM-CSF receptor genes are located here is particularly interesting because loss of either the X or the Y chromosome is seen in 25% of cases of M2 AML, suggesting that a recessive oncogene (tumour suppressor factor) might also be located in this region (Gough et al., 1990).

The M-CSF/CSF-1 receptor (c-*fms*) and PDGFβ receptor are

arranged in a tandem head-to-tail fashion on chromosome 5 (q33.3), suggesting that they evolved from the same ancestral gene which amplified and subsequently diverged (see Sherr, 1990). However, c-*kit*, the receptor for SCF, is located on chromosome 4 (Yarden *et al.*, 1987) despite its probable evolutionary relationship to the M-CSF and PDGF receptors. The gene for the IL-2 receptor β chain is located on chromosome 22q11.2–q12 in a region that is subject to non-random chromosome aberrations in several lymphoid malignancies (Gnarra *et al.*, 1990) whilst human IFN receptor genes are located on chromosome 21 (α/β) and chromosome 6q21–q22 (see Langer and Petska, 1988). The gene for the human erythropoietin receptor has been assigned to chromosome 19p but this region has not been associated with any inherited deficiencies of erythropoiesis (Winkelman *et al.*, 1990).

Signal transduction

Signal transduction is the mechanism whereby a growth factor bound to a receptor at the cell surface transmits a signal across the cell membrane and elicits the appropriate cellular response. Once transduced into the cell interior, the signal activates biochemical pathways and the mechanisms of signal transduction and the consequent cellular events are being studied in a variety of cell types. Several pathways have been identified and their roles in the stimulation of haemopoietic target cells following growth factor binding are under investigation. These studies could help to answer some of the puzzles surrounding the multitarget and multifunctional aspects of the biological effects of haemopoietic growth factors. For example, activation by a single growth factor of different intracellular pathways could lead to different responses in different cells. Also, it is possible that different mechanisms could operate within a single cell to reinforce the signal.

Three major biochemical pathways have been implicated in signal transduction in general (Michell, 1989; Farrar *et al.*, 1990) and they appear to be applicable to growth factor-mediated activation of haemopoietic progenitor cells (Fig. 1.15). One of these mechanisms is receptor-mediated protein tyrosine phosphorylation, indicating that the target molecules may be protein tyrosine kinases or phosphatases. The other two processes require guanosine triphosphate-dependent coupling proteins and involve either the activation of adenylate cyclase, which results in the formation of cyclic adenosine monophosphate, or hydrolysis of inositol lipids. The common outcome of these intracellular reactions is a change in the phosphorylation status of target proteins and this is of central importance in the regulation of cell metabolism.

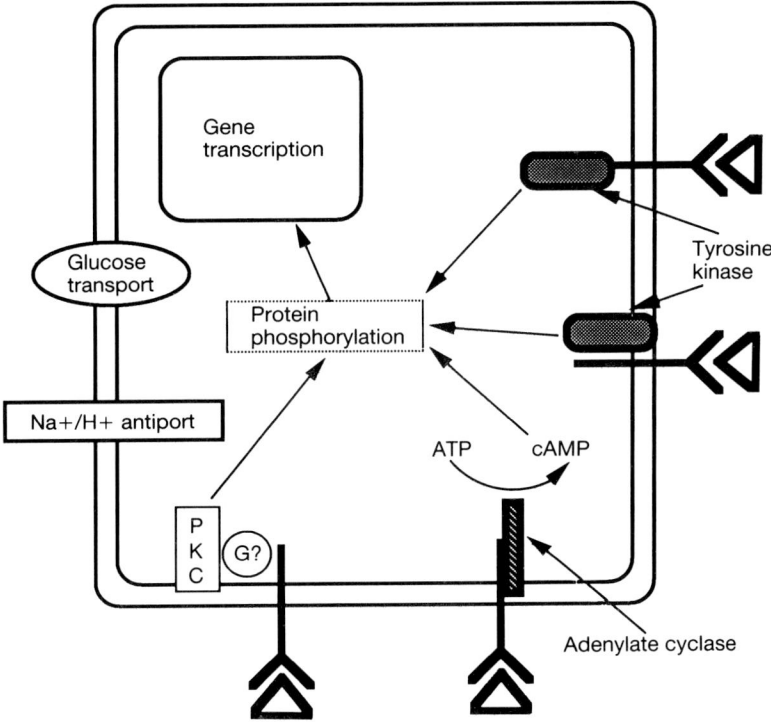

Fig. 1.15 Components of signal transduction pathways.

The signal transduction events initiated by HGFs binding to their receptors have been reviewed by Farrar *et al.* (1990) and the molecular mechanisms of transmembrane signalling in B cells by Cambier and Ransom (1987). Information in this area is incomplete and most work has been done on signal transduction by the IL-2 receptor.

The receptors can be separated into two major classes – those which have intrinsic tyrosine kinase activity and those which do not. The only HGF receptors that have been shown to have intrinsic kinase activity are the M-CSF receptor (c-*fms*) and the SCF receptor (c-*kit*) but none can be attributed to receptors such as those for GM-CSF, IL-1 or IL-2. However, the information summarized earlier in this chapter shows that growth factor-binding proteins may not constitute biologically active receptors and components that have not yet been discovered may form parts of receptors that confer tyrosine kinase activity. The commonality of the β subunit of the IL-3, GM-CSF and IL-5 receptors described earlier in this chapter, together with its role in signal transduction (Kitamura *et al.*, 1991a), are at first sight inconsistent with the different responses of cells stimulated with these growth factors. The β subunit lacks the consensus sequences of signalling molecules such as protein tyrosine kinases and may interact

Table 1.6 Signal transduction in haemopoietic cells

GM-CSF	A role for guanine nucleotide regulatory proteins indicated by effects of pertussis toxin (Sorensen et al., 1989) Phosphorylation of multiple proteins on serine and tyrosine
G-CSF	Activation of G proteins and adenylate cyclase system Protein (p68) phosphorylation (Matsuda et al., 1989)
M-CSF	Receptor-mediated internalization and degradation of M-CSF (Chen et al., 1987) Intrinsic tyrosine kinase activity
IL-3	Protein kinase C translocates from cytosol to membrane (Farrar et al., 1985; Whetton et al., 1986) Diacylglycerol replaces IL-3 (Evans et al., 1986) Intracellular Ca++ levels unchanged (Whetton et al., 1988a) Na+/H+ antiport activated and intracellular pH increased (Whetton et al., 1988b) Increased glucose transport and intracellular adenosine triphosphate (Whetton and Dexter, 1983; Palacios and Garland, 1984; Whetton et al., 1984) Serine/threonine and tyrosine phosphorylation of numerous proteins
Epo	Intracellular Ca++ increased; Ca++ adenosine triphosphatase (calcium pump) activity decreased (Sawyer and Krantz, 1984; Mladenovic et al., 1986; Lawrence et al., 1987) Decreased phosphorylation of membrane pp43 (Choi et al., 1987)
IL-1	Effects of cyclic adenosine monophosphate on B cells implicates adenylate cyclase (Shirakawa et al., 1989) Activation of phospholipase C (Kester et al., 1989) Phosphoinositide pathway implicated in T cells but not in B cells (Farrar et al., 1986; Tigges et al., 1989)
IL-2	Increased guanosine triphosphate binding and hydrolysis Activation and translocation of protein kinase C Protein phosphorylation
IL-4	No change in Ca++ concentration No change in inositol phospholipid metabolism Protein phosphorylation on tyrosine (see Paul, 1991)
IL-7	Inositol phosphate metabolism; protein tyrosine phosphorylation (Dibirdik et al., 1991; Uckun et al., 1991)

For abbreviations see Table 1.1.

with further undefined signalling molecules to elicit a response. It is of interest to note that both IL-3 and GM-CSF and their receptors use the *ras* gene product (p21) as a signal transducer (Satoh et al., 1991).

A variety of approaches can be used to implicate a particular pathway in receptor-mediated signal transduction. For example, phorbol ester treatment of cells can substitute for diacylglycerol and activate protein kinase C; translocation of protein kinase C from the cytosol to the membrane and changes in intracellular calcium concentrations can be measured; treatment with pertussis toxin prevents inhibition of cyclic adenosine monophosphate formation by blocking G proteins in the adenylate cyclase pathway and inhibitors of protein kinase C can also be used. The responses of haemopoietic cells to stromal cells have been investigated in similar ways and agents that are known to influence adenosine diphosphate-ribosylation of membrane-associated proteins have been shown to have profound effects on the growth and development of haemopoietic cells in stroma-supported systems *in vitro* (Heyworth and Dexter, 1988). Other studies have investigated the signal transduction events that accompany the stimulation of stromal cells to produce growth factors (Derigs *et al.*, 1990).

Some of the information that has been produced by studies of signal transduction pathways is summarized in Table 1.6. The pathways culminate in altered protein phosphorylation and transcription of certain genes and major efforts have been made to identify phosphorylation events and phospho-amino acid specificities. The finding that there can be several phosphorylation events following stimulation with a single growth factor suggests that several serine/threonine kinase and several tyrosine kinase systems can be activated at the same time.

Phosphatases also are important for regulating protein phosphorylation in cell signalling (see Alexander, 1990). The CD45 family of phosphotyrosine phosphatases is particularly interesting because they occur in at least five isoforms, some of which are differentially expressed on primitive haemopoietic cells (Lansdorp *et al.*, 1990). Also, the expression of CD45 cell surface antigens has been linked to haemopoietic cell stimulation by growth factors (Broxmeyer *et al.*, 1991b). The transmembrane phosphatases may function as receptors for unknown ligands and be coupled to second messenger systems involving tyrosine dephosphorylation. Potential ligands include extracellular matrix molecules because the phosphatases share common structural motifs with known cell adhesion molecules (see Alexander, 1990).

BIOLOGICAL EFFECTS OF GROWTH FACTOR–TARGET CELL INTERACTIONS

This section is concerned with the correspondence between HGFs and the target cells that respond to them. It is noteworthy that growth factors are not thought to be required for the survival of primitive progenitor cells in the G_0 period of the cell cycle (Leary *et al.*, 1989). Much of this area has been thoroughly and expertly reviewed already and it is not necessary to give a complete account here. However, several points are worth mentioning because they document advances that have been made in haemopoietic cell culture technology. One advance is the use of purified recombinant proteins for many *in vitro* studies instead of unpurified or semipurified natural proteins. In general, purified recombinant growth factors do not appear to stimulate the full range of colony-forming cells within a compartment but, rather, have been shown to stimulate subpopulations of GEMM-CFC, BFU-E and GM-CFC (Sieff et al., 1985; Strife et al., 1987). This observation suggests that the growth factors themselves interact with other activities present in serum or conditioned medium when they are used in in vitro culture systems. Efforts have been made to avoid this complication by developing serum-free culture systems.

Another variable that will influence the results is the presence in the culture system of cells which might perform an accessory function by producing a factor that may interact with the factor of interest. This problem can be circumvented by preparing enriched or purified populations of target progenitor cells. Obviously, whilst interactions with accessory cells and other growth factors are important for predicting responses in vivo, the final assignation of growth factors to specific target cells requires that these conditions are met. None the less, a great many studies have been done on unpurified progenitor cells in serum-containing cultures. The influence of refined culture systems on the observed progenitor cell response is discussed more fully later on in this section. Finally, semisolid culture systems do not take account of any role of marrow stromal cells in progenitor cell responses to growth factors. These influences can be expected to be physiologically important and, as such, relevant to the in vivo response to therapeutically administered growth factors.

Human HGFs and their targets

The effects of the haemopoietic and lymphopoietic growth factors and cytokines on their target cells may be stimulatory, inhibitory or synergistic. 'Stimulatory' and 'inhibitory' actions are self-explanatory. 'Synergy' refers to the phenomenon observed when combinations of two or more growth factors result in a greater effect than would be expected from the results of testing the factors individually. For example, some synergistic factors have no intrinsic capacity to stimulate colony formation by themselves but enhance the effects of other growth factors (Quesenberry, 1986). The synergizing activities may induce early cells to express receptors so that they can respond to other growth factors. Alternatively, they may act as competence factors which prime cells for entry into the DNA-synthetic phase of the cell cycle whilst other factors act as 'progression' factors (O'Keefe and Pledger, 1983).

Only brief comments will be made about the individual growth factors in this text.

GM-CSF

Granulocyte-macrophage colony-stimulating factor has activities throughout the haemopoietic system which qualify it as a multi-lineage haemopoietin. As well as stimulating colony formation by progenitor cells of the myeloid and erythroid lineages, it stimulates haemopoiesis in long-term bone marrow cultures (Coutinho *et al.*, 1990) and limited proliferation by blast cells, promyelocytes and promonocytes (Begley *et al.*, 1988). It stimulates the production of cytokines, such as IL-1α and β, IL-6, IFNα and TNF by neutrophils and monocytes (Lopez *et al.*, 1987; Cannistra *et al.*, 1987, 1988; Sisson and Dinarello, 1988; Dinarello *et al.*, 1989; Ciccio *et al.*, 1990; Shirafuji *et al.*, 1990) and promotes the effector functions and functional activities of monocytes, tissue macrophages, neutrophils, eosinophils and antigen-presenting cells (Lopez *et al.*, 1986, 1987; Metcalf *et al.*, 1986; Fabian *et al.*, 1987; Morrissey *et al.*, 1987; Wang *et al.*, 1987; Cannistra *et al.*, 1988; Coleman *et al.*, 1988; Socinski *et al.*, 1988). In combination with other haemopoietic growth factors, GM-CSF has synergistic effects on colony formation by progenitor cells *in vitro* (Paquette *et al.*, 1988; Zhou *et al.*, 1988; Caracciolo *et al.*, 1989; Bot *et al.*, 1990b). Outside of the haemopoietic system, GM-CSF stimulates the migration and proliferation of endothelial cells (Bussolino *et al.*, 1989).

Burst-promoting activity (BPA) was first identified as a factor that improves erythroid burst formation by BFU-E *in vitro* (see Gordon and Barrett, 1985) but it is now known to be the same factor as GM-CSF and has, therefore, the same target cells and range of activities.

IL-3

Interleukin-3 and GM-CSF affect similar target cell populations in colony assays, long-term cultures and tests of mature cell function (Lopez *et al.*, 1987; Messner *et al.*, 1987; Cannistra *et al.*, 1988; Saeland *et al.*, 1988; Sieff *et al.*, 1988; Oster *et al.*, 1989; Coutinho *et al.*, 1990). It also demonstrates similar synergistic activities (Leary *et al.*, 1988; Paquette *et al.*, 1988; Zhou *et al.*, 1988; Bot *et al.*, 1989a) and can counteract the inhibitory action of TGFβ on colony formation by BFU-E (Del Rizzo *et al.*, 1990).

G-CSF

This factor acts on relatively late granulocyte colony-forming cells (G-CFC) and is mostly lineage-restricted in its action, although it has an unexpected influence on endothelial cells (Bussolino *et al.*, 1989). It stimulates the later stages of haemopoiesis in long-term cultures

(Coutinho *et al.*, 1990) and enhances the functional activities of neutrophils (Wang *et al.*, 1988; Shirafuji *et al.*, 1990). Synergistic effects with IL-3 and GM-CSF have been observed in cultures of GM-CFC, G-CFC, eosinophil (Eo)-CFC and M-CFC (Paquette *et al.*, 1988). In blast colony assays, the colonies appear earlier in the presence of G-CSF, which is interpreted as showing that G-CSF stimulates early resting (G_0) cells to enter the cell cycle (Ikebuchi *et al.*, 1988).

M-CSF

This lineage-restricted growth factor stimulates the proliferation and differentiation of mononuclear phagocytes from M-CFC, promotes the effector functions of macrophages and stimulates cytokine production by them (see Baccarani and Stanley, 1990). It synergizes with IL-3, IL-1 and IL-6 in assays of M-CFC (Zhou *et al.*, 1988; Bot *et al.*, 1989a). In the long-term culture system, however, it inhibits the development of progenitors of the granulocyte, macrophage and erythroid lineages. This effect probably is mediated by the stromal cells producing inhibitory factors in response to the M-CSF (Mayani *et al.*, 1991).

Erythropoietin

Erythropoietin stimulates the proliferation and maturation of the later stages of erythropoiesis during colony formation by BFU-E and stimulates colony formation by CFU-E. It also promotes colony formation by megakaryocyte progenitor cells. Recently, it has been shown that erythropoietin retards DNA breakdown and prevents programmed cell death (apoptosis) in erythroid precursor cells (Koury and Bondurant, 1990). This survival effect is its major effect on late erythroid progenitor cells where it has little mitogenic activity (Spivak *et al.*, 1991).

Steel factor/SCF

Stem cell factor appears to be an early-acting cytokine that stimulates immature haemopoietic progenitor cells to enter the cell cycle, like G-CSF (Ogawa, 1991). In clonogenic assays, SCF has little stimulating activity on its own but it enhances colony formation in the presence of other haemopoietic growth factors (Bernstein *et al.*, 1991; Broxmeyer *et al.*, 1991a).

IL-1

Interleukin-1 refers to a family of polypeptide growth factors (Oppenheim *et al.*, 1986) that are essential for immunological and inflammatory responses and for tissue repair. They are produced mainly by mononuclear phagocytes and influence several cell types in different ways.

Interleukin-1 has multiple direct and indirect effects on the haemopoietic system. It stimulates blast colony formation, haemopoiesis in long-term cultures, T cell colony formation and growth factor production by stromal cells and monocytes (Lovhaug et al., 1986; Zucali et al., 1987a/b; Brandt et al., 1988; Fibbe et al., 1988; Kaushansky et al., 1988; Schindler and Dinarello, 1990). It suppresses erythropoiesis via TNFα, inhibits B lymphopoiesis in stromal cultures and inhibits IL-7-induced B cell colony formation (Schooley et al., 1987; Dorshkind, 1988; Suda et al., 1989; Furmanski and Johnson, 1990). It synergizes with M-CSF, GM-CSF or IL-3 in M-CFC cultures (Zhou et al., 1988) and with IL-4 or IL-6 in B cell activation and antibody formation (see Schindler and Dinarello, 1990).

Interestingly, exposure to IL-1 up-regulates the expression of receptors for IL-3, IL-5, GM-CSF and erythropoietin, which suggests that it has a role in regulating the growth factor responsiveness of haemopoietic cells during differentiation (Kitamura et al., 1991c). It also induces expression of GM-CSF in immature normal bone marrow cells, which indicates that autocrine stimulation of haemopoiesis is a normal regulatory mechanism (Bot et al., 1990a). In endothelial cells, increased levels of IL-1α, an autocrine negative regulator of endothelial growth, are associated with cell senescence. This can be counteracted by treating the cells with an IL-1α antisense oligomer (Cozzolino et al., 1990; Maier et al., 1990).

IL-2

Interleukin-2 was originally described as T cell growth factor and is very prominent in the regulation of this lineage. It stimulates the proliferation of activated T and B cells, induces proliferation of NK cells and enhances their effector functions, and increases oxidative burst activity in monocytes (see Schwinzer and Resch, 1990).

IL-4

This is another lymphokine with many biological activities that has been known by a variety of names relating to its effects on B cells, T cells, mast cells and macrophages. It stimulates DNA synthesis, immunoglobulin E (IgE) and IgG_1 synthesis in stimulated B cells and proliferation by mast cells and T cells but suppresses the direct effects of IL-2 on B cells (see Jansen et al., 1990 and Callard, 1991, for review). It promotes basophilic and eosinophilic growth (Favre et al., 1990) but inhibits IL-3-dependent haemopoietic colony formation (de Wolf et al., 1990; Sonada et al., 1990; Vellenga et al., 1990) and synergizes with G-CSF in G-CFC assays (Sonada et al., 1990; Vellenga et al., 1990). It also inhibits secretion of IL-1β, TNFα and IL-6 by monocytes (te Velde et al., 1990) and down-regulates the IL-2 receptor β chain (p75) by accelerating its endocytosis (Ishikawa et al., 1991).

IL-5

Interleukin 5 appears to be the factor that is important for the terminal differentiation of eosinophils (Campbell et al., 1987; Sonada et al., 1989). It stimulates murine B cells but not human B cells (Sanderson et al., 1986, 1988).

IL-6

Megakaryopoiesis and megakaryocyte development *in vitro* are enhanced by IL-6 (Ishibashi et al., 1989; Koike et al., 1990; Williams et al., 1990). It increases the cell cycle activity of GEMM-CFC, GM-CFC and BFU-E and synergizes with the HGFs in colony assays (Bot et al., 1989a; Caracciolo et al., 1989; Gardner et al., 1990; Leary et al., 1990) and with IL-1 and IL-4 in thymocyte proliferation (see van Snick, 1990).

In the blast colony assay it stimulates G_0 cells to enter the cell cycle, with the result that blast colony formation is accelerated (Ikebuchi et al., 1987). In this respect, IL-6 and G-CSF are similar.

IL-7

The influence of IL-7 appears to be restricted to lymphopoiesis. It stimulates proliferation of murine pre-B cells and is mitogenic for immature T cells. It is conceivable, therefore, that IL-7 is responsible for lymphoid differentiation at the stem cell level. Mature T cells respond to IL-7 in the presence of a second mitogenic or antigenic stimulus but this is likely to be an indirect effect because IL-7 causes the release of IL-2 and the expression of IL-2 receptors. In fact, responses to concanavalin A plus IL-7 were inhibited by antibodies against either IL-2 or the IL-2 receptor (reviewed by Henney, 1989). In cultures of human bone marrow cells, IL-7 stimulated the production of mature T cells expressing either CD4 or CD8 but CD4+CD8+ lymphocytes (i.e. earlier cells) were not found. There was no detectable B lymphopoiesis in the cultures, but this may have been a result of very low numbers of B lineage target cells in the adult bone marrow (Tushinski et al., 1991).

IL-8

The main role of IL-8 is to act as a chemo-attractant for neutrophils and induce them to migrate to sites of inflammation where they are activated, generate superoxide and degranulate. It has been implicated in inflammatory conditions such as the adult respiratory distress syndrome, idiopathic pulmonary fibrosis, rheumatoid arthritis and asthma.

IL-9

Interleukin-9 has been shown to support the maturation of adult erythroid progenitors *in vitro* and to synergize with IL-3 and GM-CSF in cultures of fetal cells (Donahue *et al.*, 1990; Holbrook *et al.*, 1991).

IL-11

Recently, IL-11 has been added to the group of factors (G-CSF, SCF, IL-6 and LIF) that act on resting blast colony-forming cells (Ogawa, 1991). It also acts on megakaryocytopoiesis, although it has no intrinsic megakaryocyte colony-stimulating activity *in vitro* (Bruno *et al.*, 1991). In murine systems, IL-11 synergizes with IL-4 (Musashi *et al.*, 1991).

LIF

The effects of leukaemia inhibitory factor (LIF/DIA/HILDA; see Table 1.1) on myeloid cells and embryonic stem cells has been reviewed by Gough and Williams (1989). It has no effect on *in vitro* colony formation by CD34+ human bone marrow cells but does accelerate the appearance of blast colonies, which indicates that it induces cells in G_0 to enter the cell cycle (Leary *et al.*, 1990). One of its activities is, therefore, similar to the actions of G-CSF, IL-6 and IL-11. It can also induce the formation of mixed lineage colonies *in vitro* but does not influence the formation of colonies by more mature progenitors (BFU-E and GM-CFC), although some studies show an increase in eosinophil colonies (Verfaillie and McGlave, 1991).

Interferons

The interferons are a family of proteins which are best known for their capacity to render cells resistant to virus growth but they can also function as growth modulators and inhibitors and have important effects on haemopoiesis. Both interferons α and γ inhibit haemopoietic colony formation and suppress haemopoiesis in long-term cultures (Broxmeyer *et al.*, 1983; Rigby *et al.*, 1985; Coutinho *et al.*, 1986; Toretsky *et al.*, 1986; Trinchieri *et al.*, 1987) but, surprisingly, IFNγ synergizes with IL-3 to stimulate the growth of immature progenitor cells (Kawano *et al.*, 1991). Interferon γ up-regulates lymphocyte binding sites on endothelial cells (Duijvestijn *et al.*, 1990), enhances GM-CSF release from monocytes (Piacibello *et al.*, 1985) and activates tissue macrophages (Black *et al.*, 1987). Interferon α restores binding by CML progenitor cells to marrow stromal layers *in vitro* (Dowding *et al.*, 1990).

TGFβ

Depending on the cell type, TGFβ can be stimulatory or inhibitory. Its inhibitory effects on haemopoiesis have received much attention. It inhibits haemopoiesis in colony assays and in long-term cultures, endomitosis in megakaryocyte development, lymphopoiesis in Whitlock-Witte cultures, IL-2-dependent B and T cell proliferation, LAK cell generation and function and immunoglobulin secretion by B cells (Ohta *et al.*, 1987; Hayashi *et al.*, 1989; Cashman *et al.*, 1990; Greenberg *et al.*, 1990; Keller *et al.*, 1990; Pfeilschrifter, 1990). It increases the synthesis of several extracellular matrix components in a variety of cell types and stimulates fibroblasts and osteoclasts, but it inhibits adipogenesis and the haemopoietic support capacity of stroma in long-term marrow cultures (see Rizzino, 1988; Hayashi *et al.*, 1989; Pfeilschrifter, 1990).

TNFα

Tumour necrosis factor α, like IL-1, protects early normal haemopoietic progenitor cells from the cytotoxic effects of 4-hydroperoxycyclophosphamide (Moreb *et al.*, 1991). Studies in colony culture systems indicate that, whereas TNF enhances colony formation stimulated by relatively early-acting factors (IL-3 and GM-CSF) it suppresses responses to G-CSF and erythropoietin (Backz *et al.*, 1991). Using purified CD34+ cells in liquid and semisolid cultures, Caux *et al.* (1991) demonstrated that TNFα stimulates early IL-3-dependent proliferation but inhibits the development of cells of the granulocyte lineage whilst potentiating monocytopoiesis.

The influence of serum-free culture conditions

A few 'endogenous' or 'spontaneous' granulocyte-macrophage colonies form in cultures that contain serum but no added growth factors.

These colonies are not seen in cultures that have been deprived of serum and do not contain growth factors, demonstrating that serum supplements do not possess the growth-promoting activities of natural serum (Migliaccio et al., 1988a). Moreover, studies using monoclonal antibodies showed that fetal calf serum contains a BPA-E that is not GM-CSF (Sonada et al., 1988). Hence, erythropoietin alone will stimulate burst formation in the presence of serum but not in serum-free cultures. In addition, Migliaccio et al. (1988a) demonstrated a need for adherent cells in the serum-free culture system.

The biological activities of IL-3 and GM-CSF overlap in serum-free as well as in serum-containing cultures (Migliaccio et al., 1988a; Sonada et al., 1988) and both require other factors to induce colony formation by GM-CFC and by BFU-E in the presence of erythropoietin. However, they do exhibit some lineage preference because GM-CSF is two to three times as effective as IL-3 in stimulating GM-CFC. Conversely, IL-3 is two to three times as effective as GM-CSF in stimulating BFU-E (Migliaccio et al., 1988a; Sonada et al., 1988). The requirement for serum in GM-CFC and BFU-E cultures stimulated by IL-3 or GM-CSF seems to be moderated by adherent cells which can play a serum-replacing role, presumably because growth factors may be produced by cells activated during the adherence process. Granulocyte CSF stimulates G-CFC half as well in serum-free compared with serum-containing cultures (Ohara et al., 1987; Migliaccio et al., 1988a). Studies in serum-free cultures have also shown that the actions of IL-1 and IL-6 on haemopoiesis are mainly indirect and mediated via the production of IL-3 and GM-CSF by accessory cells. However, additional factors in serum are necessary for this stimulation of growth factor production (Migliaccio et al., 1991).

It is relevant to our understanding of haemoglobin gene expression that the abnormally high levels of fetal haemoglobin synthesis seen in serum-supplemented BFU-E cultures of adult haemopoietic cells were not seen in serum-free cultures (Fujimori et al., 1990).

The requirement for serum has been investigated further using liquid culture systems. Progenitor cells in serum-free cultures of adherent cell-depleted marrow remain fairly constant for up to eight days but decline if T cells are removed. Interleukin-3 increased BFU-E numbers, GM-CSF maintained cells in T-depleted cultures and G-CSF had no effect (Migliaccio et al., 1988b).

Enriched progenitor cell populations and the influence of accessory cells

Enriched progenitor cell fractions have been prepared from blood or bone marrow by cell sorting (Bot et al., 1988), panning on affinity plates (Strife et al., 1987; Saeland et al., 1988) or using antibody-coated immunomagnetic beads. These studies have demonstrated that recombinant growth factors can stimulate colony formation in cell populations of which 70–90% are responding target cells (Saeland et al., 1988). However, the range of cell types stimulated by the growth factors can be modified by accessory cells. Bot et al. (1988) found that human recombinant IL-3 stimulated colony formation by BFU-E, GEMM-CFC and Eo-CFC in enriched populations of $CD34^+$ cells but did not stimulate GM-, G- or M-CFC in separated cell populations. The full spectrum of colony formation was seen only in cultures of unseparated cells. The accessory cells were identified as monocytes which can produce growth factors in response to cytokines (Warren and Ralph, 1986; Horiguchi et al., 1987).

Monocytes produce M-CSF mRNA and protein constitutively and GM-CSF and G-CSF production are induced following exposure to bacterial lipopolysaccharide (Sieff et al., 1988). Granulocyte-macrophage CSF stimulates the production of TNF, IL-1α and IL-1β by blood mononuclear cells which may play an important role in orchestrating host defence mechanisms in vivo (Cannistra et al., 1987, 1988; Dinarello et al., 1989). In addition, Oster et al. (1989) have shown that GM-CSF and IL-3 can activate G-CSF transcription and release by monocytes. This pathway of growth factor induction could be involved in granulopoietic cell maturation in vivo and colony formation in vitro because both GM-CSF and G-CSF are necessary for complete stimulation of cultured human myeloid progenitors (Ferrero et al., 1989). These observations raise the possibility that high levels of growth factors acting on immature progenitor cells can have 'feed-forward' effects on the production of growth factors required for the next stage in cell development. Circulating monocytes can instantly distribute their secretory products throughout the body and macrophage populations in the tissues provide a large pool of long-lived cells with factor-producing potential. These features of the mononuclear phagocyte system make it eminently suitable for mediating inflammatory responses.

Similar types of accessory cell effect occur in the regulation of lymphopoiesis. For example, IL-7 causes IL-2 release and the expression of IL-2 receptors which are probably responsible for the apparent effect of IL-7 on mature T cell proliferation (see Henney, 1989).

Several types of marrow stromal cells can be induced in vitro to produce HGFs and many studies have been performed using murine cells in long-term bone marrow cultures. There is now an extensive literature about the regulation of growth factor production by marrow stromal cells and other mesenchymal cell populations. Sieff et al. (1988) found that M-CSF mRNA and protein are produced constitutively by human umbilical vein endothelial cells and by dermal fibroblasts. Retrovirus-immortalized endothelial cells also constitutively produce GM-CSF and G-CSF. In another study, Mizutani et al. (1987) showed that SV-40 transfected epithelial cells from the human thymic subcapsular cortex produced M-CSF.

Exposure to IL-1 induces cultured human endothelial cells to produce GM-CSF and prostaglandin E_2 (Bagby et al., 1986; Zucali et al., 1986; Sieff et al., 1987b) and IL-1 also induces thymic stromal cells to produce GM-CSF (Ridgway et al., 1988). A variety of cell types, including normal human lung fibroblasts, vascular endothelial cells and cells from several malignant tissues, produce G-, M- and GM-CSF in response to exposure to TNF (Munker et al., 1986; Broudy et al., 1987; Seelentag et al., 1987).

Physiology of the growth factor response

The HGFs we have discussed seem best designed to stimulate the rapid output of numerous cells by a single progenitor which, in semisolid culture systems, produces a colony. This type of response *in vivo* is appropriate when large numbers of cells are required rapidly. Thus, neutrophils can be produced rapidly to combat infection and red cells to restore losses due to bleeding. However, this type of response does seem appropriate for the regulation of normal steady-state haemopoiesis when stem cell activity is finely balanced to produce equal numbers of self-replicating progeny and progeny destined for differentiation. Regulation at this level is thought to be controlled by different mechanisms in which the stromal cells of the marrow play an important role.

Colony formation *in vitro* suggests a simple model of haemopoietic regulation by growth factors which involves the interaction of soluble mediators with specific receptors on the surface of target cells. In semisolid cultures, the growth factors are freely available at a uniform concentration and any cell expressing the appropriate receptor has the opportunity to respond (Fig. 1.16). This situation provides a model for the action of diffusible growth factors *in vivo* and provides for the effect of combinations of growth factors to act on a single cell without requiring the different growth factors to be produced in the vicinity of the target. However, this simple model is unlikely to provide the tightly regulated control that is characteristic of the haemopoietic system and does not explain how responses to multiple factors by cells with multiple receptors can be controlled. The issue of growth factor receptor expression by early haemopoietic cells is not yet fully resolved since some observations indicate that multipotential cells can express receptors for several growth factors (Heyworth et al.,

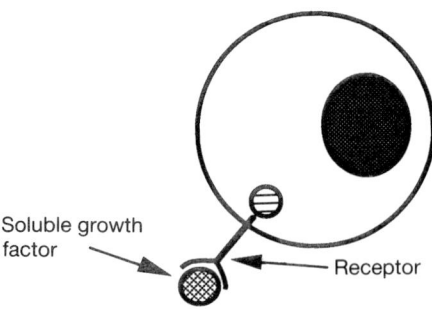

Fig. 1.16 A simple model for the regulation of target cells by soluble growth factors.

1988). Other observations, including the delayed development of blast colonies *in vitro* (see Ogawa, 1989) argue that primitive cells do not express the growth factor receptors that are found on later cells.

Clearly, the response of a progenitor cell to HGFs is determined by the availability of the growth factor and the availability of the corresponding receptors (Fig. 1.16 and see Gordon, 1991, for review). It is now apparent that both of these aspects of the growth factor response can be altered by a variety of binding interactions and modifications of the HGF and receptor proteins (Table 1.7) These alterations are likely to represent an important level of regulation of the growth factor response.

Information about the immobilization of target cells has been derived largely from studies on stroma-based culture systems *in vitro* (i.e. the long-term culture system and the Bl-CFC assay; see p. 7). It is thought that these models reflect the localization of haemopoiesis in normal adult humans which is restricted to exclusive regions of the bone marrow. Moreover, haemopoietic stem cells do not normally colonize extrahaemopoietic tissue, despite the fact that small numbers

Table 1.7 Factors affecting the availability of growth factors and their receptors

Target cells
1 Immobilization by binding to the microenvironment via surface-expressed cell adhesion molecules

Growth factors
1 Localization by binding to extracellular matrix glycosaminoglycans
2 Expression as cell surface molecules on producer cells
3 Inactivation by binding to carrier proteins
4 Activation by complexing with carrier proteins
5 Blocking by soluble receptors
6 Neutralization by autoantibodies

of stem cells circulate normally and bone marrow transplantation can be achieved by intravenous infusion of bone marrow. These observations indicate not only that haemopoiesis requires the conditions provided by the haemopoietic microenvironment, but also that stem cells can seed or 'home' to haemopoietic tissue (Gordon, 1988; Gordon and Greaves, 1989).

In long-term cultures, haemopoietic stem and progenitor cells are released into the supernatant medium but the majority of the most primitive cells are located amongst the stromal cells of the adherent layer (Cashman et al., 1985). It is likely that the relationships between stromal cells and early haemopoietic cells are maintained by binding interactions between cell adhesion molecules (CAMs) expressed by the stem and progenitor cells and the corresponding ligands which may be structures on the stromal cell surface or extracellular matrix components. The stroma-dependent blast colony assay provides a model for these binding interactions because the Bl-CFC must bind to the stromal layer before they can form colonies and be detected.

It is worth emphasizing that the different pieces of evidence for the expression of CAMs by stem cells cannot be used to imply that

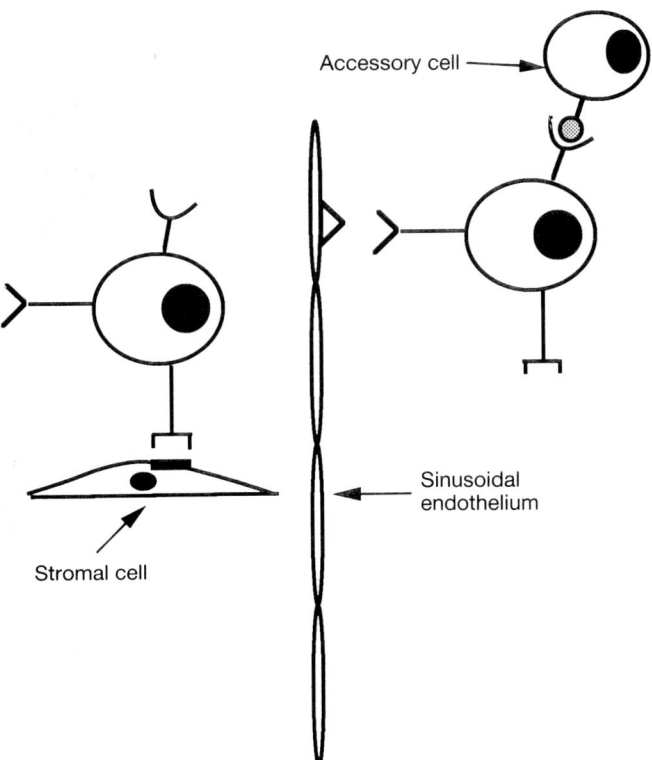

Fig. 1.17 Cell adhesion molecules and 'homing' receptors on haemopoietic cells.

the same CAM is responsible for all interactions. For example, the CAM that normally holds stem cells in the extracellular spaces of the marrow cavity may be different from the CAM that directs transplanted stem cells to haemopoietic tissue (Fig. 1.17). Also, the expression of CAMs and other properties such as migration and chemotaxis can be anticipated to alter as cells mature so that they can selectively be released into the blood stream.

A need for mechanisms to control the availability of growth factors has been indicated by experiments using mice expressing HGF transgenes or mice transplanted with cells that produce HGF as a result of infection with a retroviral construct containing an HGF gene. These experiments have shown that prolonged and high levels of exposure to the HGFs *in vivo* can have very serious toxic effects and that these occur when the HGFs are produced at high concentrations and in inappropriate locations.

Lang *et al.* (1987) produced transgenic mice expressing the murine GM-CSF transgene which resulted in an 80-fold increase in GM-CSF levels in the urine, peritoneal cavity and eye, accumulations of macrophages in the lens, retina and striated muscle and premature death. The transgene was not expressed in haemopoietic tissue and haemopoiesis was not affected significantly. Transplantation of lethally irradiated mice with bone marrow infected with GM-CSF expressing retrovirus produced even higher levels of GM-CSF (Johnson *et al.*, 1989). The mice were afflicted with a fatal disease associated with large numbers of circulating, infiltrating neutrophils, macrophages and eosinophils, massive expansion of granulocyte and macrophage populations in the peripheral blood, spleen and peritoneal cavity and infiltration of liver, lungs, skeletal muscle and eyes. Similarly, mice transplanted with retrovirus-infected IL-3 producing stem and progenitor cells develop a myeloproliferative syndrome and die (Chang *et al.*, 1989a; Wong *et al.*, 1989) but mice transplanted with cells expressing the G-CSF gene do not suffer severe tissue damage and do not die prematurely (Chang *et al.*, 1989b). Metcalf and Gearing (1989) transplanted mice with factor-dependent FDCP-1 cells that had been retrovirally-infected with the LIF gene. After 17–20 days, the mice developed a fatal syndrome involving cachexia, formation of new bone, calcification of muscle tissue, pancreatitis, atrophy of the thymus and abnormalities of the adrenal cortex, ovaries and testes.

These dramatic examples serve to emphasize the potential toxicity of very high HGF levels. Also, the contrast between the results of providing HGFs via deregulated gene expression *in vivo* and the effects of injecting them directly into the circulation suggests that physiological mechanisms exist to limit the activities of these potentially toxic agents. These mechanisms have been reviewed by Gordon (1991)

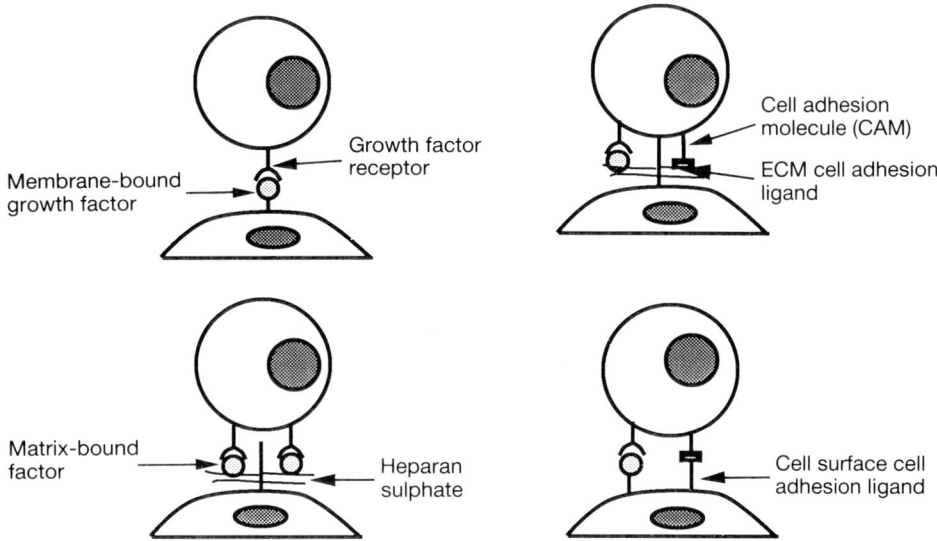

Fig. 1.18 Models for the immobilization of growth factors and their targets.

and are summarized in the following sections and in Figures 1.18 and 1.19.

Growth factor binding to components of the extracellular matrix (ECM)

Granulocyte-macrophage CSF and IL-3 bind in biologically active forms to the extracellular matrix glycosaminoglycan (GAG), heparan sulphate. Also, IFNγ binds to heparan sulphate in basement membrane ECM and there are distinct mRNAs for LIF, generated by the use of alternative promoters, that are transcribed to produce matrix-binding and diffusible glycoprotein factors. The factors appear to bind to the GAGs with relatively low affinity. This property may reflect a biological requirement for a difference in affinity for the ECM binding site and the growth factor receptor on the target cell to allow competitive removal of the growth factor from the ECM and internalization of the growth factor–receptor complex.

The finding that HGFs bind to the ECM produced in stromal cultures suggests that they could, in effect, function as CAMs and localize cells as well as stimulate their proliferation (Fig. 1.18). Alternatively, cells may 'dock' in the haemopoietic microenvironment by interaction between a dedicated CAM and its ligand and be stimulated by interaction between its growth factor receptor and matrix- or cell curface-bound growth factor (Fig. 1.18).

Growth factor modulation by binding to GAGs

Several growth factors, such as the stem cell inhibitor and a leukaemia-derived factor, have the potential to interact with heparin-like molecules *in vivo* because heparin-affinity chromatography was used in their purification. These factors may, therefore, bind to the ECM of the haemopoietic microenvironment. Equally, heparin-binding might reflect another role for GAG in the regulation of the growth factor response. Recent information from a variety of systems suggests that these roles may be of several types.

Low-affinity heparin-like binding sites for basic fibroblast growth factor (bFGF) have been shown to function as accessory molecules that are required for binding FGF to high-affinity receptors (Yayon *et al.*, 1991). Moreover, the finding that the type III receptor for TGFβ is a proteoglycan further implicates these molecules in the regulation of the growth factor response (Cheifetz *et al.*, 1988; Segarini and Seyadin, 1988). Another role for heparin-like molecules is implied by studies showing that IL-7 is a heparin-binding growth factor and that the addition of heparin to cultures inhibits IL-7-driven cell proliferation (Kimura *et al.*, 1991). In this instance, the GAG negatively regulates the activity of the growth factor.

Finally, there is evidence that M-CSF is secreted as an 80 kDa homodimer and as a multimer of more than 200 kDa that is associated with proteoglycan (Manos, 1988; Rettenmeir and Roussel, 1988). The physiological significance of this association is not known but the proteoglycan could protect the growth factor from degradation.

Membrane-bound growth factors

Several haemopoietic growth factors and other cytokines (M-CSF, SCF/c-*kit* ligand, IL-1, TGFα, TNF) can exist as membrane-bound as well as soluble molecules (see Gordon, 1991, for references). Macrophage-CSF can be expressed as an integral membrane molecule that is slowly released by proteolytic cleavage. The membrane-bound form is biologically active and stimulates the growth of mononuclear phagocytes and macrophages when it is expressed on the surface of NIH-3T3 fibroblasts. Similar activities have been demonstrated for membrane-bound SCF, IL-1, TNF and TGFα, suggesting that several growth factors may have the potential to participate in dual interactions involving cell adhesion and stimulation. Moreover, bound and soluble forms may have different effects on haemopoiesis, as shown by Williams (1991). He expressed membrane-bound and soluble SCF in stromal cell lines that do not themselves produce SCF and tested their capacity to support haemopoiesis. The stroma expressing the soluble

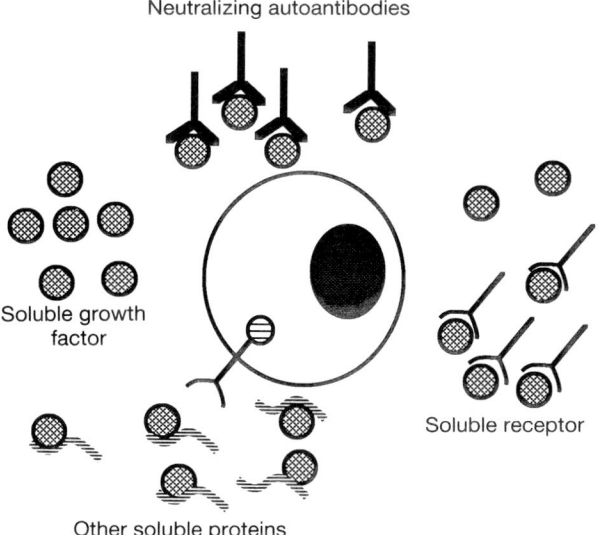

Fig. 1.19 Regulation of growth factor levels by soluble factor-binding proteins.

factor supported a short burst of haemopoiesis which subsequently failed whereas the stroma expressing the membrane-bound form supported longer-term haemopoiesis. Similarly, using stromal cells engineered to produce IL-3, Otsuka et al. (1991) showed that the concentration, duration of exposure and mode of presentation influence cellular responses to IL-3.

Growth factor binding to soluble proteins

Interactions with naturally occurring growth factor antibodies (neutralizing and non-neutralizing) and to α_2-macroglobulin have been proposed as mechanisms for regulating the effective concentrations and distributions of the HGFs. For example, latent TGFβ is complexed with α_2-macroglobulin in serum (O'Conner-McCourt and Wakefield, 1987) and the complex is dissociated by heparin (McCaffrey et al., 1989). The soluble proteins may provide carriers for growth factors, protect them from degradation or, alternatively, inactivate them (Fig. 1.19).

Growth factor binding to soluble receptors

Soluble growth factor receptors can bind to their cognate ligands in solution. The soluble IL-2 receptor has been recognized for several years and consists of the p55 (Tac antigen) chain that is part of the cell surface IL-2 receptor. Soluble forms of the IL-4 and IL-7 receptor have been detected and found to block binding of IL-4 or IL-7 to their respective target cell receptors (see Gordon, 1991, for references). Recently, a soluble human GM-CSF receptor has been identified and cloned (Raines et al., 1991) and an inhibitor of TNF has been identified as a soluble form of the TNF receptor (Fig. 1.19).

Direct producer cell-responder cell transfer

Some growth factors may be transmitted directly from producer cell to target cell, as indicated by the findings of Rich et al. (1988), who showed that marrow macrophages produce erythropoietin and are closely associated with developing normoblasts.

This discussion has demonstrated the existence of several mechanisms, with the potential to control the access of growth factors to target cells, which are likely to be physiologically important. Soluble, diffusible growth factors can act on target cells that are distant from the production site and, moreover, responses to more than one factor produced at different sites can be elicited at the same time. In comparison, immobilization of growth factors, either by binding to the ECM in haemopoietic tissue or being retained at the cell surface, may be relevant to the local control of haemopoiesis in the bone marrow. In some circumstances, it may be important to confine the range of action of potentially harmful molecules. Other potential consequences of growth factor sequestration in the ECM include deposition and storage of growth factors and protection from proteolysis.

Soluble receptors, autoantibodies and α_2-macroglobulin all have the potential to regulate growth factor interactions with their cell surface receptors. They are likely to influence the bioavailability and distribution of growth factors and may facilitate or block growth factor activities and provide carriers of growth factors in the circulation. These associations could protect the growth factors from excretion, absorption or degradation; provide a reservoir for the sustained release of active factors or prevent potentially dangerous and inappropriate effects.

REFERENCES

Aggarwal BB, Eessasu EE, Hass PE (1985) Characterization of receptors for human tumour necrosis factor and their regulation by γ-interferon. *Nature* 318, 665.

Aguet M, Dembic Z, Merlin G (1988) Molecular cloning and expression of the human interferon γ receptor. *Cell* 55, 273.

Alexander D (1990) The role of phosphatases in signal transduction. *New Biologist* 2, 1049.

Andrews RG, Singer JW, Bernstein ID (1990) Human hematopoietic precursors in long-term culture: single CD34[+] cells that lack detectable T cell, B cell and myeloid cell antigens produce multiple colony-forming cells when cultured with marrow stromal cells. *Journal of Experimental Medicine* 172, 355.

Ashman LK, Cambareri AC, To LB, Levinsky RJ, Juttner CA (1991) Expression of the YB5.B8 antigen (c-kit proto-oncogene product) in normal human bone marrow. *Blood* 78, 30.

Ashmun RA, Look AT, Roberts WM et al. (1989)

Monoclonal antibodies to the human CSF-1 receptor (c-fms proto-oncogene product) detect epitopes on normal mononuclear phagocytes and on human myeloid leukemia blast cells. *Blood* 73, 827.

Atkins HL, Broudy VC, Papayannopoulou T (1991) Characterization of the structure of the erythropoietic receptor by ligand blotting. *Blood* 77, 2577.

Auron PE. Webb AC, Rosenwasser RJ et al. (1984) Nucleotide sequence of human monocyte interleukin 1 precursor cDNA. *Proceedings of the National Academy of Sciences of the USA* 81, 7907.

Avalos BR, Gasson JC, Hedvat C et al. (1990) Human granulocyte colony-stimulating factor: biologic activities and receptor characterization on hematopoietic cells and small cell lung cancer lines. *Blood* 75, 851.

Azuma C, Tanabe T, Konishi M et al. (1986) Cloning of cDNA for human T-cell replacing factor (interleukin-5) and comparison with the murine homologue. *Nucleic Acids Research* 14, 9149.

Baccarini M, Stanley ER (1990) Colony stimulating factor-1. In: Habenicht A (ed.) *Growth Factors, Differentiation Factors and Cytokines*. Springer-Verlag, Berlin, p. 188.

Backz B, Broeders L, Bot FJ, Lowenberg B (1991) Positive and negative effects of tumor necrosis factor on colony growth from highly purified normal marrow progenitors. *Leukemia* 5, 66.

Bagby GC, Dinarello CA, Wallace P, Wagner C, Hefeneider S, McCall E (1986) Interleukin-1 stimulates granulocyte-macrophage colony-stimulating activity release by vascular endothelial cells. *Journal of Clinical Investigation* 78, 1316.

Balkwill FR (1989) *The Cytokines in Cancer Therapy*. Oxford University Press, Oxford.

Barker CR, Worman CP, Smith JL (1975) Purification and quantification of T and B lymphocytes by an affinity method. *Immunology* 29, 776.

Bazan JF (1990a) Haemopoietic receptors and helical cytokines. *Immunology Today* 11, 350.

Bazan JF (1990b) Shared architecture of hormone binding domains in type I and type II interferon receptors. *Cell* 61, 753.

Bazan JF (1990c) Structural design and molecular evolution of a cytokine receptor superfamily. *Proceedings of the National Academy of Sciences of the USA* 87, 6934.

Bazan JF (1991) Genetic and structural homology of stem cell factor and macrophage colony-stimulating factor. *Cell* 65, 9.

Begley CG, Nicola NA, Metcalf D (1988) Proliferation of normal human promyelocytes and myelocytes after a single pulse stimulation by purified GM-CSF or G-CSF. *Blood* 71, 640.

Bernstein ID, Andrews RG, Zsebo KM (1991) Recombinant human stem cell factor enhances the formation of colonies by $CD34^+$ and $CD34^+$ lin$^-$ cells, and the generation of colony-forming cell progeny from $CD34^+$ lin$^-$ cells cultured with interleukin-3, granulocyte colony-stimulating factor or granulocyte-macrophage colony-stimulating factor. *Blood* 77, 2316.

Black CM, Caterall JR, Remington JS (1987) In vivo and in vitro activation of alveolar macrophages by recombinant interferon γ. *Journal of Immunology* 138, 491.

Boraschi D, Antonio G, Perin F et al. (1990) Defining the structural requirements of a biologically active domain of IL-1β. *European Cytokine Network* 1, 21.

Bot FJ, Dorssers L, Wagemaker G, Lowenberg B (1988) Stimulating spectrum of human recombinant multi-CSF (IL-3) on human marrow precursors: influence of accessory cells. *Blood* 71, 1609.

Bot FJ, Van Eijk L, Broeders L, Aarden LA, Lowenberg B (1989a) Interleukin 6 synergises with M-CSF in the formation of macrophage colonies from purified human marrow progenitor cells. *Blood* 73, 435.

Bot FJ, Van Eijk LI, Schipper PJ, Lowenberg B (1989b) Effects of interleukin-3 on granulocytic colony forming cells in human bone marrow. *Blood* 73, 1157.

Bot FJ, Schipper P, Broeders L, Delwel R, Kaushansky K, Lowenberg B (1990a) Interleukin-1α also induces granulocyte-macrophage colony-stimulating factor in immature normal bone marrow cells. *Blood* 76, 307.

Bot FJ, Van Eijk L, Schipper P, Backx B, Lowenberg B (1990b) Synergistic effects between GM-CSF and G-CSF or M-CSF on highly enriched human marrow progenitor cells. *Leukemia* 4, 325.

Brandhuber BJ, Boone T, Kenney WC, McKay DB (1987) Three dimensional structure of interleukin-2. *Science* 238, 1707.

Brandt J, Baird N, Lu L, Srour E, Hoffman R (1988) Characterization of a human hematopoietic progenitor cell capable of forming blast cell containing colonies in vitro. *Journal of Clinical Investigation* 82, 1017.

Broudy VC, Kaushansky K, Segal GM, Harlan JM, Adamson JW (1987) Tumor necrosis factor type α stimulates human endothelial cells to produce granulocyte/macrophage colony-stimulating factor. *Proceedings of the National Academy of Sciences of the USA* 83, 7467.

Broxmeyer HE, Lu L, Platzer E, Feit C, Juliano L, Rubin BY (1983) Comparative analysis of the influences of human α, β and γ interferons on CFU-GEMM, BFU-E and CFU-GM progenitor cells. *Journal of Immunology* 131, 1300.

Broxmeyer HE, Cooper S, Lu L et al. (1991a) Effect of murine mast cell growth factor (c-kit proto-oncogene) on colony formation by human marrow hematopoietic progenitor cells. *Blood* 77, 2142.

Broxmeyer HE, Lu L, Hangoc G et al. (1991b) CD45 cell surface antigens are linked to stimulation of early human myeloid progenitor cells by interleukin-3 (IL-3), granulocyte/macrophage colony-stimulating factor (GM-CSF), a GM-CSF/IL-3 fusion protein and mast cell growth factor (a c-kit ligand). *Journal of Experimental Medicine* 174, 447.

Bruno E, Briddell RA, Cooper RJ, Hoffman R (1991) Effects of recombinant interleukin 11 on human megakaryocyte progenitor cells. *Experimental Hematology* 19, 378.

Budel LM, Touw IP, Delwel R, Lowenberg B (1989a) Granulocyte colony-stimulating factor receptors in human acute myelocytic leukemia. *Blood* 74, 2668.

Budel LM, Touw IP, Delwel R, Clark SC, Lowenberg B (1989b) Interleukin-3 and granulocyte-monocyte colony-stimulating factor receptors on human acute myelomonocytic leukemia cells and relationship to proliferative response. *Blood* 74, 565.

Bussolino F, Wang JM, Defilipi P et al. (1989) Granulocyte- and granulocyte-macrophage-colony-stimulating factors induce human endothelial cells to migrate and proliferate. *Nature* 337, 471.

Callard RE (1991) Annotation: immunoregulation by IL-4 in man. *British Journal of Haematology* 78, 293.

Cambier JC, Ransom JT (1987) Molecular mechanisms of transmembrane signalling in B lymphocytes. *Annual Review of Immunology* 5, 175.

Campbell HD, Tucker WQJ, Hort Y et al. (1987) Molecular cloning, nucleotide sequence and expression of the gene encoding human eosinophil differentiation factor (interleukin 5). *Proceedings of the National Academy of Sciences of the USA* 84, 6629.

Cannistra SA, Groshek P, Garlick R, Miller J, Griffin JD (1990) Regulation of surface expression of the granulocyte/macrophage colony-stimulating factor receptor in normal human myeloid cell. *Proceedings of the National Academy of Sciences of the USA* 87, 93.

Cannistra SA, Rambaldi A, Spriggs DR, Herrmann F, Kufe D, Griffin JD (1987) Human granulocyte-macrophage colony-stimulating factor induces expression of the tumor necrosis factor gene by the U937 cell line and by normal human monocytes. *Journal of Clinical Investigation* 79, 1720.

Cannistra SA, Vellenga E, Groshek P, Rambaldi A, Griffin JD (1988) Human granulocyte-monocyte colony-stimulating factor and interleukin-3 stimulate monocyte toxicity through a tumor necrosis factor-dependent mechanism. *Blood* 71, 672.

Caracciolo D, Clarke SC, Rovera G (1989) Human interleukin-6 supports granulocytic differentiation of hematopoietic progenitor cells and acts synergistically with GM-CSF. *Blood* 73, 666.

Carnot P, Deflandre C (1906) Sur l'activité haemopoietique du sérum au cours de la regeneration du sang. *Comptes Rendues de l'Academie de Science* 143, 384.

Cashman J, Eaves AC, Eaves CJ (1985) Regulated proliferation of primitive hematopoietic progenitor cells in long-term human marrow cultures. *Blood* 66, 1002.

Cashman JD, Eaves AC, Raines EW, Ross R, Eaves CJ (1990) Mechanisms that regulate the cell cycle status of very primitive hematopoietic cells in long-term human marrow cultures I. Stimulatory role of a variety of mesenchymal cell activators and inhibitory role of TGFβ. *Blood* 75, 96.

Caux C, Favre C, Saeland S et al. (1991) Potentiation of early hematopoiesis by tumor necrosis factor-α is followed by inhibition of granulopoietic differentiation and proliferation. *Blood* 78, 635.

Chang JM, Metcalf D, Lang RA, Johnson GR (1989a) Non-neoplastic hematopoietic myeloproliferative syndrome induced by dysregulated multi-CSF (IL-3) expression. *Blood* 73, 1487.

Chang JM, Metcalf D, Gonda TJ, Johnson GR (1989b) Long-term exposure to retrovirally expressed granulocyte colony-stimulating factor induces non-neoplastic granulocyte and progenitor cell hyperplasia without tissue damage in mice. *Journal of Clinical Investigation* 84, 1488.

Chaudhary PM, Roninson IB (1991) Expression and activity of P-glycoprotein, a multidrug efflux pump, in human hematopoietic stem cells. *Cell* 66, 85.

Cheifetz S, Weatherbee JA, Tsang ML-S et al. (1987) The transforming growth factor-β system, a complex pattern of cross-reactive ligands and receptors. *Cell* 48, 409.

Cheifetz S, Andres JL, Massague J (1988) The transforming growth factor-β receptor type III is a membrane proteoglycan. *Journal of Biological Chemistry* 263, 16984.

Chen BD-M, Chou T-H, Clark CR (1987) Delineation of receptor-mediated colony-stimulating factor (CSF-1) utilization and cell production by precursors of mononuclear phagocyte series at various stages of differentiation. *British Journal of Haematology* 67, 381.

Chiba S, Tojo A, Kitamura T, Urabe A, Miyazono K, Takaku F (1990) Characterization and molecular features of the cell surface receptor for human granulocyte-macrophage colony-stimulating factor. *Leukemia* 4, 29.

Chiu P-K, Moulds C, Coffman RL, Rennick D, Lee F (1988) Multiple biological activities are expressed by a mouse interleukin 6 cDNA clone isolated from bone marrow stromal cells. *Proceedings of the National Academy of Sciences of the USA* 85, 7099.

Choi H-S, Wojchowski DM, Sytkowski AJ (1987) Erythropoietin rapidly alters phosphorylation of pp43, an erythroid membrane protein. *Journal of Biological Chemistry* 262, 2933.

Ciardelli TL, Landgraf B, Gadski R, Strnad J, Cohen FE, Smith KA (1988) A design approach to the structural analysis of interleukin-2. *Journal of Molecular Recognition* 1, 42.

Ciccio NA, Lindemann A, Content J et al. (1990) Inducible production of interleukin 6 by human polymorphonuclear neutrophils: role of granulocyte-macrophage colony-stimulating factor and tumor necrosis factor-alpha. *Blood* 75, 2049.

Clark SC, Collins KC, Gandy MS, Webb AC, Auron PE (1986) Genomic sequence for human prointerleukin 1 beta: possible evolution from a reverse transcribed prointerleukin 1 alpha gene. *Nucleic Acids Research* 14, 7897.

Clark-Lewis I, Schrader JW (1982) Biochemical characterization of factors derived from T cell hybridomas and spleen cells. *Journal of Immunology* 128, 168.

Clark-Lewis I, Lopez AF, To LB et al. (1988) Structure–function studies of human granulocyte-macrophage colony-stimulating factor: identification of residues required for activity. *Journal of Immunology* 141, 881.

Cohen GI, Canellos GP, Greenberger JS (1980) In vitro quantitation of engraftment between purified populations of bone marrow haemopoietic stem cells and stromal cells. In: Gale RP, Fox CF (eds) *Biology of Bone Marrow Transplantation*. Academic Press, New York, p. 491.

Coleman DL, Chodakewitz JA, Bartiss AH, Mellors JW

(1988) Granulocyte-macrophage colony-stimulating factor enhances selective effector functions of tissue-derived macrophages. *Blood* 72, 573.

Cosman D, Lyman SD, Idzerda RL et al. (1990) A new cytokine receptor superfamily. *Trends in Biochemical Sciences* 15, 265.

Coulombel L, Eaves AC, Eaves CJ (1983) Enzymatic treatment of long-term human marrow cultures reveals the preferential location of primitive hemopoietic progenitors in the adherent layer. *Blood* 62, 291.

Coutinho LH, Testa NG, Dexter TM (1986) The myelosuppressive effect of recombinant interferon γ in short-term and long-term marrow cultures. *British Journal of Haematology* 63, 517.

Coutinho LH, Will A, Radford J, Schiro R, Testa NG, Dexter TM (1990) Effects of recombinant human granulocyte colony-stimulating factor (CSF) human granulocyte-macrophage CSF and gibbon interleukin-3 on hematopoiesis in human long-term bone marrow culture. *Blood* 75, 2118.

Cozzolino F, Torcia M, Aldinucci D et al. (1990) Interleukin 1 is an autocrine regulator of human endothelial cell growth. *Proceedings of the National Academy of Sciences of the USA* 87, 6487.

Curtis BM, Williams DE, Broxmeyer HE et al. (1991) Enhanced hematopoietic activity of human granulocyte/macrophage colony-stimulating factor-interleukin 3 fusion protein. *Proceedings of the National Academy of Sciences of the USA* 88, 5809.

D'Andrea A, Fasman GD, Lodish HF (1989) Erythropoietin receptor and interleukin-2 receptor β chain: a new receptor family. *Cell* 58, 1023.

D'Andrea AD, Szklut PJ, Lodish HF, Alderman EM (1990) Inhibition of receptor binding and neutralisation of bioactivity by antierythropoietin monoclonal antibodies. *Blood* 75, 874.

Deguchi Y, Kehri JH (1991) Selective expression of two homeobox genes in CD34-positive cells from human bone marrow. *Blood* 78, 323.

Deguchi Y, Moroney JF, Kehri JH (1991) Expression of the Hox-2.3 homeobox gene in human lymphocytes and lymphoid tissue. *Blood* 78, 445.

Del Rizzo RF, Eskinazi D, Axelrad A (1990) Interleukin-3 opposes the action of negative regulatory protein (NRP) and of transforming growth factor-β (TGFβ) in their inhibition of DNA synthesis of the erythroid stem cell BFU-E. *Experimental Hematology* 18, 138.

Derigs HG, Burgess GS, Klingberg D et al. (1990) Role for cyclin AMP in the postreceptor control of cytokine-stimulated stromal cell growth-factor production. *Leukemia* 4, 471.

Derynck R, Jarrett JA, Chen EY et al. (1985) Human transforming growth factor-β complementary DNA sequence and expression in normal and transformed cells. *Nature* 316, 701.

Devos R, Plaetinck G, Van Der Heyden J et al. (1991) Molecular basis of high affinity murine interleukin-5 receptor. *EMBO Journal* 10, 2133.

De Wolf JTM, Beentjes JAM, Esselink MT, Smit JW, Halie MR, Vellenga E (1990) Interleukin-4 suppresses the interleukin-3 dependent erythroid colony formation from normal human bone marrow cells. *British Journal of Haematology* 74, 246.

Dexter TM, Allen TD, Lajtha LG (1977) Conditions controlling the proliferation of haemopoietic stem cells in vitro. *Journal of Cell Physiology* 91, 335.

Dibirdik I, Langlie M-C, Ledbetter JA et al. (1991) Engagement of interleukin-7 receptor stimulates tyrosine phosphorylation, phosphoinositide turnover, and clonal proliferation of human T-lineage acute lymphoblastic leukemia cells. *Blood* 78, 564.

Dick JE (1991) Immune deficient mice as models of normal and leukemic human hematopoiesis. *Cancer Cells* 3, 39.

Dinarello CA, Clark BD, Pulen AJ, Savage N, Rosoff PM (1989) The interleukin 1 receptor. *Immunology Today* 10, 49.

DiPersio JF, Golde DW, Gasson JD (1990) GM-CSF: receptor structure and transmembrane signalling. *International Journal of Cell Cloning* 8 (suppl 1), 63.

Donahue RE, Yang YC, Clark SC (1990) Human P40 T-cell growth factor (interleukin-9) supports erythroid colony formation. *Blood* 75, 2271.

Dorshkind K (1988) Interleukin-1 inhibition of B lymphopoiesis is reversible. *Blood* 72, 2053.

Dorssers L, Burger H, Bot F et al. (1987) Characterization of a human multilineage-colony-stimulating factor cDNA clone identified by a conserved non coding sequence in mouse interleukin-3. *Gene* 55, 115.

Dowding CR, Gordon MY (1991) Physical, phenotypic and cytochemical characterisation of stroma-adherent blast colony-forming cells. *Leukemia* 6, 347.

Dowding C, Guo AP, Siczkowski M, Osterholz J, Goldman JM, Gordon MY (1990) Interferon-alpha (rIFN-α) counteracts the defective attachment of CML progenitor cells to normal marrow stromal cells. *Experimental Hematology* 18, 645 (abstract).

Dower SK, Call SM, Gillis S, Urdal DL (1986) Similarity between the interleukin 1 receptors on a murine T-lymphoma cell line and on a murine fibroblast cell line. *Proceedings of the National Academy of Sciences of the USA* 83, 1060.

Duijvestijn AM, Matsuda S, Ogura H et al. (1990) Granulocyte colony-stimulating factor stimulates human mature neutrophilic granulocytes to produce interferon α. *Blood* 75, 17.

Elliot MJ, Vadas M, Eglinton JM et al. (1989) Recombinant human interleukin-3 and granulocyte-macrophage colony-stimulating factor show common biological effects and binding characteristics on human monocytes. *Blood* 74, 2349.

Evans SW, Rennick D, Farrar WL (1986) Multilineage hematopoietic growth factor interleukin-3 and direct activators of protein kinase C stimulate phosphorylation of common substrates. *Blood* 68, 906.

Fabian I, Baldwin GC, Golde DW (1987) Biosynthetic granulocyte-macrophage colony-stimulating factor enhances neutrophil cytotoxicity toward human leukemia cells. *Leukemia* 1, 613.

Farrar WL, Thomas TP, Anderson WB (1985) Altered cytosol/membrane enzyme redistribution on interleukin-3 activation of protein kinase C. *Nature* 315, 235.

Farrar WL, Cleveland JL, Beckner SK, Bonvini E, Evans SW (1986) Biochemical and molecular events associated with interleukin 2 regulation of lymphocyte function. *Immunological Reviews* 92, 49.

Farrar WL, Brini AT, Harel-Bellan A (1990) Hematopoietic growth factor signal transduction and regulation of gene expression. In: Dexter TM, Garland JM, Tests NG (eds) *Colony-stimulating Factors: Molecular and Cellular Biology*. Marcel Dekker, New York, p. 379.

Favre C, Saeland S, Caux C, Duvert V, De Vries JE (1990) Interleukin-4 has basophilic and eosinophilic cell growth-promoting activity on cord blood cells. *Blood* 75, 67.

Ferreira SH, Lorenzetti BB, Bristow AF, Poole S (1988) Interleukin-1β as a potent hyperalgesic agent antagonised by a tripeptide analogue. *Nature* 334, 698.

Ferrero D, Tarella C, Badoni R et al. (1989) Granulocyte-macrophage colony-stimulating factor requires interaction with accessory cells or granulocyte colony-stimulating factor for full stimulation of human myeloid progenitors. *Blood* 73, 402.

Fibbe WE, Goselink HM, Van Eeden G et al. (1988) Proliferation of myeloid progenitor cells in human long-term bone marrow cultures is stimulated by interleukin-1 beta. *Blood* 72, 1242.

Flanagan JG, Leder P (1990) The kit ligand: a cell surface molecule altered in Steel mutant fibroblasts. *Cell* 63, 185.

Flanagan JG, Chan DC, Leder P (1991) Transmembrane form of the kit ligand growth factor is determined by alternative splicing and is missing in the Sl^d mutant. *Cell* 64, 1025.

Fujimori Y, Ogawa M, Clark SC, Dover GJ (1990) Serum-free culture of enriched hematopoietic progenitors reflects physiologic levels of fetal hemoglobin synthesis. *Blood* 75, 1178.

Fukunaga R, Ishizaka-Ikeda E, Seto Y, Nagata S (1990) Expression cloning of a receptor for murine granulocyte colony-stimulating factor. *Cell* 61, 341.

Furmanski P, Johnson CS (1990) Macrophage control of normal and leukemic erythropoiesis: identification of the macrophage-derived erythroid suppressing activity as interleukin-1 and the mediator of its in vivo action as tumor necrosis factor. *Blood* 75, 2328.

Furutani Y, Notake M, Fukui T et al. (1986) Complete nucleotide sequence of the gene for human interleukin 1 alpha. *Nucleic Acids Research* 14, 3167.

Gardner JD, Leichty KW, Christensen RD (1990) Effects of interleukin-6 on fetal hematopoietic precursors. *Blood* 75, 2150.

Gasson JC (1991) Molecular physiology of granulocyte-macrophage colony-stimulating factor. *Blood* 77, 1131.

Gearing DP, King JA, Gough NM, Nicola NA (1989) Expression cloning of a receptor for human granulocyte-macrophage colony-stimulating factor. *EMBO Journal* 8, 3667.

Gesner T, Mufson RA, Turner KJ, Clark SC (1989) Identification through chemical cross-linking of distinct granulocyte-macrophage colony-stimulating factor and interleukin-3 receptors on myeloid leukemic cells KG-1. *Blood* 74, 2652.

Gimble JM, Pietrangeli C, Henley A et al. (1989) Characterization of murine bone marrow and spleen-derived stromal cells: analysis of leukocyte marker and growth factor mRNA transcript levels. *Blood* 74, 303.

Gnarra JR, Otani H, Wang MG, McBride OW, Sharon M, Leonard WJ (1990) Human interleukin 2 receptor β-chain gene: chromosomal localisation and identification of 5' regulatory sequences. *Proceedings of the National Academy of Sciences of the USA* 87, 3440.

Goldwasser E, Beru N, Smith D (1990) Erythropoietin. In: Dexter TM, Garland JM, Testa NG (eds) *Colony Stimulating Factors: Molecular and Cellular Biology*. Marcel Dekker, New York, p. 257.

Goodwin RG, Friend D, Ziegler SF et al. (1990) Cloning of the human and murine interleukin 7 receptors: demonstration of a soluble form and homology to a new receptor superfamily. *Cell* 60, 941.

Gordon MY (1988) Adhesive properties of haemopoietic cells. *British Journal of Haematology* 68, 149.

Gordon MY (1991) Hemopoietic growth factors and receptors: bound and free. *Cancer Cells* 3, 127.

Gordon MY, Barrett AJ (1985) *Bone Marrow Disorders: The Biological Basis of Clinical Problems*. Blackwell Scientific Publications, Oxford.

Gordon MY, Greaves MF (1989) Physiological mechanisms of stem cell regulation in bone marrow transplantation and haemopoiesis. *Bone Marrow Transplantation* 4, 335.

Gordon MY, Hibbin JA, Kearney LU, Gordon-Smith EC, Goldman JM (1985) Colony formation by primitive haemopoietic progenitor cells in cocultures of bone marrow cells and stromal cells. *British Journal of Haematology* 60, 129.

Gordon MY, Ford AM, Greaves MF (1990) Interactions of haemopoietic progenitor cells with extracellular matrix. In: Long MW, Wicha M (eds) *The Hemopoietic Microenvironment*. Pergamon Press, Oxford.

Goto M, Murakami A, Akai K et al. (1989) Characterisation and use of monoclonal antibodies directed against erythropoietin that recognise different antigenic determinants. *Blood* 74, 1415.

Gough NM, Williams RL (1989) The pleiotropic effects of leukemia inhibitory factor. *Cancer Cells* 1, 77.

Gough NM, Gearing DP, King JA et al. (1988) Molecular cloning and expression of the human homologue of the murine gene encoding myeloid leukemia inhibitory factor. *Proceedings of the National Academy of Sciences of the USA* 85, 2623.

Gough NM, Gearing DP, Nicola NA et al. (1990) Localisation of the human GM-CSF receptor gene to the X-Y pseudoautosomal region. *Nature* 345, 734.

Greenberg SM, Chandrasekhar C, Golan DE, Handin RI (1990) Transforming growth factor b inhibits mitosis in the Dami human megakaryocytic cell line. *Blood* 76, 533.

Hamblin AS (1988) *Lymphokines*. IRL Press, Oxford.

Hanazono Y, Hosoi T, Kuwaki T et al. (1991) Structural analysis of the receptors for granulocyte colony-stimulating factor on neutrophils. *Experimental Hematology* 18, 1097.

Hatakeyama M, Tsudo M, Minamoto S et al. (1989) Interleukin-2 β receptor gene: generation of three receptor forms by cloned human α and β chain cDNAs. *Science* 244, 551.

Hauser H (1990) Interferons. In: Habenicht A (ed.) *Growth Factors, Differentiation Factors and Cytokines*. Springer Verlag, Berlin, p. 243.

Hayashi S-I, Gimble JM, Henley A, Ellingsworth LR, Kincade PW (1989) Differential effects of TGFβ on lymphohaemopoiesis in long-term bone marrow cultures. *Blood* 74, 1171.

Hayashida K, Kitamura T, Gorman DM, Arai K, Yokata T, Miyajima A (1990) Molecular cloning of a second subunit of the receptor for human granulocyte-macrophage colony-stimulating factor (GM-CSF): reconstitution of a high affinity GM-CSF receptor. *Proceedings of the National Academy of Sciences of the USA* 87, 9655.

Henney CS (1989) Interleukin 7: effects on early events in lymphopoiesis. *Immunology Today* 10, 170.

Heyworth CM, Dexter TM (1988) The development of hemopoietic cells in response to stromal cells or growth factors is modified by agents that influence ADP-ribosylation. *Leukemia* 2, 6.

Heyworth CM, Ponting ILO, Dexter TM (1988) The response of haemopoietic cells to growth factors: developmental implications of synergistic interactions. *Journal of Cell Science* 91, 239.

Hirano T, Akira S, Taga T, Kishimoto T (1990) Biological and clinical aspects of interleukin 6. *Immunology Today* 11, 44.

Hirata Y, Taga T, Hibi M, Nakaro N, Hirano T, Kishimoto T (1989) Characterization of IL-6 receptor expression by monoclonal and polyclonal antibodies. *Journal of Immunology* 143, 2900.

Holbrook ST, Ohls RK, Schibler KR, Yang Y-C, Christensen RD (1991) Effects of interleukin-9 on clonogenic maturation and cell cycle status of fetal and adult hematopoietic progenitors. *Blood* 77, 2129.

Holmes WE, Lee J, Kuang W-J, Race GC, Wood WI (1991) Structure and functional expression of a human interleukin-8 receptor. *Science* 253, 1278.

Horiguchi J, Warren MK, Kufe D (1987) Expression of the macrophage specific colony stimulating factor in human monocytes treated with granulocyte-macrophage colony-stimulating factor. *Blood* 69, 1259.

Idzerda RL, March CJ, Moseley B et al. (1990) Human interleukin-4 receptor confers biological responsiveness and defines a novel receptor superfamily. *Journal of Experimental Medicine* 171, 861.

Ikebuchi K, Wong GG, Clarke SC, Ihle JN, Hiral Y, Ogawa M (1987) Interleukin 6 enhancement of interleukin-3-dependent proliferation of multipotential hemopoietic progenitors. *Proceedings of the National Academy of Sciences of the USA* 84, 9035.

Ikebuchi K, Clark SC, Ihle JN, Souza LM, Ogawa M (1988) Granulocyte colony-stimulating factor enhances interleukin-3-dependent proliferation of multipotential hemopoietic progenitors. *Proceedings of the National Academy of Sciences of the USA* 85, 3445.

Imamura K, Spriggs D, Kufe D (1987) Expression of tumor necrosis factor receptors on human monocytes and internalisation of receptor bound ligand. *Journal of Immunology* 139, 2989.

Ishibashi T, Kimura H, Uchida T, Kariyone S, Friesep P, Burstein SA (1989) Human interleukin 6 is a direct promotor of maturation of megakaryocytes in vitro. *Proceedings of the National Academy of Sciences of the USA* 86, 5953.

Ishikawa T, Uchiyama T, Kamio M, Onishi R, Kodaka T, Okuma M (1991) IL-4 downregulates IL-2 receptor p75 by accelerating its endocytosis. *International Immunology* 3, 517.

Itoh N, Yonehara S, Schreurs J et al. (1990) Cloning of an interleukin-3 receptor gene: a member of a distinct receptor gene family. *Science* 247, 324.

Jacobs K, Shoemaker C, Rudersdorf R et al. (1985) Isolation and characterisation of genomic and cDNA clones of human erythropoietin. *Nature* 313, 806.

Jacobs CA, Lynch DH, Roux ER et al. (1991) Characterisation and pharmacokinetic parameters of recombinant soluble interleukin-4 receptor. *Blood* 77, 2396.

Jansen JH, Fibbe WE, Willemze R, Kluin-Nelemans JC (1990) Interleukin 4. A regulatory protein. *Blut* 60, 209.

Johnson GR, Gonda TJ, Metcalf D, Hariharan IK, Cory S (1989) A lethal myeloproliferative syndrome in mice transplanted with bone marrow cells infected with a retrovirus expressing granulocyte-macrophage colony-stimulating factor. *EMBO Journal* 8, 441.

Jones SS, D'Andrea AD, Haines LL, Wong GG (1990) Human erythropoietin receptor: cloning, expression and biological characterisation. *Blood* 76, 31.

Kamel-Reid S, Dick JE (1988) Engraftment of immune deficient mice with human hematopoietic stem cells. *Science* 242, 1706.

Kanakura Y, Cannistra SA, Brown CB et al. (1991) Identification of functionally distinct domains of human granulocyte-macrophage colony-stimulating factor using monoclonal antibodies. *Blood* 77, 1033.

Katz FE, Tindle R, Sutherland DR, Greaves MF (1985) Identification of a membrane glycoprotein associated with haemopoietic progenitor cells. *Leukemia Research* 9, 191.

Kaushansky K, O'Hara PJ, Berkner K, Segal GM, Hagen FS, Adamson JW (1986) Genomic cloning, characterization and multilineage growth-promoting activity of human granulocyte-macrophage colony-stimulating factor. *Proceedings of the National Academy of Sciences of the USA* 83, 3101.

Kaushansky K, O'Hara PJ, Hart CE, Forstrom JW, Hagan FS (1987) Role of carbohydrate in the function of human granulocyte-macrophage colony-stimulating factor. *Biochemistry* 26, 4361.

Kaushansky K, Lin N, Adamson JW (1988) Interleukin-1 stimulates fibroblasts to synthesise granulocyte-macrophage and granulocyte colony-stimulating factors. *Journal of Clinical Investigation* 81, 92.

Kaushansky K, Shoemaker SG, Alfaro S, Brown C (1989) Hematopoietic activity of granulocyte/macrophage colony-stimulating factor is dependent on two distinct regions of the molecule: functional analysis based on the activities of interspecies hybrid growth factors. *Proceedings of the National*

Academy of Sciences of the USA 86, 1213.

Kawano Y, Takaue Y, Hirao A et al. (1991) Synergistic effect of recombinant interferon-γ and interleukin-3 on the growth of immature human hematopoietic progenitors. *Blood* 77, 2118.

Kelleher CA, Wong GG, Clark SC, Schendel PF, Minden MD, McCulloch EA (1988) Binding of iodinated recombinant human GM-CSF to blast cells of acute myeloblastic leukemia. *Leukemia* 2, 211.

Kelleher K, Bean K, Clark SC et al. (1991) Human interleukin-9: genomic sequence, chromosomal location and sequences essential for its expression in human T-cell leukemia virus (HTLV)-1-transformed human T cells. *Blood* 77, 1436.

Keller JR, McNiece IK, Sill KT et al. (1990) Transforming growth factor β directly regulates primitive murine hematopoietic cell proliferation. *Blood* 75, 596.

Kester M, Simonson MS, Mene P, Sedor JR (1989) Interleukin-1 generates transmembrane signals from phospholipids through novel pathways in cultured rat mesangial cells. *Journal of Clinical Investigation* 83, 718.

Kimura K, Matsubara H, Sogoh S et al. (1991) Role of glycosaminoglycans in the regulation of T cell proliferation induced by thymic stroma-derived T cell growth factor. *Journal of Immunology* 146, 2618.

Kincade PW, Lee G, Pietrangelli CE, Hayashi S-I, Gimble JM (1989) Cells and molecules that regulate B lymphopoiesis in bone marrow. *Annual Review of Immunology* 7, 111.

Kitamura T, Hayashida K, Sakamaki K, Yokota T, Arai K-I, Miyajima A (1991a) Reconstitution of functional receptors for human granulocyte/macrophage colony-stimulating factor (GM-CSF): evidence that the protein encoded by the AIC2B cDNA is a subunit of the murine GM-CSF receptor. *Proceedings of the National Academy of Sciences of the USA* 88, 5082.

Kitamura T, Sato N, Arai K-I, Miyajima A (1991b) Expression cloning of the human IL-3 receptor cDNA reveals a shared β subunit for the human IL-3 and GM-CSF receptors. *Cell* 66, 1165.

Kitamura T, Takaku F, Miyajima A (1991c) IL-1 upregulates the expression of cytokine receptors on a factor-dependent human hemopoietic cell line, TF1. *International Immunology* 3, 571.

Kohama T, Handa H, Harigaya K (1988) A burst-promoting activity derived from the human bone marrow stromal cell line KM-102 is identical to the granulocyte-macrophage colony-stimulating factor. *Experimental Hematology* 16, 203.

Koike K, Nakahata T, Kubo T et al. (1990) Interleukin-6 enhances murine megakaryocytopoiesis in serum-free culture. *Blood* 75, 2286.

Koury MJ, Bondurant MC (1990) Erythropoietin retards DNA breakdown and prevents programmed death in erythroid progenitor cells. *Science* 248, 378.

Krantz SB, Sawyer ST, Sawada K-I, Wolfe F, Bocagno J (1990) Erythropoietin: receptors and clinical use in rheumatoid arthritis. *International Journal of Cell Cloning* 8 (suppl 1), 181.

Kuga T, Komatsu Y, Yamasaki M et al. (1989) Mutagenesis of human granulocyte colony-stimulating factor. *Biochemical and Biophysical Research Communications* 159, 103.

Lafage M, Maroc N, Dubreuil P et al. (1989) The human interleukin-1β gene is located on the long arm of chromosome 2 at band q13. *Blood* 73, 104.

Lang RA, Metcalf D, Cuthbertson RA et al. (1987) Transgenic mice expressing a hemopoietic growth factor gene develop accumulations of macrophages, blindness and a fatal syndrome of tissue damage. *Cell* 51, 675.

Langer JA, Petska S (1988) Interferon receptors. *Immunology Today* 9, 393.

Lansdorp PM, Sutherland HJ, Eaves CJ (1990) Selective expression of CD45 isoforms on functional subpopulations of $CD34^+$ hemopoietic cells from human bone marrow. *Journal of Experimental Medicine* 172, 363.

Larsen A, Davis T, Curtis BM et al. (1990) Expression cloning of a human granulocyte colony-stimulating factor receptor: a structural mosaic of hematopoietin receptor, immunoglobulin and fibronectin domains. *Journal of Experimental Medicine* 172, 1559.

Lawrence WD, Davis PJ, Blau SD (1987) Action of erythropoietin in vitro on rabbit reticulocyte Ca^{2+}-ATPase activity. *Journal of Clinical Investigation* 80, 586.

Leary AG, Ikebuchi K, Hirai Y et al. (1988) Synergism between interleukin-6 and interleukin-3 in supporting proliferation of human hematopoietic stem cells: comparison with interleukin-1α. *Blood* 71, 1759.

Leary AG, Hirai Y, Kishimoto T, Clark SC, Ogawa M (1989) Survival of hemopoietic progenitors in the G_0 period of the cell cycle does not require early hemopoietic regulators. *Proceedings of the National Academy of Sciences of the USA* 86, 4535.

Leary A, Wong GG, Clark SC, Smith AG, Ogawa M (1990) Leukemia inhibitory factor/differentiation-inhibiting activity/human interleukin for DA cells augments proliferation of human hemopoietic stem cells. *Blood* 75, 1960.

Le Beau MM, Lemons RS, Espinosa R, Larson RA, Arai N, Rowley JD (1989) Interleukin-4 and interleukin-5 map to human chromosome 5 in a region encoding growth factors and receptors and are deleted in myeloid leukaemias with a del (5q). *Blood* 73, 647.

Libbert M, Lindenmann H, Mantovani L, Wong GG, Mertelsman R, Hermann F (1989) mRNA for leukemia inhibitory factor is expressed by human mesenchymal cells. *Blood* 74 (suppl 1), 273a.

Lin F-K, Suggs S, Lin C-H et al. (1985) Cloning and expression of the human erythropoietin gene. *Proceedings of the National Academy of Sciences of the USA* 82, 7580.

Lindley I, Aschauer H, Siefert J-M et al. (1988) Synthesis and expression in *Escherichia coli* of the gene encoding monocyte-derived neutrophil-activating factor: biological equivalence between natural and recombinant neutrophil-activating factor. *Proceedings of the National Academy of Sciences of the USA* 85, 9199.

Loetscher H, Pan Y-CE, Lahm H-W et al. (1990)

Molecular cloning and expression of the human 55kD tumor necrosis factor receptor. *Cell* 61, 351.

Lopez AF, Williamson J, Gamble JR et al. (1986) Recombinant human granulocyte-macrophage colony-stimulating factor stimulates in vitro mature human neutrophil and eosinophil function, surface receptor expression and survival. *Journal of Clinical Investigation* 78, 1220.

Lopez F, To LB, Yang YC et al. (1987) Stimulation of proliferation, differentiation and function of human cells by primate interleukin 3. *Proceedings of the National Academy of Sciences of the USA* 84, 2761.

Lopez AF, Eglington JM, Gillis D, Park LS, Clark SC, Vadas MA (1989) Reciprocal inhibition of binding between interleukin-3 and granulocyte-macrophage colony-stimulating factor to human eosinophils. *Proceedings of the National Academy of Sciences of the USA* 86, 7022.

Lovhaug D, Pelus LM, Nordlie EM, Boyum A, Moore MAS (1986) Monocyte-conditioned medium and IL-1 induce granulocyte-macrophage colony-stimulating factor production in the adherent layer of murine bone marrow cultures. *Experimental Hematology* 14, 1037.

McCaffrey TA, Falcone DJ, Brayton CF, Agarwal LA, Welt FG, Weksler BB (1989) Transforming growth factor-β activity is potentiated by heparin via dissociation of the transforming growth factor-β/α2-macroglobulin inactive complex. *Journal of Cell Biology* 109, 441.

McCune JM, Namikawa R, Kaneshima H, Shultz LD, Lieberman M, Weissman IL (1988) The SCID-hu mouse: murine model for the analysis of human hematolymphoid differentiation and function. *Science* 241, 1632.

McGinnes K, Quesniaux V, Hitzler J, Paige C (1991) Human B lymphopoiesis is supported by bone marrow-derived stromal cells. *Experimental Hematology* 19, 294.

Magli MC, Barba P, Celetti A, De Vita G, Cillo C, Bonicelli E (1991) Coordinate regulation of HOX genes in human hematopoietic cells. *Proceedings of the National Academy of Sciences of the USA* 88, 6348.

Maier JAM, Voulalas P, Roeder D, Macaig T (1990) Extension of the lifespan of human endothelial cells by an interleukin-1α antisense oligomer. *Science* 249, 1570.

Mallett S, Barclay AN (1991) A new superfamily of cell surface proteins related to the nerve growth factor receptor. *Immunology Today* 12, 220.

Manos MM (1988) Expression and processing of a recombinant human macrophage colony-stimulating factor in mouse cells. *Molecular and Cellular Biology* 8, 5035.

March CJ, Moseley B, Larsen A et al. (1985) Cloning, sequence and expression of two distinct human interleukin-1 complementary cDNAs. *Nature* 315, 641.

Martin FH, Suggs SV, Langley KE et al. (1990) Primary structure and functional expression of rat and human stem cell factor DNAs. *Cell* 63, 203.

Massague J, Like B (1985) Cellular receptors for type β transforming factor. Ligand binding and affinity labeling in human and rodent cell lines. *Journal of Biological Chemistry* 260, 2636.

Matsuda S, Shirafuji N, Asano S (1989) Human granulocyte colony-stimulating factor specifically binds to murine myeloblastic NFS-60 cells and activates their guanosine triphosphate binding proteins/adenylate cyclase system. *Blood* 74, 2343.

Mayani H, Guilbert LJ, Clark SC, Janowska-Wieczorek A (1991) Inhibition of hematopoiesis in normal human long-term marrow cultures treated with recombinant human macrophage colony-stimulating factor. *Blood* 78, 651.

Messner HA, Yamasaki K, Jamal N et al. (1987) Growth of human hemopoietic colonies in response to recombinant gibbon interleukin 3: comparison with human recombinant granulocyte and granulocyte-macrophage colony-stimulating factor. *Proceedings of the National Academy of Sciences of the USA* 84, 6765.

Metcalf D, Gearing DP (1989) Fatal syndrome in mice engrafted with cells producing high levels of the leukemia inhibitory factor. *Proceedings of the National Academy of Sciences of the USA* 86, 5948.

Metcalf D, Begley CG, Johnson GR et al. (1986) Biologic properties in vitro of a recombinant human granulocyte-macrophage colony-stimulating factor. *Blood* 67, 37.

Michell RH (1989) Post-receptor signalling pathways. *Lancet* i, 765.

Migliaccio G, Migliaccio AR, Adamson JW (1988a) In vitro differentiation of human granulocyte/macrophage and erythroid progenitors: comparative analysis of the influence of recombinant human erythropoietin, G-CSF, GM-CSF and IL-3 in serum-supplemented and serum-deprived cultures. *Blood* 72, 248.

Migliaccio AR, Migliaccio G, Adamson JW (1988b) Effect of recombinant hematopoietic growth factors on proliferation of human marrow progenitor cells in serum-deprived liquid culture. *Blood* 72, 1387.

Migliaccio G, Migliaccio AR, Adamson JW (1991) In vitro differentiation and proliferation of human hematopoietic progenitors: the effects of interleukins 1 and 6 are indirectly mediated by the production of granulocyte-macrophage colony-stimulating factor and interleukin-3. *Experimental Hematology* 19, 3.

Mita S, Takaki S, Hitoshi Y et al. (1991) Molecular characterisation of the β chain of the murine IL-5 receptor. *International Immunology* 3, 665.

Miyajima A, Otsu K, Schreurs J, Bond MW, Abrams JS, Arai K (1986) Expression of murine and human granulocyte-macrophage-colony-stimulating factors in S cerevisiae: mutagenesis of the potential glycosylation site. *EMBO Journal* 5, 1193.

Miyake T, Kung CK, Goldwasser E (1977) Purification of human erythropoietin. *Journal of Biological Chemistry* 252, 5558.

Mizutani S, Watt SM, Robertson D et al. (1987) Cloning of human thymic subcapsular cortex epithelial cells with T-lymphocyte binding sites and hemopoietic growth factor activity. *Proceedings of* the *National Academy of Sciences of the USA* 84, 4999.

Mladenovic J, Zanjani ED, Kay NE (1986) Erythropoietin stimulates cytoplasmic calcium flux in bone marrow cells. *Clinical Research* 34, 465a.

Mochizuki DY, Eisenmann JR, Conlon PJ, Larsen AD, Tushinski RJ (1987) Interleukin-1 regulates hematopoietic activity, a role previously ascribed to hemopoietin-1. *Proceedings of the National Academy of Sciences of the USA* 84, 5267.

Moonen P, Mermod J-J, Ernst JF, Hirschi M, Delamarter JF (1987) Increased biological activity of deglycosylated recombinant human granulocyte/macrophage colony-stimulating factor produced by yeast or animal cells. *Proceedings of the National Academy of Sciences of the USA* 84, 4428.

Moore KW, Viera P, Fiorentino DF, Trounstine ML, Khan TA, Mosmann TR (1990) Homology of cytokine synthesis inhibitory factor (IL-10) to the Epstein–Barr virus gene BCRF1. *Science* 248, 1230.

Moreau JF, Donaldson DD, Bennett F, Witek-Giannotti JA, Clark SC, Wong GG (1988) Leukaemia inhibitory factor is identical to the myeloid growth factor human interleukin for DA cells. *Nature* 336, 690.

Moreb J, Zucali JR, Rueth S (1991) The effects of tumor necrosis factor-α on early human hematopoietic progenitor cells treated with 4-hydroperoxy-cyclophosphamide. *Blood* 76, 681.

Morrissey PJ, Bressler L, Park LS, Alpert A, Gillis S (1987) Granulocyte-macrophage colony-stimulating factor augments the primary antibody response by enhancing the function of antigen-presenting cells. *Journal of Immunology* 139, 1113.

Moseley B, Beckman PM, March CJ *et al.* (1989) The murine interleukin-4 receptor: molecular cloning and characterisation of secreted and membrane bound forms. *Cell* 59, 335.

Mosier DE, Guliza RJ, Baird SM, Wilson DB (1988) Transfer of a functional human immune system to mice with severe combined immunodeficiency. *Nature* 335, 256.

Munker R, Gasson J, Ogawa M, Koeffler HP (1986) Recombinant human TNF induces production of granulocyte-monocyte colony-stimulating factor. *Nature* 323, 79.

Murphy PM, Tiffany HL (1991) Cloning of a complementary DNA encoding a functional human interleukin-8 receptor. *Science* 253, 1280.

Musashi M, Clark SC, Sudo T, Urdal DL, Ogawa M (1991) Synergistic interactions between interleukin-11 and interleukin-4 in support of proliferation of primitive hematopoietic progenitors of mice. *Blood* 78, 1448.

Nagata S, Tsuchiya M, Asano S *et al.* (1986a) Molecular cloning and expression of cDNA for human granulocyte colony-stimulating factor. *Nature* 319, 415.

Nagata S, Tsuchiya M, Asano S *et al.* (1986b) The chromosomal gene structure and two mRNAs for human granulocyte colony-stimulating factor. *EMBO Journal* 5, 575.

Namen AE, Lupton S, Hjerrild K *et al.* (1988) Stimulation of B cell progenitors by cloned murine interleukin 7. *Nature* 333, 571.

Nicola NA (1987) Hemopoietic growth factors and their interactions with specific receptors. *Journal of Cellular Physiology* 5 (suppl.), 9.

Nicola NA (1991) Annotation: Receptors for colony-stimulating factors. *British Journal of Haematology* 77, 133.

Nicola NA, Peterson L, Hilton DJ, Metcalf D (1988) Cellular processing of murine colony-stimulating factor (multi-CSF, GM-CSF, G-CSF) receptors by normal hemopoietic cells and cell lines. *Growth Factors* 1, 41.

O'Conner-McCourt M, Wakefield LM (1987) Latent transforming growth factor-β in serum. A specific complex with α2-macroglobulin. *Journal of Biological Chemistry* 262, 14090.

Ogawa M (1989) Effects of hemopoietic growth factors on stem cells in vitro. *Hematology/Oncology Clinics of North America* 3, 453.

Ogawa M (1991) Cellular organisation of the hemopoietic system. *Experimental Hematology* 19, 457a.

Ohara A, Suda T, Seito M, Miura Y, Okabe T, Takaku F (1987) The effect of recombinant human granulocyte colony-stimulating factor on hemopoietic cells in serum-free culture. *Experimental Hematology* 15, 695.

Ohara A, Suda T, Tokuyama N *et al.* (1991) Generation of B lymphocytes from a single hemopoietic progenitor cell in vitro. *International Immunology* 3, 703.

Ohta M, Greenberger JS, Anklesaria P, Bassols A, Massague J (1987) Two forms of transforming growth factor β distinguished by multipotential haematopoietic progenitor cells. *Nature* 329, 539.

Okabe M, Asano M, Kuga T *et al.* (1990) In vitro and in vivo hematopoietic effect of mutant human granulocyte colony-stimulating factor. *Blood* 75, 1788.

O'Keefe EJ, Pledger WJ (1983) A model of cell cycle control: sequential events regulated by growth factors. *Molecular and Cellular Endocrinology* 31, 167.

Onetto-Pothier N, Aumont N, Haman A *et al.* (1990) Characterization of granulocyte-macrophage colony-stimulating factor receptor on the blast cells of acute myeloblastic leukemia. *Blood* 75, 59.

Oppenheim JJ, Kovacs EJ, Matsushima K, Durum SK (1986) There is more than one interleukin-1. *Immunology Today* 7, 45.

Oster W, Lindemann A, Mertelsman R, Herrman F (1989) Granulocyte-macrophage colony-stimulating factor (CSF) and multilineage CSF recruit human monocytes to express granulocyte CSF. *Blood* 73, 64.

Oster W, Herrmann F, Lindemann A, Mertelsmann R (1990) Experimental and clinical evaluation of erythropoietin. In: Habenicht A (ed.) *Growth Factors, Differentiation Factors and Cytokines.* Springer-Verlag, Berlin.

Otsuka T, Miyajima A, Brown N *et al.* (1988) Isolation and characterization of an expressible cDNA clone encoding human interleukin 3: induction of IL-3 mRNA in human T cell clones. *Journal of*

Immunology 140, 2288.

Otsuka T, Thacker CD, Eaves CJ, Hogge D (1991) Differential effects of microenvironmentally presented interleukin-3 versus soluble growth factor on primitive human hematopoietic cells. *Journal of Clinical Investigation* 88, 417.

Palacios R, Garland J (1984) Distinct mechanisms may account for the growth-promoting activity of interleukin 3 on cells of lymphoid and myeloid origin. *Proceedings of the National Academy of Sciences of the USA* 81, 1208.

Pandiella A, Massague J (1991) Cleavage of the membrane precursor for transforming growth factor α is a regulated process. *Proceedings of the National Academy of Sciences of the USA* 88, 1726.

Paquette RL, Zhou J-Y, Yang Y-C, Clark SC, Koeffler HP (1988) Recombinant gibbon interleukin-3 acts synergistically with recombinant human G-CSF and GM-CSF in vitro. *Blood* 71, 1596.

Park LS, Friend D, Gillis S, Urdal DL (1986) Characterization of the cell surface receptor for human granulocyte/macrophage colony-stimulating factor. *Journal of Experimental Medicine* 164, 251.

Park LS, Waldron PE, Friend D et al. (1989) Interleukin-3, GM-CSF and G-CSF receptor expression on cell lines and primary leukemia cells: receptor heterogeneity and relationship to growth factor responsiveness. *Blood* 74, 56.

Park LS, Gillis S, Urdal DL (1990) Hematopoietic growth factor receptors. In: Dexter TM, Garland JM, Testa NG (eds) *Colony-stimulating Factors: Molecular and Cellular Biology*. Marcel Dekker, New York, p. 39.

Parry DAD, Minasian E, Leach SJ (1988) Conformational homologies among the cytokines: interleukins and colony-stimulating factors. *Journal of Molecular Recognition* 1, 107.

Paul WE (1991) Interleukin 4: a prototypic immunoregulatory lymphokine. *Blood* 77, 1859.

Paul SR, Bennett F, Calvetti JA et al. (1990) Molecular cloning of a cDNA encoding interleukin 11, a stromal cell-derived lymphopoietic and hematopoietic cytokine. *Proceedings of the National Academy of Sciences of the USA* 87, 7512.

Pettenati MJ, Le Beau MM, Lemons RS et al. (1987) Assignment of CSF-1 to 5q33.1: evidence for clustering of genes regulating hematopoiesis and for their involvement in the deletion of the long arm of chromosome 5 in myeloid disorders. *Proceedings of the National Academy of Sciences of the USA* 84, 2970.

Pfeilschrifter J (1990) Transforming growth factor β. In: Habenicht A (ed.) *Growth Factors, Differentiation Factors*. Springer Verlag, Berlin, p. 58.

Piacibello W, Lu L, Wachter M, Rubin B, Broxmeyer HE (1985) Release of granulocyte-macrophage colony-stimulating factors from major histocompatibility complex class II antigen-positive monocytes is enhanced by human gamma interferon. *Blood* 66, 1343.

Pitha PM (1990) Interferons: a new class of suppressor genes? *Cancer Cells* 2, 25.

Ploemacher RE, Van Der Sluijs JP, Voerman JSA, Brons NHC (1989) An in vitro limiting-dilution assay of long-term repopulating hematopoietic stem cells in the mouse. *Blood* 74, 2755.

Powell JS, Berkner KL, Lebo RV, Adamson JW (1986) Human erythropoietin gene: high level expression in stably transfected mammalian cells and chromosome localisation. *Proceedings of the National Academy of Sciences of the USA* 83, 6465.

Quesenberry PJ (1986) Synergistic hematopoietic growth factors. *International Journal of Cell Cloning* 4, 3.

Raines MA, Liu L, Quan SG, Joe V, Dipersio JF, Golde DW (1991) Identification and molecular cloning of a soluble human granulocyte-macrophage colony-stimulating factor receptor. *Proceedings of the National Academy of Sciences of the USA* 88, 8203.

Rettenmeir CW, Roussel MF (1988) Differential processing of colony-stimulating factor-1 precursors encoded by two human cDNAs. *Molecular and Cellular Biology* 8, 5026.

Rettenmier CW, Sherr CJ (1989) The mononuclear phagocyte colony-stimulating factor. *Hematology/Oncology Clinics of North America* 3, 479.

Rich IN, Vogt C, Pentz S (1988) Erythropoietin gene expression in vitro and in vivo detected by in situ hybridisation. *Blood Cells* 14, 505.

Rigby WFC, Ball ED, Guyre PM, Fahger MW (1985) The effects of recombinant-DNA-derived interferons on the growth of myeloid progenitor cells. *Blood* 65, 858.

Ridgway D, Borzy MS, Bagby GC (1988) Granulocyte-macrophage colony-stimulating activity production by cultured human thymic non-lymphoid cells is regulated by endogenous interleukin-1. *Blood* 72, 1230.

Rizzino A (1988) Transforming growth factor β: multiple effects on cell differentiation and extracellular matrix. *Developmental Biology* 130, 411.

Robb RJ, Rusk CM, Yodoi J, Greene WC (1987) Interleukin 2 binding molecule distinct from Tac protein: analysis of its role in the formation of high affinity receptors. *Proceedings of the National Academy of Sciences of the USA* 84, 2002.

Saeland S, Caux C, Favre C et al. (1988) Effects of recombinant human interleukin-3 on CD34-enriched normal hematopoietic progenitors and on myeloblastic leukemias. *Blood* 72, 1580.

Sanderson CJ, O'Garra A, Warren DJ, Klaus GGB (1986) Eosinophil differentiation factor also has B-cell growth factor activity: proposed name interleukin 4. *Proceedings of the National Academy of Sciences of the USA* 83, 437.

Sanderson CJ, Campbell HD, Young IG (1988) Molecular and cellular biology of eosinophil differentiation factor (interleukin 5) and its effects on human and mouse B cells. *Immunological Reviews* 102, 29.

Saragovi H, Malek TR (1990) Evidence for additional subunits associated to the mouse interleukin 2 receptor p55/p75 complex. *Proceedings of the National Academy of Sciences of the USA* 87, 11.

Satoh T, Nakafuku M, Miyajima A, Kaziro Y (1991) Involvement of ras p21 protein in signal-transduction pathways from interleukin 2, interleukin 3 and granulocyte/macrophage colony-stimulating factor, but not from interleukin 4. *Proceedings of the National Academy of Sciences of the USA* 88, 3314.

Sawyer TS, Krantz SB (1984) Erythropoietin stimulates $^{45}Ca^{2+}$ uptake in Friend virus-infected erythroid cells. *Journal of Biological Chemistry* 259, 2769.

Schall TJ, Lewis M, Koller KJ et al. (1990) Molecular cloning and expression of a receptor for human tumor necrosis factor. *Cell* 61, 361.

Schindler R, Dinarello CA (1990) Interleukin-1. In: Habenicht A (ed.) *Growth Factors, Differentiation Factors and Cytokines.* Springer-Verlag, Berlin, p. 85.

Schooley JC, Kullgren B, Allison AC (1987) Inhibition by interleukin-1 of the action of erythropoietin on erythroid precursors and its possible role in the pathogenesis of hypoplastic anaemia. *British Journal of Haematology* 67, 11.

Schwinzer B, Resch K (1990) Interleukin 2. In: Habenicht A (ed.) *Growth Factors, Differentiation Factors and Cytokines.* Springer-Verlag, Berlin, p. 103.

Seelentag WK, Mermod J-J, Montesano R, Vasilli P (1987) Additive effects of interleukin-1 and tumor necrosis factor-alpha on the accumulation of three granulocyte and macrophage colony stimulating factor mRNAs in human endothelial cells. *EMBO Journal* 6, 2261.

Segarini PR, Seyedin SM (1988) The high molecular weight receptor to transforming growth factor-β contains glycosaminoglycan chains. *Journal of Biological Chemistry* 263, 8366.

Sehgal PB, Zilberstein A, Ruggieri R et al. (1986) Human chromosome 7 carries the $β_2$ interferon gene. *Proceedings of the National Academy of Sciences of the USA* 83, 5219.

Seigel LJ, Harper ME, Wong-Staal F, Gallo RC, Nash WG, O'Brien SJ (1984) Gene for T cell growth factor: location on human chromosome 4q and feline chromosome B1. *Science* 223, 175.

Sherr C (1990) Colony-stimulating factor-1 receptor. *Blood* 75, 1.

Shirafuji N, Matsuda S, Ogura H et al. (1990) Granulocyte colony-stimulating factor stimulates human mature neutrophilic granulocytes to produce interferon α. *Blood* 75, 17.

Shirakawa F, Chedid M, Suttles J, Pollock BA, Mizel SB (1989) Interleukin 1 and cyclic AMP induce k immunoglobulin light-chain expression via activation of an NF-kB-like DNA-binding protein. *Molecular and Cellular Biology* 9, 959.

Sideras P, Bergstedt-Lindqvist S, Macdonald HR, Severinson E (1985) Partial biochemical characterization of IgG_1 inducing factor. *European Journal of Immunology* 15, 586.

Sieff CA (1988) Haemopoietic growth factors: in vitro and in vivo studies. In: Hoffbrand AV (ed.) *Recent Advances in Haematology* 5. Churchill Livingstone, Edinburgh, p. 1.

Sieff CA, Emerson SG, Donahue RE et al. (1985) Human recombinant granulocyte-macrophage colony-stimulating factor: a multilineage hematopoietin. *Science* 230, 1171.

Sieff CA, Niemeyer CM, Nathan DG et al. (1987a) Stimulation of human hematopoietic colony formation by recombinant gibbon multi-colony-stimulating factor or interleukin-3. *Journal of Clinical Investigation* 80, 818.

Sieff CA, Tsai S, Faller DV (1987b) Interleukin-1 induces cultured human endothelial cell production of granulocyte-macrophage colony-stimulating factor. *Journal of Clinical Investigation* 79, 48.

Sieff CA, Niemeyer CM, Mentzer SJ, Faller DV (1988) Interleukin-1, tumor necrosis factor and the production of colony-stimulating factors by cultured mesenchymal cells. *Blood* 72, 1316.

Simmers RN, Weber LM, Shannon MF et al. (1987) Localization of the G-CSF gene on chromosome 17 proximal to the breakpoint in the t(15; 17) in acute promyelocytic leukemia. *Blood* 70, 330.

Sisson SD, Dinarello CA (1988) Production of interleukin-1α, interleukin-1β and tumor necrosis factor by human mononuclear cells stimulated with granulocyte-macrophage colony-stimulating factor. *Blood* 72, 1368.

Smith CA, Davis T, Anderson D et al. (1990) A receptor for tumor necrosis factor defines an unusual family of cellular and viral proteins. *Science* 248, 1019.

Socinski MA, Cannistra SA, Sullivan R et al. (1988) Granulocyte-macrophage colony-stimulating factor induces the expression of CD11b surface adhesion molecule on human granulocytes in vivo. *Blood* 72, 691.

Sonada Y, Yang Y-C, Wong GG, Clark SC, Ogawa M (1988) Erythroid burst-promoting activity of recombinant GM-CSF and interleukin-3: studies with anti-GM-CSF and anti-IL-3 sera and studies in serum-free cultures. *Blood* 72, 1381.

Sonada Y, Arai N, Ogawa M (1989) Humoral regulation of eosinophilopoiesis in vitro: analysis of the targets of interleukin-3, granulocyte/macrophage colony-stimulating factor (GM-CSF) and interleukin-5. *Leukemia* 3, 14.

Sonada Y, Okuda T, Yokota S et al. (1990) Actions of human interleukin-4/B-cell stimulating factor-1 on proliferation and differentiation of enriched hematopoietic progenitor cells in culture. *Blood* 75, 1615.

Sorensen PHB, Mui AL-F, Murthy SC, Krystal G (1989) Interleukin-3, GM-CSF and TPA induce distinct phosphorylation events in an interleukin-3-dependent multipotential cell line. *Blood* 68, 906.

Souza LM, Boone TC, Gabrilove J et al. (1986) Recombinant human granulocyte colony-stimulating factor: effects on normal and leukemic myeloid cells. *Science* 232, 61.

Spivak JL, Pham T, Isaacs M, Hankins WD (1991) Erythropoietin is both a mitogen and a survival factor. *Blood* 77, 1228.

Strife A, Lambek C, Wisniewski D et al. (1987) Activities of four purified growth factors on highly enriched human hematopoietic progenitor cells. *Blood* 69, 1508.

Suda T, Okada S, Suda J et al. (1989) A stimulatory

effect of recombinant murine interleukin-7 (IL-7) on B cell colony formation and an inhibitory effect of IL-1α. *Blood* 74, 1936.

Sutherland GR, Baker E, Callen DF et al. (1988) Interleukin-5 is at 5q31 and is deleted in the 5q-syndrome. *Blood* 71, 1150.

Sutherland GR, Baker E, Fernandez KEW et al. (1989a) The gene for human interleukin 7 (IL-7) is at 8q12–13. *Human Genetics* 82, 371.

Sutherland GR, Baker E, Hyland VJ, Callen DF, Stahl J, Gough NM (1989b) The gene for human leukemia inhibitory factor [LIF] maps to 22q12. *Leukemia* 3, 9.

Taga T, Kananishi Y, Hardy RR, Hirano T, Kishimoto T (1987) Receptors for B cell stimulatory factor 2. *Journal of Experimental Medicine* 166, 967.

Takaki S, Tominaga A, Hitoshi Y et al. (1990) Molecular cloning and expression of the murine interleukin-5 receptor. *EMBO Journal* 9, 4367.

Takatsu K, Tominaga A, Harada N et al. (1988) T cell-replacing factor (TRF)/interleukin 5 (IL-5): molecular and functional properties. *Immunological Review* 102, 107.

Tamura S, Suganara M, Tanaka H et al. (1990) A new hematopoietic cell line, KMT-2, having human interleukin-3 receptors. *Blood* 76, 501.

Tanabe T, Konishi M, Mizuta T, Noma T, Honjo T (1987) Molecular cloning and structure of the human interleukin-5 gene. *Journal of Biological Chemistry* 262, 16580.

Taniguchi T, Matsui H, Fujita T et al. (1986) Molecular analysis of the interleukin-2 system. *Immunological Review* 92, 121.

Tavernier J, Devos R, Cornelius S et al. (1991) The human high affinity interleukin-5 receptor (IL-5R) is composed of an IL-5-specific α chain and a β chain shared with the receptor for GM-CSF. *Cell* 66, 1175.

Terstappen LWMM, Huang S, Safford M, Lansdorp PM, Loken MR (1991) Sequential generations of hematopoietic colonies derived from single nonlineage-committed $CD34^+CD38^-$ progenitor cells. *Blood* 77, 1218.

Te Velde A, Huijbens RJF, Heije K, De Vries JE, Figdor CG (1990) Interleukin-4 (IL-4) inhibits secretion of IL-1β, tumor necrosis factor α and IL-6 by human monocytes. *Blood* 76, 1392.

Thatcher DR (1990) Large-scale production of hematopoietic growth factors. In: Dexter TM, Garland JM, Testa NG (eds) *Colony-stimulating Factors: Molecular and Cellular Biology*. Marcel Dekker, New York, p. 329.

Thomas KM, Taylor L, Navarro J (1991) The interleukin-8 receptor is encoded by a neutrophil-specific cDNA clone, F3R. *Journal of Biological Chemistry* 266, 14839.

Tigges MA, Casey LS, Koshland ME (1989) Mechanism of interleukin-2 signalling: mediation of different outcomes by a single receptor and transduction pathway. *Science* 243, 781.

Toretsky JA, Shahidi NT, Finlay JL (1986) Effects of recombinant interferon gamma on hematopoietic progenitor cell growth. *Experimental Hematology* 14, 182.

Trinchieri G, Murphy M, Perussia B (1987) Regulation of hematopoiesis by lymphocytes and natural killer cells. *CRC Critical Reviews in Hematology/Oncology* 7, 219.

Tsujimoto M, Feinman R, Vilcek J (1986) Differential effects of type I IFN and IFN-γ on the binding of tumor necrosis factor to receptors in two human cell lines. *Journal of Immunology* 137, 2272.

Tushinski RJ, McAlister IB, Williams DE, Namen AE (1991) The effects of interleukin-7 (IL-7) on human bone marrow in vitro. *Experimental Hematology* 19, 749.

Uckun FM, Tuel-Ahlgren L, Obuz V et al. (1991) Interleukin-7 engagement stimulates tyrosine phosphorylation, inositol phospholipid turnover, proliferation and selective differentiation to the CD4 lineage by human fetal thymocytes. *Proceedings of the National Academy of Sciences of the USA* 88, 6323.

Udomsakdi C, Eaves CJ, Sutherland HJ, Lansdorp PM (1991) Separation of functionally distinct sub-populations of primitive human hematopoietic cells using rhodamine-123. *Experimental Hematology* 19, 338.

Urdal DL, Park LS (1988) Studies on hematopoietic growth factor receptors using human recombinant IL-3, GM-CSF, G-CSF, M-CSF, IL-1 and IL-4. *Behring Institute Mitteilungen* 83, 27.

Uze G, Lutfalla G, Gresser I (1990) Genetic transfer of a functional human interferon α receptor into mouse cells: cloning and expression of its cDNA. *Cell* 60, 225.

Uzumaki H, Okabe T, Sasaki N et al. (1989) Identification and characterization of receptors for granulocyte colony-stimulating factor on human placenta and trophoblastic cells. *Proceedings of the National Academy of Sciences of the USA* 86, 9323.

Van Snide J (1990) Interleukin-6: an overview. *Annual Review in Immunology* 8, 253.

Vellenga E, De Wolf JTM, Beentjes JAM, Esselink MT, Smit JW, Halie MR (1990) Divergent effects of interleukin-4 (IL-4) on granulocyte colony-stimulating factor and IL-3 supported myeloid colony formation from normal and leukemic bone marrow. *Blood* 75, 633.

Verfaillie C, McGlave P (1991) Leukemia inhibitory factor/human interleukin for DA cells is a growth factor that stimulates the in vitro development of multipotential human hematopoietic progenitors. *Blood* 77, 263.

Verfaillie C, Blakolmer K, McGlave P (1990) Purified primitive hematopoietic cells with long-term in vitro repopulating capacity adhere selectively to irradiated bone marrow stroma. *Journal of Experimental Medicine* 172, 509.

Vieria P, De Waal-Malefyt R, Dang MN et al. (1991) Isolation and expression of human cytokine synthesis inhibitory factor cDNA clones: homology to Epstein–Barr virus open reading frame BCRF1. *Proceedings of the National Academy of Sciences of the USA* 88, 1172.

Wakefield LM, Smith DM, Masui T, Harris CC, Sporn MP (1987) Distribution and modulation of the cellular receptor for transforming growth factor-beta.

Journal of Cellular Biology 105, 965.
Walker F, Nicola NA, Metcalf D, Burgess AW (1985) Hierarchical downmodulation of hemopoietic growth factor receptors. *Cell* 43, 269.
Wang JM, Colella S, Allavena P, Mantovani A (1987) Chemotactic activity of human recombinant granulocyte-macrophage colony-stimulating factor. *Immunology* 60, 439.
Wang JM, Chen ZG, Colella S et al. (1988) Chemotactic activity of recombinant human granulocyte colony-stimulating factor. *Blood* 72, 1456.
Warren MK, Ralph P (1986) Macrophage growth factor CSF-1 stimulates human monocyte production of interferon, tumor necrosis factor and myeloid CSF. *Journal of Immunology* 137, 2281.
Wasley LC, Timony G, Murtha P et al. (1991) The importance of N- and O-linked oligosaccharides for the biosynthesis and in vitro and in vivo biologic activities of erythropoietin. *Blood* 77, 2624.
Webb AC, Collins KL, Auron PE et al. (1986) Interleukin-1 gene (IL-1) assigned to long arm of chromosome 2. *Lymphokine Research* 5, 77.
Welte K, Platzer E, Lu L et al. (1985) Purification and biochemical characterisation of pluripotent hematopoietic colony-stimulating factor. *Proceedings of the National Academy of Sciences of the USA* 82, 1526.
Whetton AD, Dexter TM (1983) Effect of haematopoietic cell growth factor on intracellular ATP levels. *Nature* 303, 629.
Whetton AD, Bazill GW, Dexter TM (1984) Haemopoietic cell growth factor mediates cell survival via its action on glucose transport. *EMBO Journal* 3, 409.
Whetton AD, Heyworth CM, Dexter TM (1986) Phorbol esters activate protein kinase C and glucose transport and can replace the requirement for growth factor in interleukin-3-dependent multipotent stem cells. *Journal of Cell Science* 84, 93.
Whetton AD, Monk PN, Consalvey SD, Huang SJ, Dexter TM, Downes CP (1988a) Interleukin-3 stimulates proliferation via protein kinase C activation without increasing inositol lipid turnover. *Proceedings of the National Academy of Sciences of the USA* 85, 3284.
Whetton AD, Valance SJ, Monk PN, Cragoe EJ, Dexter TM, Heyworth CM (1988b) Interleukin-3 stimulated stem cell proliferation: evidence for activation of protein kinase C and Na^+/H^+ exchange without inositol lipid hydrolysis. *Biochemical Journal* 256, 585.
Whitlock CA, Witte ON (1982) Long-term culture of B lymphocytes and their precursors from murine bone marrow. *Proceedings of the National Academy of Sciences of the USA* 79, 3608.
Williams DA (1991) Microenvironment regulation of hematopoiesis: the role of stromal-derived cytokines in blood cell formation. *Experimental Hematology* 19, 457a.
Williams N, De Giorgio T, Banu N, Withy R, Hirano T, Kishimoto T (1990) Recombinant interleukin 6 stimulates immature murine megakaryocytes. *Experimental Hematology* 18, 69.
Wingfield P, Graber P, Mosnen P, Craig S, Pain RH (1988) The conformation and stability of recombinant granulocyte-macrophage colony-stimulating factors. *European Journal of Biochemistry* 173, 65.
Winkelman JC, Penny LA, Deaven LL, Forget BG, Jenkins RB (1990) The gene for the human erythropoietin receptor: analysis of the coding sequence and assignment to chromosome 19p. *Blood* 76, 24.
Wognum AW, Lansdorp PM, Humphries RK, Krystal G (1990a) Detection and isolation of the erythropoietin receptor using biotinylated erythropoietin. *Blood* 76, 697.
Wognum AW, Lansdorp PM, Krystal G (1990b) Immunochemical analysis of monoclonal antibodies to human erythropoietin. *Experimental Hematology* 18, 228.
Wong PC, Chung S-W, Dunbar CA, Bodine DM, Ruscetti S, Nienhuis AW (1989) Retrovirus-mediated transfer and expression of the interleukin-3 gene in mouse hematopoietic cells results in a myeloproliferative disorder. *Molecular and Cellular Biology* 9, 798.
Yamasaki K, Taga T, Hirata Y et al. (1988) Cloning and expression of the human interleukin 6 (BSF-2/IFNβ2) receptor. *Science* 241, 825.
Yang Y-C, Ciarletta AB, Temple PA et al. (1986) Human interleukin-3 (multi-CSF): identification by expression cloning of a novel haematopoietic growth factor related to murine IL-3. *Cell* 47, 3.
Yang Y-C, Kovacic S, Kriz R et al. (1988) The human genes for GM-CSF and IL-3 are closely linked in tandem on chromosome 5. *Blood* 71, 958.
Yang Y-C, Ricciardi S, Ciarletta J, Kelleher K, Clark SC (1989) Expression cloning of a cDNA encoding a novel human hematopoietic growth factor: human homologue of murine T-cell growth factor P40. *Blood* 74, 1880.
Yarden Y, Kuang W-J, Yang-Feng T et al. (1987) Human proto-oncogene c-kit: a new cell surface receptor tyrosine kinase for an unidentified ligand. *EMBO Journal* 6, 3341.
Yayon A, Klagsbrun M, Esko JD, Leder P, Ornitz DM (1991) Cell surface, heparin-like molecules are required for binding of basic fibroblast growth factor to its high affinity receptor. *Cell* 64, 841.
Yokota T, Arai N, De Vries J et al. (1988) Molecular biology of interleukin 4 and interleukin 5 genes and biology of their products that stimulate B cells, T cells and hemopoietic cells. *Immunological Review* 102, 137.
Zhou Y-Q, Stanley ER, Clark SC et al. (1988) Interleukin-3 and interleukin-1α allow earlier bone marrow progenitors to respond to human colony-stimulating factor-1. *Blood* 72, 1870.
Zucali JR, Dinarella CA, Oblon DJ, Gross MA, Anderson L, Weiner RS (1986) Interleukin-1 stimulates fibroblasts to produce granulocyte macrophage colony-stimulating activity and prostaglandin E_2. *Journal of Clinical Investigation* 79, 48.

Chapter 2
Treatment Strategies in Bone Marrow Disorders

Haematological malignancies, 73
  Introduction, 73
  Relevance of malignant cell biology to treatment, 74
  Treatment implications, 80
  Treatment planning, 84
  Treatment strategies in individual haematological malignancies, 93
Congenital bone marrow disorders, 112
  Introduction, 112
  Bone marrow transplantation, 114

Cytokines, growth factors and other agents, 115
Gene therapy, 117
Aplastic anaemia and drug-induced cytopenias, 122
  Pathophysiology of aplastic anaemia, 122
  Treatment, 125
  Drug-induced cytopenias, 127
References, 133

HAEMATOLOGICAL MALIGNANCIES

Introduction

Fifty years ago leukaemias and most disseminated lymphomas were incurable. Today we can improve survival in most haematological malignancies and achieve cures in an increasing number. Improved treatment approaches have developed largely in an empirical manner. Nevertheless a better understanding of the underlying biology of haematological malignancies and also of normal haemopoiesis has enabled us not only to identify disease subtypes with distinct behaviour and treatment responses, but also to design rational treatment approaches. The discovery of new chemotherapeutic agents such as vincristine and the anthracyclines has contributed to treatment progress, but the most important developments derive from improved schedules and combinations of drugs that have been in existence for some time. For example, cyclophosphamide and busulphan, which are highly effective agents in bone marrow transplant preparative regimens, were among the earliest chemotherapy drugs to be developed in the 1950s. Recently there has been some progress in understanding chemotherapeutic drug resistance, but how much this problem impinges on successful treatment outcome is not clearly defined. There is now a diversity of treatments for haematological malignancies including autologous or allogeneic bone marrow transplantation (Chapter 4), use of haemopoietic growth factors (Chapter 5) and modification of the immune response (Chapter 6). Attempts are also being made to treat haematological malignancies with differentiation-inducing agents. This approach has proved useful in two particular instances: the use of all-trans-retinoic acid (ATRA) in acute promyelocytic leukaemia, and the treatment of hairy cell leukaemia with interferon α. In this chapter we examine the way in which newer treatments are used in conjunction with established modalities of chemotherapy and radiotherapy in malignant disorders, and outline strategies of treatment for individual disorders. For an account of the principles of chemotherapy and radiotherapy the reader is referred to Gordon and Barrett (1985).

Relevance of malignant cell biology to treatment

Many techniques are now available that help to characterize more fully the precise ontogeny and extent of haematological malignant processes, define their proliferative behaviour, and detect small amounts of residual disease: *in vitro* culture systems are used to determine the ability of leukaemic progenitors to self-replicate by measuring their replating efficiency. Growth factor responsiveness can be assessed, and the capacity of the cells to undergo maturation under the influence of growth and differentiation factors can be tested (Vellenga *et al.*, 1987; Reilly *et al.*, 1989; Russell and Reilly, 1989; Uckun *et al.*, 1989; McCulloch, 1990; Uckun and Heerema, 1990). Techniques for identifying the origin of malignancies include chromosome analysis and, more recently, the use of chromosome-specific probes to identify individual chromosomes or their subregions in interphase cells (fluorescent *in situ* hybridization; Poddige *et al.*, 1991). Several methods are used to detect minimal residual disease: T and B cell receptor gene rearrangement (Luzzatto and Foroni, 1986), chromosome analysis (Arthur *et al.*, 1988; Holt *et al.*, 1989), polymerase chain reaction amplification of leukaemia-specific gene fusions such as BCR/ABL in chronic myeloid leukaemia (CML) (Hughes *et al.*, 1991), and use of informative combinations of monoclonal antibodies specific for leukaemia cells (Campana *et al.*, 1991).

Ontogeny of leukaemias and lymphomas

Malignant change can affect any stage of lymphohaemopoietic development from the pluripotent stem cell precursor to differentiated but proliferating cells. It is now possible to map the development of haemopoietic and lymphopoietic cells in considerable detail using a panel of monoclonals directed against antigens expressed at different stages of maturation of lymphoid cells, myeloid cells, and stem cells (Catovsky and Foa, 1990; Civin, 1990; Janossy and Campana, 1991). Chromosome analysis and semisolid cultures for cloning malignant cells give additional information about the earliest progenitors affected by the malignant process. These techniques broadly categorize haematological malignancies into those derived from

Table 2.1 Precursor origin of lymphoid malignancies

Disorder	Phenotype	Stem cell precursor
Acute lymphoblastic leukaemia		
c-ALL of childhood	Pre-B cell	−
B-ALL	B cell	−
T-ALL	T cell	−
c-ALL t(9;22) p210 CML type	Pre-B cell	+
c-ALL t(9;22) or BCR/ABL fusion only	Pre-B cell	+
Null-ALL with t(4;11)	Pre-pre-B	+
Biphenotypic leukaemias	B or T cell	+
Other lymphoid leukaemias		
B-CLL	Mature B cell	−
T-CLL	Mature T cell	−
Hairy cell	Mature B cell	−
Lymphomas		
B-NHL	Follicular B cell	−
T lymphomas	Mature T cell	−
Other		
Myeloma	Plasma cell	+?
Waldenström's macroglobulinaemia	Memory B cell	−

ALL, Acute lymphoblastic leukaemia; c-ALL, common ALL; CML, chronic myeloid leukaemia; CLL, chronic lymphoblastic leukaemia; NHL, non-Hodgkin's lymphoma.

myeloid, lymphoid, biphenotypic (cells with features of both lines), or pluripotent stem cells.

Lymphoid malignancies (Table 2.1)

The distinct changes in surface phenotype during lymphocyte ontogeny have allowed a precise definition of the developmental origin of many lymphoid malignancies. The demonstration of clonality in B and T cell diseases by immunoglobulin heavy chain (IgH) and T cell receptor (TCR) gene rearrangements respectively is compelling evidence that the disorders have arisen at a relatively mature stage of lymphocyte development (Luzzatto and Foroni, 1986). Culture systems for lymphoid leukaemia colony-forming cells have extended our knowledge of acute lymphoblastic leukaemia (ALL) cell populations (Uckun et al., 1989; Uckun and Heerema, 1990). Good-risk childhood common (c) ALL appears to be a disease confined to an early stage of B cell development with a colony-forming progenitor that has similar surface marker characteristics to the major population of leukaemic blasts. However, many lymphoid malignancies, including some with the surface phenotype of c-ALL, have complex hierarchies: for example, the null-

Table 2.2 Myeloid disorders: phenotype and precursor origin

Disorder	Phenotype of major (and minor) population	Earliest precursor
Acute myeloid leukaemia		
M0	Undifferentiated	Stem cell
M1	Undifferentiated	Stem cell
M2	Granulocytic	?
M3	Promyelocyte	? Committed granulocyte progenitor
M4	Myelocyte and monocyte	?
M5	Monocyte	Stem cell? B cell progenitor?
M6	Erythrocyte	?
M7	Megakaryocyte (MK)	?
Myelodysplastic syndromes		
Refractory anaemia ± sideroblasts	Erythrocyte (granulocyte, MK)	Stem cell
CMML	Monocytes	Stem cell
RAEB	Erythrocytes, granulocytes, MK	Stem cell
Myeloproliferative disorders		
Primary polycythaemia	Erythrocytes (MK, granulocyte)	Stem cell
Essential thrombocythaemia	MK (granulocyte)	Stem cell
Myelofibrosis	MK, erythrocyte, granulocyte	Stem cell
CML	Granulocytes (MK)	Stem cell

CML, chronic myeloid leukaemia; CMML, chronic myelo-monocytic leukaemia; RAEB, refractory anaemia with excess of blasts.

ALL phenotype often associated with a t(4;11) karyotype has stem cell features and may express myeloid as well as lymphoid markers (Sobol et al., 1987) and the c-ALL occurring in blast crisis chronic myeloid leukaemia (CML) is part of a pluripotent stem cell abnormality (Fialkow et al., 1977). Myelomas may have more than one immunoglobulin producing clone. Furthermore the myeloma plasma cell is generated by precursors with lymphocyte morphology bearing the CD10 antigen common to pre-B cells (Millar et al., 1988; Warburton et al., 1989), and some myelomas also express myeloid antigens, suggesting a pluripotent stem cell origin of the disease (Grogan et al., 1989). It is therefore possible that apparently differentiated lymphoid malignancies in fact arise from more primitive precursors.

Myeloid disorders (Table 2.2)

Myeloid disorders arising from a pluripotent myeloid stem cell include CML (Fialkow et al., 1977), the myeloproliferative disorders (myelofibrosis (MF), essential thrombocythaemia (ET) and primary polycythaemia (PP) (Adamson et al., 1976; Jacobson et al., 1978; Fialkow et al., 1981), myelodysplastic syndromes (MDS) (Prchal et al., 1978; Raskind et al., 1984; Janssen et al., 1989) and some but not all cases of acute myeloid leukaemia (AML) (Fialkow et al., 1987). The evidence for a pluripotent precursor origin of myeloid malignancies is supported by finding early stem cell surface markers on AML blasts (Janossy and Campana, 1991), finding morphological abnormalities in more than one lineage in myelodysplastic syndromes and some AML, and demonstrating proliferative abnormalities in erythroid, granulocytic and megakaryocytic progenitors in the myeloproliferative disorders (Adams et al., 1988). The technique used by Fialkow and others to demonstrate a clonal pluripotent cell origin of haemopoiesis involves studies in female patients with myeloid disorders who are also heterozygous for the glucose-6-phosphate dehydrogenase (G6PD) isoenzyme. Random X chromosome inactivation (the Lyon hypothesis) dictates that in a single clone the varient enzyme will either be represented 0% or 100%, depending on whether it was inactivated or not at the generation of the stem cell responsible for the clone. In patients with CML, PP ET, and MF the same proportion of G6PD isoenzyme activity was found in all three myeloid lineages — erythropoiesis, granulopoiesis and megakaryocytopoiesis — but not in fibroblasts. In a patient with CML, B lymphocytes (but not T lymphocytes) were also demonstrated to be part of the same clone, suggesting a clonal origin at an early lymphomyeloid progenitor level (Fialkow et al., 1977).

Stem cell and biphenotypic leukaemias

Normal marrow cells bearing the CD34 but not the CD33 antigen have the stem cell characteristic of proliferating in blast cell assays with a high replating efficiency (see Chapter 1). CD34-bearing cells are positive for terminal deoxyribosyltransferase (TdT). More differentiated stem cells acquire the CD33 antigen as well, and in further maturation they lose CD34 and TdT. Leukaemias with this stem cell surface phenotype have been variously characterized morphologically and by surface markers as undifferentiated, lymphoid, myeloid or biphenotypic. The discovery of leukaemias sharing both lymphoid and myeloid surface antigens has been puzzling. Occasionally true mixed leukaemias (termed bilineage leukaemias) occur where two distinct populations of leukaemia are identifiable as myeloid and lymphoid. More frequently, myeloid surface antigens (CD13, CD33) are represented on cells bearing either B cell antigens (e.g. CD19, CD10), T cell antigens (e.g. CD7), or showing immunoglobulin

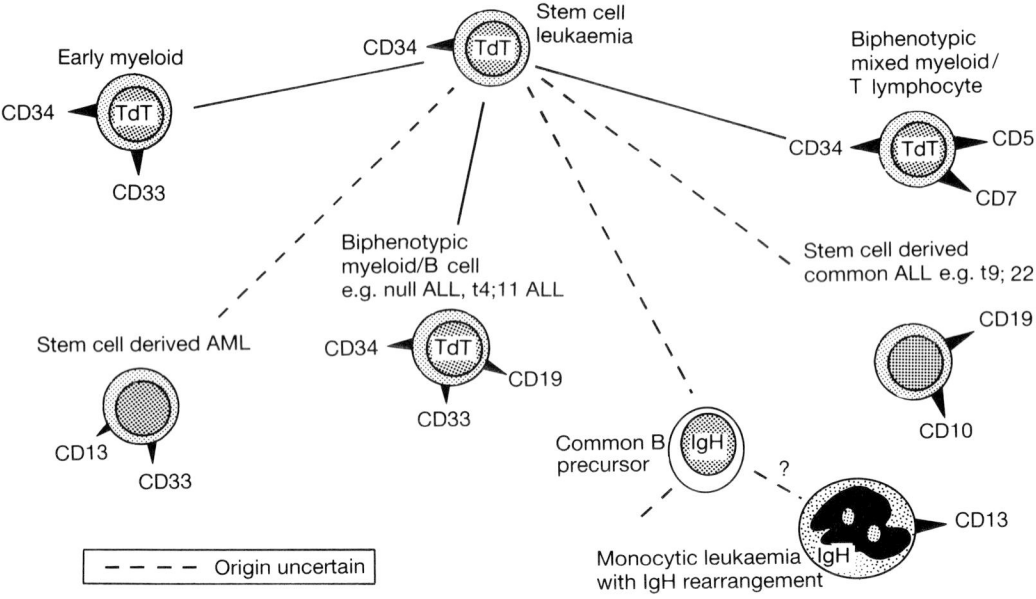

Fig. 2.1 Stem cell derived leukaemias.

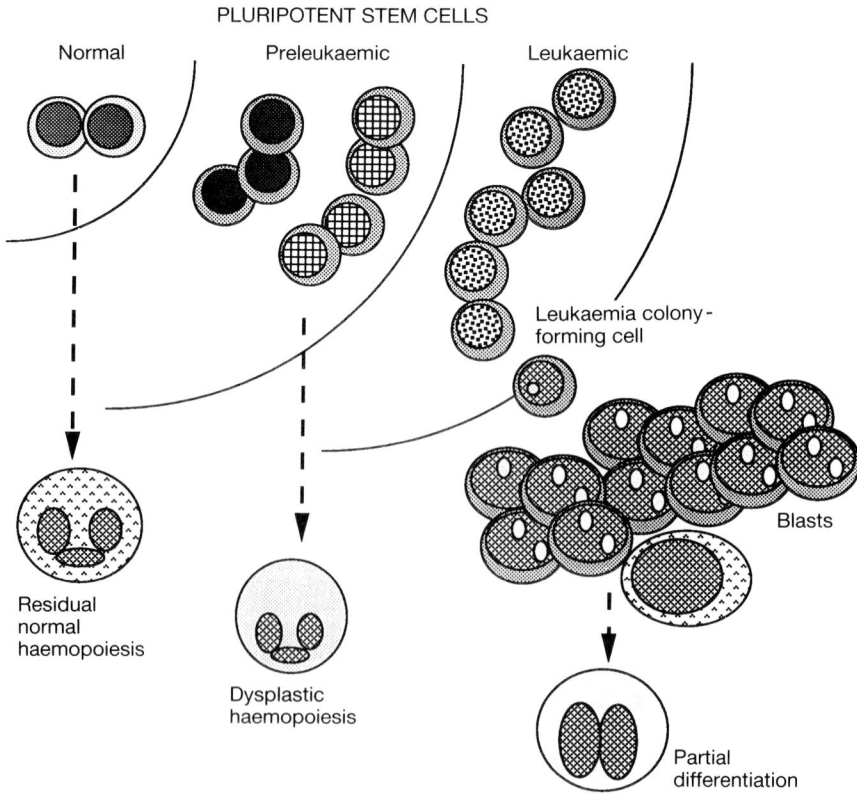

Fig. 2.2 Heterogeneity of leukaemia cell populations.

gene rearrangement (Norton *et al.*, 1987). It has been proposed that biphenotypic leukaemias represent either leukaemic dysregulation where a leukaemia arising, for example, from a committed myeloid cell aberrantly expresses a lymphoid marker (lineage infidelity), or a malignant process affecting stem cells at an undifferentiated stage in their development (lineage promiscuity) (Greaves *et al.*, 1986). The latter explanation appears to be the most likely for leukaemias of mixed phenotype showing stem cell characteristics together with either mixed T cell and myeloid, or mixed B cell and myeloid surface markers. Confirmation that a subgroup of macrophages is derived from B cells suggests the existence of a lymphoid monocyte stem cell (Paietta, 1990; Del Vecchio *et al.*, 1991). The existence of this common precursor would explain the finding of immunoglobulin gene rearrangement in some monocytic acute leukaemias (Macdonald *et al.*, 1991). The common phenotypes of mixed leukaemias are shown in Figure 2.1. Interestingly, this type of leukaemia appears to be able to change its expression under different treatment conditions. Thus CML may progress through lymphoid and myeloid transformations; and biphenotypic leukaemias diagnosed and treated as ALL may relapse as myeloid leukaemias, and vice versa (Stass *et al.*, 1984).

Diversity of cell populations in leukaemias and lymphomas

Haematological malignancies often represent complex hierarchies consisting of a mixture of precursors and more mature cells at different stages of development (Heard *et al.*, 1984; Mecucci *et al.*, 1986; Dormer *et al.*, 1987). At least four developmental stages can be identified in some leukaemias: early self-replicating progenitors (e.g. Ph^1 positive progenitor cells in CML), leukaemic colony-forming cells, morphologically identifiable leukaemia blasts, and mature or dysmature end cells showing varying degrees of differentiation (Fig. 2.2). In understanding the diversity of behaviour of leukaemias and lymphomas, their temporal development must also be taken into consideration. Myelodysplastic syndromes, for example, evolve through a series of stem cell mutations with progressive failure of differentiation to a frank leukaemic state characterized by the expansion of a blast cell population and progression to AML (Lyons *et al.*, 1988; Pierre *et al.*, 1989). At the time of leukaemic transformation a mixed population of stem cells exists derived from different stages in the evolution of the disease. The relative proportions of each stem cell type will be dictated by its survival advantage, the more recent mutations having a proliferative advantage (Russell and Reilly, 1989). Similar patterns of clonal progression probably occur in the evolution of ALL (Uckun and Heerema, 1990), lymphoma, myeloma, and some AML.

Persistence of normal haemopoiesis

The degree to which the malignant process affects normal stem cell function plays a central role in determining the likely response to treatment. Most lymphomas and some leukaemias such as chronic lymphoblastic leukaemia (CLL) affect normal marrow function only moderately, while acute leukaemias often cause marrow failure at presentation. A consideration of therapeutic importance is whether residual normal stem cells, not affected by leukaemic transformation, persist at presentation of the malignancy, and after initial treatment. Clearly, bone marrow remission following successful elimination of the leukaemic clone by chemotherapy is only possible if there are residual normal stem cells in the marrow. In fact, the demonstration of persisting clonal abnormalities in patients morphologically in remission from AML indicates that haematological recovery and clinical remission are sometimes sustained by a preleukaemic stem cell which has retained many normal differentiative properties (McCulloch, 1990). Clinical experience has shown that the chance of sustained remission and cure of AML is greater in diseases where the onset is rapid and without a preleukaemic phase. This suggests that residual normal stem cells diminish with time.

In CML the presence of a well-defined chromosome marker and its associated rearranged gene sequence has made it possible to identify separately normal and leukaemic haemopoiesis. Such investigations have shown that both in long-term culture and after interferon-α treatment, normal progenitors negative for the BCR/ABL fusion gene can be detected, indicating that normal stem cells do coexist with leukaemia cells in this disorder (Talpaz et al., 1988). The presence of residual normal cells has also been found by long-term culture in some AML (Coulombel et al., 1985).

Treatment implications

The cellular biology of haematological malignancies has a critical impact on the approach to treatment and its outcome:

Involvement of the stem cell in the malignant process

The development level at which the malignant process arises has major implications for treatment. As the relationship of the malignant process with normal ontogeny becomes better characterized, the disease features used to define prognosis have become less empirical and based more upon the underlying biology of the malignancy. While morphological and surface antigen classification of the leukaemias and

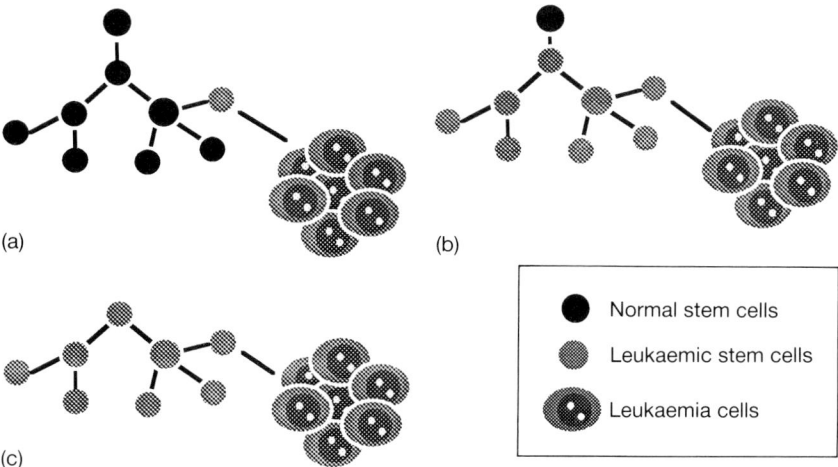

Fig. 2.3 Importance of normal stem cell presence in treatment approach and outcome. (a) Leukaemia arising from committed progenitor: normal stem cell function, selective antileukaemic treatment possible, e.g. common ALL, possibly AML M3. (b) Leukaemia arising from a pluripotent stem cell: myelotive treatments against abnormal stem cells, e.g. CML, some AML. (c) Leukaemia arising from a pluripotent stem cell. No residual normal stem cells. Remission induction leads to bone marrow failure. Cure only possible with allogeneic BMT, e.g. myelodysplastic syndromes, some AML, stem cell leukaemias.

lymphomas have been relatively successful in identifying the phenotype of the malignancy, their main defect is that they do not necessarily indicate the true precursor origin of the malignant process. This is an important consideration since diseases affecting the pluripotent stem cell are the least susceptible to cure with chemotherapy. Treatments intensive enough to eradicate malignant pluripotent stem cells induce severe marrow failure. Only diseases where a residual population of normal stem cells survive from a stage prior to the development of the malignancy could be expected to be cured. The only chance of curing disorders with no residual normal stem cells is by allogeneic bone marrow transplantation. In contrast, diseases where the malignant process spares the pluripotent stem cell include many that are curable by chemotherapy and autologous marrow transplantation (Fig. 2.3).

Proliferation rate

Haematological malignancies exhibit very different proliferation rates. Rapidly proliferating diseases are typified by T cell ALL, and Burkitt-type leukaemia or lymphoma. They often present with a high tumour load, are chemosensitive, and regress rapidly because a large proportion of the tumour is in cell cycle and vulnerable to cytotoxic agents. However, relapse can follow equally rapidly. Successful treatment requires frequent pulses of treatment designed to reduce malignant cell numbers faster than they can regenerate. These conditions may be uncontrollable if their rate of regeneration is faster than that of normal haemopoietic recovery. The high cell turnover may also facilitate the emergence of drug-resistant subclones by creating a survival advantage for chemoresistant mutations. In contrast, diseases typified by CLL and low-grade non-Hodgkin's lymphoma have a slow cell proliferation rate. Because the bulk of the tumour is not in cell cycle they respond poorly to cycle-active drugs. Reduction in tumour bulk is best achieved by repeated or continuous treatment with agents active against non-cycling cells such as alkylating agents. The large population of non-cycling cells makes complete eradication of the malignancy difficult to achieve without causing bone marrow failure.

Differentiation potential

There is a wide variation in the capacity of haematological malignancies to undergo differentiation. For example, the abnormal clones in CML, myeloproliferative diseases and myelodysplastic syndromes undergo almost complete maturation and maintain some degree of bone marrow function for a long period in the natural history of the disease. It has been appreciated for some time that certain agents such as retinoids, vitamin D_3, phorbol esters and interferon can induce maturation in leukaemia cell lines (Greenberg, 1991). This has stimulated the idea of using maturation-inducing agents to treat leukaemias in the expectation that as blast cells are induced to mature, they lose their proliferative potential and undergo clonal extinction. The shortcoming of this approach is that in only one instance (acute promyelocytic leukaemia (APML) treated with all-trans retinoic acid (ATRA) has it been possible to induce leukaemia maturation *in vivo*. Furthermore, ATRA does not cure the leukaemia, nor even control the remission for long. Failure to eradicate such leukaemias may in part be due to the persistence of progenitors not susceptible to the maturation-inducing agent (Meng-Er *et al.*, 1988; Castiagne *et al.*, 1990).

Impact of the malignancy on normal haematopoietic function

The impact of the malignant process on haemopoiesis affects the severity of the disorder, and the facility with which it can be managed. The acute leukaemias have a profound inhibitory effect on normal haemopoiesis, leading to an early presentation with clinical features of bone marrow failure. The recovery of normal bone marrow function typically requires high-intensity remission-induction chemotherapy. The chronic leukaemias, in contrast, progress slowly without life-threatening features of marrow failure to produce a large tumour burden in the reticuloendothelial system. In CLL where normal marrow function is relatively well-preserved, treatment of relatively low intensity usually allows recovery of haemoglobin, platelet and neutrophil levels to normal. Ultimately, however, bone marrow failure may supervene due both to disease progression and to cumulative stem cell damage from chemotherapy. The lack of serious marrow suppression caused by chemotherapy or radiotherapy facilitates the treatment of disorders where the bone marrow is not involved, such as Hodgkin's lymphoma.

Immunogenicity of the malignancy

The ability of the host's immune system to regulate the growth of the malignant process has an important influence upon the possibility of disease control and cure by chemotherapy. For example, it has long been appreciated that lymphocyte infiltration is a favourable feature of Hodgkin's disease. Recently the expression of class I major histocompatibility antigens by lymphoma cells has been linked to an improved survival following chemotherapy, suggesting the existence of a favourable T lymphocyte recognition and regulation of class I-bearing lymphoma cells (Swan *et al.*, 1991).

Immune response of the patient

While there is strong evidence for an inverse relationship between tumour growth and immune competence in virus-related lymphoproliferative disorders, almost nothing is known about the relationship between the natural killer (NK) cell and T lymphocyte function of the individual and the response of the leukaemia or lymphoma to treatment. Evidence for immune regulation in haematological malignancies is discussed more fully in Chapter 6. The possibility exists that the quality of the autologous immune response to the malignant process may have an important bearing on outcome.

Disease status

It is a universal observation in haematological malignancies that treatment becomes less successful as the disease becomes more advanced. Thus, primary induction failure, relapse and chemotherapy-resistant relapse confer a lower chance of survival than do diseases responding satisfactorily at the outset of treatment. Resistance to chemotherapy may be related to the evolution of drug resistance by the induction of multiple drug-resistant (MDR) genes (Kartner et al., 1985; Pastan and Gottesman, 1987; reviewed by Kaye and Kerr, 1991). The gene product P-glycoprotein is an adenosine triphosphate-driven membrane pump capable of actively exporting from the cell certain cytotoxic drugs such as vindesine, and anthracyclines. A number of agents, including the calcium channel blocker verapamil (Maruyama et al., 1989) and cyclosporin (Twentyman, 1988), have been shown to antagonize MDR in malignant cells. Combinations of anti-MDR drugs are beginning to be applied in treatment, but results at present do not indicate that overcoming drug resistance is central to the success or failure of chemotherapy treatment.

Treatment planning

The prerequisite for rational treatment of haematological malignancies is to define the *prognostic category* for a particular patient. This involves the following:
1 Accurate diagnosis of the disease and its subtype. Detailed leukaemia and lymphoma subclassifications are routinely applied to treatment decision-making.
2 Determining the extent of the disease involvement, e.g. local or disseminated disease, involvement of the central nervous system, and the degree of tumour burden.
3 The age of the patient, his or her performance status, and presence of other disorders affecting major organ systems must be taken into account in choosing appropriate treatment.

The treatment *objectives* can then be determined (Fig. 2.4). These can be categorized into disease control, remission induction and cure. Measurements capable of detecting minimal residual disease have helped considerably in understanding the nature of the remission state, relapse or cure of the disease. While the use of chemotherapy has evolved largely in an empirical fashion it is nevertheless possible to draw up a set of guidelines which relate the optimization of chemotherapy treatment schedules to improve the therapeutic action on the malignancy and reduce adverse effects on the normal haemopoietic and immune systems.

Disease control

The aim of this approach is to control symptoms and prevent the complications of unchecked expansion of the malignancy. Chemotherapy or agents such as interferon α may be used to reduce tumour bulk and malignant cell proliferation without seriously suppressing

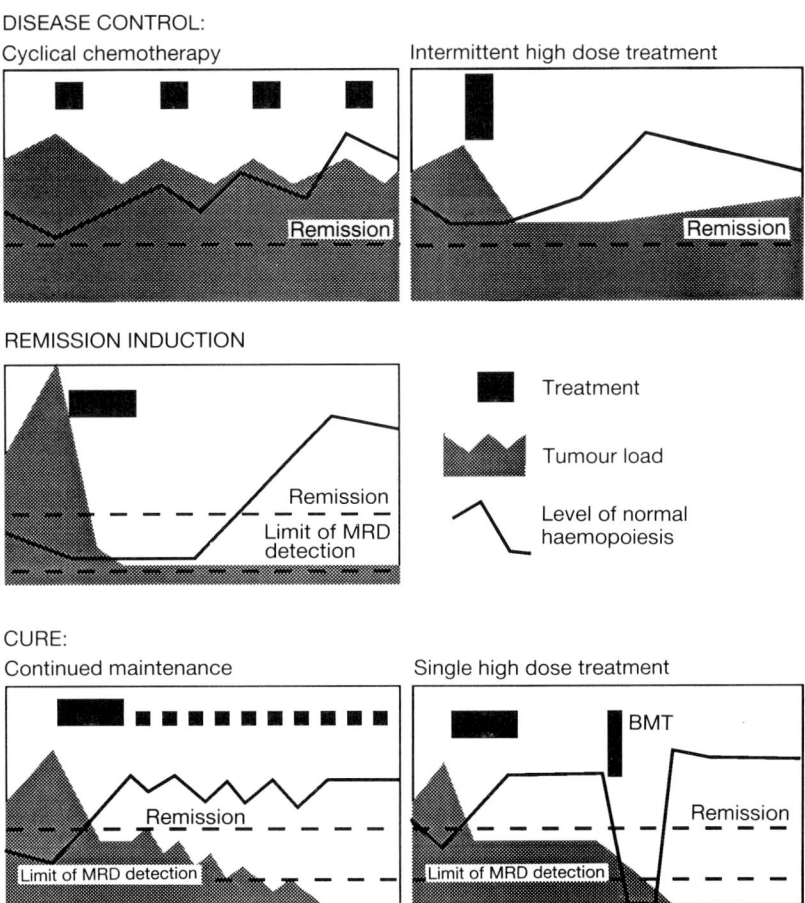

Fig. 2.4 Treatment objectives.

normal marrow function. Such treatment plays an important role in the successful management of low-grade lymphoproliferative disorders such as CLL over many years. Some disorders causing bone marrow failure, such as the myelodysplastic syndromes, and end-stage myelofibrosis are primarily managed by haematological support with blood and platelet transfusion without chemotherapy.

Remission induction

More intensive approaches to reduce tumour burden and improve bone marrow function are usually accompanied by a period of pancytopenia, but can produce remissions where bone marrow and immune function return to normal and it becomes impossible to detect residual disease by conventional means. Remission is associated with significant

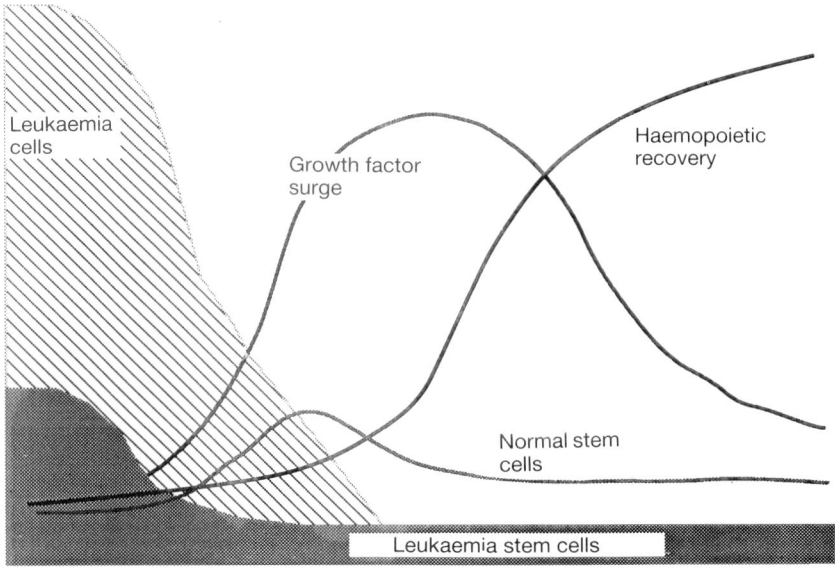

Fig. 2.5 Haematological changes during remission induction.

clinical improvement, and is therefore an important goal, even in disorders such as AML where subsequent relapse is likely.

Remission in acute leukaemia is defined as the restoration of normal haemopoiesis with less than 5% blast cells in the bone marrow. The changes in the normal and leukaemic marrow cells are illustrated in Fig. 2.5. Little is known about the interaction between leukaemic and normal cells at presentation, or during remission-induction. There is some evidence that leukaemic cells actively suppress normal haemopoiesis either by cytokine production or by interaction with the microenvironment of the bone marrow. In fact, *in vitro* studies do not convincingly demonstrate suppressive effects of acute leukaemia cells on normal haemopoiesis (Spitzer *et al.*, 1981).

Normal haemopoietic recovery after chemotherapy for leukaemia is accompanied by a surge of progenitor cells in the blood, monocytosis, and subsequently recovery of the leukocyte count to normal levels. Circulating haemopoietic stem cells have been extensively studied by researchers interested in the use of blood as a source of stem cells for autologous stem cell transplantation. Several groups have demonstrated that blood cells harvested at the peak of circulating stem cell production are capable of producing rapid early and sustained haemopoiesis and lymphopoiesis when used as autologous transplants following high-dose chemotherapy and radiotherapy (Juttner and To, 1990; Reiffers *et al.*, 1991). Thus it appears that haemopoietic recovery releases pluripotent and committed stem cells from the marrow into the blood. Remission is accompanied by changes in growth factor production. Serum of patients following chemotherapy and marrow transplantation contains increased amounts of granulopoietins and thrombopoietins (Mazur *et al.*, 1984; Adams *et al.*, 1990). The remission state is associated with a major clinical improvement: infection under partial antibiotic control resolves, undefined fevers and elevated acute-phase proteins normalize, mucositis heals, platelet production increases, and intensive transfusion support can be withdrawn.

Minimal residual disease (MRD) and relapse

The highly sensitive techniques now available have made it possible for the first time to identify patients in apparent full haematological remission with small amounts of persisting disease undetectable by morphological examination of the blood and marrow (Chapter 3). A major factor in the interpretation of the clinical significance of MRD is the sensitivity of the detection method. Table 2.3 lists the techniques that have been used to detect MRD in humans. The most sensitive technique – the polymerase chain reaction (PCR) – detects in the order of one leukaemia cell/10^6 cells but is difficult to quantitate. More easily quantifiable techniques using fluorescence, microscopy and immunocytochemistry are less sensitive, detecting down to $1/10^5$ cells. Diseases with chromosome markers are also susceptible to

Table 2.3 Techniques and application of minimal residual disease detection

Technique	Sensitivity	Application
Morphology	1/100	Defining remission in acute leukaemia
Surface markers (flow cytometry)	Up to 1/100 000	AML, B-ALL, T-ALL
Cytogenetics Blood and marrow cells	Depends on number of metaphases screened	t(15;17) AML, t(8;14), t(4;11), t(9;22)
Southern blotting IgH chain gene TCR gene	1/100 1/1 000 000	B cell malignancies T cell malignancies
Polymerase chain reaction on fusion genes	1/10 000–1 000 000	IgH, B-ALL TCR, T-ALL t(9;22) CML ALL t(15;17) AML M3
Paraprotein analysis	<100 g of tumour	Myeloma

AML, Acute myeloid leukaemia; ALL, acute lymphoblastic leukaemia; IgH, immunoglobulin heavy chain; TCR, T cell receptor; CML, chronic myeloid leukaemia.

MRD analysis but the detection sensitivity depends on how many metaphases are examined. Chromosome analysis on cultured colonies from remission patients may enhance the sensitivity by several logs, but the technique is difficult and unreliable. Several techniques have now been applied to leukaemia patients under treatment to detect disease at a stage when conventional methods are negative. T cell receptor or IgH gene rearrangements to detect MRD in lymphoid malignancies are still under evaluation. Preliminary reports suggest the technique can accurately map the slow disappearance of ALL during successful maintenance treatment, and predict the re-emergence of leukaemia several months before clinical relapse is detected (Yamada et al., 1990). In CML the PCR technique has enabled us to study the effect of bone marrow transplantation (BMT) and interferon on the leukaemia population (Hughes et al., 1991). These studies indicate that disappearance of the BCR/ABL signal corresponds with cure after BMT, while the probe still detects BCR/ABL rearrangement and therefore persisting disease in interferon-treated patients who have become negative for leukaemia by chromosome analysis (Lee et al., 1989). In AML, several techniques have been used: detection of clonal abnormalities by culture of remission marrow; detection of unique leukaemia phenotypes by double-labelling and fluorescent-activated cell sorter (FACS) analysis of remission marrow (Campana et al., 1991), and the application of chromosome analysis in diseases such as APML characterized by the presence of a chromosome translocation (Chomienne et al., 1990). Surprisingly, many patients in stable remission appear to have persisting clonal leukaemic haematopoiesis (Fialkow et al., 1987).

The detection of a low level of persisting leukaemia could be interpreted in different ways: it could represent a re-emerging, possibly resistant, clone of leukaemia that, given time, would generate clinical relapse, or a *de novo* leukaemia. Alternatively, relapse may represent a disturbance of a stable equilibrium between residual leukaemia regrowth and its suppression by haemopoietic microenvironmental influences, or the immune system. It is also necessary to consider the possibility that the residual leukaemia cell population may represent a stem cell population with different characteristics to the blast cell responsible for overt disease. Furthermore the residual population may itself be a mixture of subclones of leukaemic stem cells, as discussed in the preceding section. All these considerations have a bearing on our understanding of the nature of relapse. If MRD is actively controlled, relapse could occur if there is a temporary lapse in immune regulation, or if the haemopoietic microenvironment becomes favourable to the leukaemic stem cell. There is evidence from animals that stem cell clones are recruited successively at intervals of a few weeks following chemotherapy-induced temporary aplasia (Abkowitz et al., 1988). If this model applies to human haemopoiesis a stochastic process of stem cell selection could pertain where relapse occurs with the chance recruitment of a leukaemic stem cell from the pool. The concept of a dynamic relationship between remission and relapse lends support to the concept of treatments aimed at increasing the activity of autologous immune regulatory cells, or alloreactive lymphocytes following bone marrow transplantation (see Chapters 3 and 6).

Cure

Cure is defined as the non-recurrence of malignancy following a disease-free interval of 5 years from the remission. It should however be considered to be a statistical probability of disease non-recurrence over the lifespan of the patient and is not necessarily equivalent to the total eradication of the last malignant cell.

Cure may be achieved in a single initial eradicative treatment (for example, the use of bone marrow transplantation as primary treatment for myelodysplasia; Appelbaum et al., 1990a), but more frequently is carried out in two stages – firstly, tumour reduction by chemotherapy, radiotherapy or surgery, to achieve a remission, followed by a second phase of treatment to eradicate the disease. Three distinct approaches are used:

1 Stepwise reduction of residual disease by chemotherapy using repeated treatment cycles over many months, as in the management of lymphomas, or consolidation treatment of intensity similar to that used in remission-induction followed by maintenance treatment of low intensity over many months, as used in the treatment of childhood ALL.
2 High-intensity treatment early in remission, often involving marrow transplantation and intensive haematological support (Chapter 5).
3 Cure by control of residual disease using biological response modifiers, such as interferon α, or immunotherapy treatments which control proliferation and maturation of malignant cells (Chapter 6).

While the development of chemotherapy combinations continues to play a central role in the initial control of the disease, the newer approaches to treatment using BMT, immunotherapy, or maturation-inducing agents is gaining an increasing place in the cure of many haematological malignancies. In this regard the ability to detect minimal residual disease is of great importance in the assessment of experimental treatments to eradicate disease in remission. The mechanisms upon which cure is based are listed in Table 2.4.

Based on the work carried out by Skipper in the mouse L1210 leukaemia/lymphoma model, it has long been considered that cure

Table 2.4 Possible mechanisms of cure of haematological malignancies

1. Repeated chemotherapy cycles achieve logwise cytoreduction beyond the last surviving cell (acute lymphoblastic leukaemia, lymphomas)
2. Physiological clonal extinction (B cell malignancies)
3. Re-establishment of preleukaemic stem cell clonal dominance (acute myeloid leukaemia)
4. Introducing graft-versus-leukaemia and lymphoma control by allogeneic marrow transplantation
5. Re-establishment of immune surveillance by natural killer cells or autoreacting T cells

equates with the statistical certainty of diminution of the leukaemia population in logwise reduction steps past the point of elimination of the last leukaemia cell (Skipper, 1986). This model might not be applicable to complicated leukaemia hierarchies, and may not be relevant at all if cure is maintained by an active process of control of MRD. There is considerable evidence from studies of BCR expression following BMT for CML that MRD may reappear and then disappear at intervals after BMT. Slavin has used murine EL4 leukaemia models to show that the balance between control of MRD and relapse can be disturbed in favour of relapse by administration of cyclosporin to stable remission chimeras (Slavin *et al.*, 1990). Whether or not low levels of residual leukaemia always remain after chemotherapy-induced cures is not known, but it seems increasingly possible that cure will not be in most instances simply explained by the elimination of the last leukaemic cell, but rather by the successful diminution of the leukaemic clone to a size where it comes under powerful but poorly understood regulatory influences.

A further possibility proposed to explain cure in childhood ALL is that maintenance treatment reduces the malignant B cell clone to a size where it can undergo the physiological clonal extinction through the apoptotic process that is characteristic of its normal B cell counterpart (Gale and Butturini, 1991). After allogeneic BMT there is abundant statistical evidence in humans (Horowitz *et al.*, 1990) and considerable experimental evidence (Sosman and Sondel, 1987) to substantiate the presence of a potent graft versus leukaemia effect which is detectable following allogeneic BMT for AML, ALL, CML, lymphoma and possibly myeloma (Gahrton *et al.*, 1991; Chapter 5).

Designing chemotherapy schedules

The number of chemotherapeutic agents which have been shown to be effective in the treatment of haematological malignancies is so great that the choice itself is counterproductive to designing optimal treatment regimens. Combination chemotherapy schedules regularly employ up to five different agents. With this number it becomes impossible, however, to evaluate clearly whether the combination used is the most effective choice of drugs, doses and schedules. It is therefore not surprising that there is still debate as to whether a third agent added to the combination of daunorubicin and cytosine arabinoside confers any further treatment advantage in remission induction for AML (Rees, 1990). It is clear, however, that the outcome of treatment is largely unaffected by the precise choice of drugs used.

Three examples serve to illustrate this latter point:
1 In the treatment of disseminated diffuse large cell lymphoma, at least six variations on the basic CHOP treatment schedule have been evaluated (Miller et al., 1988). There is no evidence that any one drug combination offers a special advantage over the original treatment approach (Bonadonna and Valagussa, 1990).
2 In the treatment of AML at least six different drugs used in various combinations can induce remission. There is no evidence that any one combination is superior to the standard daunorubicin–cytosine arabinoside schedule (Rees, 1990).
3 Numerous high-dose chemotherapy and radiotherapy conditioning schedules have been used to prepare patients for marrow transplantation. There is no evidence that a particular choice of drug is of benefit in conferring a better outcome after BMT. What does appear to affect outcome is the *intensity* of the treatment used, determined by the drug doses and the duration of their treatment.

Intensification of treatment is measurable in three ways:
1 improvement in the antimalignant efficacy;
2 increased haematological toxicity;
3 increased non-haematological toxicity.

Treatments can be developed that optimize the relationship between the unwanted toxicity to normal tissues and the required action against the leukaemia or lymphoma. The principles adopted to achieve these aims are summarized in Table 2.5.

Successful treatment protocols follow patterns dictated by the limitations on dose and schedule imposed by the effect of chemotherapy on normal tissues, and the treatment aim (see above). Both single and multiple-agent treatments can be used effectively for disease control or in higher doses (with stem cell rescue if necessary) with the aim of cure. Stem cell rescue following high-dose marrow ablative treatment has for a long time been advocated as a means of altering the dose-limiting relationship between malignant cell reduction and unwanted toxicities. However, while autologous stem cell

Table 2.5 Principles of treatment schedule design

1 Achieving optimum action against the malignancy
   (a) Use high doses to achieve maximum uptake by malignant cells
   (b) Use combinations of drugs to achieve synergy
   (c) Give local treatment of sanctuary sites for disease not reached by treatment
   (d) Give prolonged treatment for slowly proliferating disease
   (e) Give short repeated cycles for rapidly proliferating disease
   (f) Use non-cycle active agents to eradicate resting malignant cell progenitors
   (g) Introduce new drugs in later cycles to avoid drug resistance
   (h) Continue treatment beyond remission to achieve cure
   (i) Consider synergy with non-cytotoxic agents (e.g. interferon α, immunotherapy)

2 Avoiding haemopoietic toxicity
   (a) Repeated pulses of treatment are better than prolonged single treatments
   (b) Use short pulses to reduce the period of neutropenia to a minimum
   (c) Cycle-active agents (e.g. methotrexate) can be given in pulsed courses, and do not cause significant stem cell marrow failure
   (d) Stem cell rescue with ABMT or BMT required for non-cycle-active agents (e.g. busulphan used in high doses)
   (e) Combinations of cycle-active and non-cycle-active agents and agents with no haemopoietic toxicity reduce haemopoietic toxicity but preserve antileukaemic effect (e.g. acute lymphoblastic leukaemia treatment)
   (f) Use haemopoietic growth factors to reduce depth and duration of marrow suppression

3 Avoiding non-haemopoietic toxicity
   (a) Use combinations of agents with different patterns of organ toxicity
   (b) Use tissue- and organ-specific protective treatments (e.g. antibiotics to reduce mucositis, experimental treatments to prevent hepatic veno-occlusive disease)

ABMT, Autologous bone marrow transplantation.

rescue with bone marrow or blood stem cells is now readily achieved, non-haemopoietic toxicity becomes a limiting factor to the widespread application of this strategy. The advent of newer treatments with interferons, immunotherapy and growth factors presents new opportunities to improve the therapeutic ratio. There are several promising developments along these lines – haemopoietic growth factors can be used to shorten the period of neutropenia and make it possible to administer more frequent cycles of chemotherapy. They also permit increased doses of cytotoxic treatment to be given without prejudicing normal marrow recovery. Alternatively, cytokines can be used to synergize with chemotherapy and achieve better tumour control (Chapter 6).

While it is possible that the advent of new chemotherapeutic drugs could still improve the outcome for various malignancies, higher cure rates for haematological malignancies are more likely to be obtained by applying non-chemotherapeutic innovations to existing treatments.

Table 2.6 Summary of treatment strategies in haematological malignancies

	Curability (disease-free survival)		Other treatment approaches
	Chemotherapy	Allogeneic BMT	
Myeloid diseases			
AML	<25%	Up to 65%	ABMT, ATRA for AML M3, ? immunotherapy/IFNα
MDS	<5%	Up to 55%	G-CSF, Epo, IL-3?, IFNα, IFNγ, maturation inducers (D3, retinoids, cytosine arabinoside) cultured stem cell autograft
CML	0%	Up to 75%	IFNα, IFNγ, IL-2/LAK cell immunotherapy? Cultured stem cell autograft
MPD	0%	Not evaluated	IFNα; ? other cytokines
Lymphoid diseases			
Childhood c-ALL	>95%	Not evaluated	Not evaluated
Poor-risk ALL	<40%	Up to 65%	ABMT
Myeloma	<5%	45%	IFNα to maintain remission/plateau, anti-IL-6
Hairy cell leukaemia	<5%	Not evaluated	IFNα, deoxycoformycin
CLL	<5%	30–40%	IFNα with chemotherapy
NHL	50%	Not evaluated	ABMT ± IL-2

BMT, Bone marrow transplantation; AML, acute myeloid leukaemia; ABMT, autologous bone marrow transplantation; ATRA, all-trans-retinoic acid; IFNα, interferon α; IFNγ, interferon γ; IL-2 interleukin 2; MDS, myelodysplastic syndromes; G-CSF, granulocyte colony-stimulating factor; Epo, erythropoietin; CML, chronic myeloid leukaemia; LAK, lymphokine activated killer; MPD, myeloproliferative disorders; C-ALL, common acute lymphoblastic leukaemia; NHL, non-Hodgkin's lymphoma.

Treatment strategies in individual haematological malignancies

Treatment strategies for haematological malignancies are summarized in Table 2.6.

Childhood ALL

The highly successful approach to the treatment of childhood ALL is a tribute to the application of randomized therapeutic trials over the last 30 years. Early successes in treatment of ALL highlighted the clinical improvement consequent upon achieving remission, and identified a high relapse rate both in the bone marrow and in extramedullary tissues. The introduction of vincristine in the early 1960s marked a turning point. Both prednisolone and vincristine used singly could produce remission in 50–60% of children but in combination with prednisolone achieved 90% remissions. With the hurdle of early death

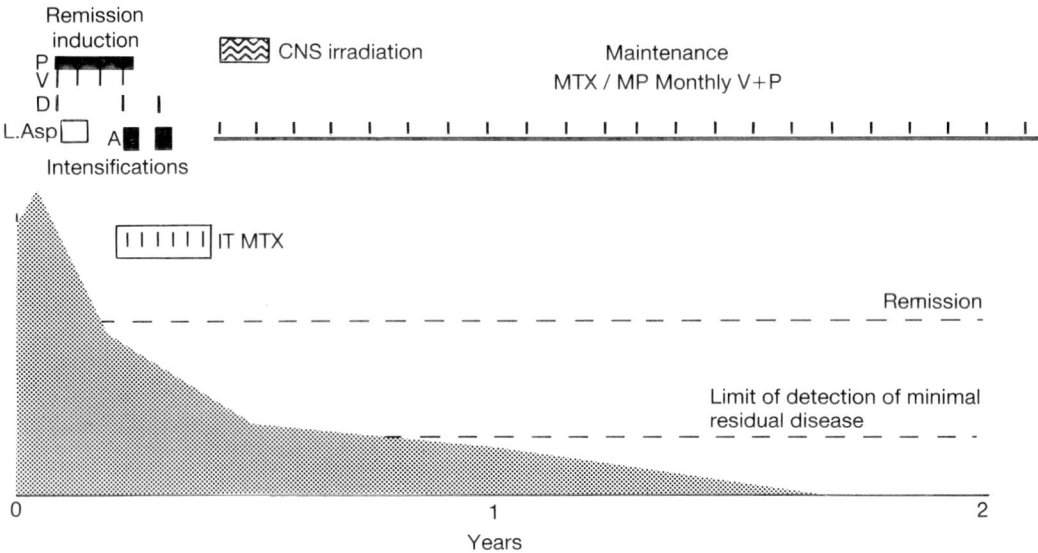

Fig. 2.6 Standard risk ALL treatment schedule: IT MTX, Intrathecal methotrexate; CNS irradiation, cranial irradiation to 18 Gy; P, prednisolone; D, daunorubicin; A, cytosine arabinoside; L.Asp, L-asparaginase; MP, mercaptopurine; V, vincristine.

from uncontrolled leukaemia and marrow failure cleared, the way was open for the trials designed to keep children in remission. Much important work was done by the Memphis team, who evolved the concept of consolidation and maintenance treatments and specific treatment of the central nervous system (CNS), to prevent CNS leukaemia and sustain remission. The principles of acute leukaemia treatment that emerged from this work, and the approach to treatment, remain essentially unchanged (Fig. 2.6).

The principles adopted in the treatment of ALL have been summarized as follows (Mauer, 1980; Pinkel, 1987):

Use of combinations of agents. The success achieved with vincristine and prednisolone was a strong indication for the use of two or more antileukaemia drugs in combination. The use of a third agent such as daunorubicin can increase remission rates to over 98% in childhood ALL.

Use of drugs with selectivity against leukaemia. Vincristine and prednisolone have no myelosuppressive effect. The search for further specific antileukaemia agents produced another drug, L-asparaginase (L-Asp), with low myelosuppression, developed to exploit the inability of lymphoid leukaemia cells to synthesize asparagine. The administration of L-Asp to the leukaemia patient would, it was argued, selectively deprive the leukaemia of asparagine. L-Asp has therefore been incorporated into many ALL treatment schedules.

Continued treatment after remission. Models of leukaemia cytoreduction, and the clinical experience that relapse occurs within weeks after remission-induction, indicates the need for further cytoreduction. It was argued that different agents would be required to avoid resistance developing. Hence, consolidation chemotherapy was introduced to initiate further reduction with agents not encountered previously by the leukaemia. A variety of agents are used, of which daunorubicin, cyclophosphamide, high-dose methotrexate, cytosine arabinoside and, more recently, etoposide are the most frequently employed, usually in combination.

Sanctuary sites. As leukaemia treatment produced longer disease-free survival, the problem of CNS relapse became a significant cause of treatment failure. The lack of success in treating established CNS leukaemia led to the development of sucessful prophylactic regimens for CNS disease. The CNS is regarded as a sanctuary site for leukaemia because of the inability of chemotherapeutic agents to cross the blood–brain barrier. The testes and ovaries and the anterior chamber of the eye are also considered as sanctuary sites. However, the diminishing frequency of testicular relapse as intensity of treatment schedule is escalated indicates that the testes present a less definite barrier to leukaemia treatment drugs.

Selection of treatment intensity according to prognostic features at presentation. Treatment of childhood ALL has continued to improve, largely through the identification of risk factors which has allowed the selection of high-intensity schedules for poor-risk patients and standard risk schedules for children with a low probability of relapse. Standard-risk ALL is regarded as a disease curable by chemotherapy alone. Most studies now demonstrate cure rates in the region of 90% for this type of ALL. Early intensification in particular appears to have improved the survival of patients with higher risk features. Such children have a cure rate of up to 70% (Clavell *et al.*, 1986; Steinberg *et al.*, 1986). Prognostic features separating standard and poor-risk features in ALL relate firstly to the tumour burden, as measured by the degree of lymphadenopathy and splenomegaly and the presenting blast cell count, but also to the proliferative capacity and the developmental origin of the leukaemia. These features are to some extent interrelated. Thus, leukaemias with a rapid doubling time, such as T-ALL and B-ALL, tend to present with high leukocyte counts and massive splenomegaly and lymphadenopathy. It is also possible to identify a very poor prognosis group of childhood ALL characterized by a myeloid cell phenotype (Urbano-Ispizna et al., 1990; Wiersma et al., 1991) and with chromosome abnormalities involving t(4;11) translocations (Pui et al., 1991), or t(9;22) translocation (Fletcher et al., 1991). These leukaemias are considered incurable by chemotherapy alone but may have a more favourable outcome after BMT (Barrett et al., 1992). These diseases behave like stem cell leukaemias, and are impossible to eradicate with standard anti-ALL drugs. Bone marrow transplantation as elective treatment for childhood ALL is reserved for this poor-risk group of patients.

The challenges now facing the treatment of childhood ALL are largely those of selecting treatment of appropriate intensity for the particular prognostic risk of the individual patient, thus avoiding unnecessary toxicity. The increasing ability to detect minimal residual disease in remission patients may also allow the use of treatment tailored to the individual patient's requirement (Yamada et al., 1990). Nevertheless, the small group of about 10% of patients with largely incurable disease presents a continuing problem.

Adult ALL

The rapid advance in the treatment of ALL in children seen over the last 30 years lent hope to the idea that similar chemotherapy strategies would eventually achieve increasing cure rates in adult acute leukaemias in general. In fact, the long-term survival for adult ALL given chemotherapy according to the treatment plan for childhood ALL remains in the region of 40% (Hoelzer and Gale, 1987). Treatment results show a steady decline in cure rate with increasing age, and ALL presenting over the age of 40 is largely incurable by chemotherapy. This is due to the increasing rarity of childhood-type c-ALL with increasing age, and the dominance of poor-prognosis ALL with biphenotypic characteristics (Sobol et al., 1987). Ph^1 chromosome positive – t(9;22) – ALL accounts for less than 5% of ALL in children, but becomes increasingly common with advancing age, accounting for up to 20% of adult ALL. There is an even greater frequency of hidden t(9;22) chromosome translocations, identified by BCR-ABL rearrangement, which are detectable in 55% of adult c-ALL (Maurer et al., 1991).

Treatment strategies for adult ALL are not satisfactorily defined – better prognostic criteria are needed to separate the 40% of patients who are potentially curable by chemotherapy alone, and the remainder who may benefit from BMT. In the absence of any completed prospective randomized trials to identify the best strategy, it is not known whether chemotherapy, autologous BMT or allogeneic BMT is the best

Table 2.7 Treatment problems and strategies in acute lymphoblastic leukaemia (ALL)

Problem	Strategy
Selecting appropriate treatment for different disease subtypes	Improved subtyping; selection of stem cell ALL for BMT
Improving remission induction for poor-risk ALL	New anthracyclines, new combinations, faster delivery of treatment, G-CSF to enhance normal marrow recovery
Determining optimum chemotherapy consolidation	Trials comparing intensity and timing of consolidation
Optimum duration of maintenance treatment	Monitoring minimal residual disease to decide on treatment length
Role of maintenance in adult ALL	Trials of long and short maintenance
How to treat poor-risk childhood ALL and adult ALL	Trials comparing ABMT and allogeneic BMT with intensive chemotherapy in remission

BMT, bone marrow transplantation; G-CSF, granulocyte colony-stimulating factor; ABMT, autologous bone marrow transplantation.

approach for a specific prognostic group. A retrospective analysis comparing ALL treatment results of a large chemotherapy database with BMT results from the International Bone Marrow Transplant Registry did not show any difference in disease-free survival between chemotherapy and BMT (Horowitz et al., 1991). The current problems and possible future strategies to improve treatment in ALL are summarized in Table 2.7.

AML

Although it is customary to use the remission-induction, consolidation and maintenance approach to AML treatment, the mechanisms involved and the results obtainable differ from those in ALL. Treatment strategies are summarized in Table 2.8.

Remission-induction. Unlike ALL, where leukaemia-specific agents are used, none of the drugs used for AML has much specificity for the leukaemia. In order to obtain remission it is therefore necessary to employ intensive and unselective chemotherapy to induce temporary marrow aplasia. Recovery and remission rely upon the presence of residual normal stem cells capable of sustaining haemopoiesis. At best, about 85% of AML patients will achieve a remission. Failure to achieve remission occurs more frequently with advancing age, which is partly due to an increasing frequency of AML arising from prior myelodysplastic syndromes. Such patients fail to achieve sustained remissions or normal haemopoietic recovery because of a lack of

Table 2.8 Treatment problems and strategies in acute myeloid leukaemia (AML)

Problem	Strategy
Improving remission rate	Two agents or three? Evaluating new drugs (e.g. idarubicin, aclarubicin) High-intensity schedules with G-CSF to enhance normal recovery
Preventing relapse	Prospective trials comparing ABMT, BMT and chemotherapy-only consolidation Experimental immunotherapy (e.g. IFNα, IL-2)
Treatment of AML M3	Establishing the place of ATRA in remission-induction and maintenance
Persisting residual disease	Minimal residual disease detection and further treatment
Treatment of elderly patients	Use of haemopoietic growth factors to reduce the cytopenic period

G-CSF, Granulocyte colony-stimulating factor; ABMT, autologous bone marrow transplantation; IFNα, interferon α; IL-2, interleukin 2; ATRA, all-transretinoic acid.

residual normal stem cells. Induction failure also occurs because of resistant disease and because of death from marrow failure, related partly to treatment and partly to the leukaemia itself. Single agents achieve remission rates in the order of 30% (Ellison et al., 1968). Combinations of an anthracycline with cytosine arabinoside have improved the remission rate to about 70% (Mayer, 1988). It is possible that the new anthracycline idarubicin may induce remission in a slightly greater proportion of patients, but in general there is little to suggest that improved results will come from better chemotherapeutic agents.

The unresolved questions surrounding remission-induction treatment for AML are whether a third agent, in addition to the combination of cytosine arabinoside and an anthracycline such as daunorubicin, may improve results further. Etoposide, mitoxantrone, idarubicin and carboplatin are under evaluation (Wiernik, 1990). Another approach is to use a third agent such as the nitrosourea CCNU, active against non-cycling leukaemia cells, with the aim of eliminating resting cells responsible for relapse at the time of the initial treatment. Improved remission-induction treatments should not only result in higher percentages of remissions but also translate into fewer subsequent relapses. There is some evidence that recent treatments, for example with idarubicin (Wiernik, 1990), etoposide (Bishop et al., 1990), and CCNU (Barrett et al., 1990), achieve this. It is clear however that developments in the scheduling of remission-inducing drugs have had a greater impact on results than has the introduction of new agents. It is now generally appreciated that the more intensive treatments induce rapid remissions and reduce early mortality from pancytopenia as a consequence (Gale et al., 1981; Rees, 1990). Using this approach better remission rates have been achieved in elderly patients who would previously have received low-intensity treatment in view of their age. Because of the lack of any useful prognostic criteria for treatment selection there have been few attempts to tailor treatment to individuals. However the bone marrow taken on the sixth day of treatment has been used to determine whether further chemotherapy should be used according to the number of residual leukaemia cells present (Browman et al., 1989).

While increasing treatment intensity may ultimately reduce the proportion of patients with resistant disease, it is likely that a corresponding increase in treatment failure from lack of normal haemopoietic recovery would become a major obstacle. The use of haemopoietic growth factors could be of value in improving recovery in this context (Buchner et al., 1990; Mertelsmann et al., 1990).

Post-remission chemotherapy. The major failure in chemotherapy approaches to the treatment of AML is the inability to maintain remission. Only 25% of patients who achieve remission become long-term survivors (Rees et al., 1986, 1987). Although the frequency of relapse drops after the first 18 months there remains a continuing risk of true relapse (as opposed to *de novo* disease) for at least 10 years. Consolidation treatment soon after remission improves survival (Preisler et al., 1987; Tricot et al., 1987) but there is little evidence to support prolongation of treatment courses. For example, Rees et al. found no advantage in using six consolidation courses rather than two (Rees et al., 1986). Likewise there is no firm evidence that prolonged maintenance treatment improves survival or cure rates. Late intensification may improve the results but has not been widely evaluated (Preisler et al., 1989). These results suggest that remission in AML is seldom associated with complete eradication of the leukaemic process.

Because of the high relapse probability in AML, treatments to maintain remission are under continuing evaluation. It is generally agreed that maintenance chemotherapy in remission does not significantly affect outcome. The central unresolved question in the treatment of AML patients up to the age of about 55 years is whether to carry out autologous BMT (ABMT), allogeneic BMT or continue chemotherapy (International Bone Marrow Transplant Registry, 1989). Although the relapse probability following allogeneic BMT (15–20%) is much lower than that observed after chemotherapy (70–80%) or

ABMT (40–60%), the higher mortality following allogeneic BMT makes it difficult to distinguish which treatment offers the best chance of survival and cure. Several prospective studies address this problem but the results so far are inconclusive (Reiffers et al., 1989).

Bone marrow transplantation. Allogeneic BMT achieves cures in AML by the efficacy of high-dose chemotherapy and irradiation, and the graft-versus-leukaemia effect of the donor immune cells. ABMT appears to cure some patients with AML. This can be attributed to the effect of the high-dose chemotherapy and irradiation used prior to BMT, and possibly an autologous graft-versus-leukaemia effect. To enhance this autoimmune effect of the autograft, interleukin 2 (IL-2) has been used to induce lymphokine activated killer (LAK) cell activity (Blaise et al., 1991), and cyclosporin has been given to induce autologous graft-versus-host disease (see Chapter 4).

Immunotherapy. Early trials using Calmette-Guérin bacillus (BCG) and adoptive transfer of irradiated leukaemia blasts failed to show conclusive benefit (Arends-Merino et al., 1983), although a long-term follow-up suggested that there was some response (Reizenstein, 1990). The availability of the potent recombinant cytokines IL-2 and interferon has renewed enthusiasm for re-evaluating immunotherapy as a means of maintaining remission in AML. Immunotherapy with IL-2 and LAK cells during remission induction is under evaluation (Boughton et al., 1991). However, IL-2 given during remission did not appear to prolong remission in a small study (Macdonald et al., 1990). Interferon α used for its antiproliferative action is also being evaluated in the UK Medical Research Council AML trials.

ATRA in APML. The demonstration that ATRA can induce remission in APML has opened up a new field of research in this leukaemia (Meng-Er et al., 1988; Castaigne et al., 1990). A specific translocation t(15;17) (q22;q11–21) has been found in every patient with APML, and the mapping of the retinoic acid receptor α (RAR-α) gene to the 17th chromosome at band q21 suggested to several workers that the RAR might be involved in APML (Mattei et al., 1988; De Thé et al., 1990). In APML it has been demonstrated that the breakpoint of the t(15;17) translocation results in the fusion of a portion of a gene from chromosome 15 (*myl*) with the RAR-α gene. This results in a hybrid gene *myl*/RAR-α, the fusion transcript of which generates an abnormal RAR. Specifically, the transactivating domain is affected. This may render the RAR less efficient at signalling when retinoic acid binds to it, resulting in a block to retinoic acid target genes. The consequence of this could be a failure of granulocyte differentiation and a maturation arrest manifest as APML. Retinoic acid derivatives are potent regulators of cell growth and embryonic development, and have been known for some time to induce neutrophil maturation in APML cells in culture. All-trans-retinoic acid appears to have a high affinity for its receptor and is particularly effective at inducing APML maturation (Chomienne *et al.*, 1990). The therapeutic action of ATRA may therefore be to overcome the inefficient handling of physiological concentrations of retinoic acid by APML cells by efficient binding and activation of maturation-inducing genes normally activated by retinoic acid.

ATRA can be used alone to induce first and second remissions in APML. The characteristic response which occurs in the majority of patients when first treated with ATRA is the rapid resolution of disseminated intravascular coagulation, followed by a progressive rise in the leukocyte count. At this stage the circulating leukocytes appear to represent the leukaemic clone with partially differentiated forms and some abnormal mature neutrophils. This first leukocytosis persists for about 30 days. Following this there is a return to normal granulopoiesis and full haematological remission. At this stage the marrow karyotype is normal (Flynn *et al.*, 1983; Castaigne *et al.*, 1990; Warrell *et al.*, 1991). However, despite continuing ATRA treatment, remission is not maintained. Attempts to induce remission for a second time with ATRA are often ineffective.

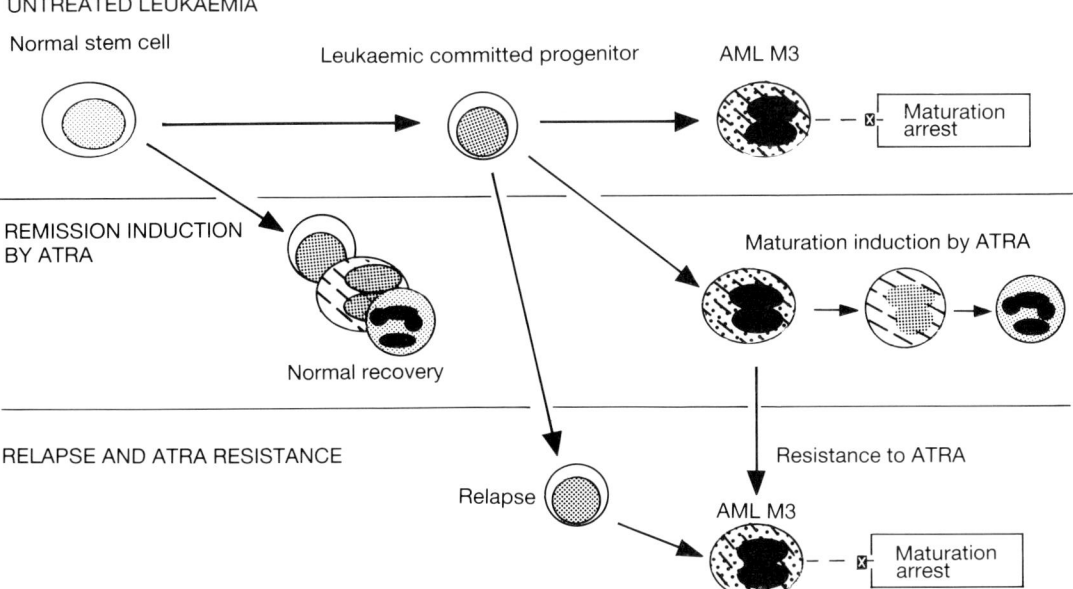

Fig. 2.7 Hypothetical model of acute promyelocytic leukaemia biology in relation to treatment.

The place of ATRA in the treatment of APML is still under evaluation. Its main value may lie in its ability to induce remission with or without additional chemotherapy. However, the tendency to relapse shows that ATRA does not eradicate the leukaemic progenitor, and therefore further treatment either with chemotherapy or BMT is necessary. The changes occurring during treatment of APML with ATRA are shown in Figure 2.7.

Myelodysplastic syndromes

Myelodysplastic syndromes are preleukaemic disorders with a myeloid stem cell abnormality (Prchal *et al.*, 1978; Raskind *et al.*, 1984; Janssen *et al.*, 1989; reviewed by Koeffler, 1986). There is a tendency to progressive pancytopenia and eventual transformation to AML in many patients (Tricot *et al.*, 1985). In the apparent absence of residual normal haemopoiesis, treatment has been directed towards supportive care with transfusions and antibiotics, induction of maturation in the defective cell lines, and recently the use of haemopoietic growth factors to stimulate erythropoiesis and granulopoiesis.

A variety of maturation-inducing agents have been used but with only modest success. They include low-dose cytosine arabinoside (Bolwell *et al.*, 1987), retinoic acid derivatives (Lishner *et al.*, 1989), dihydroxyvitamin D_3 (Koeffler *et al.*, 1984), interferon α (Galvani *et al.*, 1987; Gisslinger *et al.*, 1990), and interferon γ (Maiolo *et al.*, 1990). At best, such treatment does no more than favour the emergence of less abnormal preleukaemic clones, and does not induce true remissions. Haemopoietic growth factor production is defective in patients with MDS (Greenberg, 1986; Jacobs *et al.*, 1989), and treatment with recombinant growth factors is therefore a logical way of increasing erythropoiesis and granulopoiesis in MDS (Vadhan-Raj *et al.*, 1987; Antin *et al.*, 1988; Negrin *et al.*, 1989; Ganser *et al.*, 1990). Erythropoietin (Bessho *et al.*, 1990), GM-CSF (Vadhan-Raj *et al.*, 1987; Antin *et al.*, 1988; Ganser *et al.*, 1989), G-CSF (Negrin *et al.*, 1989) and, most recently, IL-3 (Ganser *et al.*, 1990) have been used (see Chapter 5).

Progression to AML is an indication to attempt remission-induction in younger patients. However, at this stage residual normal stem cells are functionally absent, and AML induction chemotherapy infrequently results in stable haemopoietic recovery. Following chemotherapy some patients develop prolonged aplasia without normal haemopoietic recovery, some have resistant leukaemia, and some recover partial but dysplastic haemopoiesis. Because of the poor response to chemotherapy and absence of normal haemopoiesis, allogeneic BMT has been used as a potentially curative option in the less common group of

Table 2.9 Treatment approaches in myelodysplastic syndromes

Management of cytopenia by cell replacement and prophylaxis
Red cell and platelet transfusion
Antibacterial and antifungal prophylaxis

Improving maturation of abnormal clones
Haemopoietic growth factors — IL-3, GM-CSF, G-CSF, erythropoietin
Differentiation-inducing agents — low dose ARA-C, retinoids, vitamin D_3, IFNα, IFNγ

Reinducing normal haemopoiesis
Low-dose chemotherapy for hyperproliferative MDS (e.g. CMML) etoposide, mercaptopurine, hydroxyurea
AML remission-induction chemotherapy
Autologous BMT using cultured marrow cells which selectively eliminate abnormal stem cells (Chang et al., 1988)
Allogeneic BMT

IL-3, Interleukin 3; GM-CSF, granulocyte-macrophage colony-stimulating factor; ARA-C, cytosine arabinoside; IFNα, interferon α; MDS, myelodysplastic syndromes; CMML, chronic myelo-monocytic leukaemia; AML, acute myeloid leukaemia; BMT, bone marrow transplantation.

patients under the age of 50 (Appelbaum et al., 1987, 1990a; De Witte et al., 1988). These treatment strategies are summarized in Table 2.9.

Chronic myeloid leukaemia

Fialkow et al. (1977) proved that CML is a disease of stem cell origin by studying CML in G6PD heterozygotes. In this way they were able to show that the expression of G6PD by the clone (either isoenzyme A or B, depending upon the random inactivation of one or other X chromosomes) always occurred in the same manner in red cell leucocytes and platelets. This indicated that the whole of the haemopoietic marrow was derived from the same clone. The presence of the Philadelphia chromosome and the characterization of the BCR/ABL fusion gene have facilitated highly refined marker studies of the leukaemic clone in this disease, using the PCR to amplify the signal from tiny populations of residual leukaemic cells. With PCR residual disease can be detected following interferon α treatment when cytogenetic tests for the Ph^1 chromosome are negative. The PCR seems to be a reliable means of predicting relapse or cure following ablative treatment and BMT (Hughes et al., 1991).

The chronic phase can be controlled with hydroxyurea or busulphan. There is no firm evidence that any treatment prevents transformation to the acute phase. At all times during treatment of the chronic phase, the BCR/ABL gene rearrangement can be detected by Southern blotting, even when chromosome analysis is negative for the Ph^1

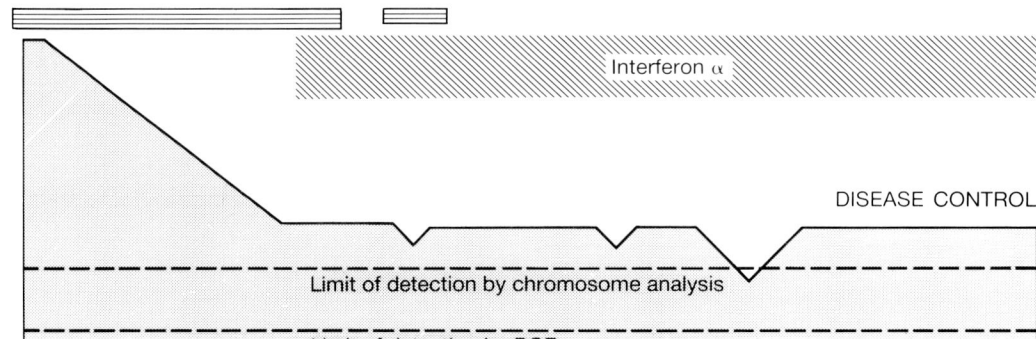

Fig. 2.8 Chronic myeloid leukaemia treatment strategies.

clone. An area of continued interest in CML treatment is the use of interferon α to regulate the proliferation of the Ph[1] clone. Chronic-phase CML is susceptible to regulation by haemopoietic growth factors and cytokines. However it is not clear that the suppression of the leukaemic clone by interferon α translates into a longer survival, or a delayed transformation to blast crisis. It is clear, however, that BMT can cure CML: long-term survivors, at least in some studies, are negative for BCR-ABL gene rearrangement using the highly sensitive PCR technique. In BMT for CML there is strong evidence for donor T cell-mediated immune regulation of residual disease. T cell depletion of donor marrow is associated with relapse (Apperley et al., 1986), and donor T lymphocyte transfusion can reverse post-transplant cytogenetic relapse to donor karyotype (Kolb et al., 1990). The impact of these various treatment approaches on the achievement of cure in CML is illustrated in Figure 2.8.

Non-leukaemic myeloproliferative disorders

The term myeloproliferative disorders (MPDs) is used here to describe the group of conditions essential thrombocythaemia (ET), primary polycythaemia (PP), and myelofibrosis (MF). There is reason to believe that these conditions are closely linked for the following reasons:
1 Patients with PP and ET may evolve into a myelofibrotic end-stage. Patients with PP often have a thrombocythaemia, and patients with ET may develop erythrocytosis. A relatively frequent pattern of evolution seen in some, but not all, patients is a presentation with ET progressing to PP and ultimately to MF.
2 Cultures of progenitor cells in MPD show several similarities. There are often higher than normal numbers of CFU-GM and CFU-E in the marrow and blood, and the proliferation of CFU-E is at least partially independent of erythropoietin in ET, PP and MF. Spontaneous production of megakaryocytes from blood in suspension culture is observed in PP, ET and MF (Adams et al., 1988).
3 A viral reverse transcriptase has been found in the platelets and megakaryocytes of patients with MPD, suggesting a common aetiology in these disorders (Boyd et al., 1989).

The MPDs are assumed to represent preleukaemic states because there is a low frequency of developing AML in MPD. Furthermore, the partial escape from control by the regulator erythropoietin and the excessive proliferation of granulopoiesis, thrombopoiesis and erythropoiesis suggests an intermediate condition between normal and leukaemic states. Unlike myeloid leukaemias however, there is no firm evidence that there is an increased risk of developing MPD after exposure to ionizing radiation. The recent finding of a retrovirus in MPD platelets reopens the possibility that the condition may represent a disordered myelopoietic state associated with the chronic infection of myeloid stem cells or their progeny by a retrovirus which modifies their proliferative behaviour. A possible mechanism is suggested by the effect of the Friend spleen focus-forming virus in mice. The virus gp55 glycoprotein binds to the erythropoietin receptor, inducing eythropoietin-independent proliferation and a form of erythroleukaemia (Li et al., 1990). However, it has to be said that the evidence for a viral aetiology of MPDs so far obtained in humans is far from conclusive. In this context it is of interest to note that NK cell activity, but not absolute numbers of circulating NK cells, is reduced in MPD (Jiang et al., 1990). Natural killer cells play a role in the regulation of normal haemopoiesis (Vinci et al., 1988), and may also regulate haemopoiesis in MPD. Defective immune surveillance could permit the emergence of abnormal MPD clones, perhaps under the influence of a transforming retrovirus. It is of course equally possible that the abnormal NK function is a consequence and not an initiator of the primary defect. There are thus several theoretical reasons to explore the antiviral potential of interferon α, and immunostimulators such as IL-2 in the MPDs.

For many years disease control has been reliably achieved in MPDs with venesection to reduce the red cell mass, and transfusion support as stem cell failure supervenes in the myelofibrotic phase. Treatment with hydroxyurea, busulphan or radioactive phosphorus controls proliferation. Hydroxyurea is preferred because it has a low potential for inducing secondary leukaemia. Recently interferon α has been shown to control excessive marrow proliferation in PP and ET (Silver, 1988; Gisslinger et al., 1990; Lazzarino et al., 1990). Remission in terms of a return to normal (non-clonal) haemopoiesis does not occur with any of these treatments. There is considerable interest in the use of interferon α to treat these disorders. Interferon α controls erythrocyte, neutrophil and platelet production in MPD but there is no evidence that the suppression induced by interferon α is associated with a remission state and return to normal haemopoiesis (Fig. 2.9). Acute

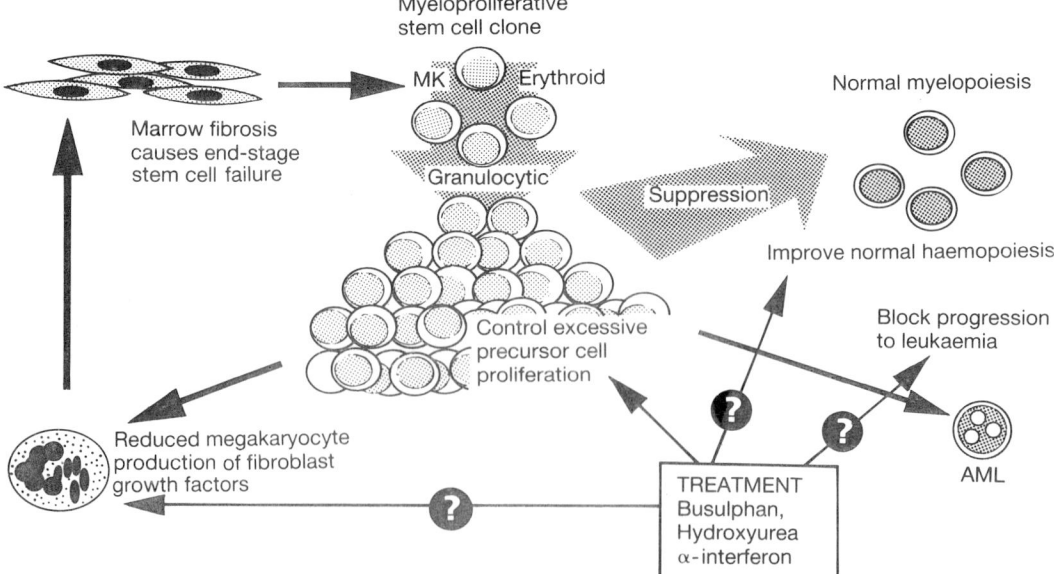

Fig. 2.9 Pathophysiology and its relation to treatment objectives in MPDs.

myelofibrosis has been successfully cured by BMT (Chapter 4), but because of the relatively benign course and elderly group of affected patients, BMT is not a therapeutic option for patients with chronic MPDs.

Chronic lymphatic leukaemia

The fact that this disease is typically benign throughout most of its course, and affects particularly the elderly, explains in part why conservative treatment strategies are employed. Chemotherapy with the alkylating agent chlorambucil is used to control the proliferation of the abnormal clone without achieving true bone marrow remission in the majority of cases. Treatment with long-term low-dose chlorambucil exerts a regulatory control on the proliferation of the malignant B cell clone without risk of causing major fluctuations in the normal blood cells. However the application of alkylating agents continually at low dose is more deleterious to bone marrow function than intermittent higher doses. Consequently chlorambucil is nowadays given in this way. Because this leukaemia is slowly progressive, occurs in older people, and is compatible with a good quality of life for many years, experimental approaches to improve disease control and achieve true cure are attempted only in the rare cases under the age of 50 or those patients with progressive disease developing cytopenia.

Progress in CLL treatment approaches is mainly due to several large national treatment studies (French Cooperative Group on CLL, 1988, 1990; Catovsky *et al.*, 1989), and to the introduction of new more specific drugs. These treatment developments are summarized below:

1 It is now clear that treatment of non-progressing stage 0 disease is not indicated and can be deleterious.

2 While chlorambucil alone or with prednisolone continues to be used as first-line treatment, patients who are resistant may benefit from more intensive treatment with the CHOP lymphoma regimen (McKelvey *et al.*, 1976; French Cooperative Group on CLL, 1990).

3 Two new drugs, 2'·deoxycorformycin and fludarabine (Catovsky and Foa, 1990; Keating *et al.*, 1991), appear to offer a much greater selectivity of action in CLL and early results suggest an improvement in disease control and achievement of remission in some patients.

4 Sensitive techniques to detect disease in remission nevertheless reveal residual leukaemia cells.

5 Bone marrow transplantation is curative in some patients but the advanced age of most patients with CLL precludes active treatment (Michallet *et al.*, 1991).

Hairy cell leukaemia (HCL)

The condition is characterized by a slowly proliferating B cell malignancy which causes profound myelosuppression, especially on granulopoiesis, through the production of inhibitors of granulocyte colony formation and to granulocyte (G-CSF) and granulocyte-macrophage colony-stimulating factor (GM-CSF). The cells are unusual in expressing large numbers of receptors for interferon α, which may relate to the potent *in vivo* suppression of the leukaemia seen with interferon α treatment.

For many years the treatment of HCL has been unsatisfactory. While splenectomy can debulk the disease and permit neutrophil recovery, not all patients respond and relapse is usual. Both low- and high-intensity treatments with single or multiple chemotherapeutic agents have proved disappointing. The demonstration by Quesada *et al.* (1984) that lymphocyte-derived interferon α could produce remission in HCL was a breakthrough in treatment. The ability of interferon α to produce remission in HCL appears to be related to its direct antiproliferative and maturation-inducing effect on the hairy cell which induces plasma cell transformation *in vitro* (see Chapter 6). Interferon α has to be continued indefinitely at a maintenance level to control the leukaemia but acquired resistance has never been described. A few patients are unresponsive to interferon α. They usually respond specifically to deoxycorformycin, an inhibitor of adenosine deaminase which is present in high levels in T cells and hairy cells (Dearden and Catovsky, 1990).

The standard treatment strategy in HCL consists of debulking by splenectomy, followed by interferon α, as disease control. Deoxycorformycin can be reserved for non-responders (Golomb *et al.*, 1989).

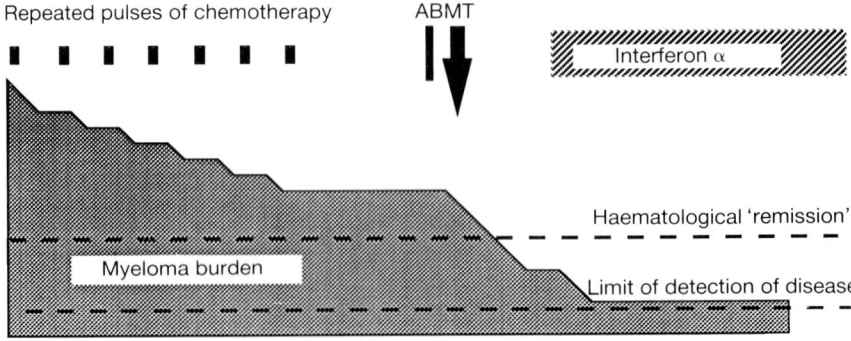

Fig. 2.10 Treatment strategy for myeloma using ABMT and interferon.

Multiple myeloma

Treatment strategies in this disease have changed considerably in the last few years (Fig. 2.10). The earlier assumption that the malignant plasma cell clone could not be eradicated has given way to the concept that the disease may be susceptible to regulation by interferon α and cured by BMT.

The alkylating agents melphalan and cyclophosphamide have been used for many years, either singly or in combination with different drugs. Typically, these schedules achieve control of the plasma cell clone for varying periods of time, as demonstrated by a plateau in the paraprotein level. The shortcoming of this approach is that disease progression with drug resistance inevitably occurs. In conjunction with the failure to control the malignant clone, there is a tendency to develop bone marrow failure due in part to the effect of long-term alkylating agents. Attempts have therefore continued to improve myeloma treatment using more intensive therapy (with high-dose melphalan; Gore et al., 1989) or more efficient drug scheduling with four-day infusions of adriamycin and vincristine and oral steroids (VAD regimen; Barlogie et al., 1987; Samson et al., 1989). With these treatments a remission state is frequently achieved, characterized by a return to normal blood count, reduction in the marrow plasma cells to less than 5%, and a much greater reduction in paraprotein levels than is usual with previous treatments. Nevertheless, the improved disease control has not stopped eventual relapse of the myeloma, which seems to recur at a median of 12 months. Attention has therefore been directed to strategies to maintain remission, either using autologous or allogeneic BMT (Gahrton et al., 1991; Chapter 4), or interferon α (Mandelli et al., 1988; see also Chapter 6). Many questions remain unanswered at present – autologous BMT inevitably involves the reintroduction of some malignant cells, but the importance of purging the marrow of myeloma cells prior to autologous reinfusion is not known. The mechanism of action of interferon α is not known. Greater understanding of the behaviour of myeloma cells in response to other cytokines may improve our ability to suppress the proliferation of the clone, for example by the use of antibodies to IL-6, which is a growth factor for myeloma cells (Kishimoto, 1989).

Non-Hodgkin's lymphoma (NHL)

Treatment strategies for NHL have undergone continuing evolution. An early confusion was the failure to appreciate that, although the lymphoma was confined to a single group of nodes, there was a high probability that it was already disseminated in the marrow. This explained the failure of local radiotherapy and surgery to prevent disease relapse, which distinguished the non-Hodgkin's lymphoma clearly from the more curable Hodgkin's disease. Staging of non-Hodgkin's lymphomas soon showed that the majority had disseminated disease (stage IV) at presentation. This led to the use of systemic chemotherapy. The most successful schedule has been the combination of cyclophosphamide, prednisolone, Adriamycin and vincristine (CHOP). This therapy regularly induces remissions or partial remissions in all but the poor-prognosis high-grade lymphomas (McKelvey et al., 1976).

The heterogeneity of NHL requires different treatment strategies for different disease types: low-grade lymphomas are less responsive to combination chemotherapy, and the same degree of disease control is achievable by single agents such as chlorambucil without the unwanted side-effect of marrow suppression. In these disorders the emphasis has been on improving response with interferon α given in conjunction with or following chemotherapy (Solal-Celigny et al., 1991). Little is known about the possible regulation of lymphoma by cytokines such as tumour necrosis factor (TNF) or LAK cells — this approach to treatment is being actively explored. In contrast, high-grade and intermediate-grade lymphomas are relatively easy to control initially with combination chemotherapy. Remission is usually achieved after three courses of CHOP. Nevertheless, drug resistance and relapse are frequent causes of treatment failure. There have been numerous modifications to the basic CHOP regimen in order to improve remission rates in less favourable disease, developed first as salvage treatments for relapsed lymphoma. There is little evidence however that the newer treatments using additional agents (ProMACE, CytaBOM etc.) achieve better results (Miller et al., 1988). Because of this, attention has been directed to eliminating residual disease either by high-dose chemotherapy and autologous or allogeneic marrow transplantation. The results of ABMT in NHL are very encouraging and are at least as favourable as the results of allografting (Armitage, 1989). Response can be largely predicted by the disease state at the time of the transplant: remission is more favourable than responding relapsed disease, which in turn has a more favourable outcome than resistant relapse. A treatment outline for NHL is shown in Figure 2.11.

Hodgkin's disease

The use of different treatment approaches according to the stage of dissemination of the lymphoma was central to the development of rational management of this largely curable disease. It was soon appreciated that Hodgkin's disease restricted to one group of nodes

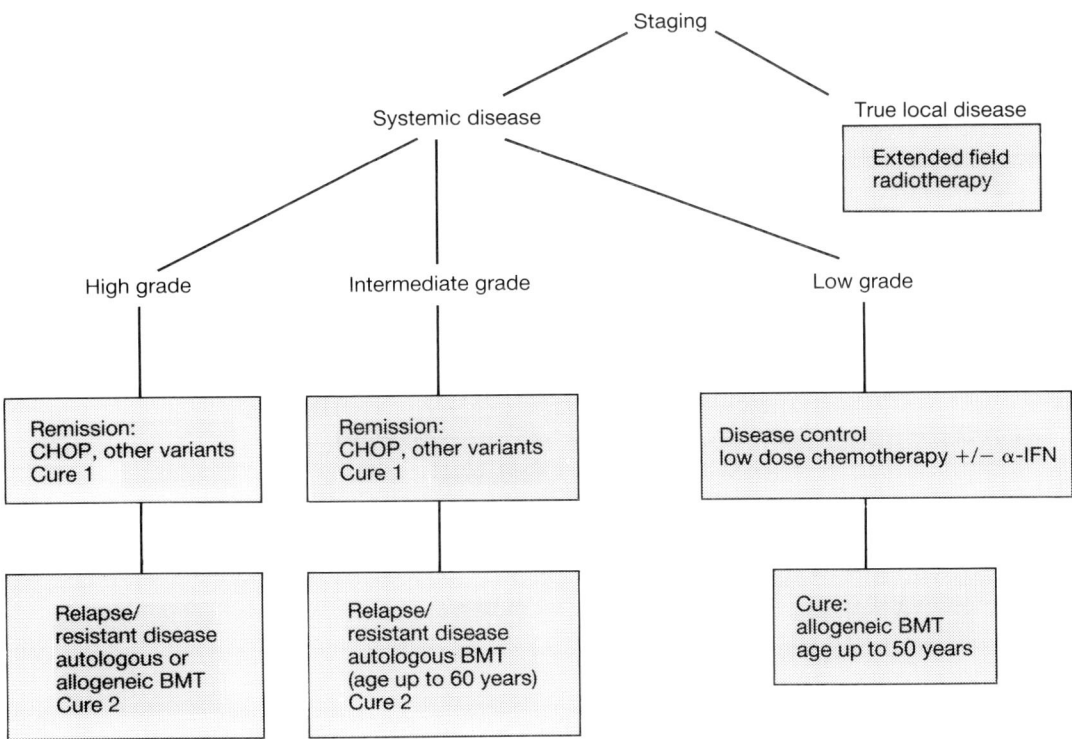

Fig. 2.11 Treatment strategies in non-Hodgkin's lymphoma.

could be eradicated by treatment of the affected group and the adjacent unaffected group. Staging the lymphoma became a central part of the management in the 1960–70s, with splenectomy being carried out at laparotomy. The availability of advanced imaging techniques has made staging much more straightforward today. The increasing reliance on chemotherapy rather than radiotherapy to treat all but stage I and II disease has largely obviated the need to distinguish between stage III (nodal) and stage IV (extranodal), and the treatment approach is now usually simplified to the use of radiotherapy for stage I and II only, and chemotherapy for stage III and IV, and also in some centres for stage II. Prognostic features of the histological appearance are helpful in predicting disease response and curability, but modern combination chemotherapy schedules now achieve spectacular disease-free survivals in the order of 90% for all but stage IV patients (Bonadonna and Valagussa, 1990). The place of BMT in Hodgkin's disease is therefore restricted to failed conventional treatment (Bezwoda and Dansey, 1989). It is debatable whether Hodgkin's disease relapsing after high-dose combination chemotherapy should be treated by ABMT or by salvage chemotherapy regimes. There is increasing use of ABMT

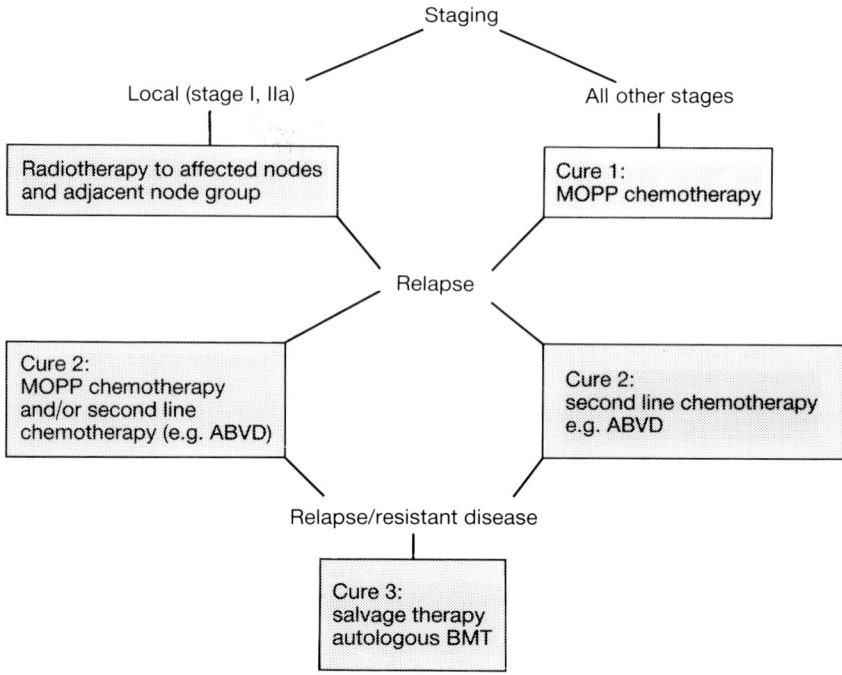

Fig. 2.12 Treatment strategies in Hodgkin's disease.

because of the promising results that can be achieved in all but the most resistant end-stage disease. The use of cytokines and interferons has not been explored in Hodgkin's disease. The treatment outline for Hodgkin's disease is shown in Figure 2.12.

CONGENITAL BONE MARROW DISORDERS

Introduction

Hereditary disorders of the bone marrow represent a large diverse group affecting either the stem cell or committed lineages, and consequently the numbers and function of the end cells they produce. Figure 2.13 shows the haemopoietic lineages and the hereditary disorders that affect them. Broadly they can be divided into conditions where the production of one or more cell lines has failed and those in which production is normal but cells are dysfunctional. The genetic basis of the disorder is well-characterized in some diseases such as the haemoglobinopathies, but is largely unknown in others such as Fanconi anaemia. Table 2.10 summarizes the aetiology of the more important congenital bone marrow disorders and the treatment approaches that have been used. Treatment involves support with

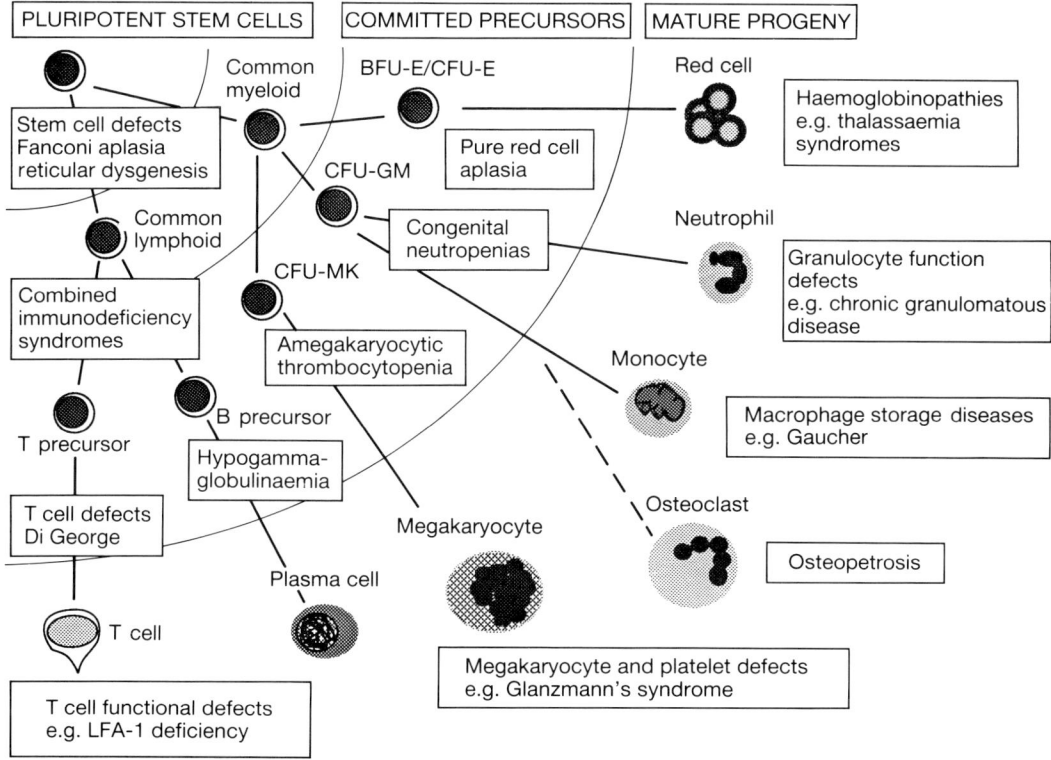

Fig. 2.13 Congenital bone marrow disorders and their relationship to normal haemopoietic development.

transfusion of red cells and platelets, prevention of infection in defects of immunity, and correction by BMT, or stimulation of cell production with growth factors or other agents. The availability of recombinant growth factors and cytokines has naturally led to investigation into their use for treating these rare and diverse disorders. Several important breakthroughs in treatment have resulted from the experimental use of growth factors and cytokines, but it is fair to say that their mode of action is not always well-understood.

Another development in the haemoglobinopathies is the use of chemotherapeutic agents such as hydroxyurea to modify the haemoglobin content of the red cell favourably. In the future there is hope that gene therapy could be used to correct haemopoietic stem cells by an autologous marrow transplant procedure where the patient's stem cells are transfected with a virus containing the missing or defective gene and retransplanted to generate corrected progeny permanently expressing the inserted gene. The place of marrow transplantation to correct these disorders, recent developments in the use of

Table 2.10 Congenital bone marrow disorders and their treatment

	Bone marrow transplantation	Other
Red cell disorders		
Severe thalassaemia syndromes	+++	Transfusion–iron chelation
Sickle cell anaemia	+	Exchange transfusion, hydroxyurea
Red cell aplasia	++	IL-3, transfusion–iron chelation
Granulocyte disorders		
Congenital neutropenia	++	Antibiotic prophylaxis, G-CSF
Chronic granulomatous disease	+	Antibiotic prophylaxis, IFNα
Chédiak–Higashi disease	+++	Antibiotic prophylaxis
Monocyte disorders		
Osteopetrosis	+++	Transfusion support? M-CSF
Gaucher's disease	+++	Liposomally packaged glucocerebrosidase
Megakaryocyte disorders		
Glanzmann's disease	+	
Lymphocyte disorders		
Severe combined immunodeficiency (SCID) syndromes	+++	Infection prophylaxis
SCID with ADA deficiency	+++	Retroviral ADA gene insertion
Wiskott–Aldrich syndrome	+++	Infection prophylaxis, platelet transfusion
Bruton-type agammaglobulinaemia	–	Regular intravenous immunoglobulin
Stem cell disorders		
Fanconi aplasia	+++	Transfusion support and infection
Reticular dysgenesis	+++	Prophylaxis

+++, Strong indication; ++, if other treatments fail; +, special cases only (e.g. severe disease); –, not indicated.
IL-3, Interleukin 3; G-CSF, granulocyte colony-stimulating factor; IFNα, interferon α; M-CSF, macrophage colony-stimulating factor; ADA, adenosine deaminase.

growth factors, cytokines, and chemotherapy, and the principles of gene therapy are discussed below.

Bone marrow transplantation

There is little debate that BMT is an effective form of correction of congenital marrow disorders whether they represent a failure of production of a particular stem cell-derived line or whether they represent a defective end cell. Bone marrow transplantation has been used extensively in these rare diseases to achieve permanent correction of the disorder or at least that component of it that is stem cell-derived (Barrett and McCarthy, 1990). Thus in Fanconi anaemia or adenosine deaminase (ADA) deficiency which affects all the cells in the body, BMT only corrects the myeloid and lymphocyte defect. From the extensive data now available from thalassaemia transplants, BMT from a fully human leukocyte antigen (HLA)-matched sibling donor into a recipient under the age of about 10 years has a procedural mortality of less than 10%. Nevertheless this mortality may still be unacceptable in disorders which are not immediately fatal but impair the quality of life, and the debate about whether to transplant or to support patients with permanent red cell production failure continues (Lucarelli *et al.*, 1990; Lucarelli and Weatherall, 1991). A further shortcoming of BMT is the lack of a suitable donor for the majority of patients. Because of this, other ways to correct and treat congenital disorders are of great importance. (See Chapter 4 for a full account of the mechanism of cure of congenital disorders by BMT.)

Cytokines, growth factors and other agents

Experimental trials with various cytokines and growth factors in congenital bone marrow disorders are beginning to reveal the therapeutic potential of these agents in a variety of rare conditions that were previously only correctable by BMT. Many of these less drastic treatments with biological response modifiers are less dangerous and therefore preferable to BMT. In general, however, lifelong treatment is necessary.

Interleukin 3 in pure red cell aplasia

This condition, first described by Diamond and Blackfan, presents as an aregenerative anaemia in the first year of life. The bone marrow shows a gross reduction in red cell progenitors but granulopoiesis and megakaryopoiesis are normal. The committed erythrocyte progenitors, BFU-E and CFU-E are correspondingly reduced or absent, but granulocyte-macrophage progenitors, CFU-GM are present in normal or increased numbers. The aetiology is not fully understood and may vary. The demonstration that cytotoxic lymphocytes or soluble factors suppress BFU-E *in vitro* has been used as evidence that there is immune dysregulation of erythropoiesis but data are conflicting (reviewed by Halpern and Freedman, 1989). Another possible mechanism is decreased sensitivity to erythropoietin (Nathan *et al.*, 1978).

It has been shown that IL-3 corrects the growth of a patient's BFU-E *in vitro*, and enhances erythropoietin sensitivity (Halpern *et al.*, 1989).

Treatment of pure red cell aplasia has relied in the past on the use of steroids which can produce a remission in about 30% of patients. More recently cyclosporin has been successfully used (Means *et al.*, 1991). Non-responders have been successfully transplanted with normal bone marrow (August *et al.*, 1976). The most promising approach is the use of erythropoietin, and more recently IL-3 (Halpern *et al.*, 1989). A rational treatment strategy in an individual patient can be planned by *in vitro* tests investigating the sensitivity of BFU-E to the growth factors IL-3 and erythropoietin, and determining whether patients' lymphocytes suppress BFU-E. In the latter case either steroid treatment or high-dose immunoglobulins may produce responses but they are often temporary (McGuire *et al.*, 1987). Interleukin 3 can however produce responses in all types of patient and may become the initial treatment approach in all patients (Dunbar *et al.*, 1991). Bone marrow transplantation should be reserved for occasional patients who do not respond to other treatments.

G-CSF in congenital neutropenia

The indications for BMT have also diminished in this disorder with the advent of molecularly engineered growth factors. Granulocyte colony-stimulating factor can induce normal granulocyte numbers, and greatly diminishes susceptibility to infection (Bonilla *et al.*, 1989). However, if BMT becomes safer, the advantage of curative therapy over long-term injections of growth factors will require reassessment.

Interferon γ in chronic granulomatous disease

There are both X-linked and rarer autosomal recessive forms of chronic granulomatous disease. Both forms affect components of the NADPH oxidase system, resulting in failure of oxidative microbicidal activity following phagocytosis. Diagnosis is made by the failure of neutrophils to reduce nitro-blue tetrazolium following stimulation of the intracellular oxidase system by phorbol myristate acetate. The autosomal recessive forms may have a tendency to be less severe clinically, but serious morbidity and mortality from bacterial and fungal infection can occur in all forms of chronic granulomatous disease. Successful HLA-matched sibling (Rappeport *et al.*, 1982) transplants have been performed.

In recent years, antimicrobial prophylaxis, principally with co-trimoxazole and itraconazole, has improved the outlook for these patients remarkably. The results of a multicentre trial suggest that recombinant interferon γ therapy further reduces susceptibility to infection. The mechanism of action of interferon γ is not fully understood (Sechler et al., 1988). There is no evidence that the cytokine improves superoxide production by the neutrophil, and the therapeutic response may be due to the activation of lymphocyte cell-mediated immune mechanisms, particularly against fungal organisms (International Chronic Granulomatous Disease Cooperative Study Group, 1991).

Androgens in Fanconi aplastic anaemia

It has been recognized for some years that patients with Fanconi aplasia are exquisitely sensitive to androgens: doses as low as 12 mg on alternate days can stimulate erythropoiesis, thrombopoiesis, and leukopoiesis in such patients, and puberty also has a beneficial effect on bone marrow function. Interestingly, androgens in low doses promote skeletal growth in Fanconi patients without causing premature fusion of the epiphyses. The effect of androgen treatment is sustained for a median of 4.5 years, after which time the effect diminishes and progressive marrow failure follows (Alter et al., 1983). The mechanism of action of androgens is unknown.

Increasing fetal haemoglobin production in sickle cell anaemia

In sickle cell anaemia treatment is mainly symptomatic and includes analgesia, hydration, prophylaxis and therapy of the infectious episodes and, following strokes, regular exchange transfusions or transfusion and iron chelation treatment. One experimental treatment approach has been to use cytotoxic drugs to increase the percentage of fetal haemoglobin, thus decreasing the tendency of sickle haemoglobin to polymerize within cells. 5-Azacytidine (De Simone et al., 1982; Ley et al., 1983) and hydroxyurea (Charache et al., 1987; Rodgers et al., 1990) can increase the red cell fetal haemoglobin content to 20% and have been used with some clinical success, but longer trials are needed to confirm the clinical benefits and establish long-term toxicities of treatment. Experiments aimed at decreasing the α/β chain imbalance by increasing the synthesis of γ chains are also under way in thalassaemia. Promising results have been reported (Ley et al., 1982), although it is not yet clear if significant clinical benefit will be obtained.

Gene therapy

The ability to introduce DNA into cells opens the possibility of correcting congenital genetic deficiencies by somatic gene therapy.

The ability to target inserted DNA to a particular site in the genome by homologous recombination also increases the specificity of the approach. A number of techniques have been used successfully to insert genes into cells. The technique most explored as a model for genetic disorder correction is to use retroviruses as the means of inserting DNA. Bone marrow disorders lend themselves to gene therapy because the pluripotent stem cell or a T lymphocyte targeted for gene insertion can establish long-term repopulation of the marrow and lymphoid system with somatically altered cells. The pluripotent stem cell frequency is in the order of 1/1000 cells in the marrow. Because of this gene therapy requires optimal methods to concentrate stem cells, and highly efficient gene transfection. Retroviral gene insertion appears to be the best approach for this at present (Lehn, 1990).

Retroviral structure (Fig. 2.14)

Retroviruses have three coding regions, gag pol and env, encoding the capsid, the reverse transcriptase and integrase, and the envelope protein respectively. There is a non-coding sequence (not built into the host genome) called the psi region which directs the packaging of the virus, and is essential for its infectivity. The whole region is bounded by a long-terminal repeat which contains promoter and enhancer elements to direct integration and replication of the genome.

The virus binds to receptors on the cell surface and enters the cell. The viral RNA is then converted by reverse transcriptase to double-stranded DNA which then integrates at multiple random sites in the host DNA. The genomic virus produces viral RNA and new viral proteins which can assemble to form new infective viral particles (Miller, 1990a).

Modification of retroviruses for gene transfer

In the construction of a virus for gene insertion the RNA coding for viral proteins gag, pol and env can be deleted and replaced by RNA coding for the required DNA sequence for insertion. Because they lack the genetic information to construct a complete virion, such viruses are not infectious and are therefore potentially safe constructs. However they cannot infect the target cell. To achieve this the viral plasmid is inserted into a packaging cell line which contains the incomplete genome of another defective virus from which the psi packaging sequence has been deleted. The DNA for insertion and its associated RNA containing the psi sequence joins with the structural proteins of the incomplete virus to form an infectious particle which is capable of

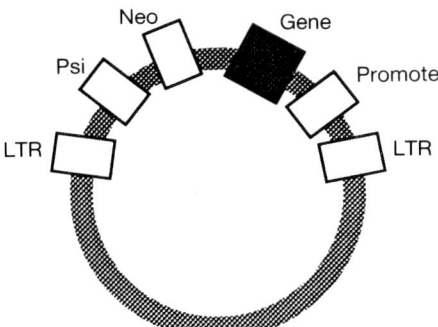

Fig. 2.14 Structure of retroviral gene construct. LTR, long terminal repeat; Psi, packaging gene sequence; Neo, neomycin resistance gene.

only a single infective event before incorporating its replication-defective genome into the target cell (Miller, 1990b).

Stem cell infection and genetic correction

The typical experimental procedure adopted by several groups has been to establish long-term marrow cultures from mice and coculture these cells with the retrovirus-producing line. Successfully transfected cells can be selected by incorporating into the viral construct the neo^r gene which confers resistance to the neomycin analogue G418. Culturing the marrow cells in the presence of G418 deletes all cells except the transfected ones which display neo^r resistance. Surviving cells are then transplanted back into an irradiated recipient mouse which is then studied for presence of the transfected DNA and its corresponding RNA and protein product.

The first successful retrovirus gene transfer was reported in 1983 by Joyner *et al.* who infected CFU-GM with the neo^r gene and conferred G418 resistance. Later Wiliams *et al.* (1984) transferred the gene into murine haemopoietic stem cells and demonstrated G418 resistance in the CFU-S of a transplanted animal. Since then, similar experiments have been carried out with the genes for hypoxanthine phosphoribosyl transferase, ADA and nucleoside phosphorylase. These genes have been widely used for gene insertion experiments because they represent permanently switched-on 'housekeeping' genes active in all cells. As a marker of gene expression, enzyme activity of the gene product can be assayed. These studies have shown that it is possible to insert genes into pluripotent haemopoietic progenitors which can be detected for several months. The problems are that the gene persists for only short periods, is present in typically less than 10% of the cells, and the gene product is not always expressed. The human β-globin gene has also been introduced into cultured animal cells, following retrovirus-mediated gene transfer, and has been

Table 2.11 Gene insertion techniques under evaluation in humans

Retroviral tagging of lymphocytes
1 Identification of homing of tumour-infiltrating lymphocytes (TILs) to tumour
2 Labelling residual leukaemic cells in autologous marrow inoculum to determine whether relapse occurs from inadequate purging of autologous marrow

Treatment
1 Correction of ADA deficiency by ADA gene insertion into circulating lymphocytes
2 Incorporation of TNF-α gene into TIL cells to enhance tumour cell killing

ADA, adenosine deaminase; TNF-α, tumour necrosis factor α.

successfully expressed in murine transplant recipients (Ledley, 1987). These reconstituted solely erythroid cells for long periods of time at significant levels (Dzierzak et al., 1988). The level of expression obtained is nevertheless much lower than that required for successful therapy. A recombinant β-globin gene has also been introduced into embryos of thalassaemic mice, creating a transgenic mouse (Constantini et al., 1986).

Gene insertion in humans

The first steps towards the use of gene insertion have now been made in humans (Table 2.11). Initial approaches have used T lymphocytes as the target cell for gene insertion. Lymphocyte populations have a high proportion of cells with the potential for clonal expansion and are readily obtainable from blood. Because of safety considerations, the first retrovirus insertions were carried out in patients with advanced malignant disease (Cornetta et al., 1991). Tumour-infiltrating lymphocytes were infected with an inert but identifiable gene marker. These tagged lymphocytes survived in the recipients and were found to home to the tumour site (Rosenberg et al., 1990). The insertion of the TNF-α gene into tumour-infiltrating lymphocytes in order to confer greater antitumour reactivity is the next logical step under investigation in the development of this technique (The TNF/TIL Human Gene Therapy Clinical Protocol, 1990).

A similar approach is being used to label genetically residual leukaemia cells in bone marrow taken for autologous retransfusion in the treatment of the leukaemia. It may be possible in this way to determine whether leukaemic relapse following autologous marrow transplantation is caused by retransfusion of (virus-tagged) leukaemia cells, or from residual cells in the recipient (Cornetta et al., 1991).

The first successful use of this approach in gene therapy of genetic disorders has been in the treatment of ADA deficiency. Once inserted, the gene confers a proliferative advantage to the lymphocyte. It is therefore not necessary to use other selection genes such as that for conferring methotrexate resistance to give the corrected cells a proliferative advantage. Three infants have received transfusions of lymphocytes corrected for ADA deficiency. They all showed a restoration of the lymphocyte count to normal, a return of normal cell-mediated immune function, and a dramatic clinical response (The ADA Human Gene Therapy Clinical Protocol, 1990).

Further progress in gene therapy

Before gene therapy can be applied successfully a number of developments in technique are required (Apperley and Williams, 1990). Only haemopoietic cells in cycle are susceptible to infection by the virus. Since most stem cells are in G_0 while less primitive cells are in cycle there is a tendency for viral infection to target non-immortalizing stem cells. Better characterization of the pluripotent stem cell, improved isolation techniques, and the use of stem cell growth factors such as IL-3, IL-1 and stem cell growth factor may improve the efficiency of stem cell infection (Nienhuis *et al.*, 1991). The studies so far have shown up surprising differences in the marrow-repopulating abilities of stem cells. Some feline stem cells appear to operate by exclusively populating the marrow for periods of about 6 weeks (clonal succession), while others have a more prolonged but less complete capacity to dominate the marrow cellularity (Abkowitz *et al.*, 1988). This means that unless a large cohort of stem cells are infected with virus the genetic correction is likely to be patchy and incomplete. However efficient the process of stem cell infection becomes it will still be necessary to give the transfected cells a growth advantage in the recipient. This can be done by high-dose chemotherapy or radiation, or by building methotrexate resistance into the inserted gene package. While methotrexate resistance can be successfully conferred it has not permitted selection of transfected cells in mice *in vivo* (Lehn, 1990). This may be because so many stem cells are out of cycle that they escape the methotrexate effect.

Another more difficult problem is the observation that while a satisfactory DNA insertion is relatively easily achieved, there is no guaranteed expression of the gene product. This may be due to the possibility that retroviral insertion is not as random as it was originally considered to be. Retrovirus insertion may target to silent areas of the genome where its genes are not transcribed. Furthermore, genes may become inactivated during the process of differentiation and maturation. One way to circumvent the problem of failure of gene expression would be to insert a much larger gene segment, including its intron

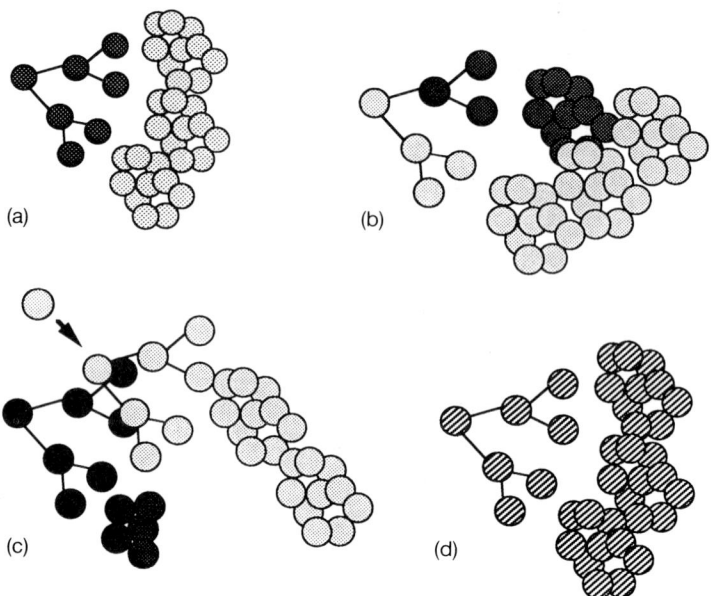

Fig. 2.15 Reasons for failure of inserted gene expression *in vivo*. (a) Failure of gene expression in mature progeny. Solution: insert complete gene mechanism with promoters and regulators. (b) Failure to correct pluripotent stem cell – reversion to untransfected cells. Solution: selection and amplification of stem cells *in vitro* prior to transfection. (c) Clonal succession replaces transfected stem cell. Solution: eliminate unmanipulated stem cells *in vivo*, increase transfection rate *in vitro*. (d) DNA inserted but not transcribed – no protein product. Solution: include promoter sequences.

sequences and promoters. This requires inserting larger segments of DNA than can be accommodated in a retrovirus. DNA viruses of the herpes group are bigger than retroviruses and would be useful candidates for transfer of complete 'protein factories' into the cell. Such techniques are of particular importance in developing successful models for globin gene insertion (Grosveld *et al.*, 1987). Before gene insertion can be used to correct genetic disorders in humans it will be necessary to understand the normal regulation of the particular gene in the cell, as well as to define *in vitro* the appropriate stem cell target and its function after retransplantation. Figure 2.15 illustrates some of the reasons for failure of inserted gene expression in the recipient.

APLASTIC ANAEMIA AND DRUG-INDUCED CYTOPENIAS

Pathophysiology of aplastic anaemia

Bone marrow failure occurs both as congenital and acquired aplastic anaemia, as a transient marrow suppression often caused by cytotoxic

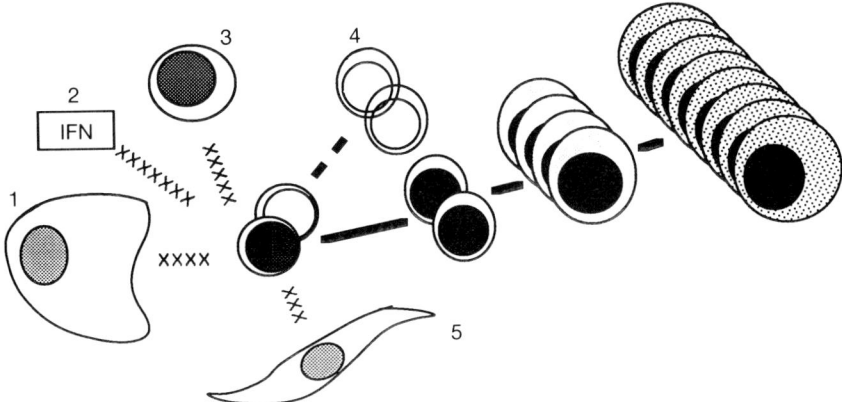

Fig. 2.16 Aetiology of aplastic anaemia: (1) stem cell suppression by abnormal macrophages and their cytokines; (2) interferon-γ production by lymphocytes; (3) lymphocyte mediated stem cell suppression; (4) defective stem cell function associated with myelodysplasia; (5) defective haemopoietic microenvironment.

drugs, or as an idiosyncratic response to a therapeutic agent. Aplastic anaemia involves the inability of the stem cell pool to produce adequate numbers of red cells, granulocytes and platelets (Gibson and Gordon-Smith, 1990; Marsh et al., 1990 review by Young, 1991). The primary aetiology might be related to the exposure to certain drugs, chemicals or viruses and the prolongation of marrow depression produced by such agents could be the consequence of abnormal response to this injury. Several components of the disorder have been identified (Fig. 2.16).

Immune-mediated myelosuppression

The most impressive evidence that immune mechanisms have some relevance in the aetiology of the stem cell failure is the observation that significant haematological recovery occurs in 50–75% of patients given antilymphocyte globulin with or without cyclosporin. Experimental data are conflicting, however, and difficult to interpret. Antibodies have occasionally been identified in the serum of patients with aplastic anaemia but their direct relevance to the stem cell failure is not established (Gordon, 1978; Barrett et al., 1979; Freedman et al., 1979). Direct cytotoxic cell-mediated suppression of progenitor cells has been described (Ascensao et al., 1976; Kagan et al., 1976; Singer et al., 1979; Nissen et al., 1980; Bacigalupo et al., 1981). Monocytes and lymphocytes from patients with aplastic anaemia have been shown to produce interferon γ and other cytokines suppressing progenitor cell proliferation (Gascon et al., 1985; Zoumbos et al., 1985; Torok-Storb et al., 1987; Gascon and Scala, 1988; Nakao et al., 1989).

The relationship of these abnormalities to the aetiology of the stem cell failure is not clear. They may represent a secondary response to the initial insult causing the aplasia.

Microenvironment and defects of growth factors

Abnormal interactions between stem cells and the environment in which they develop may play a part in the pathogenesis (Young, 1991; Knospe and Crosby, 1971) but there is little direct support for the idea that the bone marrow microenvironment is directly responsible for aplastic anaemia. Nevertheless, a microenvironmental defect has been invoked to explain the reproducible phenomenon that BMT between identical twins fails in about 30% of cases unless cyclophosphamide is given prior to marrow infusion (Champlin *et al.*, 1984). There is likewise little evidence to support the idea that aplastic anaemia is caused by a deficiency of growth factors. The serum of aplastic anaemia patients contains increased amounts of a number of haemopoietic growth factors including GM-CSF, IL-3 and erythropoietin, and aplastic serum is highly stimulatory to marrow growth in long-term cultures, causing an increase in the generation of CFU-GM and megakaryocytes (Nissen *et al.*, 1979; Adams and Barrett, 1983).

Stem cell defect

Aplastic anaemia can be induced in mice by administration of busulphan. In this model it is suggested that once reduction of the stem cell pool passes a critical limit, the remaining cells are incapable of restoring the pool to a functioning size (Boggs and Boggs, 1976). Residual stem cells are directed towards maturation and not to self-replication. As a result the stem cell pool never regains its functioning size. It is possible that busulphan in fact damages the stem cell DNA, rendering it incapable of a normal proliferative response.

The question therefore arises whether the stem cells in patients with aplastic anaemia are abnormally susceptible to certain marrow-suppressive agents. There is accumulating evidence that aplastic anaemia overlaps with myelodysplastic syndromes: the observation that the clonal PNH abnormality and myelodysplasia or frank myeloid leukaemia develop in long-term aplasia survivors treated with anti-lymphocyte globulin suggests the severe aplastic anaemia (SAA) may represent a form of stem cell myelodysplasia (Raghavachar *et al.*, 1991). A unifying hypothesis to explain these observations is that haematological responses to immunosuppressive treatments occur because immune control of abnormal stem cells is removed, permit-

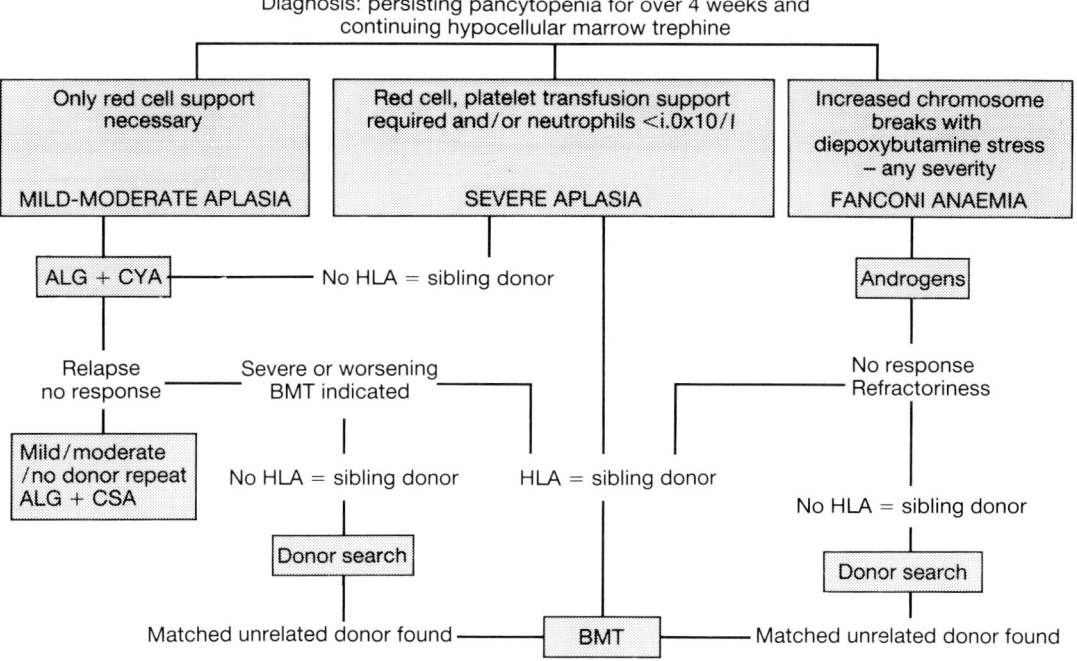

Fig. 2.17 Treatment approaches in aplastic anaemia.

ting proliferation and increasing blood cell production, but allowing further clonal evolution towards leukaemia.

Treatment

Patients die as a consequence of the pancytopenia, usually from bleeding or infection, reflecting a failure of long-term support measures for these patients. Rarely patients show spontaneous recovery but most with severe disease will die unless some degree of marrow function is restored. There are three treatment approaches currently in use: immunosuppression, BMT and growth factors. A typical treatment strategy is illustrated in Figure 2.17.

Immunosuppressive agents

Antilymphocyte globulin (Mathé et al., 1970; Speck et al., 1977; Gluckman et al., 1978; Champlin et al., 1983) and cyclosporin (Stryckmans et al., 1984) are effective. The optimum treatment appears to be the combination of antilymphocyte globulin and cyclosporin which produces up to 75% responses (Frickhofen et al., 1991; Gluckman et al., 1991). Recovery is unpredictable, but in general the more severe the marrow depression, as indicated by the peripheral blood count and the degree of hypocellularity of the marrow, the less likely is recovery (Marsh *et al.*, 1987). Even when recovery is apparently complete, the marrow remains abnormal and relapse or the development of clonal disorders in the form of PNH, myelodysplastic syndromes or acute non-lymphoblastic leukaemia may occur in as many as 25% of survivors if they are followed over a 5–10-year period (Tichelli *et al.*, 1988; de Planque *et al.*, 1988). Further evidence to support a preleukaemic aetiology of SAA is the observation in G6PD heterozygotes that the remission marrow represented a single clone (reviewed by Marsh and Geary, 1991).

The mechanism whereby immunosuppression induces haematological responses is not known. Antilymphocyte globulin treatment causes lymphopenia, reduces serum factors inhibitory to CFU-GM (Faille *et al.*, 1979), and reduces lymphocytotoxicity to CFU-GM (Young *et al.*, 1989), and interferon γ production (Young, 1991). It also has a direct stimulatory action on haemopoietic precursors (Hunter *et al.*, 1985), and repairs NK functional defects in SAA patients (Myint *et al.*, 1990). These changes may be important in improving proliferation of residual stem cells. Figure 2.18 illustrates the possible mode of action of antilymphocyte globulin.

Bone marrow transplantation

An alternative approach to the treatment of aplastic anaemia is the reintroduction of normal haemopoietic stem cells by the infusion of normal bone marrow. Bone marrow transplantation was first successfully used to correct SAA using marrow from an identical twin (Pillow *et al.*, 1966). This proved to be an isolated success and further attempts to correct SAA by marrow transplantation awaited the development of successful marrow allografts in the 1970s (Thomas *et al.*, 1972). Bone marrow transplantation from an HLA-matched sibling has a success rate in the order of 60–70% in SAA. It is the treatment of choice for patients with extremely severe aplasia who are at risk of early death from infection, and who do not respond well to immunosuppressive treatment. In other situations it may be appropriate to attempt correction of the pancytopenia with immunosuppressive therapy, and reserve BMT for non-responders or patients relapsing from treatment. While immunosuppressive treatment is the safer option in the short term, the high rate of eventual transformation to myelodysplastic syndromes makes it necessary to consider BMT for dysplasia evolving from SAA. Conditioning with cyclophosphamide alone appears to be sufficient to eradicate the PNH abnormality (Szer *et al.*, 1984). However patients with an acquired cytogenetic abnormality require whole-

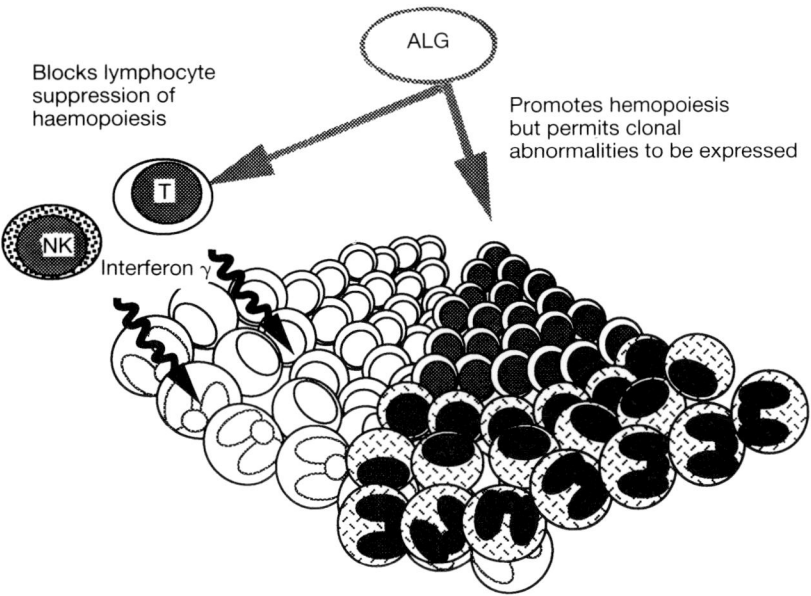

Fig. 2.18 Possible modes of action of antilymphocyte globulin.

body irradiation in addition to cyclophosphamide to prevent relapse into acute leukaemia following BMT (Appelbaum *et al.*, 1990b).

Growth factors

The introduction of GM-CSF, G-CSF, and IL-3 into clinical practice has stimulated several trials of these growth factors in SAA. The reader is referred to Chapter 5 for a detailed review. Overall the results of growth factor treatment in aplastic anaemia have been predictable: modest responses in granulocyte counts have been achieved. They are short-lived but may be useful in tiding over the patient whose major problem of marrow failure is in neutrophil production before the definitive procedure of marrow transplantation is carried out. Predictably, only those patients with some mimimal bone marrow function show any useful benefit from treatment with growth factors. There is however some suggestion that IL-3 may increase both the neutrophil count and the platelet count, and several IL-3 trials are under way in SAA.

Drug-induced cytopenias

Because the bone marrow contains a population of rapidly proliferating cells it is susceptible to the effects of agents which interfere with cell division. Drugs affecting marrow proliferation can be divided into

Table 2.12 Cytopenias caused by cytotoxic drugs and as idiosyncratic responses to drugs

	Cytotoxic drugs	Idiosyncratic responses
Drugs affecting cycling cells only Type: Cytopenia affecting one or all cell lines Onset: 7–10 days after exposure (immediate after second exposure for autoimmune type) Duration: 7–14 days	Methotrexate Hydroxyurea Mercaptopurine Cytosine arabinoside Etoposide	Thiazides, digoxin, quinidine, (thrombocytopenia) Amidopyrine (autoimmune neutropenia) Thiouracil, carbimazole, mianserin, phenothiazides (neutropenia) Chloramphenicol (red cell aplasia)
Drugs affecting non-cycling cells Type: Pancytopenia Onset: Up to 6 weeks after exposure Duration: Slow or incomplete recovery lasting months	Alkylating agents Busulphan Chlorambucil Melphalan Nitrosoureas BCNU CCNU	Gold salts Phenylbutazone Chloramphenicol Carbimazole Others

two categories: those with predictable dose and schedule cytotoxic action which are mostly anticancer agents, and those which cause unpredictable myelosuppression, whose main therapeutic action is not on the marrow. Although there is great diversity in the mode of action of drugs acting on the bone marrow their overall effect on haemopoiesis can be divided into two distinct modes of action – agents which affect proliferating cells, and agents affecting both proliferating and non-proliferating cells. This mode of action determines the duration and type of myelosuppression produced. This is because drugs which affect cells in cycle spare the pluripotent stem cell compartment, the majority of which are not undergoing cell division. These resting stem cells subsequently proliferate and cause prompt haematological recovery. In contrast, drugs that damage resting stem cells exert a profound and longer-lasting myelosuppression and can cause aplastic anaemia (Treleaven and Barrett, 1990). Table 2.12 gives examples of cytotoxic and idiosyncratic drugs and the type of marrow suppression produced.

Use of cytotoxic drugs in cancer treatment

Antiproliferative agents such as methotrexate can be used repeatedly without risk of causing marrow aplasia. However, it should be appreciated that even drugs in this category can cause prolonged aplasia if the treatment schedule is prolonged. In this situation earlier progenitors are brought into cycle by the depletion of the more mature proliferating cell compartment, and ultimately resting stem cells are recruited into cycle and become susceptible to the effect of the cycle-active agent. Thus even small doses of methotrexate given daily for more than 14 days can cause prolonged aplasia. Conversely, very high doses of methotrexate can be used with a modest period of cytopenia provided the cytotoxic effect is restricted to about 24 hours by the use of folinic acid rescue to antagonize its action. Drugs such as the alkylating agent busulphan, which affects resting stem cells, have a dose-dependent rather than schedule-dependent action on marrow function. In the treatment of CML busulphan has been traditionally used in small doses of about 2 mg daily for many weeks. Similar control of the leukaemia can be readily achieved with intermittent high doses of 100 mg given at about 6-week intervals. In fact, the intermittent high-dose schedule appears to be safer. This is because the appearance of marrow aplasia is delayed by about 6 weeks from the onset of stem cell failure provoked by cumulative stem cell suppression from an ill-defined critical busulphan dose. There is less risk

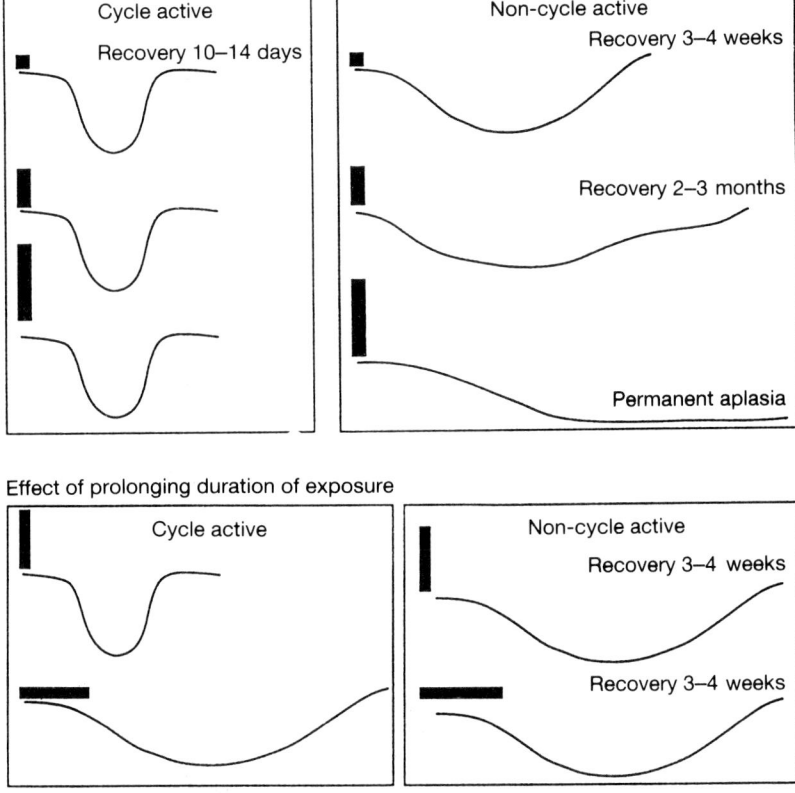

Fig. 2.19 Effect of cytotoxic drug dose and schedule on haemopoietic recovery.

of cumulative stem cell damage occurring with intermittent treatment. Very high doses of busulphan in the region of 15 mg/kg can cause permanent marrow aplasia. Such doses of busulphan are used in marrow transplant preparative regimens followed by marrow rescue. The impact of dose and schedule of cycle active and non-cycle active agents is illustrated in Fig. 2.19.

The type of action a cytotoxic drug has on the normal marrow determines the way in which the chemotherapy schedule is designed, as detailed in Table 2.12.

Idiosyncratic marrow suppression

There is a wide spectrum of drugs which occasionally have a catastrophic and unpredicted action on haemopoiesis. The characteristics of these idiosyncratic reactions can be summarized as follows (Williams *et al.*, 1973; De Gruchy, 1975):

1 The reactions are rare, affecting less than 1/10 000 of the population exposed.
2 The reactions have counterparts in the pattern of bone marrow damage with the effects of cytotoxic drugs.
3 Individual drugs may cause different cytopenias. For example, the antidepressant mianserin usually causes an idiosyncratic agranulocytosis, but less frequently can cause aplastic anaemia.

Table 2.13 Possible mechanisms involved in cytopenias from idiosyncrasy to drugs

Abnormality	Mechanism
Genetic predisposition for autoimmunity linked to human leukocyte antigen type?	Shared antigens on drug and cell surface leading to autoantibody generation, e.g. amidopyrine-induced neutropenia – commoner in northern Europeans
Unusual pharmacokinetics	1 Slow inactivation of a potentially myelotoxic agent 2 Delayed excretion – prolonged blood levels 3 Unusual degradation pathway generates myelotoxic intermediate metabolite
Stem cell defect	1 Subclinical DNA repair abnormality, e.g. Fanconi anaemia heterozygotes 2 Subclinical stem cell damage caused by same environmental factors responsible for aplastic anaemia 3 Reduced stem cell population and proliferative capacity associated with ageing 4 Defective multiple drug resistance gene allowing abnormal accumulation of toxic levels of drug or metabolite in the stem cell

4 Related drugs tend to cause similar cytopenias. For example, all thiazide diuretics may cause thrombocytopenia.
5 Rechallenge of a patient suspected of having an idiosyncratic drug reaction results in a further episode of cytopenia.
6 Individuals who have an idiosyncrasy to one type of drug have a higher risk of developing idiosyncrasy to another agent.

There is no way to identify susceptible individuals and the basis of the idiosyncratic response is largely speculative.

Two distinct idiosyncratic responses can be identified: autoimmune (e.g. agranulocytosis induced by amidopyrine) and non-immune (most reactions, e.g. aplastic anaemia induced by phenothiazides). The low frequency of both types of reaction strongly suggests either a multi-factorial origin requiring the rare association of a number of hereditary and environmental factors, or the presence of an extremely rare,

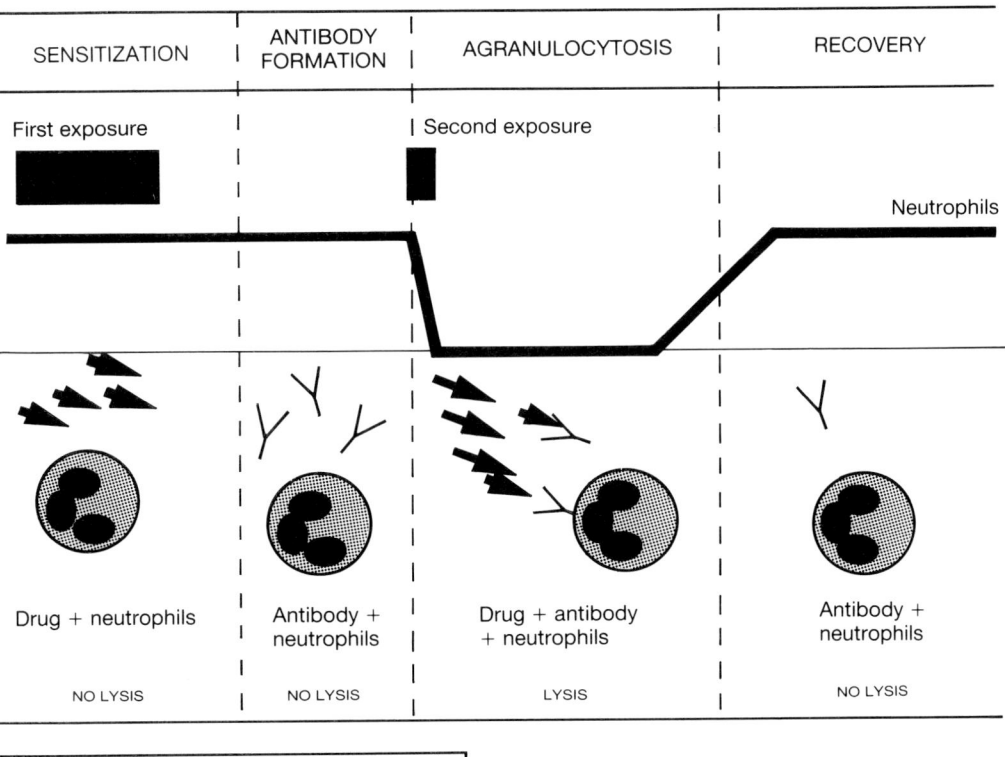

Fig. 2.20 Mechanism of immune cytopenia (amidopyrine mediated agranulocytosis).

possibly recessively inherited, gene defect. Table 2.13 lists several possible genetic bases for drug idiosyncrasy, but there is very little evidence to corroborate any of them.

The mechanisms of immune marrow suppression are illustrated in Fig. 2.20. In amidopyrine agranulocytosis the drug induces antibody formation which causes cell damage only on subsequent re-exposure to amidopyrine. This suggests that the antibody acts as a hapten binding to amidopyrine and adhering to the surface of neutrophils and their precursors (Barrett et al., 1976). Splenic sequestration of antibody-coated cells leads to the elimination of the late stages of granulopoiesis. Profound neutropenia follows, and is only reversed by recovery of earlier progenitors, which takes about 7–10 days.

Several mechanisms may cause non-immune marrow suppression. Firstly, drug metabolism may be aberrant in the type of metabolites produced, the level accumulating in the marrow, or the speed with which the agent is eliminated. Secondly, the stem cell compartment may be atypically susceptible to the effects of normally metabolized drugs with normal pharmacokinetics. For example, it is conceivable that DNA repair defects, such as occur in Fanconi anaemia, might render the haemopoietic system unusually susceptible to the action of otherwise harmless drugs. There is a suggestion that elderly patients are more likely to develop drug-induced marrow suppression. This could be caused by a greater susceptibility of ageing stem cells to cytotoxic damage (Mauch et al., 1982).

Management of drug-induced idiosyncratic cytopenias

Because of their rarity and unpredictability the prevention of these reactions is impossible. Regular blood count monitoring is expensive and impracticable. It is also likely to be unhelpful because at the time a fall in the blood count is registered the effect on the progenitor compartment may already be irreversible. Nevertheless, it would be prudent to check the blood count before starting treatment with particular classes of drugs such as the antidepressants, and to check it within 6 weeks of starting therapy. Patients who have not responded adversely by this time are not likely to do so thereafter.

If a cytopenia occurs the diagnosis of marrow suppression should be made by marrow aspirate. The suspected drugs should be stopped and appropriate supportive care with transfusions of red cells and platelets, and antibiotic cover instituted. Both G-CSF and GM-CSF can be used to shorten the period of cytopenia in reversible marrow suppression. Patients developing aplastic anaemia require treatment along the standard lines detailed above.

REFERENCES

Abkowitz JL, Ott RM, Holly RD et al. (1988) Clonal evolution following chemotherapy induced stem cell depletion in cats heterozygous for glucose-6 phosphate dehydrogenase. *Blood* 71, 1687.

Adams JA, Barrett AJ (1983) Haematopoietic stimulators in the serum of patients with severe aplastic anaemia. *British Journal of Haematology* 53, 161.

Adams JA, Barrett AJ, Beard J et al. (1988) Primary polycythaemia, essential thrombocythaemia and myelofibrosis – three facets of a single disease process? *Acta Haematologica* 79, 33.

Adams JA, Gordon AA, Jiang YZ et al. (1990) Thrombocytopenia after bone marrow transplantation for leukaemia: changes in megakaryocyte growth and growth-promoting activity. *British Journal of Haematology* 75, 195.

Adamson JW, Fialkow PJ, Murphy S et al. (1976) Polycythemia vera: stem-cell and probably clonal origin of the disease. *New England Journal of Medicine* 295, 913.

Alter BP, Rappeport JM, Parkman R (1983) The bone marrow failure syndromes. In: Nathan DG, Oski FA (eds) *Haematology of Infancy and Childhood* 2nd edn. WB Saunders, Philadelphia, pp. 168–249.

Antin JH, Smith BR, Holmes W et al. (1988) Phase I/II study of recombinant granulocyte-macrophage colony stimulating factor in aplastic anaemia and myelodysplastic syndrome. *Blood* 72, 705.

Appelbaum FR, Storb R, Ramberg RE et al. (1987) Treatment of preleukaemic syndromes with marrow transplantation. *Blood* 69, 92.

Appelbaum FR, Barrall J, Storb R et al. (1990a) Bone marrow transplantation for patients with myelodysplasia. *Annals of Internal Medicine* 112, 590.

Appelbaum FR, Barrall J, Storb R et al. (1990b) Clonal cytogenetic abnormalities in patients with otherwise typical aplastic anaemia. *Experimental Hematology* 15, 1134.

Apperley JF, Williams DA (1990) Gene therapy: current status and future directions. *British Journal of Haematology* 75, 148.

Apperley JF, Jones L, Hale G et al. (1986) Bone marrow transplantation for patients with chronic myeloid leukaemia: T-cell depletion with Campath 1 reduces incidence of graft-versus-host disease but may increase risk of leukaemic relapse. *Bone Marrow Transplantation* 1, 53.

Arends-Merino A, Sjogren AM, Reizenstein P (1983) Modifying the biological response to acute myeloid leukemia. I: BCG, allogeneic leukemic cells and spontaneous cytotoxicity. *Anticancer Research* 3, 239.

Armitage JO (1989) Bone marrow transplantation in the treatment of patients with lymphoma. *Blood* 73, 1749.

Arthur CK, Apperley JF, Guo AP et al. (1988) Cytogenetic events after bone marrow transplantation for chronic myeloid leukaemia in chronic phase. *Blood* 71, 1179.

Ascensao J, Kagan W, Moore M et al. (1976) Aplastic anaemia: evidence for an immunological mechanism. *Lancet* 1, 669.

August CS, King E, Githens JH et al. (1976) Establishment of erythropoiesis following bone marrow transplantation in a patient with congenital hypoplastic anaemia (Diamond Blackfan syndrome). *Blood* 48, 491.

Bacigalupo A, Podesta M, van Lint MT et al. (1981) Severe aplastic anaemia: correlation of in vitro tests with clinical response to immunosuppression in 20 patients. *British Journal of Haematology* 47, 423.

Barlogie B, Alexanian R, Dicke KA et al. (1987) High-dose chemoradiotherapy and autologous transplantation for resistant multiple myeloma. *Blood* 70, 869.

Barrett AJ, McCarthy DM (1990) Bone marrow transplantation for genetic disorders. *Blood Reviews* 4, 116.

Barrett AJ, Weller E, Rozengurt N et al. (1976) Amidopyrine agranulocytosis: drug inhibition of granulocyte colonies in the presence of patient's serum. *British Medical Journal* 2, 850.

Barrett AJ, Faille A, Saal F et al. (1979) Marrow graft rejections and CFU-C inhibition by serum in aplastic anaemia. *Journal of Clinical Pathology* 31, 1244.

Barrett AJ, Treleaven JG, Samson DM et al. (1990) Rapid remission induction and improved disease-free survival in acute myeloid leukaemia using daunorubicin, Ara-C and CCNU. *Leukaemia and Lymphoma* 3, 139.

Barrett AJ, Horowitz MM, Ash RC et al. (1992) Bone marrow transplantation for Philadelphia chromosome positive acute lymphoblastic leukaemia. *Blood* 79, 3067.

Bessho M, Jinnai I, Matsuda A et al. (1990) Improvement of anaemia by recombinant erythropoietin in patients with myelodysplastic syndromes. *International Journal of Cell Cloning* 8, 445.

Bezwoda WR, Dansey R (1989) High dose chemotherapy with bone marrow rescue for treatment of relapsed and refractory Hodgkin's disease. *Leukaemia and Lymphoma* 1, 71.

Bishop JF, Lowenthal RM, Jochua D et al. (1990) Etoposide in acute nonlymphoblastic leukemia. *Blood* 75, 27.

Blaise D, Viens P, Olive D et al. (1991) Recombinant interleukin-2 (rIL-2) after autologous bone marrrow transplantation: a pilot study in 19 patients. *European Cytokine Network* 2, 121.

Boggs DR, Boggs SS (1976) The pathogenesis of aplastic anaemia: a defective pluripotent haematopoietic stem cell with an inappropriate balance of differentiation and self-replication. *Blood* 48, 71.

Bolwell BJ, Cassileth PA, Gale RP (1987) Low dose cytosine arabinoside in myelodysplasia and acute myelogenous leukaemia: a review. *Leukemia* 1, 575.

Bonadonna G, Valagussa P (1990) Influence of clinical trials on current treatment strategy for Hodgkin's disease. *International Journal of Radiation Oncology Biology and Physics* 19, 209.

Bonilla MA, Gillio AP, Ruggiero M et al. (1989) Effects

of recombinant human granulocyte colony stimulating factor on neutropenia in patients with congenital agranulocytosis. *New England Journal of Medicine* 320, 1574.

Boughton BJ, O'Brien D, Simpson A (1991) Autologous IL-2/LAK cell therapy for AML in second complete remission. *Haematologica* 76 (suppl 4), 55.

Boyd MT, MacLean N, Oscier DG (1989) Detection of retrovirus in patients with myeloproliferative disease. *Lancet* 1, 814.

Browman G, Preisler H, Raza A et al. (1989) Use of the day 6 bone marrow to alter remission induction therapy in patients with acute myeloid leukaemia: a leukaemia intergroup study. *British Journal of Haematology* 71, 493.

Buchner T, Hiddemann W, Koenigsman M et al. (1990) Recombinant human granulocyte colony stimulating factor after therapy for acute leukaemias at higher age or after relapse. *Haematology and Blood Transfusion* 33, 724.

Campana D, Coustain-Smith E, Behm FG (1991) The definition of remission in acute leukaemia with immunological techniques. *Bone Marrow Transplantation* 8, 429.

Castaigne S, Chomienne C, Daniel MT et al. (1990) All trans retinoic acid as a differentiation agent in the treatment of acute promyelocytic leukaemia. *Blood* 76, 1704.

Catovsky D, Foa R (1990) Immunological markers. In: *The Lymphoid Leukaemias*. Butterworth, London, p. 1.

Catovsky D, Fooks J, Richards S (1989) Prognostic factors in chronic lymphocytic leukaemia: the importance of age, sex and response to treatment on survival. *British Journal of Haematology* 72, 141.

Champlin R, Ho W, Gale RP (1983) Antilymphocyte globulin treatment in patients with aplastic anaemia. *New England Journal of Medicine* 308, 113.

Champlin RE, Feig SA, Sparkles RS et al. (1984) Bone marrow transplantation for identical twins in the treatment of aplastic anaemia; implications for the pathogenesis of the disease. *British Journal of Haematology* 56, 455.

Charache S, Dover GJ, Moyer MA et al. (1987) Hydroxyurea-induced augmentation of fetal hemoglobin production in patients with sickle cell anaemia. *Blood* 69, 109.

Chomienne C, Ballerini P, Balitrand N et al. (1990) All trans retinoic acid in acute promyelocytic leukaemia. II: In vitro studies: structure–function relationship. *Blood* 76, 1710.

Civin CI (1990) Human monomyeloid cell membrane antigens. *Experimental Hematology* 18, 461.

Clavell LA, Gelber RD, Cohen HJ et al. (1986) Four agent induction and intensive asparaginase therapy for treatment of childhood acute lymphoblastic leukaemia. *New England Journal of Medicine* 315, 657.

Constantini F, Chada K, Magram J (1986) Correction of murine β-thalassemia by gene transfer into the germ line. *Science* 233, 1192.

Cornetta K, Morgan RA, Anderson WF (1991) Safety issues related to retroviral mediated gene transfer in humans. *Human Genetic Therapy* 2, 5.

Coulombel L, Eaves C, Kalousek D et al. (1985) Long-term marrow culture of cells from patients with acute myelogenous leukaemia. Selection in favor of normal phenotypes in some but not all cases. *Journal of Clinical Investigation* 75, 961.

Dearden C, Catovsky D (1990) Treatment of hairy cell leukaemia with 2-deoxycoformycin. *Leukaemia and Lymphoma* 1, 179.

De Gruchy GC (1975) *Drug Induced Blood Disorders*. Blackwell Scientific Publications, Oxford.

Del Vecchio L, Finizio O, Lo Pardo C et al. (1991) Co-ordinate expression of T-cell antigens on acute myelogenous leukaemia and of myeloid antigens on T-acute lymphoblastic leukaemia. Speculation on a highly balanced bilinearity. *Leukaemia* 5, 815.

de Planque MM, Bacigalupo A, Wursch A et al. (1988) Long-term follow-up of severe aplastic anaemia (SAA) patients treated with immunosuppression (IS). *Bone Marrow Transplantation* 3 (suppl 1), 239.

De Simone J, Heller P, Hall L et al. (1982) 5-Azacytidine stimulates fetal haemoglobin synthesis in anaemic baboons. *Proceedings of the National Academy of Sciences of the USA* 79, 4428.

de Thé H, Chomienne C, Lanotte M et al. (1990) The t(15;17) translocation of acute promyelocytic leukaemia fuses the retinoic acid receptor α gene to a novel transcribed locus. *Nature* 347, 558.

De Witte T, Zwaan FE, Gratwohl A et al. (1988) Allogeneic bone marrow transplantation in secondary leukaemias and myelodysplastic syndromes. *Bone Marrow Transplantation* 3 (suppl 1), 142.

Dormer P, Hershko C, Voss R et al. (1987) Myelodysplastic syndromes: evolution of overt leukaemia by one or several steps of transformation. *British Journal of Haematology* 67, 141.

Dunbar C, Smith DA, Kimball J et al. (1991) Treatment of Diamond-Blackfan anaemia with haemopoietic growth factors, granulocyte-macrophage colony stimulating factor and interleukin-3: sustained remission following interleukin-3. *British Journal of Haematology* 79, 316.

Dzierzak EA, Papayannopoulou TH, Mulligan RC (1988) Lineage-specific expression of a human β-globin gene in murine bone marrow transplant recipients reconstituted with retrovirus-transduced stem cells. *Nature* 331, 35.

Ellison RR, Holland JF, Weil M (1968) Arabinosyl cytosine: a useful agent in the treatment of acute leukaemia in adults. *Blood* 32, 507.

Faille A, Barrett AJ, Balitrand N et al. (1979) Effect of antilymphocyte globulin on granulocyte precursors in aplastic anaemia. *British Journal of Haematology* 42, 371.

Fialkow PJ, Jacobson RJ, Papayannopoulou T (1977) Chronic myelocytic leukemia: clonal origin in a stem cell common to the granulocyte, erythrocyte, platelet and monocyte/macrophage. *American Journal of Medicine* 63, 125.

Fialkow PJ, Faguet GB, Jacobson RJ et al. (1981) Evidence that essential thrombocythaemia is a clonal disorder with origin in a multipotent stem cell. *Blood* 58, 916.

Fialkow PJ, Singer JW, Raskind WH et al. (1987) Clonal development, stem-cell differentiation, and clinical remissions in acute nonlymphocytic leukemia. *New England Journal of Medicine* 317, 468.

Fletcher JA, Lynch EA, Kimball VM et al. (1991) Translocation 9;22 is associated with an extremely poor prognosis in intensively treated children with acute lymphoblastic leukemia. *Blood* 77, 435.

Flynn P, Miller W, Weisdorf D et al. (1983) Retinoic acid treatment of acute promyelocytic leukaemia: in vitro and in vivo observations. *Blood* 62, 1211.

Freedman MH, Gelfand EW, Saunders EF et al. (1979) Acquired aplastic anemia: antibody mediated hematopoietic failure. *American Journal of Hematology* 6, 135.

French Cooperative Group on Chronic Lymphocytic Leukaemia (1988) Effectiveness of 'CHOP' regimen in advanced untreated chronic lymphocytic leukaemia. *Lancet* 1, 1346.

French Cooperative Group on Chronic Lymphocytic Leukaemia (1990) Effects of chlorambucil and therapeutic decision in initial forms of chronic lymphocytic leukemia (stage A): results of a randomised clinical trial on 612 patients. *Blood* 75, 1414.

Frickhofen N, Kaltwasser JP, Schrezenmeier H et al. (1991) Treatment of aplastic anaemia with antilymphocyte globulin and methyl prednisolone with and without cyclosporine. *New England Journal of Medicine* 324, 1297.

Gahrton G, Tura S, Ljungman P et al. (1991) Allogeneic bone marrow transplantation in multiple myeloma. *New England Journal of Medicine* 325, 1267.

Gale RP, Butturini A (1991) Maintenance chemotherapy and cure of childhood acute lymphoblastic leukaemia. *Lancet* 2, 1315.

Gale RP, Foon KA, Cline MJ et al. (1981) Intensive chemotherapy for acute myelogenous leukemia. *Annals of Internal Medicine* 94, 753.

Galvani DW, Cawley JC, Nethersall A et al. (1987) Alpha interferon in myelodysplasia. *British Journal of Haematology* 66, 145.

Ganser A, Seipelt G, Lindemann A et al. (1990) Effects of recombinant interleukin-3 in patients with myelodysplastic syndromes. *Blood* 76, 455.

Gascon P, Scala G (1988) Decreased interleukin-1 production in aplastic anemia. *American Journal of Medicine* 85, 668.

Gascon P, Zoumbos N, Djeu J et al. (1985) Lymphokine abnormalities in aplastic anemia. Implications for the mechanism of action of ATG. *Blood* 65, 407.

Gibson FM, Gordon-Smith EC (1990) Long-term culture of aplastic anaemia bone marrow. *British Journal of Haematology* 75, 421.

Gisslinger H, Chott A, Linkesch W (1990) Long term interferon therapy in myelodysplastic syndromes. *Leukemia* 4, 91.

Gluckman E, Devergie A, Faille A et al. (1978) Treatment of severe aplastic anaemia with antilymphocyte globulin and androgens. *Experimental Hematology* 6, 679.

Gluckman E, Bourdeau-Esperou H, Boogaerts M et al. (1991) New approach of treatment of severe aplastic anaemia. *Bone Marrow Transplantation* 7 (suppl 2), 106.

Golomb HM, Ratain MJ, Moormeier J (1989) What is the choice of treatment for hairy cell leukemia? *Journal of Clinical Oncology* 7, 156.

Gordon MY (1978) Circulating inhibitors of granulopoiesis in patients with aplastic anaemia. *British Journal of Haematology* 39, 491.

Gordon M, Barrett AJ (1985) *Bone Marrow Disorders: The Biological Basis of Clinical Problems*. Blackwell Scientific Publications, Oxford.

Gore ME, Selby PJ, Viner C et al. (1989) Intensive treatment of multiple myeloma and criteria for complete remission. *Lancet* 2, 879.

Greaves MF, Chan LC, Furley AJ et al. (1986) Lineage promiscuity in hemopoietic differentiation and leukemia. *Blood* 67, 1.

Greenberg PL (1986) In vitro culture techniques defining biologic abnormalities in the myelodysplastic syndromes and the myeloproliferative disorders. *Clinical Haematology* 15, 973.

Greenberg PL (1991) Treatment of myelodysplastic syndromes. *Blood Reviews* 5, 42.

Grogan TM, Durie BGM, Spier CM et al. (1989) Myelomonocytic antigen positive multiple myeloma. *Blood* 73, 763.

Grosveld F, Antonio UM, van Assendelft GD et al. (1987) Regulation of expression of human beta-globin genes. *Progress in Clinical Biological Research* 251, 133.

Halpern DS, Freedman MH (1989) Diamond Blackfan anaemia: etiology, pathophysiology and treatment. *American Journal of Pediatric Hematology and Oncology* 11, 380.

Halpern DS, Estrov Z, Freedman MH (1989) Diamond Blackfan anaemia: promotion of a marrow erythropoiesis in vitro by recombinant interleukin-3. *Blood* 73, 1168.

Heard JM, Fichelson S, Sola B et al. (1984) Multistep leukemogenesis in vitro: description of a model specifying three steps within the myeloblast malignant process. *Molecular and Cellular Biology* 4, 531.

Hoelzer D, Gale RP (1987) Acute lymphoblastic leukaemia in adults. Recent progress, future directions. *Seminars in Haematology* 24, 27.

Holt C, Arensen E, Carstens B et al. (1989) Persistence of pseudodiploidy del(16q) in remission bone marrow of two children with acute lymphoblastic leukaemia. *Proceedings of the American Society of Clinical Oncology* 8, 218.

Horowitz MM, Gale RP, Sondel PN et al. (1990) Graft-versus-leukaemia reactions after bone marrow transplantation. *Blood* 75, 555.

Horowitz MM, Messerer D, Hoelzer D et al. (1991) Comparison of chemotherapy and bone marrow transplantation for adults with acute lymphoblastic leukemia in first remission. *Annals of Internal Medicine* 115, 13.

Hughes TP, Morgan GJ, Martiat P et al. (1991) Detection of residual leukaemia after bone marrow transplantation for chronic myeloid leukaemia: role of polymerase chain reaction in predicting relapse. *Blood* 77, 874.

Hunter RF, Mold NG, Mitchell RB et al. (1985) Differentiation of normal myeloid and HL-60 cells induced by anti-thymocyte globulin. *Proceedings of the National Academy of Sciences of the USA* 14, 23.

International Bone Marrow Transplant Registry (1989) Transplant or chemotherapy in acute myelogenous leukaemia. *Lancet* 1, 1119.

International Chronic Granulomatous Disease Cooperative Study Group (1991) A controlled trial of interferon gamma to prevent infection in chronic granulomatous disease. *New England Journal of Medicine* 324, 509.

Jacobs A, Janowska-Wieczorek A, Caro J et al. (1989) Circulating erythropoietin in patients with myelodysplastic syndromes. *British Journal of Haematology* 73, 36.

Jacobson RJ, Salo A, Fialkow PJ (1978) Agnogenic myeloid metaplasia: a clonal proliferation of hematopoietic stem cells with secondary myelofibrosis. *Blood* 51, 189.

Janossy G, Campana D (1991) Monoclonal antibodies in the diagnosis of leukaemia. In: Catovsky D (ed.) *The Leukemic Cell*. Methods in Hematology series, 2nd edn, Churchill Livingstone, Edinburgh, p. 168.

Janssen JW, Buschle M, Layton M et al. (1989) Clonal analysis of myelodysplastic syndromes: evidence of multipotent cell origin. *Blood* 73, 248.

Jiang YZ, Borzy MS, Macdonald D et al. (1990) Defective natural immunity in patients with essential thrombocythaemia. *Experimental Hematology* (abstracts) 18, 644.

Joyner A, Keller G, Phillips RA et al. (1983) Retrovirus mediated transfer of a bacterial gene into mouse haematopoietic progenitor cells. *Nature* 305, 206.

Juttner CA, To LB (1990) Peripheral stem cell mobilisation by myelosuppressive chemotherapy. In: Dicke KA, Armitage JO, Dicke Evinger MJ (eds), *Autologous Bone Marrow Transplantation: Proceedings of the Fifth International Symposium*. University of Nebraska Medical College, Omaha, p. 783.

Kagan WA, Ascensao JA, Pahwa RN et al. (1976) Aplastic anemia: presence in human marrow of cells that suppress myelopoiesis. *Proceedings of the National Academy of Sciences of the USA* 73, 2890.

Kartner N, Evernden-Porelle D, Bradley G et al. (1985) Detection of P-glycoprotein in multidrug resistant cell lines by monoclonal antibodies. *Nature* 316, 820.

Kaye SB, Kerr DJ (1991) Multidrug resistance: clinical relevance in haematological malignancies. *Blood Reviews* 5, 38.

Keating MJ, Kantarjian H, O'Brien S et al. (1991) Fludarabine: a new agent with marked cytoreductive activity in untreated chronic lymphocytic leukaemia. *Journal of Clinical Oncology* 9, 44.

Kishimoto T (1989) The biology of interleukin-6. *Blood* 74, 1.

Knospe WH, Crosby WH (1971) Aplastic anaemia: a disorder of the sinusoidal microcirculation rather than stem cell failure? *Lancet* 1, 20.

Koeffler HP (1986) Myelodysplastic syndromes (preleukaemia). *Seminars in Hematology* 23, 284.

Koeffler HP, Amatruda T, Ikekawa N et al. (1984) Induction of macrophage differentiation of human normal and leukaemic myeloid stem cells by 1:25 dihydroxyvitamin D3 and its fluorinated analogues. *Cancer Research* 44, 5624.

Kolb HJ, Mittermuller J, Clemm CH et al. (1990) Donor leukocyte transfusions for treatment of recurrent chronic myelogenous leukaemia in marrow transplant patients. *Blood* 76, 2462.

Lazzarino M, Vitale A, Morra E et al. (1990) Therapy of essential thrombocythemia with alpha-interferon: results and prospects. *European Journal of Haematology* 45 (suppl 52), 15.

Ledley FD (1987) Somatic gene therapy for human disease: background and prospects. Part II. *Journal of Pediatrics* 110, 167.

Lee M, Kantarjian H, Deisseroth A et al. (1989) Clinical usage of polymerase chain reaction (PCR) to analyse the BCR-ABL splicing patterns and minimal residual disease (MRD) in Philadelphia chromosome (Ph[1])-positive CML. *Blood* 74 (199a abstract), 745.

Lehn PM (1990) Gene therapy using bone marrow transplantation: a 1990 update. *Bone Marrow Transplantation* 5, 287.

Ley TJ, DeSimone J, Anagnou NP et al. (1982) 5-Azacytidine selectively increases γ-globin synthesis in a patient with β+thalassemia. *New England Journal of Medicine* 307, 1469.

Ley TJ, DeSimone J, Noguchi CT et al. (1983) 5-Azacytidine increases γ-globin synthesis and reduces the proportion of dense cells in patients with sickle-cell anaemia. *Blood* 62, 370.

Li JP, D'Andrea AD, Lodish HF et al. (1990) Activation of cell growth by binding of Friend spleen focus-forming virus gp55 glycoprotein to the erythropoietin receptor. *Nature* 343, 762.

Lishner M, Curbis JE, Minkin S et al. (1989) Interaction between retinoic acid and cytosine arabinoside affecting the blast cells of acute myeloblastic leukemia. *Leukemia* 3, 784.

Lucarelli G, Weatherall DJ (1991) For debate: bone marrow transplantation for severe thalassaemia. 1) The view from Pesaro. 2) To be or not to be. *British Journal of Haematology* 78, 300.

Lucarelli G, Galimberti M, Polchi P et al. (1990) Bone marrow transplantation in patients with thalassemia. *New England Journal of Medicine* 322, 417.

Luzzatto L, Foroni L (1986) DNA rearrangements of cell lineage specific genes in lymphoproliferative disorders. *Progress in Hematology* 14, 303.

Lyons J, Janssen JW, Bartram C et al. (1988) Mutations of Ki-ras and N-ras oncogenes in myelodysplastic syndromes. *Blood* 71, 1701.

McCulloch EA (1990) Biological characteristics of acute myeloid leukaemia contributing to management strategy. In: Freireich EJ (ed.) *New Approaches to the Treatment of Leukemia*. Springer-Verlag, Berlin, p. 87.

Macdonald DM, Jiang YZ, Gordon AA et al. (1990) Recombinant interleukin-2 for acute myeloid leukaemia in first complete remission: a pilot study. *Leukaemia Research* 14, 967.

Macdonald DM, Jiang YZ, Swirsky D et al. (1991) Acute myeloid leukaemia relapsing following interleukin-2 treatment expresses the alpha chain of the interleukin-2 receptor. British Journal of Haematology 77, 43.

McGuire WA, Young HH, Bruno E (1987) Treatment of antibody mediated pure red cell aplasia with high dose intravenous gamma-globulin. New England Journal of Medicine 317, 1004.

McKelvey EM, Gottlieb JA, Wilson HE et al. (1976) Hydroxyldaunomycin (adriamycin) combination chemotherapy in malignant lymphoma. Cancer 38, 1484.

Maiolo AT, Cortelezzi A, Calori R et al. (1990) Recombinant gamma interferon as first line therapy for high risk myelodysplastic syndromes. Leukemia 4, 480.

Mandelli F, Tribalto M, Avvisati G et al. (1988) Recombinant interferon alpha-2b (Intron A) as post-induction therapy for responding multiple myeloma patients. M84 protocol. Cancer Treatment Review 15 (suppl A), 43.

Marsh JC, Geary CG (1991) Is aplastic anaemia a pre-leukaemic disorder? British Journal of Haematology 77, 447.

Marsh JCW, Hows JM, Bryett KA et al. (1987) Survival after antilymphocyte globulin therapy for aplastic anemia depends on disease severity. Blood 70, 1046.

Marsh JC, Chang J, Testa NG et al. (1990) The hemopoietic defect in aplastic anemia assessed by long-term bone marrow culture. Blood 76, 1748.

Maruyama Y, Murohashi I, Nava N (1989) Effects of verapamil on the cellular accumulation of daunorubicin in blast cells and on the chemo-sensitivity blast progenitors in acute myelogenous leukaemia. British Journal of Haematology 72, 357.

Mathé G, Amiel JL, Schwarzenberg L et al. (1970) Bone marrow graft in man after conditioning by anti-lymphocyte globulin. British Medical Journal 2, 131.

Mattei MG, Petkovich M, Mattei JF et al. (1988) Mapping of the human retinoic acid receptor to the q21 band of chromosome 17. Human Genetics 80, 186.

Mauch P, Botnick LE, Hanam EC et al. (1982) Decline in bone marrow proliferative capacity as a function of age. Blood 60, 245.

Mauer AM (1980) Therapy of acute lymphoblastic leukemia in childhood. Blood 56, 1.

Maurer J, Janssen JW, Thiel E et al. (1991) Detection of chimeric BCR-ABL genes in acute lymphoblastic leukemia by polymerase chain reaction – frequency and clinical relevance. Lancet 337, 1055.

Mayer RJ (1988) Allogeneic transplantation versus intensive chemotherapy in first remission acute leukaemia: is there a 'best choice'? Journal of Clinical Oncology 10, 1532.

Mazur EM, De Alarcon P, South K, Micelli L (1984) Human serum megakaryocyte stimulating factor increases in response to intensive cytotoxic chemotherapy. Experimental Hematology 12, 624.

Means RT, Dessypris EN, Kranz SB (1991) Treatment of refractory pure red cell aplasia with cyclosporine A: disappearance of IgG inhibitor associated with clinical response. British Journal of Haematology 78, 114.

Mecucci C, Rege-Cambrin G, Michaux JL et al. (1986) Multiple chromosomally distinct populations in myelodysplastic syndromes and their possible significance in the evolution of disease. British Journal of Haematology 64, 699.

Meng-Er H, Yu-Chen Y, Shu-song C et al. (1988) Use of all-trans retinoic acid in the treatment of acute promyelocytic leukaemia. Blood 72, 567.

Mertelsmann R, Herrmann F, Hecht T et al. (1990) Haemopoietic growth factors in bone marrow transplantation. Bone Marrow Transplantation 6, 73.

Michallet M, Corront B, Molina L et al. (1991) Allogeneic bone marrow transplantation in chronic lymphocytic leukemia: 17 cases. Report of the EBMT. Leukemia and Lymphoma 5 (suppl 1), 127.

Millar BC, Bell JB, Lakhani A et al. (1988) A simple method for culturing myeloma cells from human bone marrow aspirates and peripheral blood in vitro. British Journal of Haematology 69, 197.

Miller AD (1990a) Retrovirus packaging cells. Human Genetics 1, 5.

Miller AD (1990b) Progress toward human gene therapy. Blood 76, 1.

Miller TP, Dana BW, Weick JK et al. (1988) Southwest oncology group clinical trials for intermediate and high-grade non-Hodgkin's lymphomas. Seminars in Hematology 25 (suppl 2), 17.

Myint AA, Malkovska V, Morgan S et al. (1990) Antilymphocyte globulin therapy enhances impaired function of natural killer cells and lymphokine activated killer cells in aplastic anaemia. British Journal of Haematology 75, 578.

Nakao S, Matsushima K, Young N (1989) Decreased interleukin 1 production by aplastic anaemia monocytes. British Journal of Haematology 71, 431.

Nathan DG, Clarke BJ, Hillman DG et al. (1978) Erythroid precursors in congenital hypoplastic (Diamond-Blackfan) anaemia. Journal of Clinical Investigation 61, 489.

Negrin RS, Haeber DH, Nagler A et al. (1989) Treatment of myelodysplastic syndromes with human recombinant granulocyte colony stimulating factor. A phase I/II trial. Annals of Internal Medicine 110, 976.

Nienhuis AW, McDonagh KT, Bodine DM (1991) Gene transfer into hemopoietic stem cells. Cancer 67 (suppl 10), 2700.

Nissen C, Iscove N, Speck B (1979) High burst-promoting activity in serum of patients with acquired aplastic anaemia. In: Baum SJ, Ledney GD (eds) Experimental Hematology Today. Springer-Verlag, New York, p. 79.

Nissen C, Cornu P, Gratwohl A et al. (1980) Peripheral blood cells from patients with aplastic anaemia in partial remission suppress growth of their own bone marrow precursors in culture. British Journal of Haematology 45, 233.

Norton JD, Campana D, Hoffbrand AV et al. (1987) Rearrangement of immunoglobulin and T-cell antigen receptor genes in acute myeloid leukaemia

with lymphoid-associated markers. *Leukemia* 1, 757.
Paietta E (1990) Ambiguous phenotypes in acute leukemia. *Leukemia and Lymphoma* 2, 17.
Pastan I, Gottesman M (1987) Multidrug resistance in human cancer. *New England Journal of Medicine* 316, 1388.
Pierre RV, Catovsky D, Mufti GJ et al. (1989) Clinical-cytogenetic correlations in myelodysplasia (pre-leukaemia). *Cancer Genetics and Cytogenetics* 2, 108.
Pillow RP, Epstein RB, Buckner CD et al. (1966) Treatment of bone-marrow failure by isogeneic marrow infusion. *New England Journal of Medicine* 275, 94.
Pinkel D (1987) Curing children of leukemia. *Cancer* 60, 1683.
Poddige PJ, Moesker O, Smeets D et al. (1991) Interphase cytogenetics of haematological cancer: comparison of classical karyotyping and in situ hybridization using a panel of eleven chromosome specific DNA probes. *Cancer Research* 51, 1959.
Prchal JT, Trockmorton DW, Carroll AJ et al. (1978) A common progenitor for myeloid and lymphoid cells. *Nature* 274, 590.
Preisler HD, Raza A, Early A (1987) Intensive remission consolidation therapy in the treatment of acute nonlymphoblastic leukaemia. *Journal of Clinical Oncology* 5, 722.
Preisler HD, Anderson K, Rai K et al. (1989) The frequency of long term remission in patients with acute myeloid leukaemia treated with conventional maintenance chemotherapy: a study of 760 patients with a minimum follow up time of six years. *British Journal of Haematology* 71, 189.
Pui CH, Fraenkel LS, Carrol AJ et al. (1991) Clinical characteristics and treatment outcome of children with acute lymphoblastic leukemia with t(4;11)(q21;q23): a collaborative study of 40 cases. *Blood* 77, 440.
Quesada JR, Reuben J, Manning JT et al. (1984) Alpha interferon for induction of remission in hairy cell leukemia. *New England Journal of Medicine* 310, 15.
Raghavachar A, Janssen JWE, Schrezenmeier H et al. (1991) Aplastic anaemia: assessment of clonality based on X-chromosome inactivation analysis. *Experimental Hematology* 19, 525(A).
Rappeport JM, Newburger PE, Goldblum RM et al. (1982) Allogeneic bone marrow transplantation for chronic granulomatous disease. *Pediatrics* 101, 952.
Raskind WH, Tirumali N, Tacobson R et al. (1984) Evidence for a multistep pathogenesis of a myelodysplastic syndrome. *Blood* 63, 1318.
Rees JHK (1990) Chemotherapy of the leukaemias. In: Freireich EJ (ed.) *New Approaches to the Treatment of Leukemia*. Springer-Verlag, Berlin, p. 1.
Rees JHK, Gray RG, Swirsky D et al. (1986) Principal results of the Medical Research Council's 8th acute myeloid leukaemia trial. *Lancet* 2, 1236.
Rees JKH, Gray R, Hayhoe FGJ (1987) The ninth British Medical Research Council trial in the treatment of acute myeloid leukaemia. *Haematology and Blood Transfusion* 30, 35.
Reiffers J, Gaspard MH, Maraninchi D et al. (1989) Comparison of allogeneic or autologous bone marrow transplantation and chemotherapy in patients with acute myeloid leukaemia in first remission: a prospective controlled trial. *British Journal of Haematology* 72, 57.
Reiffers J, Trouette R, Marti G et al. (1991) Autologous blood stem cell transplant for chronic granulocytic leukaemia in transformation. A report of 47 cases. *British Journal of Haematology* 77, 339.
Reilly IAG, Kozlowski R, Russell NH (1989) Heterogeneous mechanisms of autocrine growth of AML blasts. *British Journal of Haematology* 72, 363.
Reizenstein P (1990) Adjuvant immunotherapy with BCG of acute myeloid leukaemia – a fifteen year follow up. *British Journal of Haematology* 75, 288.
Rodgers GP, Dover GJ, Noguchi CT et al. (1990) Hematologic responses of patients with sickle cell disease to treatment with hydroxyurea. *New England Journal of Medicine* 322, 1037.
Rosenberg SA, Aebersold P, Cornetta K et al. (1990) Gene transfer into humans – immunotherapy of patients with advanced melanoma using tumor infiltrating lymphocytes modified by retroviral gene transduction. *New England Journal of Medicine* 323, 570.
Russell NH, Reilly IAG (1989) Role of autocrine growth factors in the leukaemic transformation of the myelodysplastic syndromes. *Leukemia* 3, 83.
Samson D, Gaminara E, Newland A et al. (1989) Infusion of vincristine and doxorubicin with oral dexamethasone as first-line therapy for multiple myeloma. *Lancet* 2, 882.
Sechler JMG, Malech HL, White CJ et al. (1988) Recombinant interferon gamma reconstitutes defective phagocyte function in chronic granulomatous desease. *Proceedings of the National Academy of Sciences of the USA* 85, 4874.
Silver RT (1988) Recombinant interferon-alpha for treatment of polycythaemia vera. *Lancet* 2, 403.
Singer JW, Doney KCX, Thomas ED (1979) Coculture studies of 16 untransfused patients with aplastic anemia. *Blood* 54, 180.
Skipper HE (1986) Laboratory models: the historical perspective. *Cancer Treatment Reports* 70, 3.
Slavin S, Ackerstein E, Naparstek R et al. (1990) Hypothesis: the graft-versus-leukaemia (GVL) phenomenon: is GVL separable from GVHD? *Bone Marrow Transplantation* 6, 155.
Sobol RE, Mick R, Royston I et al. (1987) Clinical importance of myeloid antigen expression in adult acute lymphoblastic leukemia. *New England Journal of Medicine* 316, 1111.
Solal-Celigny P, Lepage E, Brousse N et al. (1991) Alpha interferon and chemotherapy in patients with high tumor burden follicular lymphoma: preliminary results of the groupe d'etude des lymphomes folliculaires. *Proceedings of the American Society of Clinical Oncology* 10, 275.
Sosman JA, Sondel PM (1987) The graft-versus-leukemia effect following bone marrow transplantation – a

review of laboratory and clinical data. *Hematology Reviews* 2, 77.
Speck B, Gluckman E, Haak HL et al. (1977) Treatment of aplastic anaemia by antilymphocyte globulin with and without allogeneic bone-marrow infusions. *Lancet* 2, 1145.
Spitzer G, Verma DS, Beran M et al. (1981) Human myeloid leukaemic cell interactions with normal myeloid colonies. *British Journal of Cancer* 43, 149.
Stass S, Mirro J, Melvin S et al. (1984) Lineage switch in acute leukemia. *Blood* 64, 701.
Steinberg PG, Gaynor P, Muller DR et al. (1986) Improved disease-free survival of children with acute lymphoblastic leukemia at high-risk for early relapse with the New York regimen – a new intensive therapy protocol; a report from the Children's Cancer Study Group. *Journal of Clinical Oncology* 4, 744.
Stryckmans PA, Dumont JP, Velu T et al. (1984) Cyclosporine in refractory severe aplastic anaemia. *New England Journal of Medicine* 312, 257.
Swan F, Manning J, Ordonez N et al. (1991) The effect of MHC class 1 expression on survival in patients with large cell lymphoma (LCL). *Blood* 78 (suppl 1), 123a.
Szer J, Deeg HJ, Witherspoon RR et al. (1984) Long term survival after marrow transplantation for paroxysmal nocturnal hemoglobinuria with aplastic anemia. *Annals of Internal Medicine* 101, 193.
Talpaz AM, Kantarjian HM, Kurzrock R et al. (1988) Therapy of chronic myelogenous leukaemia: chemotherapy and interferons. *Seminars in Hematology* 25, 62.
The ADA Human Gene Therapy Clinical Protocol (1990) *Human Gene Therapy* 1, 327.
The TNF/TIL Human Gene Therapy Clinical Protocol (1990) *Human Gene Therapy* 1, 441.
Thomas ED, Buckner CD, Storb R et al. (1972) Aplastic anaemia treated by bone marrow transplantation. *Lancet* 1, 284.
Tichelli A, Gratwohl A, Wursch A et al. (1988) Late haematological complications in severe aplastic anaemia. *British Journal of Haematology* 69, 413.
Torok-Storb B, Johnson G, Bowden R et al. (1987) Gamma-interferon in aplastic anaemia: inability to detect significant levels in sera or demonstrate hematopoietic suppressing activity. *Blood* 69, 629.
Treleaven J, Barrett AJ (1990) Drugs and the bone marrow. *British Journal of Hospital Medicine* 44, 245.
Tricot G, Boogaerts MA, De Wolf-Peeters C et al. (1985) The myelodysplastic syndromes: different evolution based on sequential morphological and cytogenetic investigations. *British Journal of Haematology* 59, 659.
Tricot G, Boogaerts MA, Vlietinck R (1987) The role of intensive remission induction and consolidation therapy in patients with acute myeloid leukaemia. *British Journal of Haematology* 66, 37.
Twentyman PR (1988) Resistance modification by non-immunosuppressive cyclosporins. *British Journal of Cancer* 57, 254.
Uckun FM, Heerema NA (1990) Use of lymphoid progenitor cell assays for a more detailed analysis of the cytogenetic changes occurring during clonal evolution in acute lymphoblastic leukaemia.
Uckun FM, Muraguchi A, Ledbetter JA et al. (1989) Biphenotypic leukemic lymphocyte precursors in $CD2^+$, $CD19^+$ acute lymphoblastic leukemia and their putative normal counterparts in human fetal hematopoietic tissues. *Blood* 73, 1000.
Urbano-Ispizna A, Matutes E, Villamor N et al. (1990) Clinical significance of the presence of myeloid associated antigens in acute lymphoblastic leukaemia. *British Journal of Haematology* 75, 202.
Vadhan-Raj S, Keating M, Le Maistre A et al. (1987) Effects of human recombinant granulocyte-macrophage colony stimulating factor in patients with myelodysplastic syndromes. *New England Journal of Medicine* 317, 1545.
Vellenga E, Young DC, Wagner K et al. (1987) The effects of GM-CSF and G-CSF in promoting growth of clonogenic cells in acute myeloblastic leukaemia. *Blood* 69, 1771.
Vinci G, Vernant JP, Nakazawa M et al. (1988) In vitro inhibition of normal human hematopoiesis by marrow $CD3^+$, $CD8^+$, $HLA-DR^+$, $HNK1^+$ lymphocytes. *Blood* 72, 1616.
Warburton P, Joshua DE, Gibson J et al. (1989) CD10-(CALLA)-Positive lymphocytes in myeloma; evidence that they are a malignant precursor population and are of germinal centre origin. *Leukemia and Lymphoma* 1, 11.
Warrell RP, Frankel SR, Miller WH et al. (1991) Differentiation therapy of acute promyelocytic leukaemia with Tretinoin (all transretinoic acid). *New England Journal of Medicine* 324, 1385.
Wiernik PH (1990) Recent advances in chemotherapy for certain leukemias. In: Freireich EJ (ed.) *New Approaches to the Treatment of Leukemia*. Springer-Verlag, Berlin, p. 187.
Wiersma S, Ortega J, Sobel E et al. (1991) Clinical importance of myeloid expression in acute lymphoblastic leukemia of childhood. *New England Journal of Medicine* 324, 800.
Williams DM, Lynch RE, Cartwright GE (1973) Drug induced aplastic anemia. *Seminars in Hematology* 10, 195.
Williams DA, Lemischka IR, Nathans DG et al. (1984) Introduction of new genetic material into pluripotent haemopoietic stem cells of the mouse. *Nature* 310, 476.
Yamada M, Wasserman R, Lange B et al. (1990) Minimal residual disease in childhood acute lymphoblastic leukaemia. Persistence of leukemic cells during the first 18 months of treatment. *New England Journal of Medicine* 323, 448.
Young NS (1991) The pathogenesis and pathophysiology of aplastic anemia. In: Hoffman R, Benz EJ Jr, Shattil SJ, Furie B, Cohen HJ (eds) *Hematology: Basic Principles and Practice*. Churchill Livingstone, New York, p. 122.
Young NS, Baranski B, Kurzman G (1989) The immune system as mediators of virus associated bone

marrow failure: B19 parvovirus and Epstein–Barr virus. *Annals of the New York Academy of Sciences* 554, 75.

Zoumbos N, Gascon P, Djeu J et al. (1985) Interferon is a mediator of hematopoietic suppression in aplastic anemia *in vitro* and possibly *in vivo*. *Proceedings of the National Academy of Sciences of the USA* 82, 188.

Chapter 3
Molecular Pathology of Haematological Disorders

Introduction, 141
Methods, 143
  Morphology and cytochemistry, 143
  Phenotype, 144
  Karyotype, 144
  Southern analysis, 145
  Northern analysis, 146
  Restriction fragment length polymorphisms, 147
  The polymerase chain reaction, 147
  Altered protein products, 149
  Progenitor assays, 150
  Tracking and localizing cells *in vivo*, 150
Genes and proteins of special interest, 152
Applications to haematological disease, 156
  Chronic myeloid leukaemia, 156
  Myeloproliferative disorders, 162
  Acute myeloid leukaemia, 163
  Myelodysplasia, 167
  Bone marrow transplantation, 168
  Lymphoid neoplasia, 172
  Aplastic anaemia, 178
  Haemoglobinopathies, 179
  Other inherited deficiencies, 180
Overview, 181
References, 181

INTRODUCTION

The need to identify, classify and quantitate malignant haemopoietic cells has been apparent since the leukaemias and lymphomas were first described (Table 3.1). At the time, leukaemia could be diagnosed only in patients with very high white cell counts. By the turn of the century, methods for staining cells were being developed and by the 1930s marrow aspirations were being performed for routine examination (Plate 3.1, facing p. 148). These advances facilitated efforts to classify leukaemias and lymphomas but it was not until after the Second World War that the information became important from the patient's point of view, since up until then no effective treatments were available. Alkylating agents were introduced as treatment in the 1940s and since then chemotherapy has improved to such an extent that some leukaemias, for example about 80% of cases of childhood acute lymphoblastic leukaemia (ALL), are now considered to be curable. Clearly, accurate diagnosis has become an important factor and should ensure that patients receive the most effective treatment for their disease.

The techniques for examining human chromosomes became available in the 1950s, and in 1956 the diploid number was established correctly as 46. Refinements in technique over the years led to sophisticated analyses of banding patterns that can be used to locate the positions of chromosome translocation breakpoints. Moreover, in conjunction with *in situ* hybridization it is now possible to localize specific genes to precise regions of specific chromosomes. Karyotypic analysis has revealed strong associations between some chromosomal translocations and haematological disease. Thus, detection of the

Table 3.1 Original descriptions of haematological neoplasms

Year	Condition	Reference
1832	Hodgkin's disease	Hodgkin T. On some morbid appearances of the absorbent glands and spleen. (*Medico-chirurgical Transactions* 17, 68)
1845	Chronic myeloid leukaemia	Bennett JH. Case of hypertrophy of the spleen and liver in which death took place from suppuration of the blood. (*Edinburgh Medical and Surgical Journal* 64, 413)
1846	Chronic lymphoblastic leukaemia	Virchow R. Weisses Blut und Milztumoren. (*Medizinische Zeitung* 15, 157)
1857	Acute leukaemia	Friedreich N. Ein neuer Fall von Leukämie. (*Virchows Archiv für Pathologische Anatomie* 12, 37)

Philadelphia chromosome is virtually diagnostic for chronic myeloid leukaemia (CML) — although this abnormality is not entirely restricted to CML.

Cell phenotypes were characterized as a result of the introduction of monoclonal antibodies which have been used successfully to classify subgroups of leukaemias. More recently, molecular biology has made a great contribution to our understanding of the genetic bases of haematological diseases and is the approach most likely to reveal underlying pathogenetic mechanisms. It is now possible, for example, to use molecular techniques to analyse chromosome translocations minutely and to link altered gene structure to the production of abnormal protein products.

Finally, the quantitation of malignant cells has become more important with the likelihood that all clonogenic cells can be eradicated or that small residual numbers can be controlled physiologically or phamacologically. Increased levels of detection are therefore desirable, and the most sensitive current technique is the polymerase chain reaction (PCR) which can detect at best one cell in a million.

The use of these methods is not restricted to malignant disease and they have been applied to the study of the haemoglobinopathies and other inherited deficiencies of haemopoiesis.

METHODS

A variety of methods is available for characterizing normal and malignant haemopoiesis. They range from morphological examination to sophisticated molecular techniques and from the well-established to those that have been recently developed or are developing. The morphological and cytochemical examination of cells provides an essential background for modern developments. Recombinant DNA methods are highly sensitive and discriminating in detecting gene mutations and have rapidly been applied to the investigation of inherited and acquired conditions. Monoclonal and polyclonal antibodies can be used to detect small amounts of proteins expressed at the cell surface (e.g. by flow cytometry) or in solution (e.g. by immunoprecipitation, Western blotting or radioimmunoassay).

Morphology and cytochemistry

Some types of leukaemic cells display a characteristic morphology that can be recognized by light or electron microscopy. Hairy cell leukaemia is an obvious example because of the irregular (hairy) outline of the cells, which can be seen quite easily in stained smears of blood or bone marrow (Plate 3.2a, facing p. 148). This characteristic feature is more apparent on electron micrographs (Plate 3.2b, facing p. 148), although electron microscopy is not used in routine diagnosis. Cytochemically, the characteristic properties of hairy cells are a strong reaction to tartaric acid-resistant acid phosphatase and, when stained with α-naphthylbutyrate esterase, the appearance of fine granules and accumulations of stained material to one side of the nucleus.

Table 3.2 The French–American–British classification of the acute leukaemias

Classification	Description
Acute myeloid leukaemias	
M0	Minimal differentiation
M1	Myeloblastic without maturation
M2	Myeloblastic with maturation
M3	Hypergranular promyelocytic
M4	Myelomonocytic
M5	Monocytic
M6	Erythroleukaemic
M7	Megakaryoblastic
Acute lymphoblastic leukaemias	
L1	Small monomorphic cells
L2	Large heterogeneous cells
L3	Large homogeneous cells (Burkitt-type)

To a large extent, the French–American–British (FAB) classification of leukaemic cells rests on their cytochemical staining properties (Table 3.2). Myeloperoxidase or Sudan black stain granules in myeloid cells and monocytic differentiation is accompanied by staining with non-specific esterase. In erythroleukaemia (M6), the early erythroid cells have prominent foci of red staining when examined using the periodic acid–Schiff reagent. A new category of acute myeloid leukaemia (AML) (M0) has recently been proposed to accommodate the 2–3% of cases with minimal features of myeloid differentiation (Bennett et al., 1991). In ALL, periodic acid–Schiff, acid phosphatase and oil red O are the special stains of most value.

Phenotype

Antigenic structures on the surface or in the cytoplasm of cells can be visualized using monoclonal antibodies in conjunction with fluorescence microscopy or immunocytochemistry (see Foon et al., 1990, for review). Typically, cells are reacted with a panel of monoclonal antibodies that can be used to distinguish between subgroups of acute leukaemia (Table 3.3).

Karyotype

Numerical deviations (gains or losses) from the normal somatic cell complement of 23 chromosome pairs occur in malignant cells so that they can be hyper- or hypodiploid. These alterations are more common in ALL than in AML. One of the myeloid diseases, the 5q– syndrome (i.e. loss of part of the long arm of chromosome 5) is particularly interesting because it involves the location of several growth factor and growth factor receptor genes (see Chapter 1).

Translocations occur when there is an exchange of genetic material

Table 3.3 Antibodies used in the discrimination of leukaemia subgroups

Antibodies	Cell types defined
CD34; TdT; HLA-DR	Haemopoietic progenitor cells
CD11; CD13; CD14; CD33	Myeloid cells
CD11; CD14	Monocytic cells
Anti-glycophorin	Erythroid cells
J15	Megakaryoblastic cells
CD10; CD19; CD26; anti-IgM	c-ALL; B-ALL
CD2; CD5; CD7	T cells

c-ALL, Common acute lymphoblastic leukaemia.

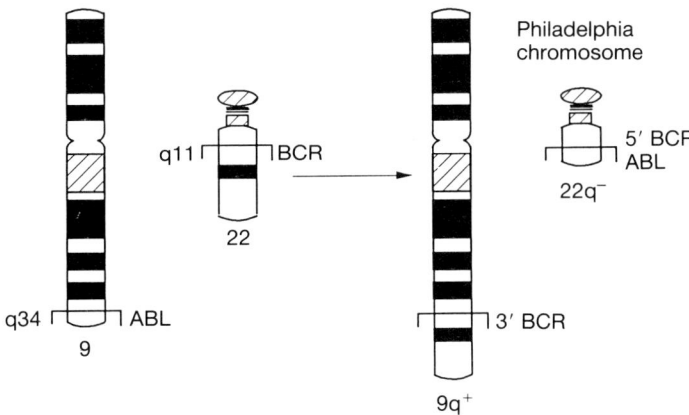

Fig. 3.1 The formation of the Philadelphia (Ph) chromosome.

between chromosomes and they may become longer or shorter than normal as a result. The best characterized of these events is the formation of the Philadelphia chromosome in CML, which can be described as t(9;22)(q34;q11) because it occurs as the result of a reciprocal exchange of material between chromosomes 9 and 22 and bands q34 and q11 (Fig. 3.1). The molecular consequences of this translocation are now well-understood and will be discussed later in this chapter. Other common translocations include t(4;11) in ALL, t(8;21) in M2 AML and t(15;17) in M3 AML.

Banding techniques rely on the differential staining of different regions of the chromosome and are valuable for detecting changes in chromosome structure that do not alter the overall size. There are various banding methods in widespread use and each technique produces a characteristic pattern of bands. Other techniques used in conjunction with cytogenetics include *in situ* hybridization, when a radioactively labelled gene probe is bound to a specific chromosomal region and visualized using autoradiography. Non-radioactively labelled probes, which are much safer than radioactive probes, are now being more widely used and have the additional advantage that permanent preparations can be made.

Routine cytogenetic analysis of 20–25 metaphases can exclude the presence of chromosomally marked cells at a frequency of more than 12–14% (Hook, 1977).

Southern analysis

The transfer technique originally described by Southern in 1975 is frequently referred to as Southern blotting and is used for detect-

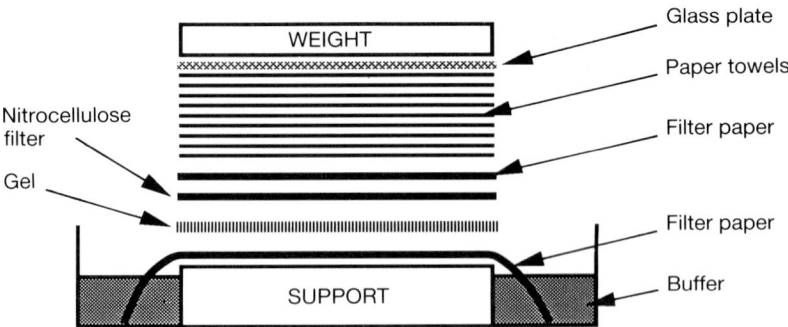

Fig. 3.2 Southern blotting by capillary transfer.

ing specific sequences in genomic DNA. This is done by extracting the DNA from cells and digesting it with restriction enzymes. The DNA fragments are then separated according to size by agarose gel electrophoresis, denatured in the gel and transferred to a solid support (a nitrocellulose filter or a nylon membrane) by blotting (Fig. 3.2). The blotting itself usually relies on capillary action, as indicated in Figure 3.2, but electrophoresis or vacuum pressure are alternatives. In the case of capillary action, the flow of water carries the DNA fragments from the gel to the filter or membrane whilst maintaining the relative positions of the different-sized fragments. Radiolabelled DNA or RNA probes are used to locate the DNA of interest by hybridizing with it and the resultant bands can be visualized by autoradiography (see Sambrook et al., 1989, for further details).

The method has been particularly valuable in demonstrating clonal genetic rearrangements in the lymphoid malignancies. This is done by choosing restriction enzymes that cut DNA to produce fragments of different sizes according to whether the gene is in its germ line configuration or is rearranged.

Southern blotting can be used to detect genetic rearrangements if the abnormal population is as small as 1–5% of the total (Roth et al., 1988).

Northern analysis

This technique is analogous to Southern blotting but is applied to the recognition of RNA sequences rather than DNA sequences. The steps in the procedure are similar to those used for the Southern technique (see Sambrook et al., 1989). It involves separation of RNA molecules according to size, denaturation, transfer to a solid support, hybridization to the labelled probe and development of the label.

Table 3.4 The use of restriction fragment length polymorphism analysis in haematology

Disease	Application
Leukaemia	Clonality of malignant populations
	Origin of relapse (original disease or *de novo* clone)
Bone marrow transplantation	Origin of repopulating cells (donor or recipient)
Haemoglobinopathies and inherited disorders	Prenatal diagnosis

Restriction fragment length polymorphisms

These DNA 'fingerprinting' methods have been useful in several areas of haematology (Table 3.4), which will be expanded upon in later sections of this chapter. The concept and use of restriction fragment length polymorphisms (RFLPs) as genetic markers have been reviewed by Botstein *et al.* (1980). The technique depends on the existence in the genome of highly variable sequences that are inherited as codominant Mendelian traits. Hence, digestion of DNA from different individuals with restriction enzymes results in DNA fragments of different lengths because of variations in sequence between the enzyme cutting sites. The lengths of the individual fragments are detected by Southern blotting using cloned DNA probes.

Vogelstein and coworkers (1985, 1987) developed a method for determining clonality based on common RFLPs of the X chromosome-linked phosphoglycerate kinase (PGK) and hypoxanthine phosphoribosyl transferase (HPRT) genes and the differential methylation of nearby cytosine residues. Methylation of the cytosines is associated with the random inactivation of one of the two X chromosomes during female embryogenesis. Digestion of DNA with a restriction enzyme, together with the use of a methylation-sensitive endonuclease (e.g. Hpa II), allows discrimination between a polyclonal and a monoclonal cell population in up to 50% of females.

The polymerase chain reaction

The PCR technique was introduced by Saiki *et al.* in 1985 and permits the amplification of a short sequence of DNA by the use of two oligodeoxynucleotide sequence-flanking primers. It is accomplished by mixing DNA with a large excess of the primers, deoxynucleotide phosphates and DNA polymerase, which are the raw materials and enzymes necessary for the reaction. The specific sequences flanked by the primers are amplified by performing repeated cycles of primer annealing and extension (Fig. 3.3).

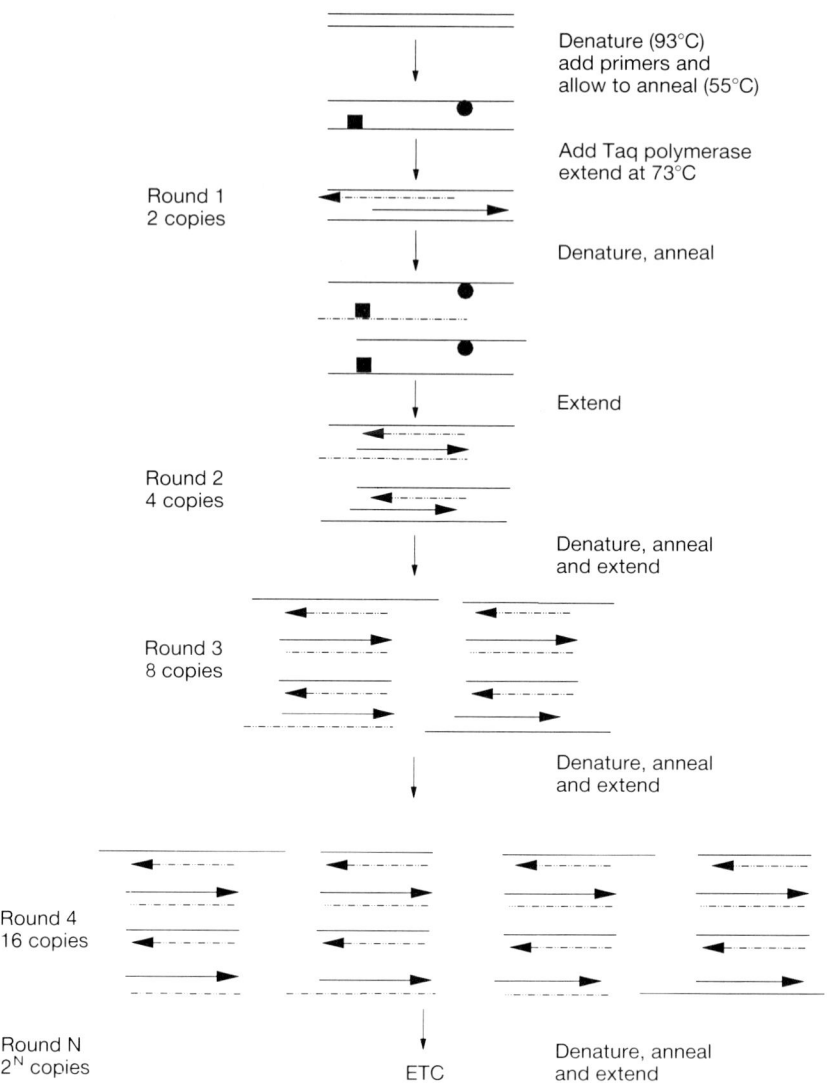

Fig. 3.3 The principle of the polymerase chain reaction.

The PCR technique is particularly appropriate for investigating malignant diseases marked by chromosomal translocations, in which case the primers are designed so that they flank the translocation junction and only sequences involved in the junction will be amplified. The technique can produce an answer in 18–24 hours, which is faster than cytogenetics. Large clinical samples are not required and, in fact, the PCR technique has been used to analyse single colonies grown *in vitro* from haemopoietic progenitor cells (Hernandez *et al.*, 1990; Gilliland *et al.*, 1991). Detection levels of one cell in a million are possible (Roth *et al.*, 1989).

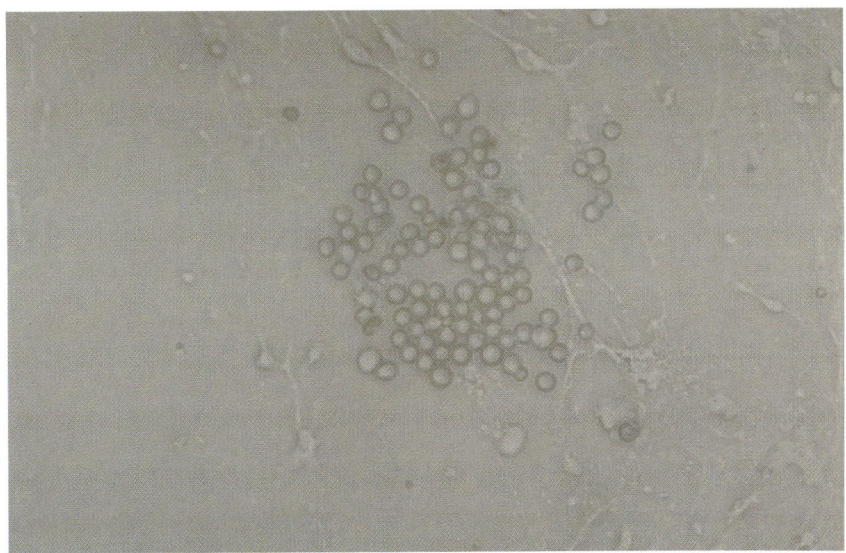

Plate 1.1 A blast colony grown on a feeder layer of cultured stromal cells.

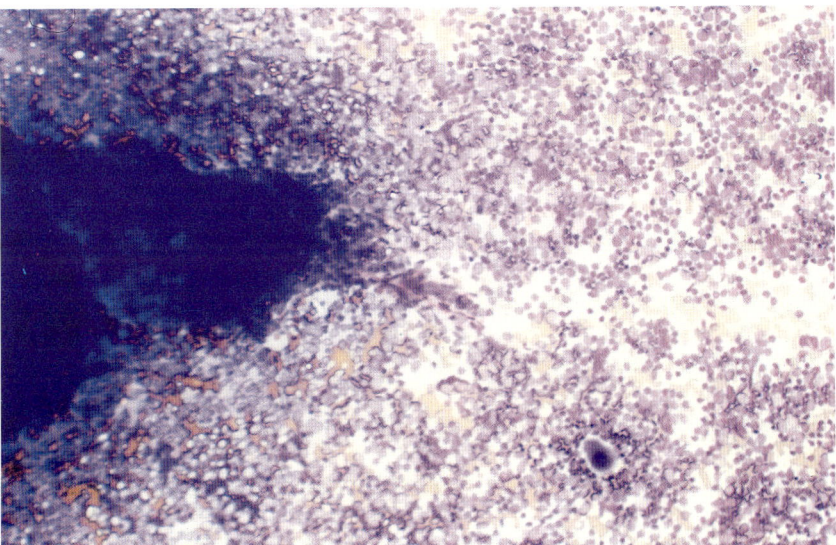

Plate 3.1 Normal aspirated bone marrow stained with May Grünwald–Giemsa.

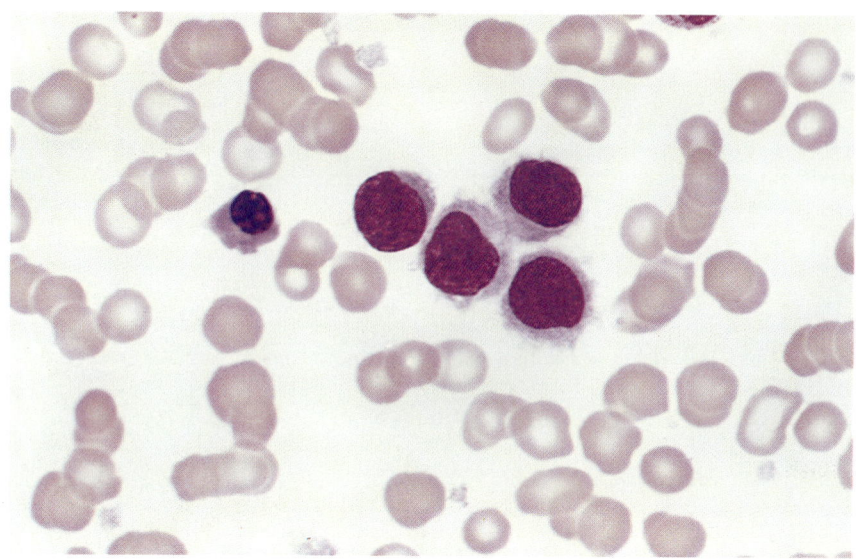

Plate 3.2a Light microscopy of hairy cell leukaemia. (Courtesy of D. Swirsky.)

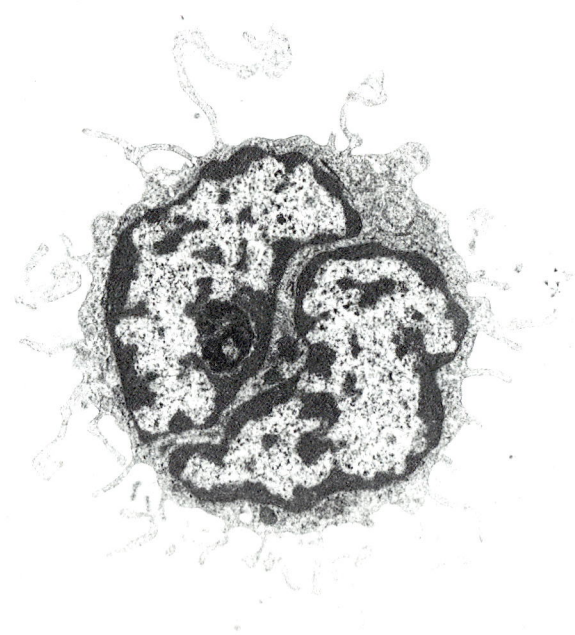

Plate 3.2b Electron microscopy of hairy cell leukaemia. (Courtesy of E. Matutes.)

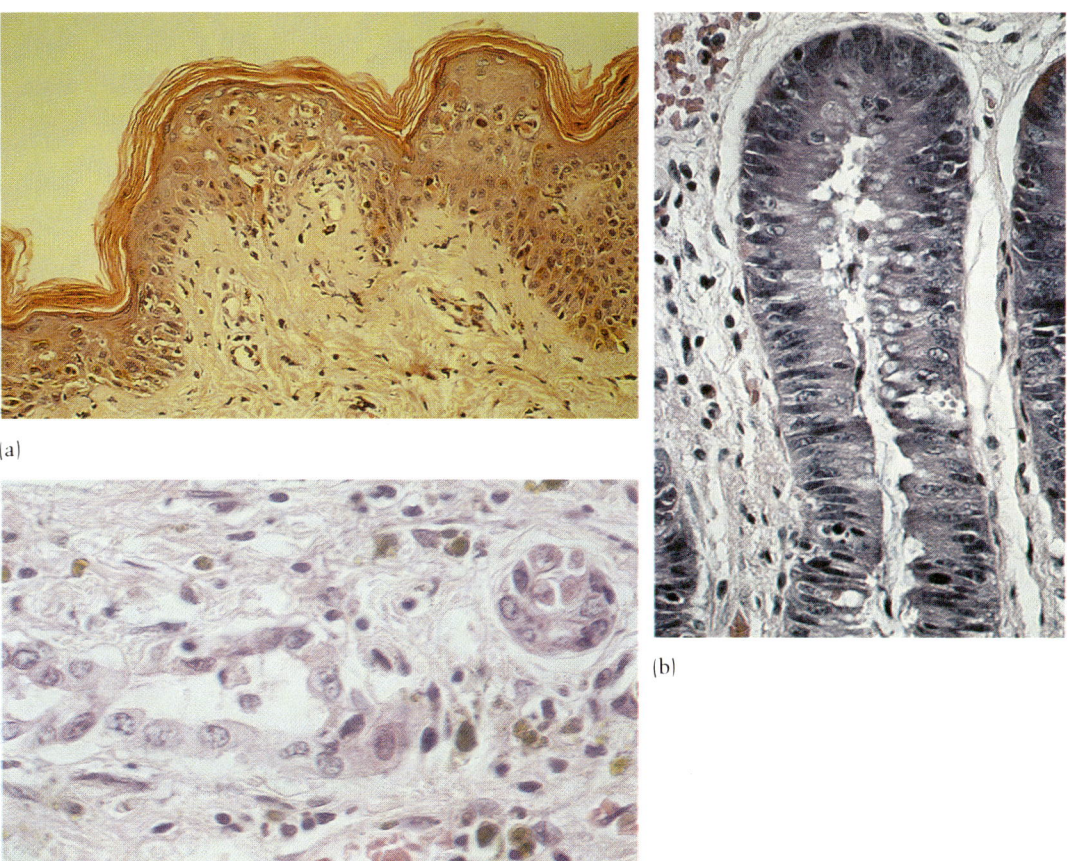

Plate 4.1 (a) Acute graft-versus-host disease of skin showing single cell necrosis of basal keratinocytes, dyskeratosis, and a mononuclear cell infiltrate. (b) Acute graft-versus-host disease of the rectum showing loss of many of the rectal glands and mucin depletion of those that remain. There is single cell necrosis and a lymphocyte infiltrate. (c) Early graft-versus-host disease of the liver showing two small bile ducts exhibiting cytological atypia and single cell necrosis of the bile duct epithelium. (Courtesy of Dr J.P. Sloane.)

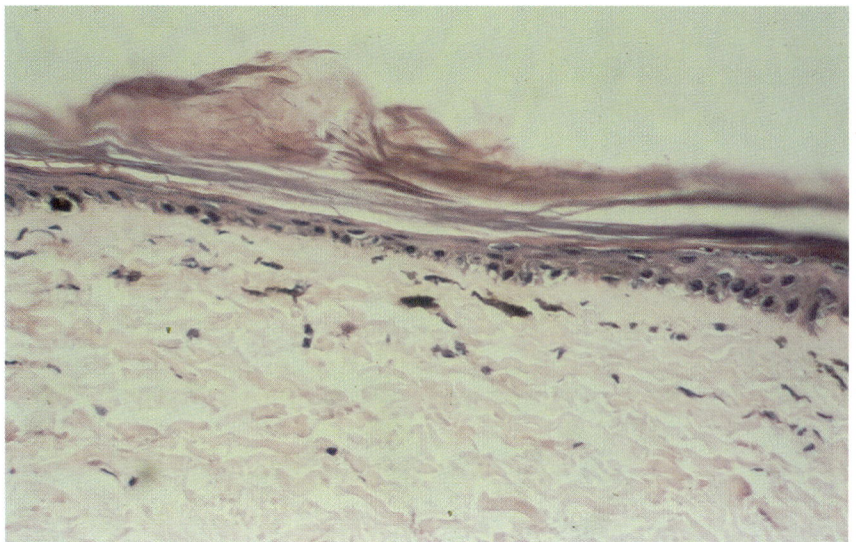
(a)

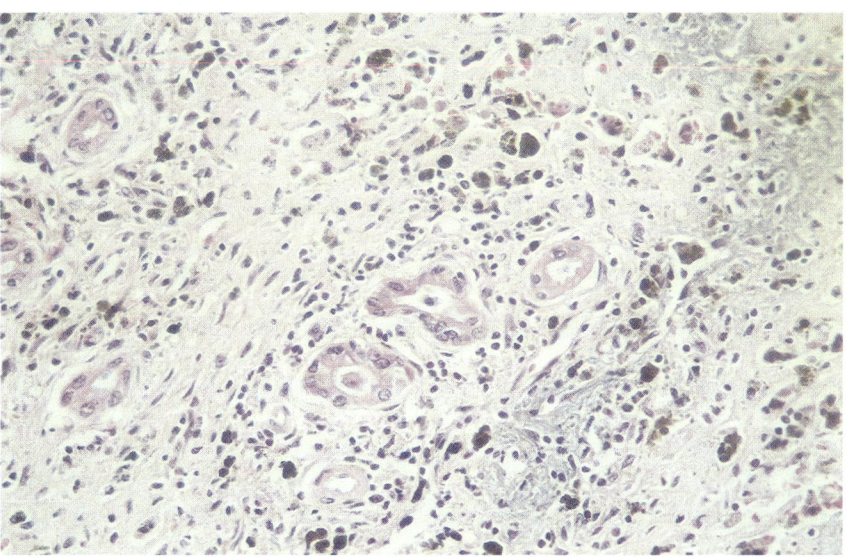
(b)

Plate 4.2 (a) Chronic graft-versus-host disease of skin showing atrophy of basal layer and dense collagen deposition in dermis. (b) Chronic graft-versus host disease of the liver showing dense fibrosis of portal tracts with persisting but damaged bile ducts. (Courtesy of Dr J.P. Sloane.)

Altered protein products

Genetic abnormalities are expressed as abnormal protein production and sometimes the normal and abnormal proteins can be distinguished by their different physicochemical properties. For example, abnormal haemoglobins or isoenzymes of glucose-6-phosphate dehydrogenase (G6PD) can be detected chromatographically or electrophoretically (Dacie and Lewis, 1984). The identification of abnormal haemoglobins is obviously important in the diagnosis of haemoglobinopathies, whilst the enzyme G6PD is a suitable marker for clonality.

The development in the 1960s of SDS-PAGE (sodium dodecyl sulphate polyacrylamide gel electrophoresis) completely revolutionized the routine analysis of proteins. The detergent SDS binds to hydrophobic regions of proteins so that they unfold and the reducing agent β-mercaptoethanol ruptures disulphide S—S bonds. As a result, polypeptide subunits of protein molecules can be analysed regardless of their inherent aqueous solubility. The method separates polypeptides according to their size and, consequently, provides information about their molecular weights when samples are run with defined marker proteins.

Western blotting

Western blotting for the characterization of proteins is the equivalent of Southern blotting for DNA and Northern blotting for RNA. In the case of proteins, the sample is separated by SDS-PAGE and the probes are antibodies that react specifically with epitopes on the target protein once it has been transferred to a solid support.

Immunoprecipitation

For this technique, radiolabelled proteins are reacted with an antibody and the antigen−antibody complexes are collected by adsorption to protein A-coated sepharose beads, heat-killed formaldehyde-fixed *Staphylococcus aureus* cells or by precipitation with an anti-immunoglobulin antibody. Once selected in this manner, the radiolabelled proteins can be further analysed.

Radioimmunoassay (RIA) and enzyme-linked immunosorbent assay (ELISA)

Radioimmunoassay is used to determine the concentration of a protein (antigen) by its ability to compete with a fixed amount of radiolabelled protein for binding to a specific antibody. Enzyme labels have replaced radioisotopes in a number of applications for reasons of safety and permanence. In ELISA antibody is added to immobilized antigen and bound antibody is quantitated by adding an enzyme (e.g. horseradish peroxidase)-labelled antibody against the first immunoglobulin. The enzyme produces a colorimetric reaction when it is allowed to react with its substrate.

Protein phosphorylation

Protein kinases phosphorylate proteins on serine/threonine or tyrosine amino acid residues and, depending on the protein, can increase or decrease their functional activities. Tyrosine phosphorylation is rare compared with phosphorylation on serine or threonine but is of particular interest because the products of oncogenes are often protein tyrosine kinases (PTKs). In particular, enhanced PTK activity is the biochemical consequence of the Philadelphia translocation in CML. Also, the binding of some growth factors to their receptors induces tyrosine autophosphorylation of the receptor as an early step in the signal transduction pathway (see Chapter 1).

Autophosphorylation is measured by incubating cytoplasmic extracts with an antibody to the PTK protein and isolating the complex using protein A-sepharose beads. The beads plus complex are incubated with $\gamma\text{-}^{32}P$ adenosine triphosphate for incorporation of the labelled phosphate. The beads are washed and denatured and the phosphorylated product is analysed by gel electrophoresis and autoradiography. The target residues for the enzyme activity (ser, thr or tyr) are determined by phospho amino acid analysis (Chan *et al.*, 1987).

Progenitor assays

Haemopoietic progenitor cell assays and clonogenic leukaemic cell assays have been used in a variety of circumstances for the investigation of bone marrow function and the estimation of residual disease. As well as providing a semiquantitative measure of the clonogenic cell populations, they can be used in conjunction with immunophenotyping, cytogenetics, isoenzyme analysis and the PCR to obtain information about the origin and nature of the colony-forming cell.

Tracking and localizing cells *in vivo*

The development of reliable methods for following the movement of cells and localizing them has become important in several approaches to treatment and in understanding disease processes. The use of tumour-infiltrating lymphocytes (TILs) in cancer therapy requires a method for demonstrating that the cells actually reach the tumour; in bone marrow transplantation, marked stem cells would facilitate studies on the course and efficiency of engraftment. Early studies followed cells labelled with ^{51}chromium or tritiated thymidine, and fluorescein isothianate has been used more recently. These methods are unsatisfactory because they can affect cell viability, function and survival and the label gradually leaches out of the cells. Newer staining methods under evaluation include the use of lipophilic fluorescent dyes that bind irreversibly to lipids in the cell membrane and do not appear to affect cell viability or survival (Slezak and Horan, 1989).

Evaluation of marrow involvement and the distribution of disease by trephine biopsies are not reliable because the small samples are not representative of the marrow as a whole. In contrast, magnetic resonance imaging (MRI) permits examination of all of the marrow and has been shown to be a sensitive method for detecting myeloma, leukaemia and lymphoma (Hinks *et al.*, 1986; Ludwig *et al.*, 1987; Dohner *et al.*, 1989). Also, progress is being made with magnetic resonance spectroscopy of biological fluids which may be used to detect changes associated with malignancy and transplantation (de Certaines, 1990; Fossel, 1991).

Table 3.5 Methods for introducing foreign DNA into cells

Calcium phosphate/DNA co-precipitation
Cells co-phagocytose/endocytose $CaPO_4$ and DNA. Most suitable for adherent phagocytic cells. Less efficient for cells in suspension. May be toxic to some types of cell

Microinjection
DNA is injected directly into the nucleus. Number and localization of injected cells can be recorded. Difficult with small cells. Non-adherent cells must be immobilized. Tedious

Pricking
Cells suspended in solution pricked with a microneedle to permit entry of DNA. Similar to microinjection

Electroporation
Application of a direct current pulse to a cell suspension induces the formation of pores for entry of DNA. Suitable for cells in suspension. Comparatively expensive

DNA packaging
DNA sealed in membranous vesicles (liposomes; fusogenic virus envelopes; bacterial plasmid protoplasts) which fuse to the cell membrane and deposit DNA directly into the cytoplasm

Retroviral vectors
Virus particle delivers DNA into cell via cell surface receptors. DNA integrated into host cell genome. High efficiency; low copy number; constraints on size of DNA

The potential value in this field of introducing genetic markers into cells has gained much attention recently. Table 3.5 lists the gene transfer techniques that have been used with varying degrees of success. Obviously, not all of them are appropriate for the manipulation of haemopoietic stem cells (microinjection, for example, requires identification of individual target cells) and the methods that have been applied most frequently and/or successfully to studies of haemopoiesis are infection with retroviral vectors and electroporation. Retroviruses provide an efficient gene delivery system but require elaborate methodology. Electroporation, on the other hand, is relatively simple, fast and convenient (see Donovan-Peluso and Bank, 1989, and references therein).

Genetic markers were used by Rosenberg and his colleagues (1990) to demonstrate that TIL cells injected intravenously migrate to the tumour and that this is associated with tumour regression. In time, this finding is likely to be extended to the introduction of an anticancer cytokine gene (e.g. tumour necrosis factor; TNF) into the TIL cells so that high TNF concentrations can be produced locally (see Culliton, 1989, 1990). Similar approaches can be used to study engraftment and lymphocyte traffic in bone marrow transplantation (see Culliton, 1990) and retrovirally inserted markers have been used to study engraftment in mice by murine (Capel et al., 1989) and recently by human (Dick et al., 1991) haemopoietic stem cells.

Transfer of foreign genes into the fertilized egg results in the production of transgenic animals with genomic integration of the foreign DNA and expression of the transgene product in their tissues. Although the regulation of gene expression in these animals is not fully understood, they are already providing model systems for pathological conditions in humans and a means of investigating *in vivo* the normal functions of a range of gene products.

GENES AND PROTEINS OF SPECIAL INTEREST

Certain genes and their products are of particular interest in the study of haematological disease, either because they are disease-specific, and therefore provide markers for abnormal cell populations as well as conferring abnormal functional properties, or because they are important for normal cellular functions and are altered in disease. Some of the genes are summarized in Table 3.6.

The tumour markers retinoic acid receptor α (RARα)/*myl* and BCR/ABL are rearranged as a result of specific chromosomal translocations that occur in all cases of acute promyelocytic leukaemia (APL;M3) and CML respectively. They are highly specific markers of these diseases and can be used as diagnostic aids and to monitor disease.

Table 3.6 Genes of interest in haematological malignancies

Classification	Putative role
Tumour markers	
Retinoic acid receptor α (RARα)/*myl*	Marker for acute promyelocytic leukaemia (M3)
BCR/ABL	Marker for chronic myeloid leukaemia (CML)
Immunoglobulin (Ig) genes	Clonally rearranged in B cell malignancy
T cell receptor (TCR) genes	Clonally rearranged in T cell malignancy
Tumour suppressor genes	
Gene encoding p53	Derepression of malignant clones in AML, CML and CLL
Retinoblastoma (RB) gene	
Multidrug-resistance gene (MDR1)	Drug resistance in leukaemia
BCL-2	Increased cell survival by preventing programmed cell death (apoptosis) in B lymphoma
Proto-oncogenes	
c-*sis* (growth factor gene)	Proliferative events involved in the pathogenesis of leukaemias, and other haematological malignancies
c-*fms* (growth factor receptor gene)	
c-*src* (cytoplasmic protein tyrosine kinase)	
ras (signal transduction)	
c-*myc/myb/fos* (nuclear proteins)	
Transcription factors/homeobox genes	Abnormalities of gene transcription in leukaemias and lymphoma

AML, acute myeloid leukaemia; CLL, chronic lymphoblastic leukaemia; CML, chronic myeloid leukaemia.

The immunoglobulin (Ig) genes and T cell receptor (TCR) genes are rearranged as part of normal B cell and T cell development. In normal cell populations, very large numbers of clones are produced but none of them is sufficiently prominent to produce a distinct band on a Southern blot. In clonal lymphoproliferative diseases, however, there is only one predominant clone and this can be detected as a specific band on a gel.

The multidrug-resistant (MDR) phenotype that has been demonstrated for a number of normal and malignant cell types is the result of increased expression of the MDR1 gene. This is a member of a multigene family where the number of genes differs between species. There are two in humans, MDR1 and MDR2, and MDR1 can be subdivided into MDR1a and MDR1b. Expression of the MDR2 gene does not confer resistance to drugs. The MDR1 gene encodes P-glycoprotein (P-gp) which is a transmembrane protein that appears to function as an energy-dependent efflux pump for a variety of lipophilic compounds (Kane et al., 1990; Roninson, 1991). Since drug-resistance is a major obstacle in the treatment of malignant disease, the expression of MDR1 has been widely studied. Certain drugs, such as cisplatin, methotrexate and 5-fluorouracil, are not pumped out by P-gp and produce marrow suppression equally in normal mice and in mice that express the human MDR1 transgene (Mickisch et al., 1991). These mice can therefore be used as a screen for new agents that bypass the effects of MDR1 gene expression. The activity of the P-gp pump can be inhibited by a variety of commonly used clinical agents such as verapamil, quinidine, quinine and cyclosporin A.

The retinoblastoma (RB) gene has been mapped to chromosome 13q14 (Sparkes et al., 1983) and encodes a nuclear phosphoprotein with a molecular weight of 105 kDa (Lee et al., 1987). Inactivation of RB seems to be critical for the development of retinoblastoma (Dryja et al., 1984) and for some solid tumours (Benedict et al., 1988; Harbour et al., 1988; Horowitz et al., 1990). It may also play a part in the development of some lymphoid neoplasms (Cheng et al., 1990; Ginsberg et al., 1991; Weide et al., 1991). Mutations of the p53 gene, which is located on chromosome 17, are now emerging as a common genetic alteration in human cancer (Levine et al., 1991). They are generally thought of as producing changes in a tumour suppressor gene but some mutants of p53 gain a function so that they become able to stimulate cell proliferation.

Translocations involving the q32 region of chromosome 14 (the location of the immunoglobulin heavy chain gene) are common in B cell non-Hodgkin's lymphoma (NHL). The t(14;18) translocation, in particular, involves the BCL-2 gene with consequent increased expression. Since high levels of BCL-2 transcription occur in normal pre-B cell development but are down-regulated in mature cells, and since lymphomas with the t(14;18) translocation produce large amounts of BCL-2 protein, dysregulation of the gene is implicated in the development of the malignancy (Cotter, 1990). It is thought that BCL-2 gene expression prolongs cell survival by preventing programmed cell death (apoptosis; Schwartz et al., 1990) and this might allow a clone to survive (McDonnell et al., 1989) until other genetic changes, such as activation of c-*myc* (Vaux et al., 1988), occur and render the cell neoplastic.

Oncogenes were first detected in RNA tumour viruses as causative agents in tumorigenesis in chicken, mice and rats. Subsequently, homologous sequences were found in normal cells and these are referred to as cellular proto-oncogenes. They are important for normal cellular functions and include genes encoding growth factors, receptors, cytoplasmic PTKs, proteins involved in signal transduction and nuclear factors involved in the control of cell proliferation and self-renewal. Therefore, alterations in the form or expression of these genes by point mutations, amplification or chromosomal translocation can be expected to play an important role in the development of malignancy (Minden, 1987).

Gene transcription is regulated by DNA-binding transcription factors which *transactivate* gene expression by interacting with specific *cis-acting* promotor elements. Transcription factors can be divided into families according to the way in which they interact structurally with DNA. Some of the terminology gives an instant impression of the way in which such DNA-binding interactions might be accomplished. Thus, transcription factors may be characterized conformationally as 'zinc finger' proteins, 'leucine zipper' proteins or 'helix–loop–helix' proteins, according to the secondary structure which is thought to govern sequence-specific binding to DNA. The genes that encode some of these proteins are known oncogenes such as *jun* and *fos* (leucine zipper) and *myc* (helix–loop–helix; Busch and Sassone-Corsi, 1990). The homeobox genes encompass a highly conserved sequence of 60 residues (the homeobox domain) which encodes a protein sequence with helix–turn–helix secondary structure and is found throughout the animal kingdom. The corresponding proteins act as transcriptional regulators during embryogenesis (Hunt and Krumlauf, 1991) and in adults the genes are expressed in specific tissues. In the haemopoietic system, they may be involved in the control of haemopoietic cell differentiation.

Knowledge about the normal functions of certain proteins (Table 3.7) and of the behaviour of malignant cells suggests that they might be altered in malignancy. For example, the nature of cell adhesion molecules (CAMs) and 'homing' receptors suggests that abnormal expression could have considerable impact on the dissemination and spread of malignant cells. The lymphocyte 'homing' receptors play a central role in the physiology of lymphocyte recirculation and, in humans, CD44 is responsible for interaction with high endothelial venules (HEVs), a necessary step for their migration from the blood

Table 3.7 Proteins of interest in haematological disorders

Cell adhesion molecules/'homing' receptors	CD44; CD11a/18; CD54
Growth factors and soluble receptors	IL-1β; TNFβ; IL-2-receptor
Shed tumour-associated antigens	CD9; CD30
Enzymes/enzyme inhibitors	TIMP-1; PAI-2
Myeloma protein	
Haemoglobin	

IL-1β, Interleukin 1β; TNFβ, tumour necrosis factor; TIMP, tissue inhibitor of metalloproteinases; PAI, plasminogen activator inhibitor.

into the surrounding tissues (Picker et al., 1989). Recent studies indicate that the role(s) of these molecules in the progression of ALL are amenable to study by transplantation into severe combined immunodeficiency (SCID) mice (Cesano et al., 1991).

The lymphocyte function-associated antigen-1 (LFA-1; CD11a/18) and its ligand (ICAM-1; CD54) are important for cell–cell interactions required for the initiation of the immune response (Springer et al., 1987; see Chapter 6).

The levels of growth factors or soluble growth factor receptors in serum of cancer patients may reflect production and release by tumour cells or may be caused by an indirect tumour-mediated activity on normal cells. In both cases, however, these molecules can provide an indication of tumour bulk. In hairy cell leukaemia, for example, measurements of soluble interleukin 2 (IL-2) receptor have been used as a measure of leukaemic cell burden and may be informative in a variety of other lymphoid malignancies (Pizzoli et al., 1987). Monoclonal myeloma protein provides a marker for the disease and abnormal haemoglobins are central to the investigation of the haemoglobinopathies.

Secretion of a variety of other products, particularly enzymes or enzyme inhibitors, may influence the behaviour of malignant cells or act on normal tissue. Examples include plasminogen activator inhibitor (PAI), an inhibitor of urokinase, and inhibitors of metalloproteinases (TIMP) (Kossakowska et al., 1991; Scherrer et al., 1991). Also, there is some evidence that leukaemic cells, at least *in vitro*, can secrete enzymes that degrade collagen and proteoglycans in extracellular matrix. Such activities can be expected to influence matrix turnover and be associated with metastasis and tissue invasiveness.

APPLICATIONS TO HAEMATOLOGICAL DISEASE

Chronic myeloid leukaemia

At the molecular level, the chronic phase of CML is probably the most thoroughly studied haematological neoplasm. This is largely a consequence of the unique chromosome marker, the Philadelphia (Ph^1) chromosome, that is present in all patients with the disease.

Diagnosis

At presentation, patients with CML usually have a grossly elevated leukocyte count ($100-500 \times 10^9$/l), including eosinophilia and basophilia, and an enlarged spleen. There is a marked deficiency in neutrophil (leukocyte) alkaline phosphatase (LAP) which serves to

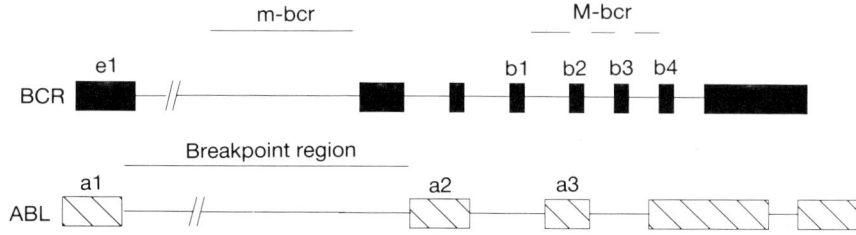
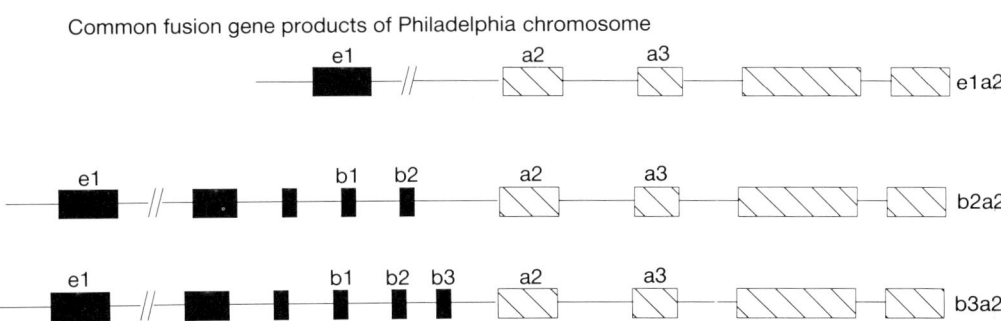

Fig. 3.4 Genetic rearrangements involved in the formation of the BCR/ABL fusion gene in CML and ALL.

distinguish the disease from reactive neutrophilia when the LAP score is high. The Ph[1] chromosome translocation (t(9;22)) is present in virtually all cases of CML and diagnosis can be confirmed by karyotyping the patient's cells. The translocation results in juxtaposition of the BCR gene (so-called because of its identification as the region of the major breakpoint cluster region) and the cellular proto-oncogene ABL (Fig. 3.4). The breakpoint on chromosome 9 occurs in a relatively large (approx 200 kb) region at the 5' end of the ABL gene, whereas the breakpoint on chromosome 22 occurs within the 5.8 kb major breakpoint cluster region (M-BCR). The breakpoints within M-BCR can be even more finely mapped to different positions so that they may be relatively 5' or 3'. Thus, the ABL gene can be linked downstream of exon 2 of M-BCR (b2a2 junction) or of exon 3 of M-BCR (b3a2 junction).

The rearrangement results in the production of hybrid messenger RNA and a hybrid BCR/ABL protein tyrosine kinase (p210) with activity that is greater than that of the normal p145 ABL gene product (Chan *et al.*, 1987). The gene and its products have been defined molecularly and can be detected using the methods described in the previous section.

Classical CML can occur without karyotypically detectable Ph[1] chromosome, which resulted in considerable debate about the molecular nature of these cases. However, BCR rearrangements were found on Southern analysis of Ph^1 chromosome-negative leukaemias, together with production of the characteristic p210 PTK (Wiedemann et al., 1988).

Molecular techniques have also been used to distinguish between Ph^1-positive cases of ALL and a lymphoid blast crisis of CML. Six per cent of children and 17–25% of adults with ALL are Ph^1-positive on karyotyping and, at this level, the translocations in CML and ALL are indistinguishable. However, rearrangement of BCR occurred in only one of the four cases of Ph^1-positive ALL investigated by Chan et al. (1987), indicating that a karyotypic Ph^1 translocation can occur without involving BCR. In these cases, the ABL gene is affected by the translocation because the cells express a p190 PTK which can be distinguished from the p210 expressed by CML cells and the p145 expressed by normal cells. The role of this protein in the aetiology of ALL will be discussed in the section on acute leukaemia.

Clonality

The clonal origin of CML in a progenitor that is common to the granulocytic, eosinophilic, basophilic, monocytic, erythroid, megakaryocytic and B lymphoid lineages is well-accepted (Canellos and Griffin, 1985; Champlin and Golde, 1985). The involvement of the T lymphoid lineage has been less clear. Giannone et al. (1988) reported a case who relapsed after bone marrow transplantation with a T cell supraclavicular lymphadenopathy that had the same BCR rearrangement as the bone marrow prior to bone marrow transplantation. Another case demonstrates that the blast cells in T lymphoblastic crisis can express the p210 PTK that characterizes CML rather than lymphoblastic leukaemias (Schuh et al., 1990). These cases indicate that CML can originate in precursor cells that are common to the T lymphoid and myeloid cells.

Pathogenesis

Although the molecular pathology of CML is known in detail (Morgan and Wiedemann, 1989) there is very little information about the function of p210 in the leukaemic cells. Lymphoid cells expressing p210 proliferate in retrovirally infected murine long-term cultures (Young and Witte, 1988) but, until recently, no *in vivo* model of CML was available. However, Daley et al. (1990) achieved retrovirus-mediated transfer of the p210 BCR/ABL gene into mouse bone marrow and obtained a myeloproliferative disease resembling CML in some animals transplanted with the infected cells. These model systems, plus elucidation of the effects of BCR/ABL antisense oligonucleotides

(Szczylik *et al.*, 1991) and progress with gene transfer into normal haemopoietic stem cells (Miller, 1990), should help to answer questions about the role of p210 protein in the pathogenesis of CML and mechanisms of disease progression.

Prognosis

The management of patients with CML is governed by the triphasic course of the disease. The chronic phase is of variable duration (median 3–4 years) and is followed by either an abrupt transformation to an acute blastic phase or an intermediate accelerated stage followed by blast transformation. Survival in the acute blast phase of the disease is limited to months. Prediction of the onset of transformation would be valuable for patient management but no universally applicable test has emerged.

Blast crisis cells in 80% of Ph[1]-positive cases of CML display additional chromosomal abnormalities (Rowley, 1978), commonly double Ph[1] chromosomes, isochromosome 17 and/or trisomy 8. Southern blot analyses have shown that multiple Ph[1] chromosomes can occur in all lineages at the time of transformation (Collins and Groudine, 1987). These cytogenetic changes, which presumably were acquired during the chronic phase, are a significant determinant of short survival following transformation (Coleman *et al.*, 1980; Kantarjian *et al.*, 1987). The transformed cells in CML may be lymphoid, myeloid or undifferentiated and Bernstein and Gale (1990) suggested that the actual phenotype expressed was determined by the additional cytogenetic changes acquired before transformation.

Several studies (see Birnie *et al.*, 1989 for review) suggested that the precise location of the breakpoint on chromosome 22 predicted the length of the chronic phase, which was longer in cases with 5' breakpoints and shorter in cases with 3' breakpoints. Other studies reached the opposite conclusion (Jaubert *et al.*, 1990; Tefferi *et al.*, 1990a). The results are quite difficult to interpret because it is difficult to identify the onset of the chronic phase and, therefore, to measure its duration. A recent series of case reports on the molecular genetics of CML patients who have survived in chronic phase for remarkably long periods of time (14–31 years) sheds some light on the puzzle (Birnie *et al.*, 1990; Johansson *et al.*, 1990; Price *et al.*, 1990; Sproul *et al.*, 1990). The noteworthy features of these patients were: first, a 3' rearrangement in M-BCR in one case and 5' rearrangements in two others; second, complete absence of the Ph[1]-positive clone in one case and confinement of the leukaemic clone to the bone marrow in another. Subsequently, Najean *et al.* (1991) reported a further unusual case in which a 27-year-long complete haematological and cytogenetic remission was followed by an acute leukaemia (M1) that had no rearrangement of BCR. Mills et al. (1991) have recently reviewed this area again and conclude that a prospective study is required to clarify the significance of the position of the breakpoint in M-BCR.

Lee et al. (1989) suggested that the type of BCR/ABL junction also influenced clinical responses to interferon α (IFNα). However, subsequent studies have shown that the position of the breakpoint does not affect the sensitivity of CML progenitor cells to treatment with IFN-α in vitro (Dowding et al., 1991) or the clinical course, conversion to blast crisis or survival of IFN-α-treated patients (Opalka et al., 1991). In a study of the causes of the development of drug-resistance in accelerated phase and blast crisis, Weide et al. (1991) examined the role of MDR-1/P-glycoprotein. They found that 5–30% of granulocytic cells in 4/11 patients expressed P-gp and 7/15 patients on treatment during chronic phase expressed similar levels. However, there was no correlation between the level of expression and response or resistance to therapy.

Activating point mutations in the *ras* gene family have been sought in cases of CML in blast crisis but have been found in only a minority of patients and do not provide a widespread marker (Ahuja et al., 1989; LeMaistre et al., 1989). The location of the p53 gene on chromosome 17 and the occurrence of isochromosome 17q and rearrangements in blast crisis have stimulated interest in the role of p53 in the evolution of CML (Ahuja et al., 1989; Kelman et al., 1989; Mashal et al., 1990; Feinstein et al., 1991). Although rearrangements of the p53 gene are found in blast crisis, they only occur in around 30% of patients.

The methylation status of genes relates to their availability for transcription so that increased methylation suppresses gene expression. Recent studies on calcitonin gene methylation have revealed that it is hypermethylated in CML blast crisis, as it is in AML (Malinken et al., 1991; Nelkin et al., 1991). It is possible that these changes reflect more widespread methylation changes in genes located on the short arm of chromosome 11, which is the location of the calcitonin gene and a region containing certain tumour suppressor genes.

Clearly, alterations in *ras*, p53 or calcitonin gene expression are not CML-specific; neither do they occur in all cases of acceleration towards blast crisis. However, if such changes are monitored in combination they might predict blast crisis in the majority of patients.

Detection and management of residual disease

Improvements in the therapy of CML, especially the use of allogeneic bone marrow transplantation (Goldman et al., 1988), have led to the possibility that Ph^1-negative, non-clonal haemopoiesis can be restored and the leukaemic cell population can be reduced below clinically detectable levels. Relapse, however, remains a major problem and is most likely to originate in residual diseased cells.

The PCR is the most sensitive available method for detecting extremely small numbers of cells with chromosomal translocations and has been applied to the measurement of residual disease in patients treated for CML. Some of the earlier literature in this area might be misleading as a result of technical problems, such as sampling errors and contamination with previously amplified material. Also, procedures have not been standardized and different authors use, for example, different numbers of cycles, one- or two-stage procedures and may or may not use nested primers. These factors help to explain the discord among some of the published results (Hughes et al., 1990).

Notwithstanding some of the reservations about the use of PCR, the technique will ultimately help to determine the significance of small numbers of leukaemic cells in patients who appear to be in remission. It has been known for some time that patients with a few cytogenetically detectable Ph^1-positive cells after bone marrow transplantation do not necessarily relapse (Goldman, 1988) and that transient cytogenetic relapses apparently occur. More recent studies using PCR have confirmed that BCR/ABL message can be detected in transplanted CML patients for the first month after normal marrow infusion. Thereafter, some remain positive, some become negative and the rest remain positive but in remission for prolonged periods of time (Roth et al., 1989). Hughes et al. (1991) have concluded from their study of 23 patients transplanted in chronic phase that the PCR result may be positive for as long as 6 months after transplantation in patients who can still expect a long-lasting remission. A positive PCR result later on, however, indicates that the likelihood of a cure may be reduced. Some workers have been unable to detect any leukaemic messenger RNA in any patients who had been given a bone marrow transplant 5–7 years previously, which suggests that patients who survive this long are in fact cured of their disease (Morgan et al., 1989). Martiat et al. (1990) found those patients in remission for more than 2 years lacked any detectable BCR/ABL message whilst Pignon et al. (1990) detected BCR/ABL transcripts up to 5 years after transplantation. In a prospective study, molecular relapse on PCR grounds preceded cytogenetic relapse in those patients who relapsed clinically but not all patients with molecular relapse relapsed clinically (Sawyers et al., 1990).

The probability of relapse is increased in patients who have been transplanted with T cell-depleted marrow in an effort to reduce graft-versus-host disease (Goldman et al., 1988). Some studies using PCR suggest that there is a higher rate of detection in patients who have received T-depleted marrow, but others see no difference between the two groups of patients (Bartram *et al.*, 1989; Gabert *et al.*, 1989; Lange *et al.*, 1989; Delfau *et al.*, 1990).

Haematological responses to IFN-α have been reported by a number of groups (see Goldman, 1988) and there is some evidence that the leukaemic clone is preferentially suppressed by IFN therapy. However, the leukaemic stem cell may not be eradicated. Lee *et al.* (1988) performed sequential studies on blood samples from two IFN-α-treated patients who were in complete haematological and cytogenetic remission but in whom molecular relapse was detected using PCR.

Myeloproliferative disorders

Clonality

Raskind *et al.* (1985) derived Epstein–Barr virus-transformed B lymphoblastoid cell lines from G6PD heterozygotes with either polycythaemia vera (PV) or essential thrombocythaemia (ET). They demonstrated that 108 of the 117 polycythaemia lines and 104 of the 109 thrombocythaemia lines expressed the single isoenzyme type found in the abnormal clone of haemopoietic cells. Thus, in the majority of cases, both PV and ET involve a pluripotent lympho-myeloid stem cell.

Restriction fragment length polymorphisms of the X chromosome genes PGK and HPRT have been used to study clonality in a variety of myeloproliferative disorders and have been informative in about 40–50% of cases (Lucas *et al.*, 1989; Anger *et al.*, 1990). Again, the majority of patients have clonal haemopoiesis and, since this feature distinguishes PV and ET from increases in red cell or platelet mass due to other causes, it can contribute to the early diagnosis of the myeloproliferative conditions.

Gilliland *et al.* (1991) used PCR to allow RFLP analysis of single haemopoietic colonies cultured from the blood of patients with PV and found that erythroid clonality was a consistent feature of the disease, whereas myeloid involvement in the disease clone was variable. This suggests that some cases of PV can originate either in a common myeloerythroid progenitor or in a progenitor already committed to erythroid differentiation. Also, results of a study of two sisters suggested that ET can arise at different levels of haemopoietic cell development. In one sister, the abnormal clone included granulocytes, monocytes and T cells in addition to megakaryocytes; in the other, only the granulocyte lineage was additionally involved (Janssen *et al.*, 1990).

Pathogenesis and prognosis

Some cases of myeloproliferative disease are marked by the Philadelphia chromosome. Molecular studies of DNA and RNA from Ph^1-positive ET patients have shown abnormalities that are indistinguishable from those in CML, which may explain the poor prognosis of Ph^1-positive ET and its increased risk of terminating in acute leukaemia (Martiat et al., 1989).

Acute myeloid leukaemia

Clonality

The prevailing view of AML is one of a monoclonal neoplasm originating from a single transformed haemopoietic cell which proliferates uncontrollably to produce the leukaemic blast cell population. However, detailed cytogenetic and phenotypic analyses have revealed some unexpected results with respect to the occurrence of disparate clones and to the cell populations that can turn out to be members of the leukaemic clone.

In a review of the literature, Heim and Mitelman (1989) found that about 1% of patients with AML had cytogenetically unrelated abnormal clones whilst Hayashi et al. (1989) reported two children with originally monoclonal disease who relapsed with two independent clones (one of which was typical of therapy-related disease). In another study, Hiorns et al. (1989) reported the restriction of an N-*ras* mutation to blast and monocytic cell fractions associated with a K-*ras* mutation in cells of all lineages. This observation indicates that the K-*ras* mutation occurred earlier than the N-*ras* mutation. Thus, whilst monoclonality may be the general rule in AML, it is not universal and may be obscured by progressive clonal evolution of the malignant cell population.

In addition, there is new evidence showing that some parts of the leukaemic clone in AML can mature relatively normally. Basophils, for example, can be part of the clone in cases involving the breakpoint 9q34 (Bodger et al., 1990), multiple lineages are involved in erythroleukaemia (Cuneo et al., 1990) and granulocyte precursors are involved in megakaryocytic (M7) leukaemia (Najfeld et al., 1988).

Pathogenesis

Recently, the role of autocrine stimulation in AML cells has received much attention as a possible pathogenetic mechanism. Blast cells from some AML patients are able to proliferate *in vitro* without the addition of growth factors and themselves secrete cytokine activities into culture medium. Earlier studies using Northern analysis and bioassays to detect growth factor production by AML cells implicated granulocyte-macrophage colony-stimulating factor (GM-CSF), M-CSF, G-CSF and IL-1β as autocrine stimulators of blast cell proliferation (Sakai *et al.*, 1987; Young *et al.*, 1987; Rambaldi *et al.*, 1988; Shirafuji *et al.*, 1988). In another study, spontaneous GM-CSF expression was rare but could be induced by exposure to TNF. Spontaneous expression of messenger RNA for IL-6 was more common. Rearrangement of a growth factor gene (in this instance, G-CSF) was found only in a single case, which emphasizes the rarity of this particular type of abnormality in AML (Fiedler *et al.*, 1990a). However, nucleic acid hybridization techniques cannot discriminate between factor production by leukaemic cells and production by any contaminating normal cells. Neither do they give any information about the numbers of cells contributing to factor production. The first problem can be avoided by purifying blast cells but these procedures, in some way, can induce or increase factor production by the leukaemic cells (Kaufman *et al.*, 1988; Young *et al.*, 1988). *In situ* hybridization, on the other hand, permits detection of RNA transcripts in single cells and has been used recently to show that up to 40% of blast cells from most cases of AML express transcripts for IL-1β. In spite of the association between AML and the production of growth factors, it is not entirely certain that autocrine growth factor production and stimulation by haemopoietic cells is pathological. It may be a physiological event in early cells, since a limited number of studies have detected induced growth factor (GM-CSF; IL-6) production in human (Bot *et al.*, 1990) or murine (Lotem *et al.*, 1987; Schneider *et al.*, 1991) blast cells exposed to IL-1α or IL-3.

Receptor abnormalities could also be involved in the pathogenesis of leukaemia and mutations of the M-CSF receptor (the c-*fms* gene) have been detected in some cases of myeloid leukaemia (Ridge *et al.*, 1990; Tobal *et al.*, 1990). The codons affected were numbers 302 and 969 which have been shown to be oncogenic in *in vitro* experiments (Roussel *et al.*, 1988). Also, *fms* gene expression has been documented in a number of AML subtypes (Dubreil *et al.*, 1988; Rambaldi *et al.*, 1988).

Rearrangements of the RARα chain as a consequence of the t(15;17)(q22;q11–21) translocation (Rowley *et al.*, 1977) have emerged as specific molecular markers in APL (M3; Chomienne *et al.*, 1990a; Lo Coco *et al.*, 1991) and are associated with clinical responses to all-trans-retinoic acid (Chomienne *et al.*, 1990b; Castaigne *et al.*, 1990). The breakpoint on chromosome 17 involves the RARα gene, whilst that on chromosome 15 involves the *myl* gene. Since rearrangements of RARα occur in 92% of cases, and rearrangements of *myl* in 73% of cases and of one or the other in 100% of cases, it is now possible to identify and monitor disease in all patients with APL (Biondi et al., 1991).

The p53 gene also is located on chromosome 17 (17p13). There is a high incidence of p53 point mutations in AML patients with monosomy of chromosome 17p but a very low incidence in patients with a normal 17p (Fenaux et al., 1991; Slingerland et al., 1991). Since the p53 gene is thought to be a tumour suppressor gene, these changes could be involved in the pathogenesis of the disease. Moreover, the association between monosomy of 17p and p53 mutations supports a recessive, rather than a dominant, model of tumour suppression.

Ahuja et al. (1990) have analysed 161 patients with haematological malignancies for mutations in ras genes and compared their findings with the published literature. They concluded that only mutations of the N-ras genes occurred with any significant frequency whilst mutations of K-ras and Ha-ras were rare. The mutations involved amino acid substitutions in codons 12 or 13 and were found in 25% of cases of AML. A similar frequency occurred in the myelodysplastic syndromes and a lower frequency (14%) in ALL. These mutations seem to be restricted to the acute leukaemias and related disorders since none were found in chronic-phase CML, lymphomas or myelomas. They may be particularly associated with therapy-related secondary leukaemias (Inokuchi et al., 1991) and those resulting from environmental exposure but otherwise do not identify clearly a subset of patients with AML.

Diagnosis and prognosis

Morphological examination of the blood and bone marrow remains important for the diagnosis of AML and the FAB classification is widely followed. Examination of cells by light microscopy can be supplemented by electron microscopy, ultrastructural cytochemistry and surface marker studies, which can be used to refine the diagnosis and obtain prognostic information (see Catovsky, 1991). Between 60 and 70% of patients enter complete remission following induction chemotherapy but 75% of them relapse. Only 15–20% of patients achieve a long-term disease-free survival and efforts have been made to identify patients with good or poor prognoses.

Some 60% of all patients with AML have at least one chromosome abnormality detectable on karyotypic analysis. Most studies find that there is a correlation between cytogenetic observations and the complete remission (CR) rate in response to therapy. In general, there is agreement that patients with t(8;21), t(15;17) and inv(16) achieve high CR rates whereas patients with complex rearrangements or rearrange-

Table 3.8 Correlations between cytogenetics and prognosis in treated AML patients

	CR rate (%)	Median CR duration (months)	Median survival (months)
All patients	59–75	15–19	Not reported
Inv/del (16)	80–100	10–23+	23
t(8;21)	75–95	8–27	15.3
t(15;17)	52–80	9.5–28	14.5–20
11q23	40–84	3–5	9–23
+8	35–80	8.5–24	10–28

See Fenaux et al. (1989) for references.
AML, Acute myeloid leukaemia; CR, complete remission.

ments involving chromosomes 5 and/or 7 achieve a low CR rate (Table 3.8 and see Fenaux et al., 1989, for references). Some groups have documented high remission rates for patients with trisomy of chromosome 8 and abnormalities of 11q23, but others have not.

The disease-free survival (DFS) of patients achieving CR can in some cases be related to karyotypic rearrangements. For example, inv(16) seems to be related to a good prognosis in this respect but opinions about the impact of t(15;17) and t(8;21) are divided. Of course, the correlations between karyotype and response to therapy are heavily influenced by the type of treatment given to the patients but, overall, cytogenetics have provided some valuable prognostic indices in AML.

Expression of the multidrug-resistance gene MDR-1 might be another determinant of difficulty in remission-induction because Sato et al. (1990) reported high levels of MDR-1 expression in patients who were relatively resistant to chemotherapy. Marie et al. (1991) found a significant inverse association between the level of MDR-1 expression and complete remission, such that the remission rate in patients with low MDR-1 expression was more than twice that of patients with high levels of expression.

The influence of proto-oncogene expression on treatment outcome in AML has been evaluated by Preisler and colleagues (1989). In particular, a high level of c-*myc* expression is associated with a low probability of achieving CR. In contrast, c-*fms* expression is positively associated with a complete remission rate. Also, there may be an inverse correlation between the levels of IL-1β transcripts and remission duration (Preisler et al., 1989).

Detection and management of minimal residual disease

Using an *in situ* immunological phenotyping technique, Gerhartz and Schmetzer (1990) were able to distinguish between clones of normal and leukaemic origin in colony cultures of patients' cells. They were able to demonstrate the persistence of leukaemic progenitors in the majority of cases who were in complete haematological remission. Miller et al. (1991) measured the sensitivity of these occult progenitors to 4-hydroperoxycyclophosphamide and showed that it correlated with the probability of relapse following autologous bone marrow transplantation.

Myelodysplasia

Myelodysplasia refers to a group of well-defined disorders which are characterized by qualitative and quantitative abnormalities of haemopoiesis, progressive bone marrow failure and a tendency to develop AML.

Clonality

The clonality of haemopoiesis in the myelodysplastic syndromes (MDS) has been established by G6PD isoenzyme analysis, which shows that the target cell affected by the disease process is a lymphomyeloid stem cell and that subsequent clonal evolution might involve a committed myeloid progenitor cell (Raskind et al., 1984). This impression has been confirmed using RFLP analysis of HPRT and PGK genes (Janssen et al., 1989). Tefferi et al. (1990b) analysed separate T lymphocyte, neutrophil and monocyte fractions and found a similar monoclonal pattern in each, further demonstrating that the abnormal clone is capable of lymphoid and myeloid differentiation. In this particular study, one patient with refractory anaemia had a polyclonal marrow population, which could reflect an early stage in the development of MDS.

Pathogenesis

The 5q− syndrome (i.e. an interstitial deletion of the long arm of chromosome 5) is a distinctive MDS characterized by refractory anaemia and poorly lobulated megakaryocytes (Van den Berghe et al., 1974). Several genes for the haemopoietic growth factors and their receptors, including the *fms* gene which encodes the M-CSF receptor, have been localized to the long arm of chromosome 5, and it has been postulated that their loss may play a part in the pathogenesis of myeloid disorders. In all of the largest group of 5q− patients studied to date, Boultwood et al. (1991) found hemizygous (6/10) or homozygous (4/10) loss of the M-CSF receptor gene. This finding supports the idea that loss of haemopoietic growth factor and receptor genes is a critical event that might result in abnormal cellular maturation. Alternatively, 5q− deletion could result in the loss of an unidentified tumour suppressor gene, analogous to the RB gene, especially in those cases with homozygous gene loss. Mutations of the c-*fms* gene have also been implicated in the pathogenesis of MDS as well as in the pathogenesis of AML (Ridge *et al.*, 1990; Tobal *et al.*, 1990), suggesting that this event could be an early step in the development of human myeloid leukaemia.

Mutations of N-*ras* genes are found, in most studies, in about 24% of cases of MDS, which is the same as their frequency in AML (Ahuja *et al.*, 1990). In other studies, the incidence has been higher. Also, Ha-*ras*, c-*myc* and c-*fos* have been implicated. It is of interest that transfection of these genes confers a multidrug-resistant phenotype (Bhushan *et al.*, 1989; Kadoyama *et al.*, 1989) since multidrug resistance is detected more commonly in MDS than in *de novo* AML. Also, certain chemical carcinogens are potent inducers of MDR1 gene expression (Burt and Thorgeirsson, 1988) and an epidemiological survey of MDS patients has revealed a very high incidence of exposure to petrochemicals and other potential mutagens (Farrow *et al.*, 1989).

Prognosis

Generally, MDS responds poorly to chemotherapy. Studies of the multidrug resistance gene (MDR1) that encodes P-gp have shown that the gene is overexpressed in MDS and may contribute to clinical drug resistance (Holmes *et al.*, 1989; List *et al.*, 1991).

Depending on the technique used for analysis, mutations in codons 12 or 13 of the N-*ras* gene occur in up to 40% of patients. These point mutations result in activation of the *ras* gene which has been implicated in the progression of MDS to AML (Lyons *et al.*, 1988; Bar-Eli *et al.*, 1989).

Studies of *in vitro* colony formation have been found to predict progression to AML by some groups (Raymakers *et al.*, 1991) but not by others (Schipperus *et al.*, 1988). The FAB classification (Bennett *et al.*, 1982), the Bournemouth score grading the severity of cytopenia in different lineages (Mufti *et al.*, 1985) and the numbers of cytogenetic abnormalities (Yunis *et al.*, 1986) all correlate with prognosis, as might be expected from the clinical features and natural history of the disease.

Bone marrow transplantation

Donor selection

The selection of a family member as a donor of bone marrow for transplantation can quite safely rely on serological human leukocyte antigen (HLA)-DR and DQ matching, which has a 98% positive correlation with a negative result in the mixed lymphocyte reaction (MLR). This correlation falls to 25% when the potential donor is not related to the patient and other ways have been sought to improve the selection process. These include the use of RFLP analysis, which has been evaluated by Bidwell *et al.* (1987) and Clay *et al.* (1989). Their results suggest that, whilst RFLP analysis of DR and DQ cannot predict a negative MLR response, it should provide a useful preliminary screen because RFLP non-identity always accompanied MLR reactivity. Thus, it is possible to reduce the number of MLR tests required for donor selection from an unrelated panel. The technique can also be used to confirm monozygosity in donor–recipient pairs who are assumed to be identical twins (Jones *et al.*, 1987).

Donations of blood from cytomegalovirus (CMV)-infected individuals is of major significance in clinical transplantation but current serological tests to detect infection are inaccurate, time-consuming and costly. The PCR approach, using three sets of primers, was tested on 420 normal donors at a blood donation centre (Bevan *et al.*, 1991). Although some problems remain, PCR may provide a practical solution to rapid screening for CMV amongst potential donors. It has also been used to detect human immunodeficiency virus 1 and human T lymphotropic virus I in blood donations (Sunzeri *et al.*, 1991) and may prove to be useful in the automated screening for a variety of pathogens.

Chimerism

Documentation of the donor or host origin of haemopoiesis in transplant recipients is important in situations associated with an increased risk of graft failure, rejection or leukaemic relapse. Several methods

Table 3.9 Methods for documenting early engraftment, graft failure and leukaemic relapse in bone marrow transplant recipients

Method	Description
Erythrocyte antigen typing	Applicable only to erythroid lineage; obscured by transfusion
HLA typing	Requires HLA non-identity
Leukocyte isoenzymes	Leukocytes only
Immunoglobulin isotypes	Lymphoid only
Karyotyping, Barr body and sex chromatin	Rarely applicable if donor and recipient are of the same sex

HLA, Human leukocyte antigen.

are available for this purpose, but none of them is generally applicable for one reason or another (Table 3.9).

Lineage-specific chimerism can be determined by combining phenotypic analysis, cell separation and *in situ* hybridization for the Y chromosome (which can be applied to interphase cells). This approach has been used to demonstrate that host cells decrease rapidly in patients who engrafted (Przepiorka *et al.*, 1990). Alternatively, karyotypic analysis of lymphoid and myeloid colonies grown from the marrow of transplanted patients has been used to distinguish donor- and host-derived haemopoiesis (Schmitz *et al.*, 1991).

In comparison with the earlier methods, RFLP analysis has several advantages. Probes that hybridize to polymorphic regions outside the HLA complex can be used; all nucleated cells can be studied; cell division is not necessary, and it does not depend on sex differences between donor and recipient. Granulocytes, T cells, B cells and monocytes can be analysed separately to distinguish between complete engraftment and mixed lymphomyeloid chimerism (Ginsberg *et al.*, 1985; Petz *et al.*, 1987). Follow-up studies using minisatellite probes have shown that engraftment can be detected as soon as 10 days after transplantation and that a single hybridization is informative in 100% of cases (Mareni *et al.*, 1990).

The use of RFLP probes in this context is, however, complicated by the fact that the donor and recipient are often siblings and cannot, therefore, be distinguished by a single genetic marker in 25% of cases. Even the use of a highly polymorphic sequence cannot guarantee success. This constraint can be overcome to a large extent by using multiple probes (Ginsberg *et al.*, 1985; Knowlton *et al.*, 1986), but this is cumbersome and time-consuming. Improved results have been obtained using hypervariable minisatellite DNA probes (Jeffreys *et al.*, 1985; Thein *et al.*, 1986) or specific 'designer' oligonucleotide probes (Yam *et al.*, 1987). Ugozzoli *et al.* (1991) used PCR to amplify polymorphic loci targeted by synthetic oligonucleotide probes and were able to detect mixed or complete chimerism, endogenous repopulation of haemopoiesis and recurrent leukaemia. This method had the advantages over RFLP analysis of high sensitivity, a requirement for small amounts of DNA, simplicity and speed.

Graft failure

Analysis of RFLPs has been used to document early failure to engraftment, late graft failure and autologous marrow regeneration (Blazar *et al.*, 1985; Weitzel *et al.*, 1988). In aplastic anaemia, for example, late graft failure followed by autologous reconstitution was documented in some 20% of transplanted patients. Use of *in situ* hybridization for the Y chromosome plus phenotyping revealed an association between persistence of recipient non-major histocompatibility complex-restricted T cells (CD8+CD57+ and CD3+CD56+) and graft failure.

Relapse

The presence of Ph-positive metaphases in colonies grown from the marrow of patients transplanted for CML has been studied by Schmitz et al. (1991). Their results indicate that relapse is accompanied by additional cytogenetic abnormalities at the progenitor cell level. Patient-specific RFLP patterns have been used to confirm the host origin of leukaemic cells at relapse in transplanted patients (Ginsberg et al., 1985; Minden et al., 1985) and, in rare cases, to identify tumours of donor origin (Schubach et al., 1982; Witherspoon et al., 1985).

Other complications

The PCR has been used to detect human CMV infection very soon after transplantation (Einsele et al., 1991). A rise in serum levels of TNFα may herald the onset of major transplant-related complications such as interstitial pneumonitis and acute graft-versus-host disease (Holler et al., 1990). Also, raised levels of soluble IL-2 receptor are associated with acute graft-versus-host disease and may help to distinguish it from, for example, a drug-sensitivity rash (Siegert et al., 1990).

Purging

In autologous transplantation, the reintroduction of malignant cells contaminating the bone marrow has always caused concern. This has been reinforced by the detection by methods of increasing sensitivity of residual leukaemic cells in patients who are, clinically and haematologically, in complete remission. Efforts to remove these cells *ex vivo* before the marrow is reinfused are referred to as 'purging' in the bone marrow transplant-related literature. Molecular knowledge and technology have contributed to innovations in purging procedures and also allow improved monitoring of the procedures themselves.

Appreciation of the influence that multidrug-resistance might have on purging methods dependent on cytotoxicity has led to tests of the effect of complement-mediated cytolysis using an antibody directed against the MDR-1 gene product, P-gp (Kulkarni et al., 1989; Aihara et al., 1991). This removed virtually all leukaemic cells and the purging efficiency was further enhanced by the addition of etoposide (VP-16).

Gene therapy

Bone marrow transplantation provides a vehicle for gene therapy, i.e. the insertion of a normal gene into an organism to correct a genetic defect. Bone marrow stem cells are ideal for this purpose because of their capacity to self-renew and produce expanded populations of progeny. Recombinant retroviruses have been the most commonly used system for introducing genes into haemopoietic cells (Lehn, 1990; Miller, 1990) and expression of integrated genes has been detected in animal models (Wilson *et al.*, 1990; Apperley *et al.*, 1991; Lothrop *et al.*, 1991) and, for human cells, in long-term bone marrow cultures (Hughes *et al.*, 1990). Although problems of efficiency of retroviral infection and long-term expression following transplantation remain to be solved, it seems likely that clinical treatment of several haematological deficiency disorders by gene therapy is on the horizon (Cournoyer and Caskey, 1990).

Lymphoid neoplasia

Diagnosis/clonality

The classification of tumours of the B or T cell lineages is now commonly based on rearrangements of the immunoglobulin or TCR genes. These genes rearrange during normal cellular development to generate the immensely variable antigen-receptor specificity that is essential for the immune response. Also, since each lymphoid precursor performs its own rearrangement of the genetic sequence, the structure of the immunoglobulin (or TCR) gene in a lymphocyte population provides a clonotypic marker.

Antibodies consist of four polypeptides, two heavy chains and two light chains which are held together in a complex by disulphide bridges (Fig. 3.5). Each chain consists of a variable region, which is responsible for antibody diversity, and a constant region. The genes that encode the heavy and light chains are found on chromosomes 14(q32), 22(q11) and 2(p12). The genes consist of variable (V), joining (J) and constant (C) regions (light chains) with additional diversity (D) regions in the heavy chain genes (Fig. 3.6) The genes are rearranged in a specific sequence under the agency of recombinase enzymes to produce unique immunoglobulin gene structures that typify clonal populations. Hence, rearrangements of immunoglobulin genes can be detected by Southern blot hybridization and used as diagnostic and clonal markers in B cell neoplasms. Congenital and infant leukaemias differ from the majority of ALLs because they are characterized by multiple heavy chain J region bands, which may be a primary feature

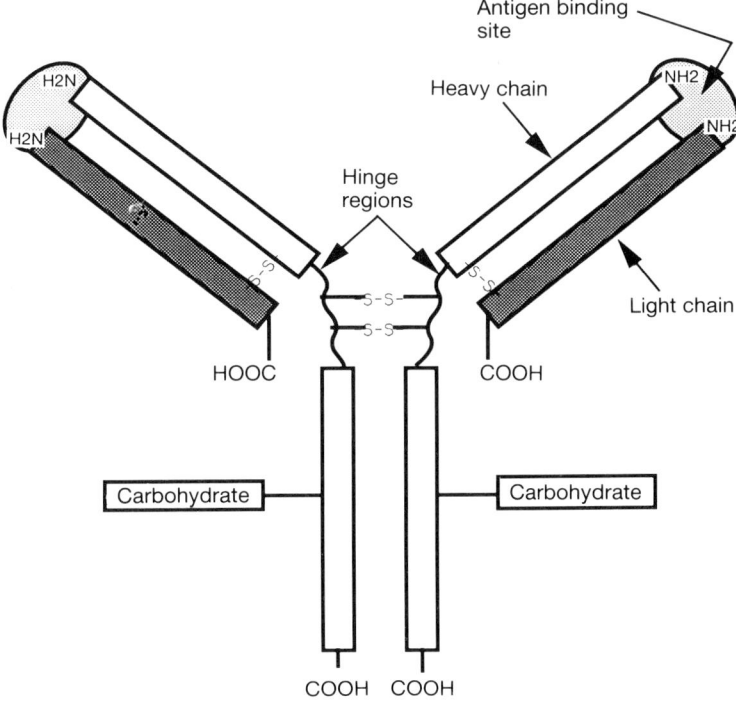

Fig. 3.5 Schematic drawing of a typical antibody molecule.

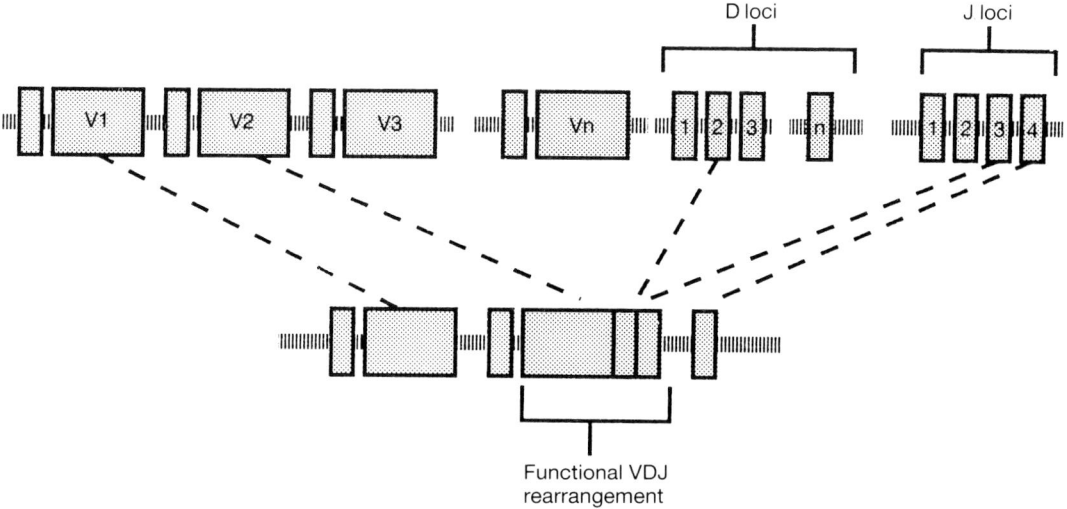

Fig. 3.6 Diagrammatic representation of VDJ recombination during immunoglobulin heavy chain formation.

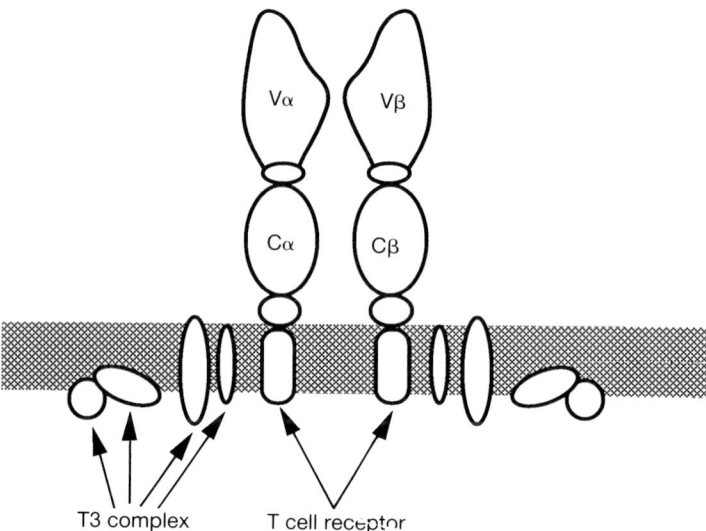

Fig. 3.7 Simplified diagram of the structure of the T cell receptor and associated T3 complex.

of the disease or a consequence of clonal evolution (Rechavi et al., 1988).

Recently, PCR has been used to detect monoclonal B cell populations in B-ALL and lymphomas (Deane and Norton, 1990; McCarthy et al., 1990; Trainor et al., 1990) because it is faster and requires less DNA than gene-probing techniques.

The TCR recognizes antigen. It is a heterodimer of α and β chains which is associated with the T3 complex of four chains (Fig. 3.7). Rearrangement of the TCRα and TCRβ chain genes appears to be very similar to the rearrangement of the immunoglobulin genes and it has even been suggested that common recombinase enzymes are involved. Southern analysis of TCRβ gene rearrangement has been widely used to establish the clonality of T lymphoid cell populations.

Pathogenesis

Translocations involving chromosomes 14, 22 and 2 (the loci corresponding to the immunoglobulin genes) have excited particular interest and have been cloned and characterized in the search for clues about pathogenetic mechanisms. These studies have implicated the proto-oncogene c-*myc* in the pathogenesis of Burkitt's lymphoma through its involvement in the t(8;14) translocation. The t(11;14) translocation has been reported in CLL, myeloma and lymphoma and is thought to result in activation of the *bcl*-2 gene (Cleary et al., 1989) and a distinct subgroup of ALL associated with eosinophilia and t(5;14)(q31;q32) involves joining the IL-3 gene to the immunoglobulin heavy chain gene (Grimaldi and Meeker, 1989).

The involvement of IL-6 in the autocrine or paracrine stimulation of myeloma cell proliferation is controversial. Myeloma cells express IL-6 receptors and respond to exogenous IL-6 *in vitro* (Kawano *et al.*, 1988). Kawano and colleagues proposed an autocrine mechanism but others (Klein *et al.*, 1989) suggest that stimulation is paracrine, possibly by IL-6 derived from marrow stromal cells. Occasionally, rearrangement of the IL-6 gene is found in patients with constitutive production by myeloma cells but the IL-6 receptor genes are unaltered (Fiedler *et al.*, 1990b). On balance, it is likely that a few myeloma patients may have IL-6 gene rearrangement with constitutive IL-6 production and autocrine myeloma cell stimulation.

The Philadelphia (Ph^1) translocation is found in some cases of B cell ALL and some of them have rearrangements in BCR. This distinguishes two types of Ph^1+ ALL (BCR+ and BCR−). The BCR+ cases can probably be equated with lymphoid blast crisis of CML occurring without a clinically detectable chronic phase since they express the protein product p210. The BCR− cases express a p190 PTK that is distinct from p210 and the normal gene product p145. These latter cases are likely to be true cases of ALL in which the target cell was a restricted B cell progenitor.

Weide *et al.* (1991) studied a cell line established from a B cell NHL with a deletion at band q14 on chromosome 13. No p105 (RB gene product) could be detected by Western blotting and no messenger RNA by Northern blots. The loss of one RB allele was confirmed by Southern blotting. Other studies on cell lines by Cheng *et al.* (1990) and Ginsberg *et al.* (1991) suggest that RB gene inactivation can be associated with a broad range of lymphoid neoplasms but this remains to be confirmed by studies of RB in primary lymphoma samples. Mutations in the coding region of the p53 tumour suppressor gene have also been detected in B cell ALL, Waldenström's macroglobulinaemia, B cell CLL and Burkitt's lymphoma (Gaidano *et al.*, 1991; Sugimoto *et al.*, 1991).

The *bcl*-2 gene is abnormally expressed in non-Hodgkin's lymphomas with the t(14;18) translocation and is implicated in the pathogenesis of the disease by its ability to confer a cell survival advantage and allow continued cell proliferation (Cotter, 1990). Also, most follicular and diffuse lymphomas without *bcl*-2 rearrangement express high levels of the protein. Small lymphocytic malignancies (small lymphocytic lymphoma, mantle zone lymphoma and CLL) express intermediate levels and levels varied in plasma cell dyscrasias (Zutter *et al.*, 1991). Thus, extension of cell survival by blocking programmed cell death (apoptosis) may provide a survival advantage in a broad range of lymphoid neoplasms, including those lacking rearrangement of the *bcl*-2 gene.

Recent studies on cell lines from patients with pre-B-ALL, marked by the t(1;19) translocation, have shown that this rearrangement results in juxtaposition of the E2A gene and a new gene, *prl*, characterized by homeobox sequences (Kamps *et al.*, 1990; Nourse *et al.*, 1990). The E2A gene, on chromosome 19, codes for the immunoglobulin enhancer-binding transcription factors E12 and E47. The translocation results in the loss of sequences coding the helix–turn–helix DNA-binding motif and its replacement by homeobox-like sequences of a gene from chromosome 1, *prl*. The chimeric messenger RNA encodes a fusion protein and it is suggested that the E2A-*prl* fusion gene is an oncogene.

Prognosis

A number of interrelated factors contribute prognostic information for patients with B-ALL within the context of a given treatment protocol but, overall, there is a general trend for the prognosis to worsen in parallel with the stage of cell development that the leukaemia represents (early pre B → pre B → mature B). The congenital and infant leukaemias, characterized by multiple Ig heavy chain J region bands on Southern analysis, have a particularly poor prognosis (Rechavi *et al.*, 1988). The importance of the various predictors is influenced by the efficacy of treatment and may diminish as treatment improves. These aspects have been reviewed by Champlin and Golde (1985).

In general, ALL in children is considered to be responsive to chemotherapy, but overexpression of the MDR-1 gene has been detected in relapsing patients and occasionally at presentation (Rothenberg *et al.*, 1989).

In B cell lymphoma, rearrangement of the *bcl*-1 gene, which is involved in the t(11;14)(q13;q32) translocation, appears particularly associated with a subset of patients with primary refractory disease and gastrointestinal involvement. Around one-third of myelomas at diagnosis have a multidrug-resistant phenotype that can be substantially counteracted with verapamil (Dalton *et al.*, 1989; Solary *et al.*, 1991).

A recent multivariate analysis of factors influencing survival in multiple myeloma identified blood urea and serum albumin (Blade *et al.*, 1989), whilst Cimino *et al.* (1990) identified three groups of patients by their serum β_2-microglobulin and IL-2 levels. The correlation between high IL-2 levels and prolonged survival is consistent with that between elevated Tγ cells and effective control of myeloma.

The expression of cell adhesion molecules influences the behaviour and distribution of malignant cells and may influence prognosis. This association has been suggested by studies of CD11a/18, CD44 and CD54 adhesion molecules in lymphoid malignancies (Horst *et al.*, 1990a,b; Jalkanen *et al.*, 1990; Maio *et al.*, 1990). Quantitation of bone marrow involvement and neoplastic cell distribution is important for the clinical staging of lymphoma and can help with treatment decisions about, for example, the use of autologous bone marrow transplantation. Evaluation of marrow involvement by biopsy is more or less restricted to the iliac crests but MRI can detect focal deposits in other areas. However, biopsy examination detects a lower degree of involvement, suggesting that a combination of the two techniques provides the best staging in lymphoma (Hoane *et al.*, 1991).

Detection and management of minimal residual disease

Detection of minimal residual disease is considered to be potentially important in determining the duration of treatment in ALL. Several techniques have been proposed but their practical value in a clinical setting is still uncertain. For example, there are quantitative limits to the value of Southern analysis of immunoglobulin and TCR gene rearrangement. Colony formation by ALL cells in remission marrow has been proposed as a detection system for minimal residual disease and has a sensitivity of about one clonogenic leukaemic cell in a thousand bone marrow cells (Estrov *et al.*, 1986).

Campana *et al.* (1990) compared results obtained using immunological detection methods and PCR and concluded that their combined use improved the accuracy of detection. The advantages of immunofluorescence included the absence of false-positive results but PCR was more sensitive. However, it is possible that PCR could amplify sequences from dead cells, which could be a particular problem soon after treatment, and further genetic rearrangements could potentially escape detection by a clone-specific probe.

Zehnbauer *et al.* (1986) used recombinant DNA probes for Southern analysis of the IgH J regions in patients with ALL in remission and established a detection level of one leukaemic cell in 500 normal cells. Jonsson *et al.* (1990) exploited the creation of the hypervariable region (HVR3) during IgH gene rearrangement. These are flanked by conserved variable (V_H) and joining (J_H) regions. Oligonucleotides to V_H and J_H were used to amplify the intervening HVR3 sequences by PCR and this allowed detection of 10 ALL cells in 10^6 normal leukocytes. The fusion gene *bcl-2*/IgH formed by the t(14;18) translocation is ideal for detection by the PCR technique since the breakpoints occur in short segments of the *bcl-2* gene. Therefore, this provides a marker for detecting malignant cells in blood and bone marrow from a subgroup of NHL patients (Cotter, 1990). Amplification by PCR of rearranged

TCR sequences has been used to assess residual disease in T cell ALL and follicular lymphoma and has been shown to predict impending relapse (Davis and Bjorkman, 1988; Stetler-Storensen et al., 1988; D'Auriol et al., 1989; Hansen-Hagge et al., 1989; Neale et al., 1991).

Serum levels of soluble IL-2 receptor (Ambrosetti et al., 1989) and IL-1β (Cimino et al., 1991) correlate with neoplastic bulk in hairy cell leukaemia and may provide a marker for monitoring disease. Similarly, soluble CD9 and CD30 could be useful for the detection of ALL and Hodgkin's disease respectively (Komada et al., 1990; Gause et al., 1991).

Aplastic anaemia

Diagnosis

Severe aplastic anaemia is diagnosed by the presence of at least two of the following features: fewer than 500 granulocytes per mm^3 in the blood; a reticulocyte count lower than 1% (corrected for haematocrit); fewer than 20 000 platelets per mm^3 and a hypocellular bone marrow. The vacant spaces in the bone marrow become filled by fat cells but there is no infiltration by leukaemic or other malignant cells.

Pathogenesis

The underlying cause of stem cell failure in aplastic anaemia could reside in the stem cell population or in the stromal or immunological microenvironment. More than one of these aspects may be involved since aplastic anaemia can be congenital or acquired. Idiopathic aplastic anaemia describes conditions for which no specific aetiological agent can be identified and idiosyncratic aplastic anaemia describes patients whose disease results from an unexpected and severe reaction to a substance that is generally considered safe for the population at large.

Evidence has been sought to support each of the theories which have been proposed to account for the pathogenesis of aplastic anaemia and much of the earlier work relied on colony and stromal culture techniques (see Gordon and Barrett, 1985). Most of these studies suggest that the most important defect in the majority of aplastic anaemia patients is in the stem cell population (see Marsh and Geary, 1991). Although several forms of aplastic anaemia and other cytopenias are constitutional (Fanconi anaemia; dyskeratosis congenita; Diamond–Blackfan anaemia; Schwachmann–Diamond syndrome), the underlying genetic defects are not known.

Clonal abnormalities in aplastic anaemia have been recognized for a long time and, in particular, clones resembling those that typify paroxysmal nocturnal haemoglobinuria (PNH). Moreover, a small number of aplastic patients develop acute leukaemia, and disease entities such as hypoplastic myelodysplasia and hypoplastic presentation of AML have been recognized. Thus, there may be a link between aplastic anaemia, clonal haemopoiesis and leukaemia (see Marsh and Geary, 1991, for references and discussion).

Clonality in aplastic anaemia has been investigated using a variety of techniques. About 5–10% of aplastic patients acquire a PNH-like clone and bone marrow progenitors from a high proportion of patients have an abnormal sensitivity to complement and a positive sucrose-lysis test (Nissen et al., 1986). Ten per cent of survivors following treatment with antilymphocyte globulin have clonal abnormalities (de Planque et al., 1989); G6PD heterozygosity has been used to demonstrate monoclonal haemopoiesis in cats (Abkowitz et al., 1984) and a patient has been investigated by RFLP analysis of X-linked DNA polymorphisms (Marsh et al., 1990).

Haemoglobinopathies

Diagnosis

Diagnosis by DNA analysis is the method of choice for many genetic disorders, including the haemoglobinopathies. Sickle cell anaemia and α-thalassaemia can be readily detected by these methods. Identification of the mutation in the sixth codon of the β haemoglobin gene in sickle cell anaemia (an A → T substitution) permits precise diagnosis by DNA hybridization using the restriction enzyme MstII to generate fragments. Subsequently, the development of oligonucleotide probes for detecting the point mutation further improved the accuracy of diagnosis. Most recently, PCR has been used to amplify β-globin gene sequences, with consequent improvements in sensitivity and the possibility of making a diagnosis on small numbers of cells (see Caskey, 1987 for review). Monk and Holding (1990) succeeded in amplifying β-globin gene sequences from single unfertilized human eggs or the first polar body isolated from them. This means that unaffected eggs can be selected for fertilization and, potentially, removes the need for diagnostic procedures on embryos.

Most of the severe α-thalassaemias are a result of gene deletion and, therefore, the absence of α-globin genes is diagnostic for the disease. However, because the β-thalassaemias are not due to gene deletion but to point mutations affecting critical parts of the β-globin gene, and only rarely involve gross gene rearrangements, many different β gene mutations have been described worldwide. Fortuitously, a restricted number of molecular defects occur in each affected population (Cao and Murru, 1989). Cai *et al.* (1988) took advantage of this fact and, in southern China, found six mutations in a localized area. Having prepared the necessary oligonucleotide probes they were able to diagnose cases before birth using PCR and dot blot hybridization. Also, new β-globin gene mutations have been identified in Italian patients by PCR and direct sequencing of the amplified DNA (Murru *et al.*, 1991).

Pathology

Whilst the molecular basis for sickle cell anaemia is well-known, the events leading to painful crisis are not clearly defined. Polymerization of haemoglobin S, reduced blood flow and tissue ischaemia are believed to occur. Dense irreversibly sickled erythrocytes decrease during painful crisis (Fabry *et al.*, 1984) and rheological studies suggest that they are sequestered in the microcirculation in ischaemic tissue (Fabry and Kaul, 1991). Imaging of tissues has been used in an effort to understand the pathophysiology of painful crisis, most recently using MRI which avoids radiography and radionuclide exposure. This technique reveals abnormally patchy marrow during the steady state and increases in this parameter correlated with the reduction in number of dense erythrocytes (Mankad *et al.*, 1990).

Other inherited deficiencies

Molecular techniques are now being applied to a wide variety of inherited disorders and studies include the use of PCR and RFLP analysis in improved prenatal diagnosis as well as efforts directed

Table 3.10 Inherited deficiency disorders under molecular investigation

Inherited disorder	Reference
von Willebrand disease	Peake *et al.* (1990)
X-linked chronic granulomatous disease	Pelham *et al.* (1990); Babior and Woodman (1990)
Haemopoiesis in Down's syndrome	Kurahashi *et al.* (1991)
Hereditary persistence of fetal haemoglobin	Bollekens and Forget (1991)
Genetic defects in DNA-repair (Fanconi's anaemia; xeroderma pigmentosum; ataxia telangiectasia)	Gordon-Smith and Rutherford (1991)
Glanzmann's thrombasthenia	Bennett (1990)
Leukocyte adhesion deficiency	Bennett (1990)
Adenosine deaminase deficiency	Carson and Carrera (1990)
Haemophilia	Furie and Furie (1990)

towards defining the molecular genetic foundation of the disorders and developing treatments and, hopefully, cures. Some of the disorders are listed in Table 3.10.

Overview

The addition of molecular techniques to the investigation of haemopoiesis has led to increased appreciation of the complexity of haematological disease. As a result of new information, it should become possible to identify with some precision the defective mechanism(s) in abnormal cells. This type of information is already available in the haemoglobinopathies such as the thalassaemias and sickle cell anaemia. Some types of leukaemia and lymphoma can now be characterized molecularly and notable examples include the involvement of the RARα/*myl* genes in promyelocytic leukaemia (M3) and p210 BCR/ABL in CML. At the other end of the scale are disorders such as acquired aplastic anaemia for which almost no genetic or molecular insight exists.

The impact of molecular biology has not, with rare exceptions, extended to developing new therapeutic strategies but can be expected to do so in the near future. With the identification of more abnormal gene products, approaches such as the therapeutic use of antisense oligonucleotides will become possible. However, a major impact has been made through the development of new tools and tests for monitoring disease and its response to treatment. In particular, the ability to measure minimal residual disease with greater sensitivity and accuracy will be invaluable in the design of new treatment protocols and will contribute to the debate concerning the need to eradicate the very last leukaemic cell (see Chapter 2).

REFERENCES

Abkowitz JL, Fialkow PJ, Niebrugge DJ, Raskind WH, Adamson JW (1984) Pancytopenia as a clonal disorder of a multipotent hemopoietic stem cell. *Journal of Clinical Investigation* 73, 258.

Ahuja H, Bar-Eli M, Advani SH, Benchimol S, Cline MJ (1989) Alterations in the p53 gene and the clonal evolution of the blast crisis of chronic myelocytic leukemia. *Proceedings of the National Academy of Sciences of the USA* 86, 6783.

Ahuja HG, Foti A, Bar-Eli M, Cline MJ (1990) The pattern of mutational involvement of RAS genes in human hematologic malignancies determined by DNA amplification and direct sequencing. *Blood* 75, 1684.

Aihara M, Aihara Y, Schmidt-Wolf G et al. (1991) A combined approach for purging multidrug-resistant leukemic cell lines in bone marrow using a monoclonal antibody and chemotherapy. *Blood* 77, 2079.

Ambrosetti A, Semenzato G, Prior M et al. (1989) Serum levels of soluble interleukin-2 receptor in hairy cell leukemia: a reliable marker of neoplastic bulk. *British Journal of Haematology* 73, 181.

Anger B, Janssen JWG, Schrezenmeier H, Hehlmann R, Heimpel H, Bartram CR (1990) Clonal analysis of chronic myeloproliferative disorders using X-linked DNA polymorphisms. *Leukemia* 4, 258.

Apperley JF, Luskey BD, Williams DA (1991) Retroviral gene transfer of human adenosine deaminase in murine hematopoietic cells: effect of selectable marker sequences on long-term expression. *Blood* 78, 310.

Babior BM, Woodman RC (1990) Chronic granulomatous disease. *Seminars in Hematology* 27, 247.

Bar-Eli M, Ahuja H, Gonzalez-Cadavid N, Foti A, Cline

MJ (1989) Analysis of N-RAS exon-1 mutations in myelodysplastic syndromes by polymerase chain reaction and direct sequencing. *Blood* 73, 281.

Bartram CR, Janssen JWG, Schmidberger M, Lyons J, Arnold R (1989) Minimal residual disease in chronic myeloid leukaemia patients after T-cell depleted bone-marrow transplantation. *Lancet* i, 1260.

Benedict WT, Fung YKT, Murphree AL (1988) The gene responsible for the development of retinoblastoma and osteosarcoma. *Cancer* 62, 1691.

Bennett JM, Catovsky D, Daniel MT et al. (FAB cooperative group) (1982) Proposals for the classification of the myelodysplastic syndromes. *British Journal of Haematology* 51, 189.

Bennett JM, Catovsky D, Daniel MT et al. (1991) Proposal for the recognition of minimally differentiated acute myeloid leukaemia (AML-M0). *British Journal of Haematology* 78, 325.

Bennett JS (1990) The molecular biology of platelet membrane proteins. *Seminars in Hematology* 27, 186.

Bernstein R, Gale RP (1990) Hypothesis: Do chromosome abnormalities determine the type of acute leukemia that develops in CML? *Leukemia* 4, 65.

Bevan IS, Daw RA, Day PJR, Ala FA, Walker MR (1991) Polymerase chain reaction for detection of human cytomegalovirus infection in a blood donor population. *British Journal of Haematology* 78, 94.

Bhushan A, Abramson R, Tritton TR (1989) c-fos gene expression in multidrug resistance. *Proceedings of the American Association for Cancer Research* 30, 504a.

Bidwell JL, Bidwell EA, Klouda PT, Goffin RB, Bradley BA, Brenner M (1987) DNA-RFLP typing in the selection of related bone marrow donors. *Bone Marrow Transplantation* 1, 413.

Biondi A, Rambaldi A, Alcalay M et al. (1991) RAR-α gene rearrangement as a genetic marker for diagnosis and monitoring in acute promyelocytic leukemia. *Blood* 77, 1418.

Birnie GD, Mills KI, Benn P (1989) Does the site of the breakpoint on chromosome 22 influence the duration of the chronic phase in chronic myeloid leukaemia? *Leukemia* 3, 545.

Birnie JD, MacKenzie ED, Goyns MH, Pollack A (1990) Sequestration of Philadelphia chromosome-positive cells in the bone marrow of a chronic myeloid leukemia patient in very prolonged remission. *Leukemia* 4, 452.

Blade J, Rozman C, Cervantes F, Reverter J-C, Montserrat E (1989) A new prognostic system for multiple myeloma based on easily available parameters. *British Journal of Haematology* 72, 507.

Blazar BR, Orr HT, Arthur DC, Kersey JH, Filipovich AH (1985) Restriction fragment length polymorphisms as markers of engraftment in allogeneic marrow transplantation. *Blood* 66, 1436.

Bodger MP, Morris CM, Kennedy MA, Bowen JA, Hilton JM, Fitzgerald PH (1990) Basophils (Bsp-1+) derive from the leukemic clone in human myeloid leukemias involving the breakpoint 9q34. *Blood* 73, 777.

Bollekens JA, Forget BG (1991) δβ-thalassemia and hereditary persistence of fetal hemoglobin. *Hematology/Oncology Clinics of North America* 5, 399.

Bot FJ, Schipper P, Broeders L, Delwel R, Kaushansky K, Lowenberg B (1990) Interleukin-1α also induces granulocyte-macrophage colony-stimulating factor in immature normal bone marrow cells. *Blood* 76, 307.

Botstein D, White RL, Skolnick M, David RW (1980) Construction of a genetic linkage map in man using restriction fragment length polymorphisms. *American Journal of Human Genetics* 32, 314.

Boultwood J, Rack K, Kelly S et al. (1991) Loss of both CSF1 (FMS) alleles in patients with myelodysplasia and chromosome 5 deletion. *Proceedings of the National Academy of Sciences of the USA* 88, 6176.

Burt RK, Thorgeirsson SS (1988) Coinduction of MDR-1 multidrug resistance and cytochrome P-450 genes in rat liver by xenobiotics. *Journal of the National Cancer Institute* 80, 1383.

Busch SJ, Sassone-Corsi P (1990) Dimers, leucine zippers and DNA-binding domains. *Trends in Genetics* 6, 36.

Cai S-P, Zhang J-Z, Huang D-H, Wang Z-X, Kan YW (1988) A simple approach to prenatal diagnosis of β-thalassemia in a geographic area where multiple mutations occur. *Blood* 71, 1357.

Campana D, Yokota S, Coustan-Smith E, Hansen-Hagge TE, Janossy G, Bartram CR (1990) The detection of residual acute lymphoblastic leukemia cells with immunologic methods and polymerase chain reaction: a comparative study. *Leukemia* 4, 609.

Canellos GP, Griffin JD (1985) Chronic granulocytic leukemia: the heterogeneity of stem cell differentiation within a single disease entity. *Seminars in Oncology* 12, 281.

Cao A, Murru S (1989) Molecular pathology and detection of beta-thalassemias. In: Buckner CD, Gale RP, Lucarelli G (eds) *Advances and Controversies in Thalassemia Therapy: Bone Marrow Transplantation and other Approaches.* Alan R Liss, New York, p. 3.

Capel B, Hawley R, Covarrubias L, Hawley T, Mintz B (1989) Clonal contributions of small numbers of retrovirally marked hematopoietic stem cells engrafted in unirradiated neonatal W/Wv mice. *Proceedings of the National Academy of Sciences of the USA* 86, 4564.

Carson DA, Carrera CJ (1990) Immunodeficiency secondary to adenosine deaminase deficiency and purine nucleoside phosphorylation deficiency. *Seminars in Hematology* 27, 260.

Caskey CT (1987) Disease diagnosis by recombinant DNA methods. *Science* 236, 1223.

Castaigne S, Chomienne C, Daniel MT et al. (1990) All-trans retinoic acid as a differentiation therapy for acute promyelocytic leukemia. I. Clinical results. *Blood* 76, 1704.

Catovsky D (ed.) (1991) *The Leukemic Cell* 2nd edn. Churchill Livingstone, Edinburgh.

Cesano A, O'Conner R, Lange B, Finan J, Rovera G, Santoli D (1991) Homing and progression patterns of childhood acute lymphoblastic leukemias in severe

combined immunodeficiency mice. *Blood* 77, 2463.
Champlin R, Gale RP (1989) Acute lymphoblastic leukemia: recent advances in biology and therapy. *Blood* 73, 2051.
Champlin RE, Golde DW (1985) Chronic myelogenous leukemia: recent advances. *Blood* 65, 1039.
Chan LC, Karhi KK, Rayter SI et al. (1987) A novel abl protein expressed in Philadelphia chromosome positive acute lymphoblastic leukaemia. *Nature* 325, 635.
Cheng J, Scully P, Shew JY, Lee WH, Vila V, Haas M (1990) Homozygous deletion of the retinoblastoma gene in an acute lymphoblastic leukemia (T) line. *Blood* 75, 730.
Chomienne C, Ballerini P, Balitrand N et al. (1990a) The retinoic acid receptor α gene is rearranged in retinoic acid-sensitive promyelocytic leukemias. *Leukemia* 4, 802.
Chomienne C, Ballerini P, Balitrand N et al. (1990b) All-trans retinoic acid in acute promyelocytic leukemia II. In vitro studies: structure–function relationship. *Blood* 76, 1710.
Cimino G, Avvisati G, Amadori S et al. (1990) High serum IL-2 levels are predictive of prolonged survival in multiple myeloma. *British Journal of Haematology* 75, 373.
Cimino G, Annino L, Giona F et al. (1991) Serum interleukin-1 beta levels correlate with neoplastic bulk in hairy cell leukemia. *Leukemia* 5, 602.
Clay TM, Jones HP, Bidwell JL, Darke C, Harvey J, Bradley BA (1989) A comparison of DNA-RFLP typing with serology and mixed lymphocyte reaction in the selection of matched unrelated bone marrow donors. *Bone Marrow Transplantation* 4, 493.
Cleary ML, Ngan B-Y, Chen-Levy Z, Nourse J (1989) The Bcl-2 proto-oncogenic protein associated with 4(14;18) translocations: biochemical properties and expression in non-Hodgkin's lymphoma. In: Furth M, Greaves M (eds) *Molecular Diagnostics of Human Cancer*. Cold Spring Harbor Laboratory Press, Cold Spring Harbor, p. 41.
Coleman M, Silver RT, Pajek TF et al. (1980) Combination chemotherapy for terminal phase chronic granulocytic leukemia: Cancer and leukemia group B studies. *Blood* 55, 29.
Collins SJ, Groudine MT (1987) Chronic myelogenous leukemia. Amplification of a rearranged c-abl oncogene in both chronic phase and blast crisis. *Blood* 69, 893.
Cotter FE (1990) The role of the bcl-2 gene in lymphoma. *British Journal of Haematology*, 75, 449.
Cournoyer D, Caskey CT (1990) Gene transfer into humans. *New England Journal of Medicine* 323, 601.
Culliton BJ (1989) News and comment: Gene transfer test: so far so good. *Science* 44, 1325.
Culliton BJ (1990) News and comment: Gene therapy: into the home stretch. *Science* 249, 974.
Cuneo A, Van Orshoven A, Michaux JL et al. (1990) Morphologic, immunologic and cytogenetic studies in erythroleukaemia: evidence for multilineage involvement and identification of two distinct cytogenetic-clinicopathological types. *British Journal of Haematology* 75, 346.

Dacie JV, Lewis SM (1984) *Practical Haematology* 6th edn. Churchill Livingstone, Edinburgh.
Daley GQ, Van Etten RA, Baltimore D (1990) Induction of chronic myelogenous leukemia in mice by the p210 bcr/abl gene of the Philadelphia chromosome. *Science* 247, 824.
Dalton WS, Grogan TM, Meltzer PS et al. (1989) Drug-resistance in multiple myeloma and non-Hodgkin's lymphoma: detection of P-glycoprotein and potential circumvention by addition of verapamil to chemotherapy. *Journal of Clinical Oncology*, 7, 415.
D'Auriol L, Macintyre E, Galibert F, Sigaux F (1989) In vitro amplification of T cell γ gene rearrangements: a new tool for the assessment of minimal residual disease in acute lymphoblastic leukemias. *Leukemia* 3, 155.
Davis MM, Bjorkman PJ (1988) T cell antigen receptor genes and T cell recognition. *Nature* 334, 395.
Deane M, Norton JD (1990) Detection of immunoglobulin gene rearrangement in B lymphoid malignancies by polymerase chain reaction gene amplification. *British Journal of Haematology* 74, 251.
DeCertaines JD (1990) High resolution magnetic resonance spectroscopy in clinical biology. *Leukemia* 4, 667.
Delfau M-H, Kerkhaert J-P, D'Hooghe MC et al. (1990) Detection of minimal residual disease in chronic myeloid leukemia patients after bone marrow transplantation by polymerase chain reaction. *Leukemia* 4, 1.
De Planque MM, Van Krieken HJ, Kluin-Nelemans MC et al. (1989) Bone marrow histopathology of patients with severe aplastic anaemia before treatment and at follow-up. *British Journal of Haematology* 72, 439.
Dick JE, Kamel-Reid S, Murdoch B, Doedens M (1991) Gene transfer into normal human hematopoietic cells using in vitro and in vivo assays. *Blood* 78, 624.
Dohner H, Guckel F, Knauf W et al. (1989) Magnetic resonance imaging of bone marrow in lymphoproliferative disorders: correlation with bone marrow biopsy. *British Journal of Haematology* 73, 12.
Donovan-Peluso M, Bank A (1989) Transfection of DNA into mammalian cells. In: Benz EJ (ed.) *Molecular Genetics*. Churchill Livingstone, Edinburgh, p. 181.
Dowding C, Guo A-P, Maisin D, Gordon MY, Goldman JM (1991) The effects of interferon-α on the proliferation of CML progenitor cells in vitro are not related to the precise position of the M-BCR breakpoint. *British Journal of Haematology* 77, 165.
Dryja TP, Cavanee WK, White R et al. (1984) Homozygosity of chromosome 13 in retinoblastoma. *New England Journal of Medicine* 310, 550.
Dubreil P, Torres H, Courcoul MA, Birg F, Mannoni P (1988) c-*fms* expression is a molecular marker of human acute myeloid leukemias. *Blood* 72, 1081.
Einsele H, Steidle M, Vallbracht A, Saul JG, Ehninger G, Muller CA (1991) Early occurrence of human cytomegalovirus infection after bone marrow transplantation as demonstrated by the polymerase chain

reaction technique. *Blood* 77, 1104.
Estrov Z, Grunberger T, Dube ID, Wang Y-P, Freedman MH (1986) Detection of residual acute lymphoblastic leukemia cells in cultures of bone marrow obtained during remission. *New England Journal of Medicine* 315, 538.
Fabry ME, Kaul DK (1991) Sickle cell vaso-occlusion. *Hematology/Oncology Clinics of North America* 5, 375.
Fabry ME, Benjamin L, Lawrence C, Nagel RL (1984) An objective sign in painful crisis in sickle cell anemia: the concomitant reduction of high density red cells. *Blood* 64, 559.
Farrow A, Jacobs A, West RR (1989) Myelodysplasia, chemical exposure and other environmental factors. *Leukemia* 3, 33.
Feinstein E, Cimono G, Gale RP et al. (1991) p53 in chronic myelogenous leukemia in acute phase. *Proceedings of the National Academy of Sciences of the USA* 88, 6293.
Fenaux P, Preudhomme C, Lay JL, Beuscart R, Bauters F (1989) Cytogenetics and their prognostic value in de novo acute myeloid leukaemia: a report on 283 cases. *British Journal of Haematology* 173, 61.
Fenaux P, Jonveaux P, Quiquandron I et al. (1991) P53 gene mutations in human acute myelogenous leukemia with 17p monosomy. *Blood* 78, 1652.
Fiedler W, Suciu E, Wittlief C, Ostertag W, Hossfeld DK (1990a) Mechanism of growth factor expression in acute myeloid leukemia (AML). *Leukemia* 4, 459.
Fiedler W, Weh HJ, Suciu E, Wittlief C, Stocking C, Hossfeld DK (1990b) The IL-6 gene but not the IL-6 receptor gene is occasionally rearranged in patients with multiple myeloma. *Leukemia* 4, 462.
Foon KA, Gale RP, Todd RF (1990) Immunologic advance in the classification of leukemia. In: Mauer AM (ed.) *The Biology of Human Leukaemia*. Johns Hopkins, Baltimore, p. 44.
Fossel ET (1991) The NMR blood test for cancer: current status. *Cancer Cells* 3, 173.
Furie B, Furie BC (1990) Molecular basis of hemophilia. *Seminars in Hematology* 27, 270.
Gabert J, Lafage M, Maraninchi D, Thuret I, Carcassonne Y, Mannoni P (1989) Detection of residual bcr/abl translocation by polymerase chain reaction in chronic myeloid leukaemia patients after bone-marrow transplantation. *Lancet* ii, 1125.
Gaidano G, Ballerini P, Gong JZ et al. (1991) p53 mutations in human lymphoid malignancies: association with Burkitt lymphoma and chronic lymphocytic leukemia. *Proceedings of the National Academy of Sciences of the USA* 88, 5413.
Gause A, Pohl C, Tschiersch A et al. (1991) Clinical significance of soluble CD30 antigen in the sera of patients with untreated Hodgkin's disease. *Blood* 77, 1983.
Gerhartz HH, Schmetzer H (1990) Detection of minimal residual disease in acute myeloid leukemia. *Leukemia* 4, 508.
Giannone L, Whitlock JA, Kinney MC, Wolff SN, Dev VG (1988) Use of the BCR probe to demonstrate extramedullary recurrence of CGL with a T cell lymphoid phenotype following bone marrow transplantation. *Bone Marrow Transplantation* 3, 631.
Gilliland DG, Blanchard KL, Levy J, Perrin S, Bunn HF (1991) Clonality in myeloproliferative disorders: analysis by means of the polymerase chain reaction. *Proceedings of the National Academy of Sciences of the USA* 88, 6848.
Ginsberg D, Antin JH, Smith BR, Orkin SH, Rappeport JM (1985) Origin of cell populations after bone marrow transplantation. Analysis using DNA sequence polymorphisms. *Journal of Clinical Investigation* 75, 596.
Ginsberg AM, Raffeld M, Cossman J (1991) Inactivation of the retinoblastoma gene in human lymphoid neoplasms. *Blood* 77, 833.
Goldman JM (1988) Chronic myeloid leukaemia: pathogenesis and management. In: Hoffbrand AV (ed.) *Recent Advances in Haematology*. Churchill Livingstone, Edinburgh, p. 131.
Goldman JM, Gale RP, Horowitz MM et al. (1988) Bone marrow transplantation for chronic myelogenous leukemia in chronic phase. *Annals of Internal Medicine* 108, 806.
Gordon MY, Barrett AJ (1985) *Bone Marrow Disorders: The Biological Basis of Clinical Problems*. Blackwell Scientific Publications. Oxford.
Gordon-Smith EC, Rutherford TR (1991) Fanconi anemia: constitutional aplastic anemia. *Seminars in Hematology* 28, 104.
Grimaldi CJ, Meeker TC (1989) The t(5;14) chromosomal translocation in a case of acute lymphocytic leukemia joins the interleukin-3 gene to the immunoglobulin heavy chain gene. *Blood* 73, 2081.
Hansen-Hagge TE, Yokota S, Bartram C (1989) Detection of minimal residual disease in acute lymphoblastic leukemia by in vitro amplification of rearranged T-cell receptor δ chain sequences. *Blood* 74, 1762.
Harbour JW, Lai SL, Whang-Peng J, Gazdar AF, Minna JD, Kaye FJ (1988) Abnormalities in structure and expression of the human retinoblastoma gene in SCLC. *Science* 241, 353.
Hayashi Y, Raimondi SC, Behm FG et al. (1989) Two karyotypically independent leukemic clones with the t(8;21) and 11q23 translocation in acute myeloblastic leukemia at relapse. *Blood* 73, 1650.
Heim S, Mitelman F (1989) Cytogenetically unrelated clones in hematological neoplasms. *Leukemia* 3, 6.
Hernandez A, Osterholz J, Price CM et al. (1990) Detection of the hybrid BCR/ABL messenger RNA in single CFU-GM colonies using the polymerase chain reaction. *Experimental Hematology* 18, 1142.
Hinks RS, Dunlap HJ, Poon PY, Curtis J, Henkelman RM (1986) Quantitative MRI of normal and leukaemic bone marrow. *Radiology* 161, 313.
Hiorns LR, Cotter FE, Young BD (1989) Co-incident N and K ras gene mutations in a case of AML, restricted to differing cell lineages. *British Journal of Haematology* 73, 165.
Hoane BR, Shields AF, Porter BA, Shulman HM (1991) Detection of lymphomatous bone marrow involvement with magnetic resonance imaging. *Blood* 78, 728.
Holler E, Kolb HJ, Moller A et al. (1990) Increased

levels of tumor necrosis factor α precede major complications of bone marrow transplantation. *Blood* 75, 1011.

Holmes J, Jacobs A, Carter G, Janowska-Wieczorek A, Padua RA (1989) Multidrug resistance in haemopoietic cell lines, myelodysplastic syndrome and acute myeloblastic leukaemia. *British Journal of Haematology* 72, 40.

Hook HB (1977) Exclusion of chromosomal mosaicism: tables of 90%, 95% and 99% confidence limits and comments on use. *American Journal of Human Genetics* 29, 94.

Horowitz JM, Park SH, Bogenmann E et al. (1990) Frequent inactivation of the retinoblastoma antioncogene is restricted to a subset of human tumour cells. *Proceedings of the National Academy of Sciences of the USA* 87, 2775.

Horst E, Meijer CJL, Radaszkiewicz T et al. (1990a) Expression of a human homing receptor (CD44) in lymphoid malignancies and related stages of lymphoid development. *Leukemia* 4, 383.

Horst E, Meijer CJL, Radaszkiewicz T, Ossekoppele GJ, Van Krieken JHJM, Pals ST (1990b) Adhesion molecules in the prognosis of diffuse large-cell lymphoma: expression of a lymphocyte homing receptor (CD44), LFA-1 (CD11a/18) and ICAM-1 (CD54). *Leukemia* 4, 595.

Hughes T, Janssen JWG, Morgan G et al. (1990) False-positive results with PCR to detect leukaemia-specific transcripts. *Lancet* i, 1037.

Hughes TP, Morgan GJ, Martiat P, Goldman JM (1991) Detection of residual leukaemia after bone marrow transplant for chronic myeloid leukemia: role of polymerase chain reaction in predicting relapse. *Blood* 77, 874.

Hunt P, Krumlauf R (1991) Deciphering the Hox code—clues to patterning branchial regions of the head. *Cell* 66, 1075.

Inokuchi K, Amuro N, Futaki M et al. (1991) Transforming genes and chromosome aberrations in therapy-related leukemia and myelodysplastic syndrome. *Annals of Hematology* 62, 211.

Jalkanen S, Joensuu H, Klemi P (1990) Prognostic value of lymphocyte homing receptor and S phase fraction in non-Hodgkin's lymphoma. *Blood* 75, 1549.

Janssen JWG, Buschle M, Layton M et al. (1989) Clonal analysis of myelodysplastic syndromes: evidence of multipotent stem cell origin. *Blood* 73, 248.

Janssen JWG, Anger BR, Drexler HG, Bartram CR, Heimpel H (1990) Essential thrombocythaemia in two sisters originating from different stem cell levels. *Blood* 75, 1633.

Jaubert J, Martiat P, Dowding C, Ifrah N, Goldman JM (1990) The position of the M-BCR breakpoint does not predict the duration of chronic phase or survival in chronic myeloid leukaemia. *British Journal of Haematology* 74, 30.

Jeffreys AJ, Wilson V, Thein SL (1985) Hypervariable 'minisatellite' regions in human DNA. *Nature* 314, 67.

Johansson B, Mertens F, Fioretos T et al. (1990) Remarkably long survival of a patient with Ph'-positive chronic myeloid leukemia and 5' bcr rearrangement. *Leukemia* 4, 448.

Jones L, Thein SL, Jeffreys AJ, Apperley JF, Catovsky D, Goldman JM (1987) Identical twin marrow transplantation for five patients with chronic myeloid leukaemia: role of DNA fingerprinting to confirm monozygosity in three cases. *European Journal of Haematology* 39, 144.

Jonsson OG, Kitchens RL, Scott FC, Smith GR (1990) Detection of minimal residual disease in acute lymphoblastic leukemia using immunoglobulin hypervariable region specific oligonucleotide probes. *Blood* 76, 2072.

Kadoyama C, Birrer M, Dosaka S, Lai D, Gazdar V, Gazdar A (1989) Transfection with H-ras or c-myc proto-oncogenes results in induction of the multidrug resistant phenotype. *Proceedings of the American Association for Cancer Research* 30, 501a.

Kamps MP, Murre C, Sun X-H, Baltimore D (1990) A new homeobox gene contributes the DNA binding domain of the t(1;19) translocation protein in pre-B ALL. *Cell* 60, 547.

Kane SE, Pastan I, Gottesman MM (1990) Genetic basis of multidrug-resistance of tumor cells. *Journal of Bioenergetics and Biomembranes* 22, 593.

Kantarjian HM, Keating MJ, Talpaz M et al. (1987) Chronic myelogenous leukemia in blast crisis. Analysis of 242 patients. *American Journal of Medicine* 83, 445.

Kaufman DC, Baer MR, Gao XZ, Wang Z, Priesler HD (1988) Enhanced expression of granulocyte-macrophage colony-stimulating factor gene in acute myelocytic leukemia cells following in vitro blast cell enrichment. *Blood* 72, 1329.

Kawano M, Hirano T, Matsuda T et al. (1988) Autocrine generation and requirement of BSF-2/IL-6 for human multiple myeloma. *Nature* 332, 83.

Kelman Z, Prokocimer M, Peller S et al. (1989) Rearrangements of the p53 gene in Philadelphia chromosome positive chronic myelogenous leukemia. *Blood* 74, 2318.

Klein B, Zhang XG, Jourdan M et al. (1989) Paracrine rather than autocrine regulation of myeloma cell growth and differentiation by interleukin-6. *Blood* 73, 517.

Knowlton RG, Brown VA, Braman JC et al. (1986) Use of highly polymorphic DNA probes for genotypic analysis following bone marrow transplantation. *Blood* 68, 378.

Komada Y, Ochiai H, Shimizu K, Azuma E, Kamiya H, Sakurai M (1990) Shedding of CD9 antigen into cerebrospinal fluid by acute lymphoblastic leukemia cells. *Blood* 76, 112.

Kossakowska AE, Urbanski SJ, Edwards DR (1991) Tissue inhibitor of metalloproteinases-1 (TIMP-1) RNA is expressed at elevated levels in malignant non-Hodgkin's lymphomas. *Blood* 77, 2475.

Kulkarni SS, Wang Z, Spitzer G et al. (1989) Elimination of resistant myeloma tumor cell lines by monoclonal anti-P-glycoprotein antibody and rabbit complement. *Blood* 74, 2244.

Kurahashi K, Hara J, Yamura-Yagi Y et al. (1991) Monoclonal nature of transient abnormal myelopoiesis in Down's syndrome. *Blood* 77, 1161.

Lange W, Snyder DS, Casro R, Rossi JJ, Blume KG (1989) Detection by enzymatic amplification of bcr-abl mRNA in peripheral blood and bone marrow cells of patients with chronic myelogenous leukemia. *Blood* 73, 1735.

Lee WH, Shew JY, Sery TW et al. (1987) The human retinoblastoma gene encodes a nuclear phosphoprotein associated with DNA binding activity. *Nature* 329, 642.

Lee M-S, Chang K-S, Friereich EJ et al. (1988) Detection of minimal residual bcr/abl transcripts by a modified polymerase chain reaction. *Blood* 72, 893.

Lee M, Kantarjian H, Deisseroth A, Frierreich E, Trujillo J, Stass A (1989) Clinical usage of polymerase chain reaction (PCR) to analyze the BCR/ABL splicing patterns and minimal residual disease (MRD) in Philadelphia chromosome (PH')-positive chronic myelogenous leukemia. *Blood* 74 (suppl), 745a.

Lehn PM (1990) Gene therapy using bone marrow transplantation: a 1990 update. *Bone Marrow Transplantation* 5, 287.

LeMaistre A, Lee M-S, Talpaz M et al. (1989) RAS oncogene mutations are rare late stage events in chronic myelogenous leukemia. *Blood* 73, 889.

Levine AJ, Momand J, Finlay CA (1991) The p53 tumour suppressor gene. *Nature* 351, 453.

List AF, Spier CM, Cline A et al. (1991) Expression of the multidrug resistance gene product (P-glycoprotein) in myelodysplasia is associated with a stem cell phenotype. *British Journal of Haematology* 78, 28.

Lo Coco F, Avvisati G, Diverio D et al. (1991) Rearrangements of the RAR-α gene in acute promyelocytic leukemia: correlates with morphology and immunophenotype. *British Journal of Haematology* 78, 494.

Lotem J, Shabo Y, Sachs L (1987) Role for different normal hematopoietic regulatory proteins in the differentiation of myeloid leukemia cells. *International Journal of Cancer* 32, 101.

Lothrop CD, Al-Lebban ZS, Niemeyer GP et al. (1991) Expression of a foreign gene in cats reconstituted with retroviral vector infected autologous bone marrow. *Blood* 78, 237.

Lucas GS, Padua RA, Masters GS, Oscier DG, Jacobs A (1989) The application of X-chromosome gene probes to the diagnosis of myeloproliferative disease. *British Journal of Haematology* 72, 530.

Ludwig H, Fruhwald F, Tscholakoff D, Rasool S, Neuhold A, Fritz E (1987) Magnetic resonance imaging of the spine in multiple myeloma. *Lancet ii*, 364.

Lyons J, Janssen JWG, Bartram C, Layton M, Mufti GJ (1988) Mutation of Ki-ras and N-ras oncogenes in myelodysplastic syndromes. *Blood* 71, 170.

McCarthy KP, Sloane JP, Wiedemann LM (1990) Rapid method for distinguishing clonal from polyclonal B cell populations in surgical biopsy specimens. *Journal of Clinical Pathology* 43, 329.

McDonnell TJ, Deane N, Platt FM et al. (1989) bcl-2-immunoglobulin transgenic mice demonstrate extended B cell survival and follicular lymphoproliferation. *Cell* 57, 79.

Maio M, Pinto A, Carbone A et al. (1990) Differential expression of CD54/intercellular adhesion molecule-1 in myeloid leukemias and in lymphoproliferative disorders. *Blood* 76, 783.

Malinken T, Palotie A, Pakkala L, Ruutu T, Jannson SE (1991) Acceleration of chronic myeloid leukemia correlates with calcitonin gene hypermethylation. *Blood* 77, 2435.

Mankad VN, Williams JP, Harpden MD et al. (1990) Magnetic resonance imaging of bone marrow in sickle cell disease: clinical, hematologic and pathologic correlations. *Blood* 75, 274.

Mareni C, Origone P, Sessarego M et al. (1990) Early and long term followup with minisatellite probes in bone marrow transplanted patients. *Leukemia* 4, 704.

Marie J-P, Zittoun R, Sikic BI (1991) Multidrug resistance (mdr1) gene expression in adult acute leukemias: correlations with treatment outcome and in vitro drug sensitivity. *Blood* 78, 586.

Marsh JCW, Geary CJ (1991) Annotation: Is aplastic anaemia a preleukaemic disorder? *British Journal of Haematology* 77, 447.

Marsh JCW, Chang J, Cowling GJ, Testa NG, Hows JM, Dexter TM (1990) Clonality studies and long-term marrow culture to assess haemopoiesis in aplastic anaemia. *Experimental Hematology* 18, 306a.

Martiat P, Ifrah N, Rasool F et al. (1989) Molecular analysis of Philadelphia positive essential thrombocythaemia. *Leukemia* 3, 563.

Martiat P, Maisin D, Philippe M et al. (1990) Detection of residual BCR/ABL transcripts in chronic myeloid leukaemia patients in complete remission using the polymerase chain reaction and nested primers. *British Journal of Haematology* 75, 355.

Mashal R, Shtalrid M, Talpaz M et al. (1990) Rearrangement and expression of p53 in the chronic phase and blast crisis of chronic myelogenous leukemia. *Blood* 75, 180.

Mickisch GH, Merlino GT, Galski H, Gottesman MM, Pastan I (1991) Transgenic mice that express the human multidrug-resistance gene in bone marrow enable a rapid identification of agents that reverse drug resistance. *Proceedings of the National Academy of Sciences of the USA* 88, 547.

Miller AD (1990) Progress toward human gene therapy. *Blood* 76, 271.

Miller CB, Zehnbauer BA, Piantadosi S, Rowley SD, Jones RJ (1991) Correlation of occult clonogenic leukemia drug sensitivity with relapse after autologous bone marrow transplantation. *Blood* 78, 1125.

Mills KI, Benn P, Birnie GD (1991) Does the breakpoint within the major breakpoint cluster region (M-bcr) influence the duration of the chronic phase in chronic myeloid leukemia? An analytical comparison of current literature. *Blood* 78, 1155.

Minden MD (1987) Oncogenes. In: Tannock IF, Hill RP (eds) *The Basic Science of Oncology*. Pergamon Press, New York.

Minden MD, Messner HA, Belch A (1985) Origin of leukemic relapse after bone marrow transplantation

detected by restriction fragment length polymorphism. *Journal of Clinical Investigation* 75, 91.
Monk M, Holding C (1990) Amplification of a β-haemoglobin sequence in individual human oocytes and polar bodies. *Lancet* 335, 985.
Morgan GJ, Wiedemann LM (1989) Molecular biology of the Philadelphia positive leukaemias. *Recenti Progressi Medicina* 80, 508.
Morgan GJ, Janssen JWG, Guo A-P et al. (1989) Polymerase chain reaction for detection of residual leukaemia. *Lancet* i, 928.
Mufti G, Stevens J, Oscier D, Hamblin T, Machin D (1985) Myelodysplastic syndromes: a scoring system with prognostic significance. *British Journal of Haematology* 59, 425.
Murru S, Loudianos G, Deiana M et al. (1991) Molecular characterization of β-thalassemia intermedia in patients of Italian descent and identification of three novel β-thalassemia mutations. *Blood* 77, 1342.
Najean Y, Millea M, Tanzer T, Lessard M, Sigaux F (1991) Chronic myelocytic leukaemia with unusual (27 years) complete remission terminating in acute undifferentiated leukaemia: a clinical and karyotypic study. *Leukemia* 5, 621.
Najfeld V, Zucker-Franklin D, Adamson J, Singer J, Troy K, Fialkow PJ (1988) Evidence for clonal development and stem cell origin of M7 megakaryocytic leukemia. *Leukemia* 2, 351.
Neale GAM, Menarguez J, Kitchingman GR et al. (1991) Detection of minimal residual disease in T-cell acute lymphoblastic leukemia using polymerase chain reaction predicts impending relapse. *Blood* 78, 739.
Nelkin BD, Przepiorka D, Burke PJ, Thomas ED, Baylin SB (1991) Abnormal methylation of the calcitonin gene marks progression of chronic myelogenous leukemia. *Blood* 77, 2431.
Nissen C, Gratwohl A, Speck B, Würsch A, Moser Y, Weis J (1986) Acquired aplastic anaemia: a PNH-like disease? *British Journal of Haematology* 64, 355.
Nourse J, Mellentin JD, Galili N et al. (1990) Chromosomal translocation t(1;19) results in synthesis of a homeobox fusion mRNA that codes for a potential chimeric transcription factor. *Cell* 60, 535.
Opalka B, Wandl U, Beer U, Roggenbuck U, Kloke O, Niederle N (1991) Breakpoint localization within the M-bcr and clinical course do not correlate in patients with chronic myelogenous leukemia undergoing alfa interferon therapy. *Leukemia* 5, 452.
Peake IR, Bowen D, Bignell P et al. (1990) Family studies and prenatal diagnosis in severe von Willebrand disease by polymerase chain reaction amplification of a variable number tandem repeat region of the von Willebrand factor gene. *Blood* 76, 555.
Pelham A, O'Reilly M-AJ, Malcolm S, Levinsky RJ, Kinnon C (1990) RFLP and deletion analysis for X-linked chronic granulomatous disease using a cDNA probe: potential for improved prenatal diagnosis and carrier determination. *Blood* 76, 820.
Petz LD, Yam P, Wallace RB et al. (1987) Mixed hematopoietic chimerism following bone marrow transplantation for hematologic malignancies. *Blood* 70, 1331.
Picker LJ, De Los Toyos J, Telen MJ, Haynes BF, Butcher EC (1989) Monoclonal antibodies against the CD44 (In(Lu)-related p-80) and Pgp-1 antigens in man recognizes the Hermes class of lymphocyte homing receptors. *Journal of Immunology* 142, 2046.
Pignon JM, Henni T, Amselem S et al. (1990) Frequent detection of minimal residual disease by the use of polymerase chain reaction in long-term survivors after bone marrow transplantation for chronic myeloid leukemia. *Leukemia* 4, 83.
Pizzoli G, Chilosi M, Semenzato G (1987) The soluble interleukin receptor in haematological disorders. *British Journal of Haematology* 67, 377.
Preisler HD, Raza A, Larson R et al. (1989) Protooncogene expression and the clinical characteristics of acute nonlymphocytic leukemia: a leukemia intergroup pilot study. *Blood* 73, 255.
Price CM, Foadi MD, Morgan GJ, Wiedemann LM (1990) Molecular analysis of a CML patient with a long duration of chronic phase before and after lymphoid blast crisis. *Leukemia* 4, 455.
Przepiorka D, Gonzales-Chambers R, Winkelstein A, Rosenfeld C, Shadduck RK (1990) Chimerism studies using in situ hybridization for the Y chromosome after T cell-depleted bone marrow transplantation. *Bone Marrow Transplantation* 5, 253.
Rambaldi A, Wakamiya N, Vellenga E et al. (1988) Expression of macrophage colony-stimulating factor and c-fms genes in human acute myeloblastic leukemia cells. *Journal of Clinical Investigation* 81, 1030.
Raskind WH, Tirumali N, Jacobson R, Singer J, Fialkow PJ (1984) Evidence for a multistep pathogenesis of a myelodysplastic syndrome. *Blood* 63, 1318.
Raskind WH, Jacobsson R, Murphy S, Adamson JW, Fialkow PJ (1985) Evidence for the involvement of B lymphoid cells in polycythaemia vera and essential thrombocythaemia. *Journal of Clinical Investigation* 75, 1388.
Raymakers R, De Witte T, Joziasse J, Van Der Lely N, Boezeman J, Haanen C (1991) In vitro growth pattern and differentiation predict for progression of myelodysplastic syndromes to acute nonlymphocytic leukemia. *British Journal of Haematology* 78, 35.
Rechavi G, Brok-Simoni F, Katzir N et al. (1988) More than two immunoglobulin heavy chain J regions in the majority of infant leukemia. *Leukemia* 2, 347.
Ridge SA, Worwood M, Oscier D, Jacobs A, Padua RA (1990) FMS mutations in myelodysplasia, leukemia and normal subjects. *Proceedings of the National Academy of Sciences of the USA* 87, 1377.
Roninson IB (1991) *Molecular and Cellular Biology of Multidrug Resistance in Tumor Cells.* Plenum, New York.
Rosenberg SA, Aebersold P, Cornetta K et al. (1990) Gene transfer into humans – immunotherapy of patients with advanced melanoma using tumor-infiltrating lymphocytes modified by retroviral gene transduction. *New England Journal of Medicine* 323, 570.
Roth MS, Schnitzer B, Bingham EL, Harnden CE, Hyder DM, Ginsberg D (1988) Rearrangement of

immunoglobulin and T cell receptor genes in Hodgkin's disease. *American Journal of Pathology* 131, 33.

Roth MS, Antrim JH, Bingham EL, Ginsberg D (1989) Detection of Philadelphia chromosome-positive cells by polymerase chain reaction following bone marrow transplant for chronic myelogenous leukemia. *Blood* 74, 882.

Rothenberg ML, Mickley LA, Cole DE et al. (1989) Expression of the mdr-1/p170 gene in patients with acute lymphoblastic leukemia. *Blood* 74, 1388.

Roussel MF, Downing JR, Rettenmeir CW, Sherr CJ (1988) A point mutation in the extracellular domain of the human CSF-1 receptor (c-fms proto-oncogene product) activates its transforming potential. *Cell* 55, 979.

Rowley JD (1978) Chromosome abnormalities in the acute phase of CML. *Virchows Archiv B Cell Pathology* 29, 57.

Rowley JD, Golomb HM, Dougherty C (1977) 15/17 translocation, a consistent chromosomal change in acute promyelocytic leukaemia. *Lancet* i, 549.

Saiki RK, Scharf SJ, Faloona F et al. (1985) Enzymatic amplification of β globin genomic sequences and restriction site analysis for diagnosis of sickle cell anaemia. *Science* 230, 1350.

Sakai H, Hattori T, Matsuoka M et al. (1987) Autocrine stimulation of interleukin-1β in acute myelogenous leukemia cells. *Journal of Experimental Medicine* 166, 1597.

Sambrook J, Fritsch EF, Maniatis T (1989) *Molecular Cloning: A Laboratory Manual* 2nd edn. Cold Spring Harbor Laboratory Press, Cold Spring Harbor.

Sandberg AA (1980) *The Chromosomes in Human Cancer and Leukemia*. Elsevier, New York.

Sato H, Preissler H, Day R et al. (1990) MDR1 transcript levels as an indication of resistant disease in acute myelogenous leukaemia. *British Journal of Haematology* 75, 340.

Sawyers CL, Timson L, Kawasaki ES, Clark SS, Witte ON, Champlin R (1990) Molecular relapse in chronic myelogenous leukemia patients after bone marrow transplantation detected by polymerase chain reaction. *Proceedings of the National Academy of Sciences of the USA* 87, 563.

Scherrer A, Kruithof EKO, Grob J-P (1991) Plasminogen activator inhibitor-2 in patients with monocytic leukemia. *Leukemia* 5, 479.

Schipperus M, Hagemeijer A, Ploemacher R, Lindemana J, Voerman J, Abels J (1988) In myelodysplastic syndromes progress into leukemia is directly related to PHA dependency for colony formation and independent for in vitro maturation capacity. *Leukemia* 2, 433.

Schmitz N, Schleselberger B, Oberboster K, Golchert K, Suttorp M, Loffler H (1991) Lymphohaemopoietic chimaerism after bone marrow transplantation for chronic myeloid leukaemia: results of simultaneous cytogenetic analysis on T-cell colonies, myeloid and erythroid progenitor cells. *British Journal of Haematology* 78, 334.

Schneider E, Ploemacher RE, Navarro S, Van Buerden C, Dy M (1991) Characterization of human hematopoietic progenitor cell subsets involved in interleukin-3-induced interleukin-6 production. *Blood* 78, 329.

Schubach WH, Hackman R, Neiman P, Miller G, Thomas ED (1982) A monoclonal immunoblastic sarcoma in donor cells bearing Epstein Barr virus genomes following allogeneic marrow grafting for acute lymphoblastic leukemia. *Blood* 60, 180.

Schuh AC, Sutherland DR, Horsfall W et al. (1990) Chronic myeloid leukemia arising in a progenitor common to T cells and myeloid cells. *Leukemia* 4, 631.

Schwartz LM, Kosz L, Kay BE (1990) Gene activation is required for developmentally programmed cell death. *Proceedings of the National Academy of Sciences of the USA* 87, 6594.

Shirafuji N, Asano S, Kozai K et al. (1988) Production of granulocyte colony-stimulating factor by acute myelomonocytic leukemia cells. *Leukemia Research* 12, 745.

Siegert W, Josimovic-Alasevic O, Schwerdtfeger R et al. (1990) Soluble interleukin 2 receptors in patients after bone marrow transplantation. *Bone Marrow Transplantation* 6, 97.

Slezak SE, Horan PK (1989) Fluorescent in vivo tracking of hematopoietic cells. Part I. Technical considerations. *Blood* 74, 2172.

Slingerland JM, Minden MD, Benchimol S (1991) Mutation of the p53 gene in human acute myelogenous leukemia. *Blood* 77, 1500.

Solary E, Bidan J-M, Calvo F et al. (1991) P-glycoprotein and in vitro reversion of doxorubicin resistance by verapamil in clinical specimens from acute leukemia and myeloma. *Leukemia* 5, 592.

Southern EM (1975) Detection of specific sequences among DNA fragments separated by gel electrophoresis. *Journal of Molecular Biology* 98, 503.

Sparkes RS, Murphree AL, Lingua RW et al. (1983) Gene for hereditary retinoblastoma assigned to chromosome 13 by linkage to esterase DD. *Science* 219, 971.

Springer TA, Dustin ML, Kishimota TK, Marlin SD (1987) The lymphocyte function-associated LFA-1, CD2 and LFA-3 molecules: cell adhesion receptors of the immune system. *Annual Review of Immunology* 5, 223.

Sproul AM, Mills KI, McDonald GA, Burnett AK (1990) Absence of bcr rearrangement and bcr/abl RNA in a patient with a 31-year survival of CML. *Leukemia* 4, 450.

Stetler-Stevenson M, Raffeld M, Cohen P, Cossman J (1988) Detection of occult follicular lymphoma by specific DNA amplification. *Blood* 72, 1822.

Sugimoto K, Toyoshima H, Sakai R et al. (1991) Mutations of the p53 gene in lymphoid leukemia. *Blood* 77, 1153.

Sunzeri FJ, Lee T-H, Brownlee RG, Busch MP (1991) Rapid simultaneous detection of multiple retroviral DNA sequences using the polymerase chain reaction and capillary DNA chromatography. *Blood* 77, 879.

Szczylik C, Skorski T, Nicolaides NC et al. (1991) Selective inhibition of leukemia cell proliferation by BCR-ABL antisense oligodeoxynucleotides. *Science*

253, 562.

Tefferi A, Bren GD, Wagner KV, Schaid DJ, Ash RC, Thibodeau SN (1990a) The location of the Philadelphia chromosomal breakpoint site and prognosis in chronic granulocytic leukemia. *Leukemia* 4, 839.

Tefferi A, Thibodeau SN, Solberg LA (1990b) Clonal studies in the myelodysplastic syndrome using X-linked restriction fragment length polymorphism. *Blood* 75, 1770.

Thein SL, Jeffreys AJ, Blacklock HA (1986) Identification of post-transplant cell populations by DNA 'fingerprint' analysis. *Lancet* ii, 37.

Tobal K, Pagluica A, Bhatt B, Bailey N, Layton DM, Mufti GJ (1990) Mutation of the human FMS gene (M-CSF receptor) in myelodysplastic syndromes and in acute myeloid leukemia. *Leukemia* 4, 486.

Trainor KJ, Briscoe MJ, Story CJ, Morley AA (1990) Monoclonality in B-lymphoproliferative disorders detected at the DNA level. *Blood* 75, 2220.

Ugozzoli L, Yam P, Petz LD *et al.* (1991) Amplification by the polymerase chain reaction of hypervariable regions of the human genome for evaluation of chimerism after bone marrow transplantation. *Blood* 77, 1607.

Van Den Berghe H, Cassiman JJ, David G, Fryns JP, Michaux JL, Sokal G (1974) Distinct haematological disorder with deletion of long arm of No 5 chromosome. *Nature* 251, 437.

Vaux DL, Cory S, Adams JM (1988) Bcl-2 gene promotes haemopoietic cell survival and co-operates with c-myc to immortalize pre B cells. *Nature* 335, 440.

Verma RS, Babu A (1989) *Human Chromosomes.* Pergamon, New York.

Vogelstein B, Fearon ER, Hamilton SR, Feinberg AP (1985) Use of restriction fragment length polymorphisms to determine the clonal origin of human tumors. *Science* 227, 642.

Vogelstein B, Fearon ER, Hamilton SR *et al.* (1987) Clonal analysis using recombinant DNA probes from the X-chromosome. *Cancer Research* 47, 4806.

Weide R, Dowding C, Sucai B, Bungey J, Chase A, Goldman JM (1991) Inactivation of the retinoblastoma susceptibility gene in a human high grade non-Hodgkin's lymphoma cell line. *British Journal of Haematology* 78, 833.

Wietzel JN, Hows JM, Jeffreys AJ, Ling Min G, Goldman JM (1988) Use of a hypervariable minisatellite DNA probe (33.15) for evaluating engraftment two or more years after bone marrow transplantation for aplastic anaemia. *British Journal of Haematology* 70, 91.

Wiedemann LM, Karhi KK, Shivji MKK *et al.* (1988) The correlation of breakpoint cluster region rearrangement and p210 phl/abl expression with morphological analysis of Ph-negative chronic myeloid leukaemia and other myeloproliferative diseases. *Blood* 71, 349.

Wilson JM, Danos O, Grossman M, Raulet DH, Mulligan RC (1990) Expression of human adenosine deaminase in mice reconstituted with retrovirus-transduced hematopoietic stem cells. *Proceedings of the National Academy of Sciences of the USA* 87, 439.

Witherspoon RP, Schubach W, Nieman P, Martin P, Thomas ED (1985) Donor cell leukemia developing six years after marrow grafting for acute leukemia. *Blood* 65, 1172.

Yam P, Petz LD, Ali S, Stock AD, Wallace RB (1987) Development of a single probe for documentation of chimerism following bone marrow transplantation. *American Journal of Human Genetics* 41, 867.

Young JC, Witte ON (1988) Selective transformation of primitive lymphoid cells by the BCR/ABL oncogene expressed in long-term lymphoid or myeloid cultures. *Molecular and Cellular Biology* 8, 4079.

Young DC, Wagner K, Griffin JD (1987) Constitutive expression of granulocyte-macrophage colony-stimulating factor gene in acute myeloblastic leukemia. *Journal of Clinical Investigation* 79, 100.

Young DC, Demitri CD, Ernst TJ, Cannistra SA, Griffin JD (1988) In vitro expression of colony-stimulating factor genes by human acute myeloblastic leukemia cells. *Experimental Hematology* 16, 378.

Yunis JJ, Rydell RE, Oken MM, Arnesen MA, Mayer MG, Lobell M (1986) Refined chromosomal analysis as an independent prognostic indicator in de novo myelodysplastic syndromes. *Blood* 67, 1721.

Zehnbauer BA, Pardoll DM, Burke PJ, Graham ML, Vogelstein B (1986) Immunoglobulin gene rearrangements in remission bone marrow specimens from patients with acute lymphoblastic leukemia. *Blood* 67, 835.

Zutter M, Hockenbury D, Silverman GA, Korsemeyer SJ (1991) Immunolocalization of the Bcl-2 protein within hematopoietic neoplasms. *Blood* 78, 1062.

Chapter 4
Bone Marrow Transplantation

Historical introduction, 190
Current results of BMT, 194
Animal models of BMT, 195
Stem cells and engraftment, 200
Recovery of haemopoiesis after BMT, 204
Immune recovery, 208
Tissue typing and matching, 211
Clinical outcome and its relationship to the source of stem cells used for transplantation, 224
Cure of leukaemia by allogeneic BMT, 225
Cure of haematological malignancies by ABMT, 233
Cure of non-malignant disorders by BMT, 238
GVHD, 242
Pathophysiology of acute GVHD, 245
Prevention and treatment of GVHD, 248
Graft failure, 253
Infections after BMT, 258
Non-haematological complications after BMT, 266
References, 271

HISTORICAL INTRODUCTION

The history of clinical bone marrow transplantation (BMT) in humans is conveniently divided into three eras: before 1970, the decade of the 1970s, and 1980 to the present.

Before 1970

The early history of BMT has been reviewed (Pegg, 1966; Bortin, 1970; Santos, 1983). Following the realization that the radioprotective effect of bone marrow transfusion in rodents was due to the engraftment of viable bone marrow cells (Lorenz et al., 1951), attempts to use autologous bone marrow grafts to rescue patients from the effects of high-dose chemotherapy were made as early as 1958 (Kurnick et al., 1958). Attempts at allogeneic BMT met with failure either from graft rejection or from graft-versus-host disease (GVHD) – 'secondary disease' – and the approach was little used until the advent of human leukocyte antigen (HLA) typing facilitated the selection of histocompatible donors. Of 49 allogeneic transplants reported before 1960, none were durably successful (Bortin, 1970). The only exception to this depressing picture were reports documenting successful correction of severe aplastic anaemia by marrow transplants between identical twins in four out of seven patients (Pegg, 1966). In the absence of any reliable typing procedure the mixed lymphocyte reaction (Bain et al., 1964) was the only means of testing compatibility, and marrow transfusions from multiple donors were often performed in the hope that the most compatible marrow would take. In 1959, Mathé et al., for example, used marrow infusions from multiple donors to treat six victims of accidental irradiation following the Vinca nuclear accident in

Yugoslavia. Transient take was documented in some, but all ultimately recovered autologous marrow function (Mathé et al., 1959).

The development of modern clinical BMT techniques owes much to the methodical work of E. Donnal Thomas who used the dog as a preclinical model, introducing methotrexate as a form of prophylaxis against GVHD, and developing improved techniques for administering total body irradiation. The characterization of the HLA system towards the end of the decade and the possibility of selecting histocompatible donors led to a renewal of interest in allogeneic BMT. The realization that some immune deficiency diseases were derived from bone marrow stem cell defects led to spectacular cures for severe combined immune deficiency (SCID; Gatti et al., 1968) and the first successful transplant for Wiskott–Aldrich disease (Bach et al., 1968). While such results were the exception, they indicated a real therapeutic potential for BMT.

1970–1980

From 1970 the pace of progress increased. With greater confidence in the success of BMT relatively large series of studies were carried out. The Seattle BMT group, led by Thomas, reported a series of 100 BMTs for relapsed leukaemia in 1977 (Thomas et al., 1977). Such attempts to treat end-stage leukaemia by BMT were largely doomed to failure because of the high initial mortality from infection, pneumonitis, relapse or resistant disease. Nevertheless 10 patients became long-term cured survivors, indicating that BMT had a potent antileukaemic effect. More encouraging results were achieved in severe aplastic anaemia – for example, Storb et al. (1974) described a 50% survival for BMT in a series of 24 such patients.

The need to share information about the complicated technology of BMT brought together a group of transplanters who formed the European Cooperative Group for Bone Marrow Transplantation (EBMT). In Milwaukee USA, Bortin and Rimm established the International Bone Marrow Transplant Registry (IBMTR) which is now a major resource for BMT statistical analyses. An important change in emphasis which improved survival figures was the application of BMT as an elective procedure for poor-risk leukaemia incurable by chemotherapy alone, rather than as a salvage attempt at the end-stage of the disease. Once reliable and effective myeloablative regimens for allogeneic BMT were established there was a resurgence of interest in autologous BMT for leukaemia using similar high-dose chemoradiotherapy. By the end of the decade BMT had progressed from an experimental procedure to become an established technique with defined clinical indications.

After 1980

The 1980s saw a huge expansion in the number and variety of autologous and allogeneic BMTs performed worldwide (Bortin and Rimm, 1986; Barrett, 1991). Data from the IBMTR indicate a progressive increase in the number of allogeneic transplants carried out yearly. This increase is mainly due to a rise in BMT for leukaemia, and for chronic myeloid leukaemia (CML) in particular. The IBMTR has reported a progressive rise in the number of new BMT teams registering, as well as an increase in the number of BMTs carried out each year by each team. In addition there has been a rise in the number of autografts for leukaemia in Europe, and for solid tumours and lymphomas particularly in North America. There have been important changes in the characteristics of patients and donors reported to the IBMTR over the last 10 years:

1 An increase in the upper age limit for allotransplant recipients with a rise in the median age at BMT from 25 to 35 years.
2 An increase in BMT from incompletely matched family donors, and from matched but unrelated donors.
3 Application of BMT to malignant disorders not previously transplanted: since 1980 BMT has been carried out in significant numbers for the first time in multiple myeloma, lymphomas, myelodysplastic syndromes, and solid tumours.
4 Application of BMT to non-malignant disorders: new disorders transplanted for the first time since 1980 include thalassaemia and sickle cell anaemia, and inherited metabolic disorders such as the mucopolysaccharidoses, and neurolipidoses. Although BMT has been used in at least 25 genetic disorders they account for only 9% of the transplants reported to the IBMTR (see Chapter 2).

New treatment agents

New drugs of great potential importance for BMT have been introduced in the last decade. Perhaps the most important innovation has been the introduction of cyclosporin for the prevention and treatment of GVHD. Control of infectious complications has been improved with the introduction of the antiviral agents acyclovir and gancyclovir, imidazole antifungal agents, and new generations of penicillins, cephalosporins, and aminoglycoside antibiotics, as well as new antibiotic types such as ciprofloxacin.

Monoclonal antibodies have been employed successfully to purge bone marrow of T lymphocytes or malignant cells, and have also been used *in vivo* in the treatment of GVHD and rejection. Latterly, trials of recombinant growth factors granulocyte-macrophage colony-stimulating factor (GM-CSF), G-CSF, interleukin 3 (IL-3) and IL-2 have been used to improve haematological recovery and stimulate immune responsiveness (see Chapter 5). It has yet to be demonstrated that any of these new agents has made a measurable impact on the outcome after BMT.

New strategies

Removal of T lymphocytes from donor marrow has proved a highly effective way to prevent GVHD, but it is now clear that the abolition of GVHD is accompanied by a corresponding rise in the rates of relapse and graft rejection. Marrow transplants depleted of T lymphocytes have nevertheless improved the results in two situations: mismatched parental grafts for severe combined immune deficiency, and matched or partially matched unrelated BMT for leukaemia.

New conditioning regimens have been developed in the last 10 years with the aim of reducing toxicity, improving the antileukaemia effect and increasing graft take. It is not yet clear whether such new regimens result in significant improvements in disease-free survival.

Changes in transplant outcome

Against the background of increased use of BMT it is appropriate to determine whether the technique itself has become safer and more effective at curing the underlying disorder.

A study by the IBMTR has identified a very small but real improvement in BMT for leukaemia: the analysis concerned 3785 leukaemia patients (1276 acute lymphoblastic leukaemia (ALL), 1393 acute myeloid leukaemia (AML), 1166 CML), transplanted between 1978 and 1987. The association between year of transplant and outcome was measured using Cox proportional hazard regression analysis. The variables included in the model were disease type and status, patient age, performance score, organ involvement, splenomegaly, infection pregraft, and interval between diagnosis and treatment. The data were also analysed to include or exclude T-depleted BMT. Between 1978 and 1987 the risk of relapse increased significantly for CML patients. This was partly related to T cell depletion. However the relative risk of relapse was also higher, but not statistically so for all patients after excluding T-depletion data. Transplant-related mortality decreased significantly for the whole group. The relative increase in survival probability translates into a 5–10% decrease in BMT-related mortality (Bortin *et al.*, 1992).

The transplant-related mortality of autologous and identical-twin BMT is comparatively low – between 5 and 10%. Thus the main contribution to transplant-related mortality is related to the effect of an allograft. It should be possible therefore to reduce BMT mortality considerably if the adverse effects of the allograft could be prevented. There is evidence that this can be achieved: for example, the Pesaro group who have pioneered BMT in thalassaemia have optimized the conditioning regime and post-transplant care and eliminated much of the transplant-related risk. They report a transplant survival of 94% in good-risk patients (Lucarelli et al., 1990). The introduction of a very low dose cyclophosphamide conditioning regimen for Fanconi anaemia by Gluckman has also resulted in lower immediate mortality and superior survival for these patients (Gluckman et al., 1984).

One challenge facing the technique of BMT is to devise ways of using the biological response modifiers now available to enhance selectively normal haematological and immune recovery, including antileukaemia activity, while reducing BMT mortality from infection and GVHD.

CURRENT RESULTS OF BMT

Despite the fact that there is a wide diversity in the techniques used for BMT, the outcome can be largely defined by a relatively small number of patient-related and treatment-related features. Treatment outcome can be considered under three headings: disease control/cure, transplant-related complications, and the combined effect of these features measured as disease-free survival. Several generalizations can be made about the results of BMT:

1 Survival following BMT depends upon the clinical state of the patient. Best results are obtainable in younger individuals, those in excellent general health as measured by the Karnofsky performance score, and those in whom the transplant was carried out electively at an early stage in the disease progression. Outcome is therefore best for malignant diseases in remission, intermediate for disease that has relapsed but is still responsive to further treatment, and worst for resistant disease either manifest as primary treatment failure or as treatment-resistant relapse.

2 Survival after allogeneic BMT is generally better for patients transplanted for non-malignant diseases.

3 Treatment-related mortality increases with increasing disparity between the recipient and the donor. Thus for autologous BMT and syngeneic BMT, procedural mortality is in the order of 5%. In fully HLA-matched donor–recipient pairs this rises to about 25% and is above 40% for HLA mismatches. This indicates that the main complications arising after BMT can be ascribed to immunological disparity between donor and recipient.

Table 4.1 Effects of modification to the bone marrow transplantation (BMT) procedure on outcome

Transplant manoeuvre	Benefit	Disadvantage
T lymphocyte depletion	Less GVHD	Increased risk of relapse and rejection
Increased intensity of antileukaemic schedule	Less relapse	Higher procedural mortality
Increased GVHD prophylaxis post-BMT	Less GVHD	Increased rate of relapse and infection
Use of autologous marrow or identical twin	Low procedural mortality	Increased rate of relapse
Use of unrelated matched donor or family donor other than sibling	More GVL	Increased risk of severe GVHD and rejection

GVHD, Graft-versus-host disease; GVL, graft versus leukaemia.

4 The ability to cure malignant diseases by BMT is linked to a poorly characterized graft versus leukaemia (GVL) effect which increases with increasing severity of GVHD and donor–recipient HLA disparity.

5 Many factors which increase the chance of cure increase the likelihood of death from transplant complications. Thus disease-free survival for transplantation in a given disease tends to vary little despite radically different BMT approaches. For example, increased intensity of the preparative regimen is associated with a decrease in the chance of rejection and relapse of a malignant process. This potential improvement in the results is however offset by an increase in procedural mortality. Other examples are shown in Table 4.1.

The results of BMT in various disorders analysed for major outcome variables obtained from collected data of the IBMTR are summarized in Table 4.2.

ANIMAL MODELS OF BMT

Animals are used to study basic transplantation biology, or as preclinical models for conditioning regimens and GVHD prevention and treatment (Table 4.3). Histocompatibility antigen systems have been determined in detail for several mammals, including the mouse and the dog. The broad similarity between the histocompatibility complexes in diverse mammalian species makes general comparisons between human and animal data possible, but the highly selected inbred strains used do not compare with the diversity of inherited tissue types occurring in the clinical arena. Rodents are sensitive to

Table 4.2 Overview of results for allogeneic bone marrow transplantation (BMT) in a variety of situations (Gorin and Aegerter, 1986; Advisory Committee of the IBMTR, 1989)

Disease	Relapse (%)	Rejection (%)	Disease free survival (%)
Leukaemias with matched sibling donors			
Elective in remission	15–30	<5	40–65
Responding disease	40–50	<5	25–40
Resistant advanced disease	50–70	<10	10–15
Leukaemias – autologous BMT			
Elective in remission	40	<5	60
Responding disease	50	<5	30–40
Resistant advanced disease	>50	5	<10
Non-malignant disorders with matched sibling donors			
Immune deficiency diseases		<5	95
Inborn errors		5–10	80
Aplastic anaemia		10–20	70

many of the cytokines and growth factors currently being evaluated, but human cells are generally non-responsive to rodent growth factors. Primates such as the baboon and the marmoset are much closer to the human both in their growth factor responses and the surface phenotype of their lymphoid and myeloid cells. Because of this they have been used in preclinical models of growth factor treatment and stem cell transplantation studies (Chapter 5). Dogs, although more radio-resistant than humans, have been widely used for many years in the development of preparative regimens for BMT. Miniature swine (which have the advantage of size and ease of handling) have similar skin responses to humans, and are useful in GVHD studies (Sachs et al., 1991).

The following section covers some of the more important recent developments in animal BMT models.

SCID mice

The phenomenon of xenograft resistance which prevents the engraftment of human cells into irradiated rodent recipients has hitherto prevented attempts to study human haematopoiesis in animal recipients. Xenograft resistance is due to several factors: T cell, natural killer (NK) and lymphokine activated killer (LAK) cell function,

Table 4.3 Animal models of bone marrow transplantation (BMT) and their applicability to human BMT

Histocompatibility
MHC broadly similar in all mammals. Mouse, dog and primate antigen systems well-characterized. Problem: inbred strains do not share the antigenic diversity that occurs in human BMT. Impact of class I or class II MHC differences on rejection, GVHD, and leukaemic relapse can be studied

Cytotoxic chemotherapy and radiation
Dose–responses to chemotherapy and radiation and non-haemopoietic side-effects can be determined. Dogs are radioresistant. Mice are radiosensitive in comparison to humans

GVHD
Syndrome is similar in its tissue distribution and pathology. Best model for human skin GVHD is the pig

Stem cell studies and purging
Early haemopoietic progenitors (CFU-S) can be studied. Primate haemopoietic progenitors carry surface antigens cross-reactive with human antigens and can be used in purging experiments

Growth factors
Most human growth factors are active in rodents and primates. However their precise actions may differ

Antileukaemia effect of BMT
Numerous leukaemia models exist in rodents. They can be used to quantitate precisely the antileukaemic efficacy of chemoradiotherapy treatment and immune manipulations. Their disadvantage is the artificiality of the leukaemia lines used

Late effects
The short natural lifespan of rodents makes them useful for the study of the effects of BMT on longevity. Non-haemopoietic toxicity from BMT is similar in rodents and humans

Congenital disorders
Several animal models of congenital disorders correctable by BMT have been studied

MHC, major histocompatibility complex; GVHD, graft versus host disease; CFU-S, spleen colony-forming units.

possible incompatibilities in the haemopoietic inductive microenvironment and lack of response of human stem cells to mouse growth factors. Recently, however, several groups have succeeded in achieving engraftment of human cells in immune-deficient mouse strains. Mosier and others (1988) used mice doubly recessive for the xid gene — SCID mice — as recipients for human peripheral blood lymphocytes. Significant levels of human lymphocytes persisted in lymphoid organs and blood and were capable of heterotopic skin graft rejection. Dick and Kamel-Reid (1991) used the triple recessive strain bg/nu/xid.

These mice are athymic (nu gene), and deficient in functioning NK/LAK cells and B cells (bg/xid gene).

Engraftment of 10^7 marrow cells was achieved in irradiated recipients as measured by granulocyte progenitor CFU-GM numbers in bone marrow which rose 40-fold by day 14 after transplantation. Erythroid and megakaryocyte engraftment was not achieved. The SCID model was also successfully used by these workers to transplant human common ALL cells which showed the same pattern of tissue distribution as seen in humans. McCune and others (1988) used transplanted human fetal thymus followed by human fetal liver to reconstitute successfully human T4 and T8 cells in SCID mouse recipients.

Many problems relating to engraftment remain. However, these studies show that human lymphoid engraftment with functioning T cells can be achieved, but that lymphoid development requires the presence of human thymic tissue. In contrast it appears that human haemopoiesis is at least partially independent of host growth factor production. These models lend themselves to many experimental applications such as the study of early events in human marrow engraftment, and the establishment of human leukaemia models for experimental treatments with adoptive immunotherapy and cytokines.

Tolerance

Mice grafted with MHC-incompatible bone marrow exhibit sustained engraftment without lethal GVHD and tolerance to donor skin grafts. Such animals are relatively immune-deficient. This immune defect appears to be related to failure of the host thymus to process donor-derived prethymic T cells. The defect can be corrected by additional host antigen presenting cells (Rayfield and Brent, 1963).

Sachs et al. (1991) evaluated mixed marrow transplants of MHC-incompatible donor cells with T lymphocyte-depleted syngeneic marrow cells to avoid rejection of the donor. Such mice showed stable mixed haemopoietic and lymphoid chimerism with no GVHD and tolerance to donor skin grafts. Across major histocompatibility differences, as typified by transplants of the strain combination B10/D2 into B10 recipients, syngeneic host cells only protected against acute GVHD and the animals succumbed later to chronic GVHD. The administration of intraperitoneal IL-2 in the first 5 days after BMT conferred protection against acute and chronic GVHD. They went on to show that their approach could be applied to mice given sublethal irradiation provided additional irradiation was given to the thymus. Such animals receiving T-depleted syngeneic marrow with donor marrow achieved stable chimerism and tolerance without GVHD. This model points the way towards the use of BMT to confer tolerance in the context of organ transplants. An important question that can be answered by this model is whether a GVL effect is conserved in the tolerant state: mice given the experimental leukaemia EL4 could be protected against progressive leukaemia by the combination of mismatched marrow and spleen cells together with IL-2 and T-depleted syngeneic marrow. No GVHD developed and tolerance was demonstrable. Another method of inducing tolerance has been investigated by Sprent et al. (1991). They used strains of mice that differ from C57 BL/6 mice either by their class I antigens (bn1 mice) or by their class II antigen (bn12 mice) to study the GVHD process initiated either by T8 lymphocyte subsets working through class I differences, or T4 subsets working through class II. Class I GVHD was not related to the dose of T8 cells given but was enhanced by small numbers of T4 cells and reduced if a large number of T4 cells were added in. In these animals tolerance to host cells was demonstrated by the lack of chronic GVHD and the ability of spleen cells from the transplanted animals to take without GVHD in further recipients. Class II GVHD was acute in onset and affected the gastrointestinal tract. The GVHD was T4 cell dose-related. The modifying effect of high doses of T4 cells on class I type GVHD was attributed to the beneficial effect of helper activity enhancing the recovery of B cells and reducing mortality from gut pathogens, but the mechanism of tolerance is not fully determined. Such experiments help to define the initiation of the GVHD reaction and show that beneficial patterns of immune reconstitution by selec-

Table 4.4 Animal models of genetic disorders evaluable by bone marrow transplantation (Vellodi et al., 1992)

Genetic disorder	Animal model
Red cell disorders	
Sickle mouse (Greaves et al., 1990)	Mouse
Leukocyte disorders	
Chédia–Higashi syndrome	Mouse
Lysosomal storage disorders	
Maroteaux–Lamy	Cat
Twitcher mouse (Krabbé)	Mouse
Hurler–Scheie	Dog
Fucosidosis	Dog
Niemann–Pick	Mouse
S-glucuronidase	Mouse
Other metabolic diseases	
Osteopetrosis (Walker, 1975)	Mouse, rat

tive repopulation with controlled numbers of T cell subsets may be achieved.

Leukaemia models

Transplantable leukaemias are restricted to rodent models. The most relevant are the slower growing leukaemias with kinetic behaviour closest to human leukaemia, such as the Brown Norway (BN) rat AML (Van Bekkum and Hagenbeek, 1977; Hagenbeek et al., 1991). More recently, leukaemias resembling Ph^1-positive CML in chronic phase (Daley et al., 1990), and in Ph^1-positive ALL (Heisterkamp et al., 1990), have been produced in mice by insertion of the relevant BCR/ABL gene sequence. Leukaemia models can be used in BMT research to study the antileukaemic effect of conditioning regimens and immune manipulation to enhance the elimination of minimal residual disease.

Models of genetic diseases

There are a variety of useful models of genetic disorders which have been used to establish the efficacy of marrow transplantation in correcting metabolic disorders, and to establish whether central nervous system metabolic disorders, such as the lipidosis resembling Krabbé disease, can be corrected by BMT (Yeager et al., 1984). The demonstration that osteopetrosis in the op/op mouse (Walker, 1975) could be corrected by BMT led to the first successful attempts at correcting the human disorder. Table 4.4 summarizes the animal genetic disorders studied as BMT models.

STEM CELLS AND ENGRAFTMENT

Characteristics of the transplantable human stem cell (HSC)

The original observation by Till and McCulloch (1961) that transplanted marrow generated mixed colonies of maturing granulocytes, erythrocytes, and megakaryocytes in the spleens and femurs of irradiated mice, and the subsequent demonstration through chromosomal markers that a single cell could repopulate the entire lymphohaemopoietic system (Metcalf and Moore, 1971), gave credence to the concept that an early pluripotent bone marrow stem cell was the basic unit required for transplantation. Recently improved assay techniques have made it possible to study the proliferation of very early stem cells in humans characterized by their surface phenotype CD34 (Egelund et al., 1990; Haylock et al., 1990; Wolf et al., 1990; and see also Chapter 1). Because the CD34 antigen is also expressed on marrow cells of baboons it has been possible to carry out transplantation experiments with pure CD34+ve populations which demonstrate that full haematopoietic reconstitution can be achieved with these cells alone (Berenson et al., 1988).

In humans, CD34+ve cells generate blast cell colonies with a high secondary plating efficiency giving rise to committed progenitor cells (Ogawa, 1991). CD34+ve cells are responsible for sustaining haemopoiesis in long-term suspension cultures of human bone marrow (Egelund et al., 1990) and are believed to be the circulating cells responsible for haemopoietic reconstitution by peripheral blood autografts (Haylock et al., 1990), cultured CML autografts (Barnett et al., 1989), as well as bone marrow transplants. The frequency of CD34+ve cells is approximately 1×10^4 nucleated bone marrow cells, thus it appears that engraftment is readily achieved in clinical practice with approximately $1-2 \times 10^6$ stem cells. There is some evidence, however, that reconstitution by CD33+ve committed stem cells is responsible for the rapid, early recovery after blood-derived stem cell

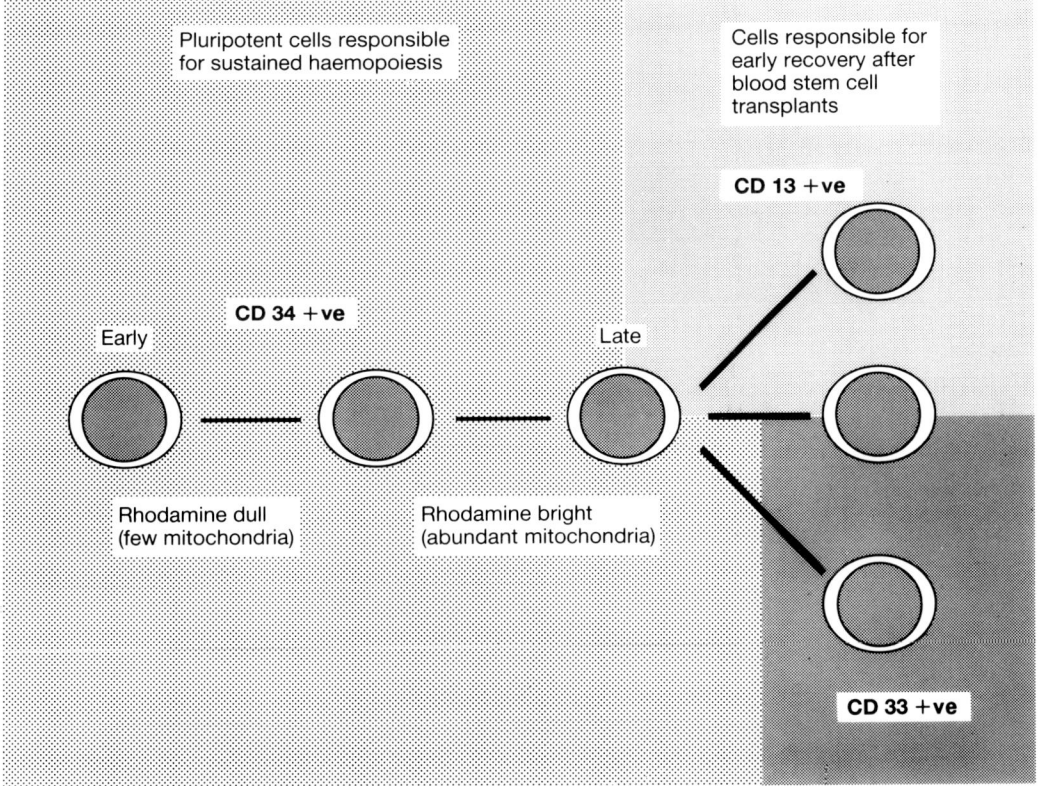

Fig. 4.1 Stem cell compartments and engraftment.

transplants, and this may be related to the presence of more differentiated progenitors of the CFU-GM class (To et al., 1990). The relationship of haemopoietic cell development with engraftment potential of progenitor populations is shown in Figure 4.1.

Sources of stem cells for BMT

Table 4.5 summarizes the important differences in the content and characteristics of stem cells derived from various sources.

Bone marrow

The process of aspirating marrow by multiple puncture breaks down the barrier between the extrasinusoidal marrow and the blood in the venous sinusoids. The cells obtained are therefore a mixture of bone marrow cells and peripheral blood cells containing a varying number of lymphocytes. Various techniques have been adopted to reduce blood cell contamination but apart from the practice of obtaining multiple small-volume aspirates from different sites, no approach results in any significant reduction in blood cell contamination. The percentage of lymphocytes in the marrow infusion has been statistically related to the risk of developing GVHD. Marrow transplants contain not only the whole range of marrow myeloid cells from stem cells to mature cells but also stromal cells, including fibroblast precursors, fat cells,

Table 4.5 Sources of stem cells for transplantation (see text for references)

	Stem cell content	T lymphocyte content	Special features
Bone marrow	+++	+	Contains fibroblasts and stroma-forming cells
Peripheral blood	+	+++	Insufficient numbers for practical application unless circulating stem cell numbers are increased by mobilization
Peripheral blood recovering from chemotherapy	++	+++	
Cord blood	+++	+++	Stem cell content similar to adult marrow. Small total volume restricts use to infants and children
Fetal liver	+++	+	High stem cell content but small volume restricts use to infants
T lymphocyte-depleted bone marrow	+++	−	Selective readdition of myeloid and stem cell component. Two log lymphocyte depletion
Cultured marrow	+++	−	Selection of purified normal stem cell fraction in autologous bone marrow transplantation for leukaemia

+ low levels, ++ intermediate levels, +++ high levels.

endothelial cells, macrophages and their precursors. There is no clear evidence that the non-stem cell components of the bone marrow infusion (with the exception of post-thymic cells and B cells) contribute permanently grafted populations in the recipient.

Peripheral blood

Peripheral blood is increasingly used as a source of stem cells for engraftment (Kessinger et al., 1988). The practical problem with this approach is the difficulty of obtaining sufficient numbers of stem cells by leukapheresis. It has been estimated that about 12 litres of blood has to be processed by leukapheresis to obtain sufficient cell numbers for engraftment (as measured by CFU-GM content). Several techniques can increase the yield of stem cells: one method is to carry out several leukaphereses following chemotherapy to coincide with the surge of recovering CD34+ve stem cells in the blood that immediately precedes monocyte and neutrophil recovery (Juttner et al., 1985; Körbling et al., 1986; Williams et al., 1990). Agents such as steroids and GM-CSF or G-CSF mobilize stem cells from the marrow and can significantly increase circulating progenitor cell numbers whose quality in terms of transplantation and their capacity to sustain haemopoiesis indefinitely is unimpaired (Körbling et al., 1990).

Fetal liver

The fetal liver is a haematopoietic organ until the third trimester. Stem cells derived from fetal liver are capable of reconstituting full lymphoid and myeloid function in human recipients, and fetal liver transplants have been used in the treatment of immune deficiency states, aplastic anaemia and leukaemia. The potential advantage of fetal liver is that the relative immaturity of the immune system permits transplantation across HLA barriers. However, there are several important limitations to its use. Firstly there are practical difficulties of obtaining fetuses of a suitable gestational age. The trend towards early termination of pregnancy means that most fetuses available are below 14 weeks. Fetal liver from fetuses below 12 weeks of gestation often fails to generate full immune reconstitution, while older fetuses have a tendency to cause GVHD. A further limiting factor is the small size of the liver which precludes obtaining enough stem cells for transplantation in adults (Gale, 1980). Fetal liver transplantation has mainly been used to treat infants with SCID. Touraine and colleagues (1981) have reported some remarkable successes, but the pace of immune recovery is exceptionally slow and frequently incomplete. The successful use of T-depleted parental haplotype-matched marrow for infants without a matched sibling donor has made the use of fetal liver transplants outmoded.

Umbilical cord blood

The possibility that umbilical cord blood (CB) might serve as a practical source of HSC comes from earlier observations that CB contains large numbers of committed precursors. Additionally, CB contains largely virgin T cells that have not yet encountered antigen. It has been argued that GVHD might be less likely to occur with CB transplants. On this basis Gluckman et al. transplanted a 4-year-old child with Fanconi anaemia using CB derived from an HLA-matched sibling. There was sustained engraftment without GVHD (Gluckman et al., 1989). These results have encouraged research into the optimum methods of collecting and storing CB, characterizing its immune function and GVHD potential, and further determining its applicability for transplantation.

Cultured marrow cells

In humans suspension cultures of marrow can only be reliably maintained for 4–6 weeks. Nevertheless autologous marrow cultured for 2 weeks from patients with acute myeloid leukaemia in remission (Chang et al., 1989) and CML (Barnett et al., 1989) can regenerate haematopoiesis when transfused into the recipient. The goal of using cultured stem cells as a pure (lymphocyte-depleted) source of CD34+ve stem cells remains some way off.

RECOVERY OF HAEMOPOIESIS AFTER BMT

Engraftment

Intravenous administration of bone marrow results in rapid clearance of CFU associated with lung sequestration, followed by a second more sustained recirculation lasting about 24 hours (Barrett et al., 1980). Mouse experiments suggest that there is no selective acquisition of HSC by the bone marrow, but rather that there is an even distribution of stem cells in the reticuloendothelial system resulting in significant haemopoiesis in the spleen. The in vivo role of intracellular adhesion molecules and specific stroma–stem cell interactions in the attachment of HSC to marrow stroma is not known. Early after BMT, circulating CFU-GM are absent but re-emerge into the blood shortly before haemopoietic recovery. The factors necessary for engraftment are the presence of a threshold number of stem cells in a favourable marrow microenvironment, the production of appropriate growth factors, and in the case of allografts, absence of cells capable of causing immediate rejection. The origin of growth factors necessary for early engraftment remains a subject of debate. There is considerable evidence that host marrow stroma itself provides all the support required. However, there is also evidence for the contribution of donor T cells to engraftment, and the possibility that the grafted myeloid cells produce stem cell growth factors (Martin, 1990).

Haematological recovery

Following BMT the first change observed is a fall in circulating leukocytes and platelets, reaching a nadir of less than $0.1 \times 10^9/l$ about 7 days after the BMT. The appearance of the bone marrow aspirate in the first 10 days is almost acellular, with occasional foci of developing erythropoiesis and granulopoiesis. By day 14 trilineage engraftment is seen in the majority of patients but the marrow remains extremely hypocellular. Marrow cellularity returns only slowly to normal and even 1 year post-transplant the recovery remains incomplete in a minority of patients. The first change in the blood count after marrow transplantation usually occurs between days 14 and 21.

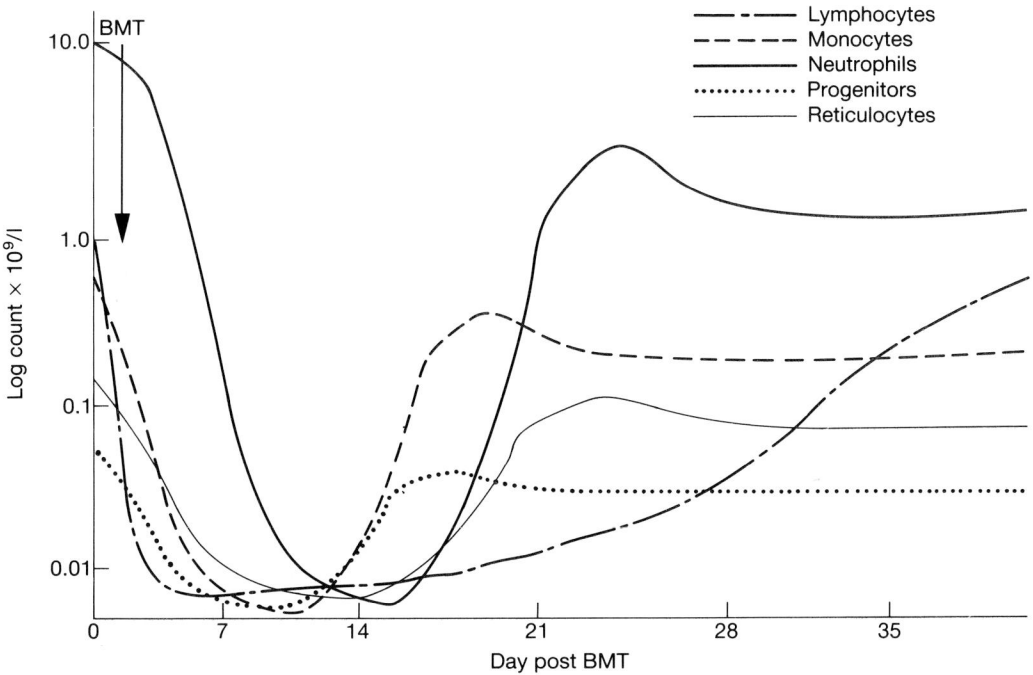

Fig. 4.2 Pattern of haematological recovery after BMT.

There is often an initial monocyte recovery accompanied by the emergence of circulating colony-forming progenitors. Subsequently the neutrophil count rises, reaching normal values by about 1 month post-BMT. Reticulocytes appear in the blood at about the same time but do not usually increase above normal absolute values. Slowest to recover are the platelets. Platelet transfusion support may be required for up to 1 month after BMT and normal counts are only achieved after several months (Fig. 4.2; Atkinson, 1990a).

Regulatory factors

The alterations in the bone marrow regulatory environment promoting stem cell recovery are not known in any detail. Animal studies indicate that early-acting stem cell growth factors are produced in response to marrow hypocellularity (Sallefors et al., 1991). Such studies did not define the nature of the growth factors involved. In humans, mRNA for IL-3, GM-CSF is detectable in blood mononuclear cells following BMT (Atkinson, 1991b). Increase in circulating growth factors G-CSF (Sheridan et al., 1989), erythropoietin (Ireland et al., 1990) and megakaryocyte-stimulating factors (Adams et al., 1990) occurs in the first 2 weeks. Thus the available evidence indicates that the recovery of haemopoiesis after BMT is not limited by a lack of growth factors.

Functional studies

There have been several studies indicating that granulocyte (Atkinson, 1990a), and platelet function is defective for some months after BMT. Red cell recovery is characterized by a phase of dyserythropoiesis and a raised level of fetal haemoglobin (Alter et al., 1976).

Factors affecting haematological recovery

The situations affecting the speed and quality of haematological recovery can be separated into host-related and donor-related factors (Table 4.6).

Host factors

The underlying disease requiring BMT has an influence on engraftment in two circumstances—severe aplastic anaemia (SAA) and myelofibrosis. The failure of a proportion of identical-twin donor marrows to engraft in an aplastic recipient without prior conditioning treatment is evidence that the marrow environment may be unsup-

Table 4.6 Factors affecting the pattern of haemopoietic recovery (Atkinson, 1990a)

Stem cell variables
Number of donor stem cells infused
Viability of stem cells after cryopreservation, storage or *in vitro* manipulation
Type of donor progenitor infused (CFU-GM are responsible for early recovery)
Chemotherapy damage to autologous stem cells delays recovery

Host factors
Splenomegaly delays engraftment
Viral infection retards engraftment

Treatment
Additional haemopoietic growth factors (G-CSF, GM-CSF accelerate recovery)
Methotrexate delays recovery

Established haemopoietic recovery impaired by
Viral infection
Graft-versus-host disease
Cytotoxic chemotherapy
Donor autoimmune processes

CFU-GM, granulocyte-monocyte colony forming units; G-CSF, granulocyte colony-stimulating factor; GM-CSF, granulocyte-macrophage colony-stimulating factor.

portive to stem cell engraftment in at least some patients with SAA (Champlin *et al.*, 1984). There is no evidence that chemoradiotherapy conditioning regimes themselves have a negative effect on marrow engraftment. In fact it is possible that the effect of the conditioning is to stimulate growth factor production by stromal cells in response to the effect of marrow hypocellularity. However, methotrexate given after the transplant to prevent GVHD significantly retards blood count recovery.

Donor factors

Experimental and clinical results support the concept that marrow engraftment is an all-or-none process with a threshold (as yet undefined) minimum stem cell number required to secure engraftment. The number of marrow cells required to achieve engraftment is related to the degree of histocompatibility between donor and recipient (Anasetti *et al.*, 1989). Conversely, ABMT and BMT between identical twins achieve satisfactory rates of engraftment with about two to three times fewer cells than are required for HLA-matched sibling transplants. The pace of recovery of a successfully engrafted marrow is not, however, affected by the degree of donor–recipient compatibility. Numerous studies have attempted to relate the number of infused nucleated cells (Arnold *et al.*, 1986), but other studies have failed to show an association (Atkinson *et al.*, 1985) or the number of committed progenitors to the speed of recovery following BMT. There is some evidence to support a relationship between the number of CFU-GM and the time to achieve a neutrophil count over $1 \times 10^9/l$ (Arnold *et al.*, 1986) but other studies have failed to show a correlation (Atkinson *et al.*, 1985). Recovery after autologous BMT is in some circumstances more rapid than after allogeneic BMT, but platelet recovery is often delayed in such recipients, possibly related to the effect of previous chemotherapy on the function of the retransplanted marrow (Gorin and Aegerter, 1986; Gorin *et al.*, 1986a). After blood stem cell autografts there is an early rise in neutrophils, often with a biphasic recovery pattern, due possibly to the presence of more mature stem cells with a faster repopulating ability than bone marrow progenitors (To *et al.*, 1990).

IMMUNE RECOVERY

While haematological recovery is prompt after BMT, recovery of the immune system is much more prolonged. Following BMT there is a combined immune deficiency state which persists for some months.

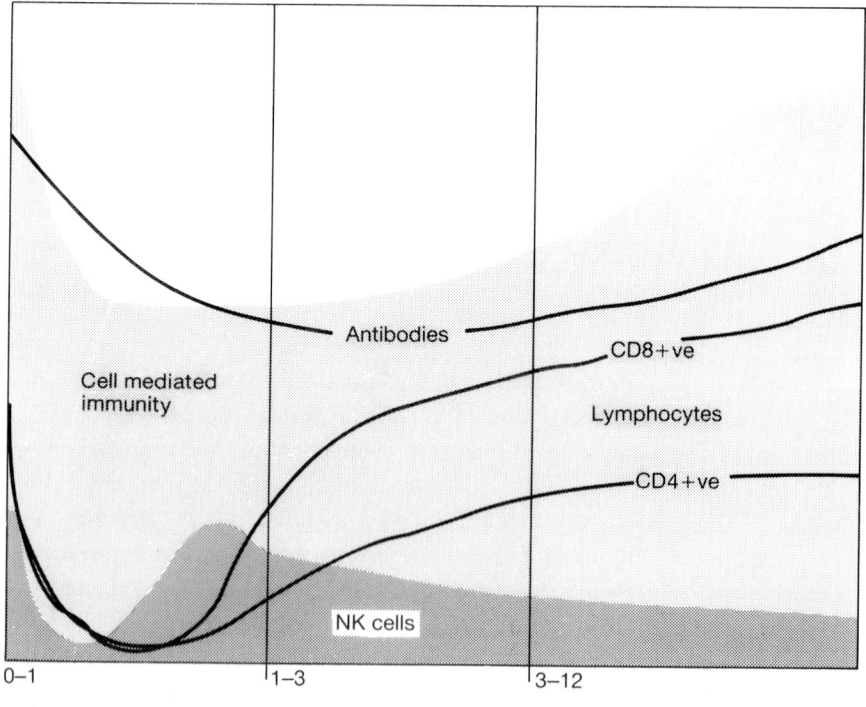

Fig. 4.3 Immune recovery after BMT.

The defect relates partly to the time taken for lymphocyte progenitors to repopulate the lymphoid system with functioning mature cells, partly because of the almost universal administration of immune suppressive agents following BMT, and partly to a phase of immune dysregulation exacerbated by viral infection and GVHD (Atkinson, 1990a).

Lymphocyte counts rise to normal by 12 weeks after BMT. However, irrespective of the source of the transplant there is a disproportionate rise in CD8+ve suppressor cells, leading to an inverted T4:T8 ratio. Natural killer cells bearing the HNK1 marker rise rapidly in the first 2–3 weeks and may exceed the normal range (Ault et al., 1985; Reittie et al., 1989). A small population of cells of unusual phenotype circulate early after BMT. They include primitive uncommitted CD3+, CD4−, CD8− lymphocytes, some of which express the γ/δ T cell receptor. Morphologically the lymphocytes circulating in the first few weeks after BMT include a population of large granular lymphocytes and atypical mononuclear cells, some of these expressing activation markers (DR+ve T cells) (Azogui et al., 1983). B lymphocytes expressing CD19 recover to normal levels in the blood by 4 weeks. The changes in lymphoid populations and immune recovery are shown in Figure 4.3.

Functional abnormalities

Numerous functional defects in lymphocyte responsiveness occur following BMT. In the first few weeks the presence of NK cells and a disproportionate increase in CD8 cells is associated with an increase in NK and LAK cell function. The early recovery of suppressor cells of the CD3+ve γ/δ cells and CD8+, CD11+ subsets may be directly responsible for a suppressive effect on the immune response (Witherspoon et al., 1986). Proliferative responses to pokeweed mitogen, phytohaemagglutinin (PHA), and allogeneic lymphocyte targets are defective for up to 6 months after uncomplicated transplants but GVHD prolongs recovery considerably (Lum, 1987). A consequence of reduced helper cell activity is impaired T/B lymphocyte cooperation, leading to defective immunoglobulin production. Immunoglobulin G (IgG) and IgM levels recover to the normal range by 6 months after BMT but IgA production and serum levels remain low for many months and may never fully recover (Izutsu et al., 1983). B lymphocytes may aberrantly bear the CD5 marker during recovery after BMT, and there is evidence that they are functionally defective, failing to switch from IgM to IgG production (Atkinson, 1990a).

The dysregulated immune recovery is associated with abnormalities of lymphokine production. Only after BMT is there a rise in interferon γ (IFNγ) and tumour necrosis factor (TNF) attributable to the increase in NK cells (Brenner *et al.*, 1986), whilst production of IL-2 is decreased related to the low number of IL-2 producing CD4+ helper cells (Atkinson, 1990a).

The role of the thymus in the recovery of immunity after BMT remains a puzzle. Circulating thymic hormone levels are surprisingly normal despite the presence of only small thymic remnants in BMT recipients. It has been suggested that other tissues, notably epithelial cells, may serve as an additional site for T lymphocyte development (Atkinson *et al.*, 1982).

The clinical consequence of these functional abnormalities coupled with quantitatively poor immune recovery is a prolonged defect of specific immunity to DNA viruses such as cytomegalovirus, herpes simplex and varicella-zoster virus as well as a persisting increased risk of bacterial and fungal infections (Winston and Gale, 1991).

Factors affecting immune recovery (Table 4.7)

The most powerful suppressive influence on immune recovery is the presence of clinical GVHD – acute and chronic GVHD are associated

Table 4.7 Factors affecting immune recovery after bone marrow transplantation (Atkinson, 1990a)

Factor	Effect
Related to the transplant inoculum	
Presence of mature T lymphocytes	GVHD
T4 and T8 lymphocyte depletion	More balanced recovery of T4 and T8
NK functional activity	More GVHD
Donor–recipient histocompatibility disparity	Better specific immune responses, but greater risk of viral reactivation and GVHD
Pre-existing primary immune response to infectious agents	
Host factors	
Residual immune function	Mixed chimerism and rejection
Pre-existing exposure to microorganisms and viruses	Enhanced specific immune responses, but greater risk of viral reactivation and GVHD
Treatment	
GVHD prophylaxis with CSA or MTX	Immune suppression
GVHD treatment with steroids or antilymphocyte antibodies	
Viral infection or reactivation	
Interleukin 2 administration	Rapid lymphocyte recovery but more GVHD

NK, Natural killer; GVHD, graft-versus-host disease; CSA, cyclosporin; MTX, methotrexate.

with prolonged and incomplete recovery of immune function. The immune defect of GVHD is further exaggerated by immunosuppressive agents used to treat GVHD, and the immunosuppressive effect of infection from DNA viruses. The administration of T cell-depleted bone marrow leads to a lower incidence of GVHD and therefore a higher frequency of ultimately normal immune recovery. However, the nature of the T-depletion process may reduce the early rise in NK cells responsible for non-specific immune reactivity.

The state of the donor's immunity has a significant impact on the pattern of recovery of specific responses in the recipient. Transfer of both protective immune function against viruses, and autoimmune responses from the donor to the recipient, have been well-documented. Specific donor responses from mature B cells are present early after BMT and persist for many months (Wimperis *et al.*, 1986).

Treatment approaches to improve immune recovery

It has proved extremely difficult to influence the pattern and rate of immune recovery after BMT. The administration of thymic hormones has not affected the recovery. Interleukin 2 is potentially of benefit, but may exacerbate GVHD and is unlikely to influence the immune dysregulation (Malkovsky *et al.*, 1986). Other growth factors, such as IL-3 and IL-4, have not been evaluated. The complicated interactions between cytokines and their targets make it unlikely that the administration of single factors could predictably influence the immune recovery favourably. In future, the combined or sequential use of lymphoid growth factors and cytokines might optimize the speed and quality of immune recovery, but at present not enough is known about the interactions between emerging lymphocyte populations after BMT to modify successfully the recovery pattern to optimize anti-infective immunity and minimize GVHD reactions. In practice, therefore, the management of the cellular immune deficient state after BMT involves prophylaxis against infection from herpes viruses with acyclovir, co-trimoxazole prophylaxis against *Pneumocystis carinii*, and immunosuppression to prevent GVHD (see below). Vaccination with live attenuated viruses is safe beyond six months after BMT and deliberate immunization of the donor against hepatitis B has been effective (Ivinondo *et al.*, 1986).

TISSUE TYPING AND MATCHING

Transplantation antigens

This term was originally used to describe antigens on transplanted tissues that could induce immune rejection by the recipient. The

Table 4.8 The human leukocyte antigen (HLA) system

MHC class I

HLA A	1	2	3	9	10	11	w19	23	24	26	28	w36	w43
				23	25		29				w68		
				24	26		30				w69		
					w34		31						
					w66		32						
							w33						
							w74						

HLA B	w4	5 w6 7 8 12 13	14	15 16 17 18 21 w22 27 35 37	40 w41 w42 w47 w48 w53 w59
	51		44	w64 w62 38	w54	w60	w67 w70
	w52		45	w65 w63 39	w55	w61	w71
				w75	w56		w72
				w76			
				w77			

MHC class II

HLA D   1 2 3 4 5   6   7 8 9 10 12 13 14 15 16 20 21 22 23 24 25 26
                         18 11
                         19 17

HLA DR 1 2 3 4   5 w6 7 w8 9 w10 w52 w53
                      w11
                      w12

HLA DQ w1 w2 w3 w4
        w5   w7
        w6   w8
                w9

HLA DP w1 w2 w3 w4 w5 w6

HLA types are arranged to show alleles with serological similarities; w denotes workshop number. MHC, major histocompatibility complex.

concept can be extended in the context of BMT to include those antigens responsible for all the immune-related phenomena associated with the procedure: rejection, GVHD and GVL reactions. These responses are mirror images and tend to be mutually exclusive (Gale and Reisner, 1986). Transplantation antigens include the major histocompatibility system, HLA A and B (MHC class I) and HLA DR (MHC class II), and the minor histocompatibility system (Table 4.8).

Genetics of the MHC complex

The human MHC is located on chromosome 6. It comprises a region of over 100 kb (Fig. 4.4). The region is divided into three domains – A, B/C, and D. The A and B regions determine the so-called class I histocompatibility locus; the D region determines the class II domain. The C region determines several complement proteins but no histocompatibility antigens and its situation between the class I and II

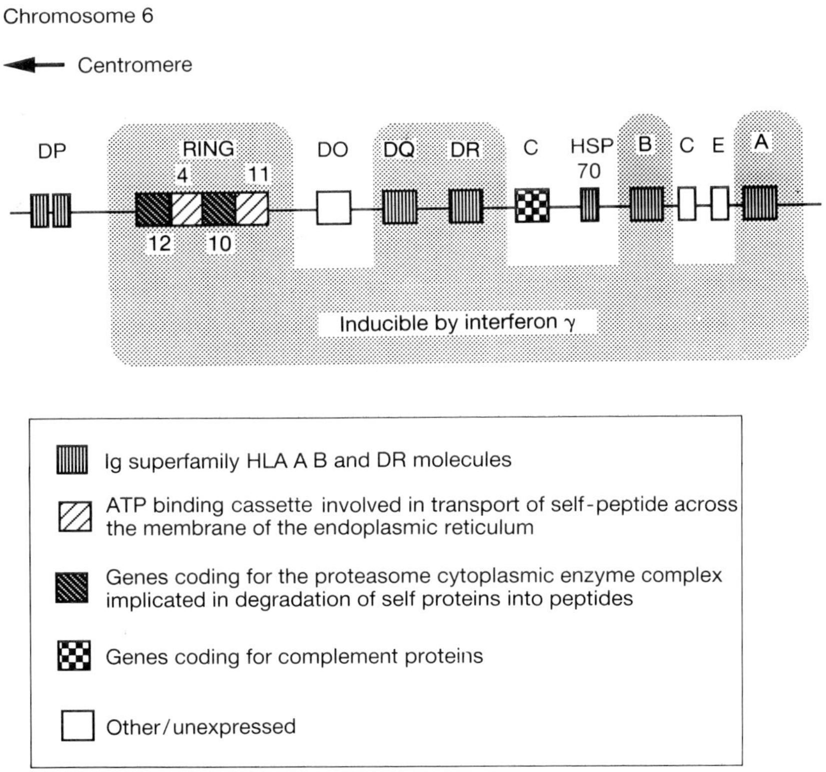

Chromosome 6

◄── Centromere

DP　　RING　　DO　DQ　DR　　C　HSP　B　C E　A
　　　4　11　　　　　　　　　　70
　　12　10

Inducible by interferon γ

▦ Ig superfamily HLA A B and DR molecules

▨ ATP binding cassette involved in transport of self-peptide across the membrane of the endoplasmic reticulum

▧ Genes coding for the proteasome cytoplasmic enzyme complex implicated in degradation of self proteins into peptides

▩ Genes coding for complement proteins

☐ Other/unexpressed

Fig. 4.4 Genetics of the MHC complex.

regions makes it a useful marker for identifying the site of crossovers. The genes for the HLA system share considerable homology with other mammalian histocompatibility genes. Both the class I and II genes appear to have arisen by gene reduplication with several closely similar genes situated adjacent to each other. The class I area contains 17 genes with at least six functioning exons producing gene products expressed on the cell surface as HLA molecules (Holmes, 1989). Class I molecules are formed by the fusion of a highly variable α chain, and a constant β chain ($β_2$-microglobulin) derived from a gene on the chromosome 15. The molecule is assembled together with endogenous peptide in the endoplasmic reticulum under the control of a specialized assembly protein controlled by the ring gene sequences situated in the class II region.

Class II genes have been mapped to five distinct subregions, each comprising several paired α and β sequences. There are six α genes, of which three produce functional proteins. Of the nine β genes, five are functional. Paired α and β genes code for highly variable proteins of the immunoglobulin superfamily. Three gene products are known to be important histocompatibility antigens – DR, DQ, and DP. Of these, DR is the most important. There are five DR genes – one α and four β. The β gene is the more variable (Holmes, 1989). DQ and DP gene products are also recognized by T lymphocytes (Zeevi and Duquesnoy, 1985; Cesbron et al., 1990). However, because the DQ locus is in tight linkage disequilibrium with the DR genes, the DQ type is usually inherited along with the DR type. The DN and DO regions are not expressed as proteins (Travers et al., 1984; Trowsdale and Campbell, 1988).

A third group of genes (ring 4, 10, 11, 12) situated in the D region appears to be responsible for antigen processing (Robertson, 1991). Rings 10 and 12 produce a large enzyme complex, termed the proteasome, responsible for intracellular peptide generation from larger proteins. The peptides generated by the proteasome are transported into the endoplasmic reticulum by an adenosine triphosphate (ATP)-driven pump (ATP-binding cassette) generated by the ring 4 and 11 genes. These self-peptides are incorporated into class I HLA molecules and are presented at the cell surface in the HLA molecule as minor histocompatibility antigens. Allelic variation in the ring gene complex may give rise to inheritable diversity in minor histocompatibility antigens presented by class I molecules.

Function of MHC molecules

Class II molecules function as antigen presenters for exogenous antigens. They are recognized by the CD4 receptor on the helper lymphocyte subset. Their major physiological role is in the presentation of viral and bacterial antigens to lymphocytes to initiate cell-mediated immune responses against microorganisms.

Class I molecules present largely endogenous antigen and have a role in the process of self-recognition during lymphocyte development. They are recognized by the CD8 structure on the surface of CD8 suppressor/cytotoxic lymphocytes. Class I molecules present self-antigens and viral antigens in the form of small peptides to CD8 T lymphocytes. These self-peptides complexed with the class I molecules form the poorly characterized minor histocompatibility antigen system.

MHC molecules and minor histocompatibility antigens

MHC molecules are members of the immunoglobulin superfamily (Fig. 4.5). They are dimers possessing a characteristic groove structure, the lips composed of two parallel α helices, and the floor composed of a series of β pleated sheet protein strands (Fig. 4.6) (Bjorkman et al., 1987; Brown et al., 1988). This molecular configuration (which is also

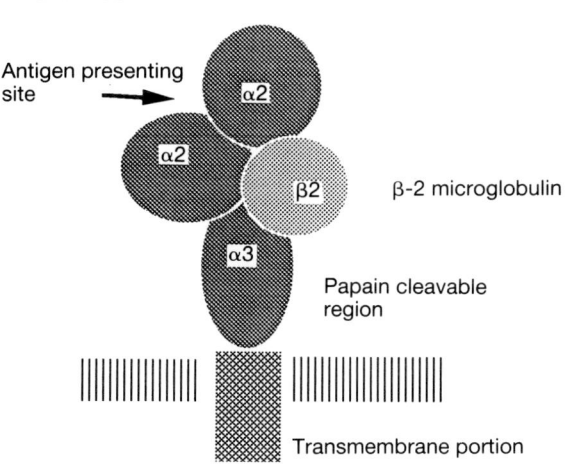
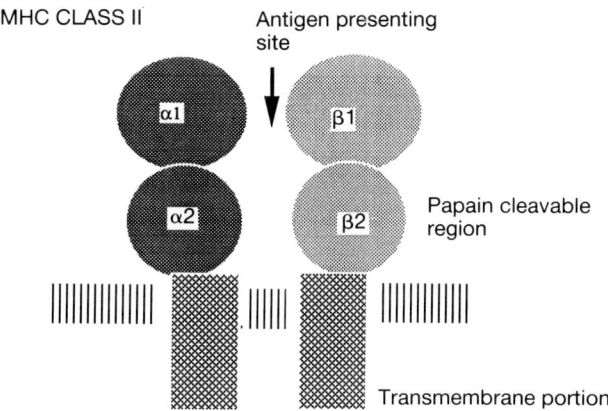

Fig. 4.5 Structure of the MHC molecules.

represented in some growth factor receptors, heat shock proteins and intracellular chaperonins; Gething and Sambrook, 1992) functions as a peptide binding site which allows small peptides to be bound in a form that can be presented as an antigen to T lymphocytes. Such peptides are not capable of stimulating an antibody response, presumably because they are hidden inside the MHC molecule and are consequently not 'seen' by B lymphocytes. It is now clear that peptides presented by MHC molecules function as minor histocompatibility antigens. The term 'minor' is in some ways inappropriate since mismatching for these non-MHC antigens in marrow transplantation is responsible for powerful rejection, GVHD and GVL phenomena (Loveland and Simpson, 1986).

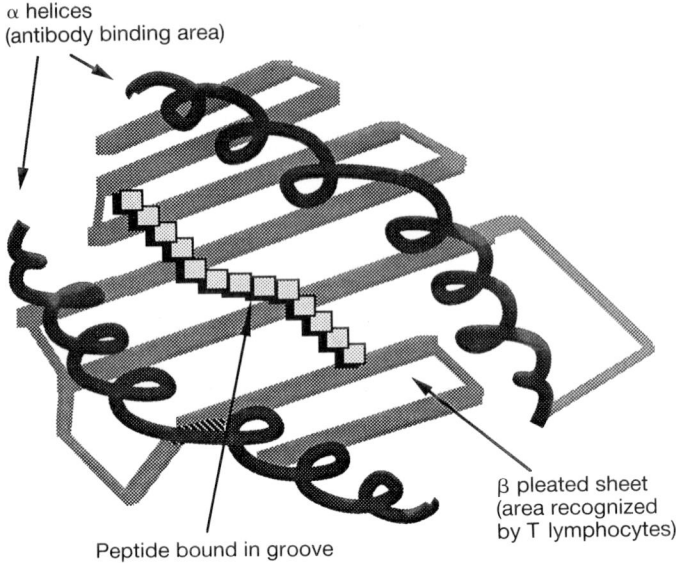

Fig. 4.6 Structure of the MHC class I peptide binding region.

The MHC system has been well-characterized by antibodies which recognize various external regions of the α helices of the class I or II molecules. In contrast, minor antigens are poorly characterized. They cannot be detected by antibodies but they are recognized by T cells. Clones can be raised with high specificity against minor antigens, provided they are presented by a class I or II molecule that is common to the antigen-presenting cell and the T lymphocyte (Goulmy et al., 1986). This gives rise to the phenomenon of restricted antigen recognition within the context of specific HLA types. Minor antigens may be peptides derived from intracellular processing of self-proteins (presented through MHC class I molecules), or extracellularly derived antigens (as well as other self-peptides) presented through class II molecules. In mice, transplantation antigens outside the class I and II loci are termed Hh antigens. Biologically they represent self-antigens that can be tissue-specific, and may include tumour antigens. Experiments with congenic mouse strains indicate that there are several hundred loci with low polymorphism scattered over a wide area of the genome (Perrault et al., 1990). They are probably all non-serologically determined peptides recognized only by MHC restricted T cells. This HLA restriction is explicable if they are considered as cellular antigens processed and presented to the cell surface in the groove of the class I or II molecule. They include the Y chromosome determined antigens (H-Y) but the origin of most has not been identified.

Even less is known about the human minor histocompatibility

antigen system. The H-Y antigen is the best characterized, and can be responsible for graft rejection in mice (Hurme et al., 1978) and sex-mismatched HLA-matched donor recipient pairs (Goulmy et al., 1986). The observation that during graft rejection T-cell clones are generated against multiple donor minor histocompatibility antigens indicates that the minor antigen system is likely to be as diverse as it is in the mouse (Perrault et al., 1990). Transplantation immunology represents a highly artificial situation where T cells recognize as foreign unmatched HLA molecules (and not the minor antigens they carry) on cells from other individuals. Conversely T cells from another individual will also recognize minor antigens if the presenting HLA molecule shares identity with that of the responding cell. Thus, haploidentical donor–recipient pairs will stimulate both anti-MHC and anti-minor histocompatibility T cell responses.

The structure of class I and class II molecules is closely linked to their function of antigen presentation to the lymphocyte. The constant structural regions are the two lips of the molecule which conform to the LFA-1 adhesion molecule of the lymphocyte. Genetic variations in the β pleated sheet which makes the antigen-presenting groove determine the antigenicity of the HLA molecule itself. The HLA molecules are situated in close proximity to important intracellular adhesion molecules. Congenital defects, either in the expression of the class I specific antigen-presenting sites, or the non-specific binding LFA-1 area, result in severe immune deficiency syndromes (see review by Kourilsky and Claverie, 1989).

Diversity of tissue antigens

Inheritance

The close proximity of the A, B and D domains on the genome means that there is a strong likelihood that during meiosis the whole complex is transferred into the zygote. The probability of a crossover occurring during meiosis is less than 1% but certain areas rich in guanosine–cytosine (GC) pairs are more prone to crossovers. Between GC-rich regions are domains where the genetic sequence is unlikely to be rearranged and haplotypes are conserved. Nevertheless, experience with large unrelated bone marrow donor panels shows that there is increasing disparity of HLA types and haplotypes between different ethnic groups. As well as matched siblings, non-sibling family members may be phenotypically identical with the patient if there is sharing of parental haplotypes or homozygosity for a particular haplotype, often associated with consanguinity within the family. The chances of finding an unrelated donor matched for HLA A, B and DR are in the region of 1/10 000. However, the likelihood of finding a donor depends upon the frequency of the haplotype. This means in practice that relatively small panels of 10 000–20 000 volunteer donors will provide matches for up to 20% of patients, but disproportionately greater panel sizes are needed to double the number of successful matches, and ultimately the extreme rarity of some HLA types renders it impossible for any panel to match all patients (Beatty et al., 1988).

Mutations in MHC molecules

As the HLA system becomes better characterized, increasing numbers of defined HLA molecules are found to show minor variations due to point mutation. They are detected by the fact that certain antisera recognize only a subfamily of a particular HLA antigen previously defined using well-characterized antisera. These 'splits' represent the detection of antigenic variation in the molecule. Such disparity is of clinical significance, being responsible for GVHD and rejection phenomena.

Diversity of minor antigens

The enormous diversity of minor histocompatibility antigens and their wide genomic distribution makes it improbable that even fully matched siblings will share complete minor antigen identity. The corollary of this is that some minor antigens may not be important transplantation antigens, or that tolerance to them is more easily acquired than to major antigens. Since there is about a 50% chance of GVHD occurring between matched siblings, and the incidence is higher if no GVHD prophylaxis is used, it is likely that minor antigen incompatibility is the rule, not the exception.

Expression of MHC molecules

Class I antigens are represented on most cells (Daar et al., 1984). Notable exceptions are central nervous system neurons, corneal endothelium, villous trophoblasts and some endocrine and exocrine cells (Sviland et al., 1988). Some are present on the surface of red cells. In contrast, class II molecules only occur on endothelial and epithelial cells, macrophages and dendritic cells, B lymphocytes, activated T lymphocytes and early myeloid cells. They are noticeably absent on the surface of the urothelium. The expression of HLA molecules on the cell surface is variable. Both IFNα and IFNγ, as well as TNFα, increase the expression of class I and II molecules. Unregulated class II expression is restricted to activated T cells, B lymphocytes, and early myeloid cells. Epidermal and endothelial cells can be induced to express class II by IFNγ (Pober et al., 1983; Volc-Platzer et al., 1985). Minor histocompatibility antigens are only represented on cells bearing MHC molecules but there is evidence that some minor antigens are tissue-restricted. T cell clones can, for example, recognize antigens on myeloid cells that are not found on lymphocytes (Marrack and Kappler, 1988; Jiang et al., 1991b).

HLA serotyping

The first description of the HLA system relied upon serological typing of the class I antigens using antibodies derived from individuals sensitized to HLA antigens by blood products or pregnancy. The pioneering work of characterizing leukocyte antigens initiated by Dausset and Terasaki was followed by a series of workshops set up to characterize antisera and define the antigens they recognized. The technique is carried out in a miniaturized system where test cells are exposed to a panel of several hundred antisera in microwells. Complement is added and the proportion of cells killed is assessed in each well using the dye exclusion property of eosin which stains dead but not living cells. Class II antigens are only expressed on B cells or activated T cells and the test requires a separation step to isolate the B cells. Subsequently serological typing methods for D, DR, DQ, and DP were developed.

Serotyping identifies 24 HLA-A antigens, 52 HLA-B antigens and 61 D, DR, DP, and DQ antigens. The nomenclature has been standardized such that the suffix w (for workshop) is added to all HLA types not universally agreed upon. Splits are denoted by the number of the antigen (usually a workshop antigen) followed in brackets by the number of the parent antigen.

New typing techniques

While monoclonal antibodies are not yet available for a wide enough range of HLA antigens for use in typing, and serotyping does not distinguish antigenically silent areas of the class I or II antigen, non-serological typing approaches are revealing further sources of heterogeneity in the system. These are: isoelectric focusing (IEF) to detect small biochemical differences in the protein sequences, and DNA analysis by oligonucleotide probing and restriction fragment length polymorphism (RFLP) analysis.

Isoelectric focusing

Isoelectric focusing reveals considerable polymorphism within serologically defined types. In this procedure HLA antigen–antibody complexes migrate in a gel under the influence of an electric current (Yang, 1989). Even single amino acid substitutions in the HLA molecule bound by the same antibody translate into large differences in polarity and migration of the molecule. There is evidence that at least some of these differences are of immunological importance – they can generate specific cytotoxic T cell clones for example Fleischhauer et al. (1990) demonstrated that graft rejection was caused by a single amino acid difference in HLA-B 44 between donor and recipient.

RFLP

The heterogeneity and size of the class II gene complex lends itself to typing with cDNA probes. Whole genomic or cDNA probes have been used to study genetic heterogeneity in the D region. Highly polymorphic sites (not only confined to the functioning exons themselves) extend throughout the HLA region. Wake and colleagues (1982) were the first to apply RFLP analysis to HLA typing using a long cDNA fragment of the DRb1 gene. The DNA sample is digested with a series of endonucleases to obtain a multiple band pattern after hybridization with the radioactive probe, this being visualized after exposure to an X-ray film. The method can be improved upon by using shorter exon-specific probes complementary to specific encoding regions (DRb, DQa and DQb). The enzyme cleaving sites will then be within the exon (Bidwell et al., 1988).

Oligonucleotide probes

Once the DNA sequence of an exon is known, it is possible to synthesize short probes 20–30 bases long, to sequence specific regions within the gene. Using synthetic primer probes that flank the area of interest, the DNA from the HLA region to be tested is amplified by the polymerase chain reaction (PCR) technique. These fragments are then radiolabelled and used in slot blots against a panel of DNAs of known specificity. This approach is still under development but is revealing further genetic heterogeneity (sometimes called micropolymorphism), particularly within the DR3 gene. The methods available for typing various HLA molecules are summarized in Table 4.9.

Compatibility testing

While tissue-typing techniques are yielding more and more detailed information about the genetics of the HLA antigens, the procedure cannot distinguish which incompatibilities are of immunological

Table 4.9 Tissue typing and compatibility testing (see text for references)

Typing
Serotyping
  HLA A, B DR, DP, DQ
Isoelectric focusing
  Splits of HLA A and B
Restriction fragment length polymorphism
  DNA analysis
Oligonucleotide typing
  DNA analysis

Compatibility testing
Mixed lymphocyte reaction
  Unreliable; becoming outmoded
Cytotoxic or helper T lymphocyte precursor frequency assay
  Highly predictive for BMT outcome; still under evaluation
Mixed epidermal–lymphocyte culture
  One way (only predictive for GVHD); requires skin biopsies
Skin explant culture
  One way (predictive for GVHD); requires skin biopsies; subjective interpretation of results

HLA, Human leukocyte antigen; BMT, bone marrow transplantation; GVHD, graft-versus-host disease.

significance. For this some form of functional compatibility test is required (Fig. 4.7). The mixed lymphocyte culture (MLC) was the first compatibility test developed (Bain et al., 1964). The MLC detects transformation and proliferation of T lymphocytes in response to HLA differences on cells from other individuals. Donor and recipient lymphocytes are incubated together for 6 days to permit a proliferative response of donor against recipient cells (prevented from proliferating by mitomycin or radiation), or a recipient response to the mitomycin-blocked donor cells. Because the MLC detects class II differences it was for a long time the only means to confirm compatibility between HLA A- and B-matched sibling pairs. A, B and DR-matched siblings show non-reactivity in both directions in the MLC in approximately 90% of cases. With the advent of DR typing the MLC can be dispensed with in practice as a test of compatibility between matched siblings (Lim et al., 1988). Mixed lymphocyte culture between HLA-matched but unrelated individuals shows a wide variation from unresponsiveness in rare cases to highly proliferative responses characteristic of a completely HLA-mismatched random pairing. There is however little evidence that the MLC is informative in this circumstance – the clinical outcome does not appear to relate to the degree of MLC reactivity (Cesbron et al., 1990). Several approaches more recently introduced promise to be more accurate predictors of GVHD and rejection.

Mixed lymphocyte reaction

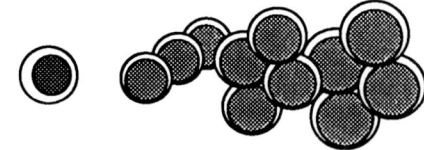

Proliferation in response to class II antigens on stimulator lymphocytes measured by tritiated thymidine uptake

Matched siblings: non-reactive
Matched unrelated: variable reactivity

Mixed epidermal cell lymphocyte reaction

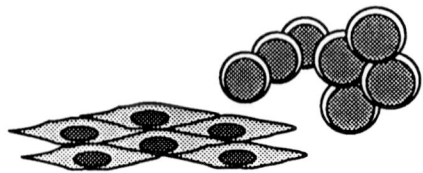

Proliferation in response to stimulator keratinocytes. GVHD detection only. Measure by tritiated thymidine uptake

Matched siblings: reactive

Skin explant assay

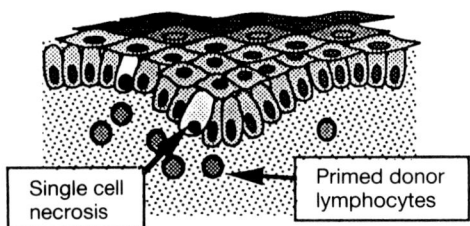

Lymphocytes from 6 day MLR incubated with recipient skin explant. Examined histologically for single cell necrosis after 48 hours. GVHD detection only

Matched siblings and matched unrelated donors

CTLp assay

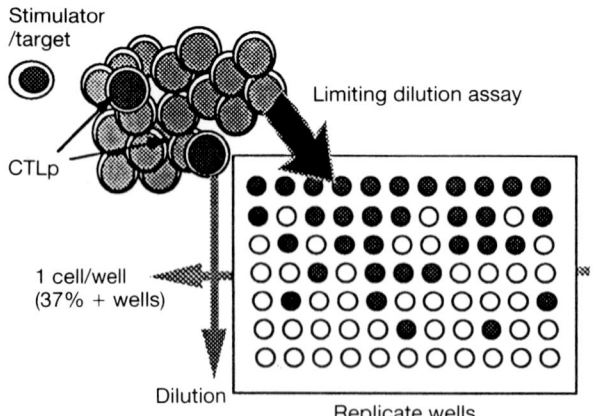

Positive wells measured as 51Cr release from stimulator/target lymphocytes

Cytotoxicity assay. Detects a minor effector population. Can predict GVHD and rejection

Unreactive for matched siblings
Reactive in matched unrelated BMT

Fig. 4.7 Compatibility testing – methods.

The recognition that the skin is a major target of the GVHD reaction suggested that keratinocytes may express antigens of particular relevance to compatibility in BMT. This has led to the development of tests in which skin biopsies are used as targets for predicting GVHD. Bagot et al. (1988) substituted keratinocytes for the recipient lymphocytes as the targets for a donor response in a mixed epidermal lymphocyte culture (MECLR). They found that epidermal cells are powerful stimulators of alloreactions by T cells, and demonstrated good correlation between positive MECLR reactions and the occurrence of GVHD in transplants between matched siblings. Latterly, several investigators have used skin explants as the target for lymphocyte reactivity. Punch biopsies of skin are reacted with lymphocytes previously cultured for 10 days with patient-derived lymphocytes. After 3 days of culture, the skin biopsy is sectioned and examined histologically for features of GVHD. A high correlation of *in vitro* changes with clinical GVHD can be achieved. A study of 32 patients predicted the occurrence of GVHD on 16 out of 18 occasions, but also reported three false positives out of 14 patients who did not develop GVHD (Berkman et al., 1982; Vogelsang et al., 1985; Dickinson et al., 1988). The limitations to the procedure are the subjective nature of the skin biopsy interpretation, the lengthy time scale and a tendency for false-positive results. It is possible that some of the changes observed in culture represent non-specific damage caused by cytokine release in this complex system.

A more biologically relevant response than measuring proliferation of lymphocytes in mixed lymphocyte culture is to test for donor cells which are cytotoxic to the recipient cells. The assay measures cytotoxic T lymphocyte precursors (CTLp). Within the immune response repertoire of the individual there are CTLp capable of responding and proliferating directly with allogeneic targets. The responder cells are incubated with irradiated stimulator cells in the presence of low levels of IL-2 for 10 days and the CTL generated in culture are tested against the target in a standard chromium release assay. To determine the CTLp frequency, a limiting dilution assay is performed using a series of different responder cell dilutions ranging over two logs, and carrying out each dilution in at least 20 replicate tests. Each well will give a positive or negative result according to the presence or absence of a CTLp. The frequency of positive wells is noted for each responder cell dilution. Applying Poisson frequency distribution analysis determines that a cell concentration of one CTLp is reached when 37% of the wells at any dilution are scored positive. By plotting the frequency distribution at each responder cell concentration the CTLp frequency in the initial population can be determined.

The ability to generate CTLp against the recipient seems to correlate very closely with GVHD in matched unrelated donor transplants, but the very low frequency of CTLp found in matched sibling BMT makes it unpredictive in this situation (Kaminsky et al., 1988). Further developments in devising accurate *in vitro* models of GVHD and rejection may make it possible in the future to define clearly potential transplant risks and allow suitable modifications of the protocol to avoid the predicted complication.

CLINICAL OUTCOME AND ITS RELATIONSHIP TO THE SOURCE OF STEM CELLS USED FOR TRANSPLANTATION

Autologous BMT (ABMT) is distinct from allogeneic BMT in having a more benign post-transplant course and low early BMT mortality, in the region of 5%. This is attributable to the lack of histoincompatibility, permitting rapid uncomplicated immune recovery, and similar results are achieved with BMT between identical twins. Both ABMT and identical-twin BMT share a similar risk of leukaemic relapse following BMT (Gale and Butturini, 1991). Increasing HLA disparity leads on the one hand to an increase in the risk of rejection and graft failure, and on the other to an increase in the incidence and severity of GVHD and intensity of the GVL effect. Donor responses to the recipient leading to GVHD are separable from recipient responses to the donor leading to rejection. Increasing disparity between major and minor histocompatibility antigens appears to be equally responsible. Studies on large patient cohorts have attempted to determine the relative importance of mismatching at different loci. The results suggest that the number of locus disparities is the main arbiter of the BMT outcome. Thus one-antigen differences have an outcome not statistically distinct from fully matched sibling donor transplants; two-locus mismatches have an intermediate outcome, and three-locus–full haplotype–mismatches have the worst outcome, with death occurring from rejection or GVHD. There is some evidence to suggest that D locus disparity is more significant than A or B locus disparity, and that single mismatches on the A locus are better tolerated than other single locus mismatches (Beatty et al., 1985). Attempts to define particular HLA types that confer either a high risk of complications, or are associated with a favourable outcome, have not been successful. The increasing use of unrelated volunteer donors has opened up the possibility of exploring further the role of minor histocompatibility antigen matching on outcome. In addition, the significance of phenotypic variation within a defined HLA type (splits) will ultimately be evaluable when sufficient numbers of BMT have been carried out.

The importance in animal studies of minor histocompatibility antigen mismatches on the GVL effect raises the possibility that some disparities may be favourable to the GVL response. Bone marrow transplantation between HLA A, B and DR-matched unrelated individuals may confer an increased GVL effect. Too few BMTs from volunteer donors have been performed so far to be definite but a preliminary comparison of relapse rates from Seattle suggests that unrelated volunteer BMTs have a lower relapse probability (Beatty et al., 1991; Gajewski and Champlin, 1991).

CURE OF LEUKAEMIA BY ALLOGENEIC BMT

It is clear that BMTs are more effective than chemotherapy in eradicating leukaemia, whether the treatment is employed early in the disease course (Goldman et al., 1988; Barrett et al., 1989a; Gale et al., 1989) or late (Thomas et al., 1977).

As discussed in Chapter 2, leukaemia cure does not necessarily equate with the eradication of all leukaemia cells; therefore, it is necessary to consider not only the role of high-dose chemotherapy and radiotherapy prior to BMT in achieving cytoreduction of leukaemia, but also mechanisms whereby relapse or recurrence of leukaemia may be suppressed by processes such as GVHD linked to GVL effects. Animal BMT experiments have identified both a high-dose chemoradiotherapy component of the preparative regimen and a GVL component responsible for leukaemia eradication and cure (Slavin et al., 1990; Hagenbeek et al., 1991).

Since identical-twin BMTs are not associated with the allogeneic interaction leading to GVL and GVHD, the various components of leukaemia cure by BMT in humans can be determined by comparing relapse rates following chemotherapy with those in identical-twin BMT. In a recent review, Gale and Butturini (1991) indicated that there is a 10–20% impact of intensive treatment on achieving cure in AML and ALL, and a greater effect in CML where identical-twin BMT achieves a 50% leukaemia relapse-free probability, compared with a zero probability of cure with conventional low-dose chemotherapy approaches.

Many questions about the efficacy of high-dose chemotherapy and radiotherapy regimens remain unanswered. The major variables examined in clinical trials have been alterations in the radiation schedule, investigating different chemotherapy and radiotherapy combinations and comparing high-dose chemotherapy schedules alone with radiotherapy-containing schedules. A major constraint in designing and comparing preparative regimens for their antileukaemia efficacy is the relatively narrow therapeutic window between insufficient leukaemia cytoreduction and unacceptable non-haemopoietic toxicity. While there has been some success in decreasing toxicity (for example, with the use of fractionated rather than single-dose irradiation; Serota *et al.*, 1983), or the use of chemotherapy-only preparative regimens, there is no evidence that greater antileukaemia efficacy can be achieved (Kanfer and McCarthy, 1989). Numerous reports of alterations to the total body irradiation (TBI) schedule or in the choice of high-dose chemotherapy continue to be published, but it is fair to say that there are no convincing data that any particular preparative regimen has been proved to be superior to the standard cyclophosphamide–TBI approach.

GVL

The idea that an allogeneic BMT might confer immunological anti-leukaemia activity in leukaemia transplant recipients was first suggested by Mathé *et al.* (1959). Some time elapsed before experimental models and clinical transplant results substantiated the existence of GVL following marrow transplantation. The GVL effect is closely related to the deleterious GVHD reaction. A major challenge therefore is to determine whether GVL reactivity can be separated from GVHD. Leukaemia and lymphoma cells may express antigenic structures or adhesion molecules on their surface which render them susceptible to

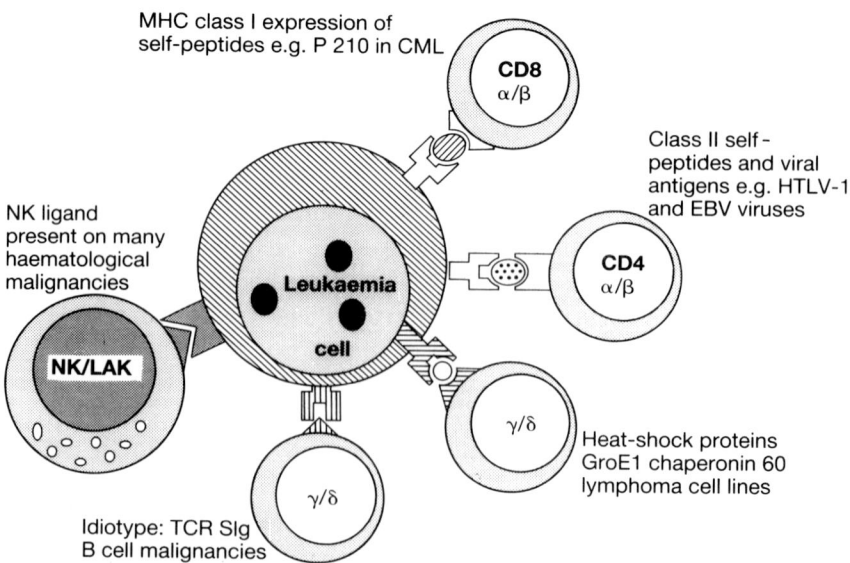

Fig. 4.8 Possible leukaemia-specific antigens and the corresponding cellular immune response.

Table 4.10 Evidence for graft versus leukaemia (GVL)

Experimental observations
Cytotoxic donor T lymphocytes with specific reactivity to patients' leukaemia circulate after BMT
Specific T lymphocyte clones with antileukaemia reactivity can be generated after BMT
Several well-established animal models of GVL

Clinical results
High relapse rate in BMT from identical twins
Acute and chronic GVHD reduces the relapse risk
Donor marrow T lymphocyte depletion increases leukaemic relapse
Donor T lymphocyte transfusions can reinduce remission in CML relapsing after BMT
Leukaemic relapse sometimes reversible by stopping GVHD prophylaxis

BMT, Bone marrow transplantation; GVHD, graft versus host disease; CML, chronic myeloid leukaemia.

immune attack (Fig. 4.8). With a greater understanding of the mechanisms involved, it may be possible to select and amplify this property of BMT for therapeutic advantage (see also Chapter 6).

Evidence for GVL (Table 4.10)

Animal studies

OKunewick and coworkers (1990) used the Rauscher virus leukaemia model to determine whether transplanted cells from B10S strain mice exerted a GVL effect in SJL/J recipients without at the same time inducing GVHD. Marrow cells conferred GVL with good survival and a low incidence of GVHD. Addition of spleen cells, however, caused early death from GVHD. In contrast these and other studies emphasized that GVL but not GVHD reactivity could be conferred by minor histocompatibility antigen differences between donor and host. Several studies attempted to identify whether GVL-reacting lymphocytes were distinct from GVHD effector cells. Truitt and colleagues (1986) used a limiting dilution technique to generate single clones of donor T cells from transplanted animals with the EL4 experimental leukaemia which they then reinfused into recipient, partially mismatched, mice bearing the EL4 leukaemia. They were able to demonstrate that such lymphocyte clones possessed distinct reactivities, some predominantly antileukaemic, some with GVHD potential, and some mixtures of the two.

In further experiments with the Rauscher leukaemia model, OKunewick used T cell-deficient C57BL/10/nude mice as donors, and compared the results of transplantation with non-T cell-deficient mice of the same strain on the proliferation of leukaemia in SLJ/J mouse recipients. Normal bone marrow conferred 40% survival in the leukaemic mice, but with the same GVHD incidence as non-leukaemic mice. Marrow from nude mice (T-deficient) donors produced no GVHD but conferred a smaller but definite GVL effect. These results showed on the one hand that there was a GVL component of GVHD, and on the other that there was a non-T cell-dependent component conferred by nude mouse bone marrow. Similar results could be produced by grafting marrow depleted of T helper cells by Lyt-1 antibody treatment. This produced a detectable but smaller GVL effect than that conferred by non-T-depleted marrow. However, the T-depleted transplants did not develop GVHD (OKunewick et al., 1987). There is also evidence for a GVL effect exerted by MHC-unrestricted NK and LAK cells (Charak et al., 1990). In order to determine whether GVL reactivity was conferred by specific T lymphocyte subsets, Korngold and Sprent (1978) carried out BMT in a leukaemia mouse model and compared the GVL potential of mice reconstituted with bone marrow and helper subsets or suppressor subsets. They showed that the major GVL effect was conferred by the helper subset, and that GVHD was mild in this instance. Lastly, several groups have demonstrated that leukaemia-specific T cell clones can be generated, which distribute widely and persist in the recipient, and exert an antileukaemia effect (Cheever et al., 1986; Klarnet et al., 1987).

In summary, therefore, animal experiments show that GVL may have two components: firstly reactivity conferred by alloreactive T helper lymphocytes which may be partially separable into GVHD and GVL-reacting clones, and secondly, a non-T cell component possibly mediated by NK cells. It is also possible that both components are involved cooperatively in establishing a GVL effect (Slavin et al., 1990).

Clinical results

There is a strong body of evidence (summarized in Table 4.10) supporting the existence of GVL in clinical BMT data. It has for some time been evident that BMT from identical-twin donors conferred a higher risk of relapse than an allograft from a matched sibling (Fefer et al., 1982). In a survey of a large number of BMTs for leukaemia, the Seattle group showed that patients developing acute or chronic GVHD had a lower probability of relapse (Weiden et al., 1979, 1981; Sullivan et al., 1989a). The favourable effects of both acute and chronic GVHD on relapse were confirmed in another large multicentre study by the IBMTR (Bortin, 1987; Butturini et al., 1987). With increasing numbers of successful BMTs for leukaemia performed worldwide, it has become possible to examine the GVL effect in more detail. In a recent analysis

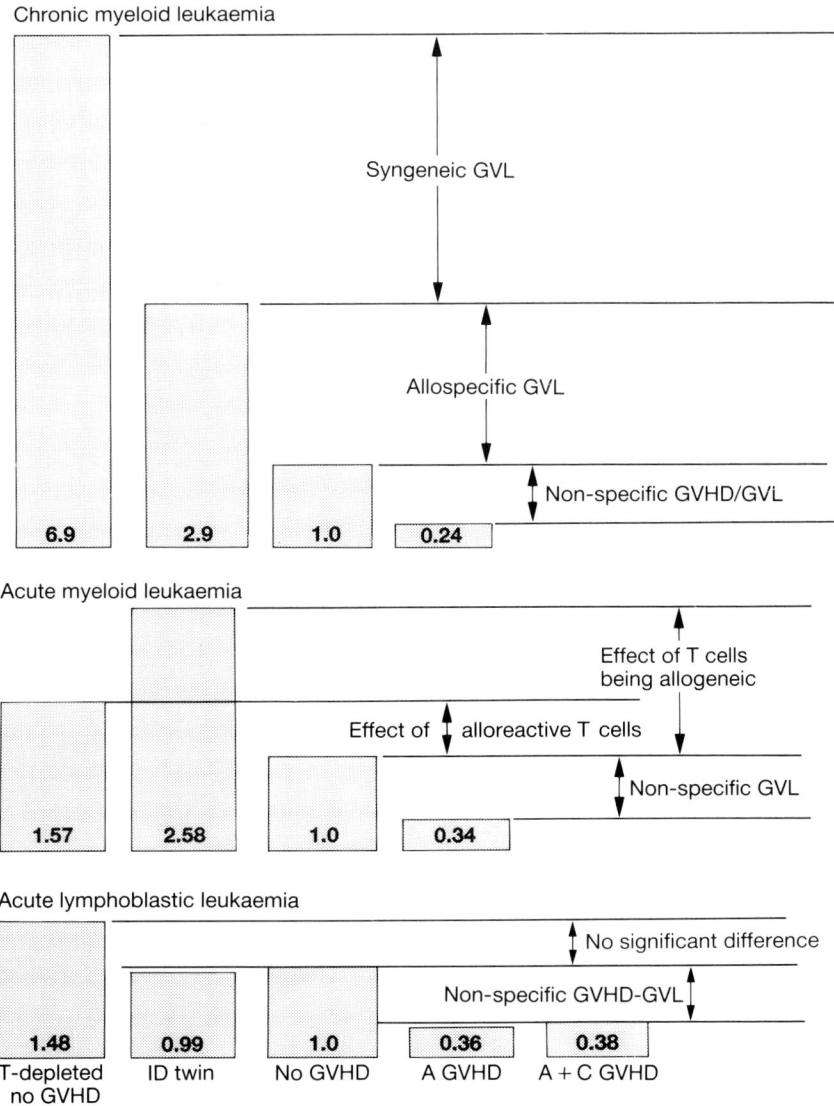

Fig. 4.9 Graft versus leukaemia effects in clinical BMT. Results shown as relative relapse risk.

from the IBMTR, relapse risk was compared between a total of 2254 transplanted patients with ALL, AML and CML (Horowitz et al., 1990). The figures were adjusted to exclude bias from competing variables, and a relative relapse risk was calculated. Patients who received an unmanipulated BMT and who did not develop GVHD were assigned a relapse risk of 1.0. Figure 4.9 shows the results. Several features emerge:

1 In all three leukaemias there is a high rate of relapse in BMT from identical twins (approximately 45%).

2 There is a favourable influence of acute and chronic GVHD on relapse, but there are differences between the effect in each leukaemia. The overall influence of GVHD is greatest in CML and least in ALL. In ALL acute GVHD is the main contributor to the effect, while in AML and CML chronic GVHD has a more powerful influence.

3 T lymphocyte depletion confers a high relapse rate in all leukaemia types, but the effect is greatest in CML and least in ALL. Three distinct components of the GVL response emerge: GVL associated with GVHD (GVHD versus no GVHD); GVL occurring in patients without GVHD (no GVHD versus identical-twin data), and in the case of CML, a powerful GVL effect that appears to be conferred by the presence of non-alloreactive T lymphocytes (twin versus T-depletion data).

The introduction of T cell depletion of donor marrow has produced convincing and important reductions in the incidence and severity of acute and chronic GVHD. However, it soon became apparent that T-depleted BMT recipients were more prone to relapse. This was convincingly shown first in BMT for CML where relapse rates increased from 15% to greater than 40% (Apperley et al., 1986; Goldman et al., 1988). A smaller but definite relapse effect was also seen in AML and ALL patients receiving T-depleted transplants (Maraninchi et al., 1988).

Further confirmation that alloreacting T lymphocytes have an antileukaemic potential comes from the results of treating patients relapsing after BMT for CML with donor lymphocyte infusions. Kolb et al. (1990) were able to achieve a further remission in three patients with cytogenetic relapse after T-depleted BMT. Similar results have been reported by the Hammersmith group who showed that donor T cell transfusions not only successfully reinduced donor haemopoiesis but reduced residual leukaemia to a level undetectable by PCR analysis (Cullis et al., 1992). There is a report of regression of relapse after BMT for ALL when immunosuppressive treatment for GVHD was withdrawn (Higano et al., 1990).

These results support the data from animal experiments that suggest that GVL is an alloimmune phenomenon requiring recognition of minor histocompatibility differences between HLA-A, B and DR-matched siblings. Patients receiving BMT from matched but unrelated donors are less likely to share minor antigens with the donor. The lower relapse probability conferred in BMT between matched but unrelated donors is consistent with the concept that minor antigens play an important role in GVL (Gajewski and Champlin, 1991). The results also suggest that GVL has several components in terms of its specificity: GVL associated with GVHD being due to the shared expression of minor antigens on leukaemia cells and tissues which are targets for GVHD, while GVL occurring without GVHD in CML and

AML suggests the presence of myeloid-restricted minor antigens. Lastly, the demonstration of a contribution of syngeneic lymphocytes to the GVL effect is enticing but not conclusive evidence supporting the possibility that identical twins recognize a specific leukaemia antigen on the recipient CML.

GVL effector cells

Several cell types may exert a GVL effect: the alloreactive component may involve both T4 and T8 lymphocyte subclasses. The process may be more or less selective depending on whether the alloantigens are

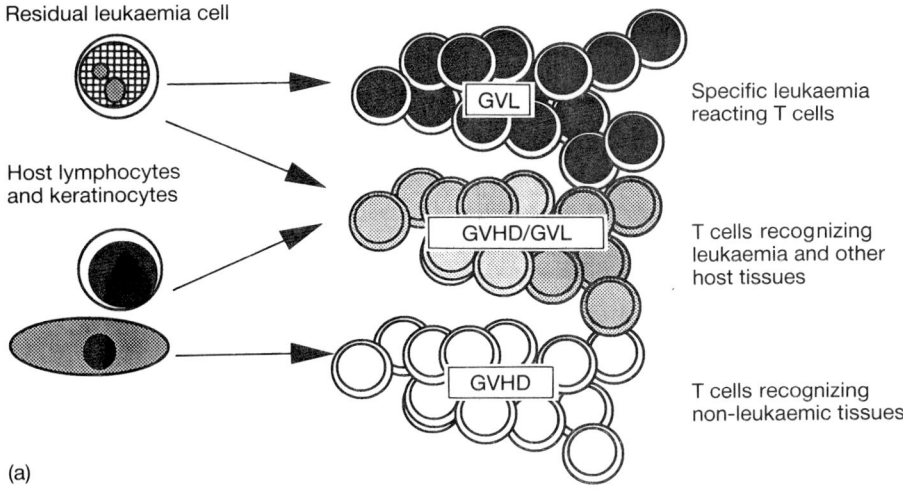

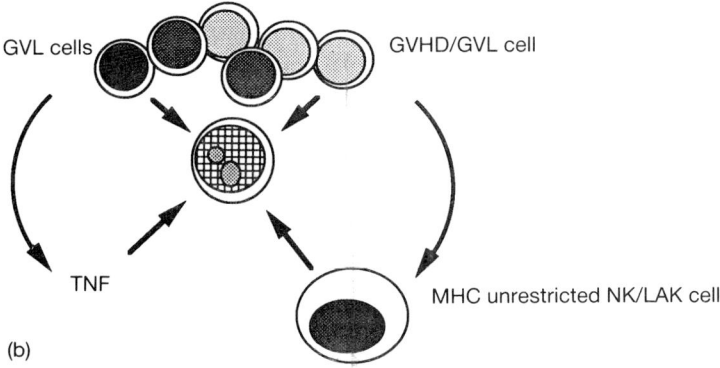

Fig. 4.10 Graft versus leukaemia mechanisms: (a) MHC restricted leukaemia recognition; (b) direct and indirect antileukaemic mechanisms resulting in cytotoxicity or suppression of proliferation.

restricted to leukaemia cells or normal cells of the same lineage, or are present on GVHD targets such as keratinocytes and enterocytes. Secondly, there may be a non-MHC-restricted, non-specific component of GVL mediated by NK cells and by LAK cells which are cytotoxic to a wide variety of host targets. It is likely that both specific and non-specific mechanisms operate together (Fig. 4.10).

Cytotoxic T lymphocytes (CTLs)

Several animal studies have demonstrated an important role for leukaemia-specific, MHC-restricted cytotoxic T lymphocyte clones in exerting a GVL effect in experimental BMT systems (Cheever et al., 1986; Truitt et al., 1986; Klarnet et al., 1987). In humans CD4+ve T cell clones which show specific cytotoxicity to the patients' leukaemia have been grown from patients after BMT (Sosman et al., 1990; reviewed by Sosman and Sondel, 1987; Brenner and Heslop, 1991). Cytotoxic T lymphocyte clones exhibiting specific colony-inhibition of recipient CML cells have been identified after BMT by Falkenburg and others (1990). This group have also succeeded in generating donor T cell clones specific to the recipient's leukaemia in vitro (Van Lochem et al., 1992). After BMT for CML a low but persisting frequency of CTLps with antileukaemic activity (Ly-CTLp) have been detected (Jiang et al., 1991a). The frequency of Ly-CTLp is always lower than the frequency of precursors with cytotoxicity to the patient's lymphocytes, suggesting that circulating donor lymphocytes have different host tissue specificities. At the level of individual clones some cells may therefore exert specific antileukaemic reactivity.

NK cells

Natural killer cells are some of the first cells to recover after both autologous and allogeneic BMT (Ault et al., 1985; Rooney et al., 1986). After BMT these cells are highly activated and behave like LAK cells in their ability to kill a wide range of tumour targets. Mackinnon and colleagues (1990) have shown that LAK cells induced in vitro following allogeneic BMT for CML exhibit strong cytotoxicity to the recipient's leukaemia. These observations suggest that NK cells may not only contribute to the GVL process in allograft recipients (Slavin et al., 1988, 1990) but also constitute a potential mechanism of GVL in autologous BMT (Brenner and Heslop, 1991).

Manipulating BMT conditions to optimize GVL

Although the mechanisms of GVL are becoming more clearly identified, our ability to select this type of alloreaction is at present limited.

Several approaches are, however, possible: certain techniques of T cell depletion may select against GVHD reactions while conserving GVL (Butturini and Gale, 1990). T depletion using countercurrent elutriation is associated with a lower relapse risk than other methods, possibly because NK function is preserved (Wagner et al., 1990). Alternatively, since CD4 (helper) cells appear to have a greater impact on GVL than CD8 lymphocytes while both are responsible for GVHD, depletion of CD8 lymphocytes from the marrow may allow some selection of GVL reactivity (Maraninchi et al., 1988).

Separation of GVH from GVL – future developments

The demonstration of specific antileukaemia T cell clones in mice (Truitt et al., 1986), and possibly in humans (Jiang et al., 1991b), lends encouragement to the possibility that leukaemia and lymphoma cells exhibit distinct tumour-specific antigens which make them targets for GVL reactions. As discussed in Chapter 6, leukaemia- and lymphoma-specific peptide antigens may be presented through MHC molecules and generate a specific GVL response. Such GVL candidate antigens are listed in Table 6.6. On this basis it might be possible in the future to generate specific antileukaemia T cell clones to give to patients after BMT to enhance GVL. An alternative approach would be to remove GVH reacting cells from the donor lymphocytes obtained by leukapheresis by clonally deleting lymphocytes responding to donor lymphocytes and keratinocytes (GVHD targets), and reinfusing lymphocytes conserving more specific antileukaemia responsiveness. It has been shown that treatment of donor cells cultured with recipient lymphocytes with an antibody to the IL-2 receptor ablates lymphocytes responding to the recipient lymphocytes, but preserves a proliferative response to the patient's leukaemia (Jiang et al., 1991a).

CURE OF HAEMATOLOGICAL MALIGNANCIES BY ABMT

The use of autologous stem cells to restore marrow function after eradicative treatment for malignant diseases is a logical solution to the problem of the unavailability of matched donors for the majority of patients. Furthermore, the use of autologous stem cells avoids many of the complications associated with the immune response of the allograft. Because of this the mortality from ABMT following preparative regimens identical to those used for allografts is significantly lower – in the region of 5% compared with 20–30% for allografts. The disadvantages of ABMT are, however, the high disease relapse rate observed and occasionally poor haematological recovery in patients whose stem cells have been previously damaged by stem cell toxic chemotherapy and radiotherapy.

There are three explanations for the occurrence of relapse after ABMT: firstly, inadequacy of the eradicative treatment; secondly, failure to eliminate residual disease by an alloimmune GVL process, and thirdly because malignant cells have been reseeded in the stem cell inoculum.

Because relapses occur in allogeneic BMT recipients given identical preparative regimens to those used in ABMT, it is clear that eradication of residual disease with the current high-dose combinations of drugs and radiotherapy is not completely effective. Nevertheless there is ample evidence that part of the failure to control disease with ABMT is related to the absence of an allogeneic GVL effect demonstrated in the higher relapse rate following marrow transplants between identical twins and after ABMT when compared with allotransplants. Too few BMTs between identical twins are carried out to make the critical comparison between the relapse rates for particular diseases after ABMT and twin BMT. It is therefore not possible to answer the question whether relapse due to reinfusion of malignant cells after ABMT makes a significant contribution to the risk of relapse.

Whether it is useful to purge autologous marrow of malignant cells before reinfusing it has never been satisfactorily resolved. This has not, however, deterred the burgeoning of a technology devoted to marrow-purging (Gee, 1991). This section examines the way in which malignant disorders are cured by ABMT: the evidence for autologous GVL effects, the techniques and role of marrow-purging in treatment, and the special problems associated with stem cell function in ABMT.

Autologous GVL

Several approaches to enhance a GVL reaction after autologous BMT are being explored: IL-2 has been administered early after ABMT to enhance NK function and increase cytotoxicity against autologous leukaemia cells. At present the value of IL-2 in this situation is unclear: initial reports suggest that some poor-risk patients given IL-2 after ABMT have shown remarkable relapse-free intervals (Foa et al., 1990). Other studies are too small for proper evaluation or are still in progress (Blaise et al., 1990; Macdonald et at., 1991).

A second approach has been to induce autologous GVHD in the hope that a GVL process will be correspondingly enhanced. A skin rash identical histologically to GVHD following allogeneic BMT has been described after identical-twin BMT as well as after autologous BMT (Rappeport et al.,1979; Thein et al., 1981). This has raised the possibility that GVHD induced after ABMT could also confer a GVL action. Tutschka et al. (1983) have shown that a GVH-like skin reaction is readily inducible in rats given cyclosporin after syngeneic BMT. They have not however shown that this GVHD syndrome equates to the allogeneic reaction in its pattern of tissue specificity. In fact, GVHD occurring in ABMT only affects the skin and is readily responsive to steroids. Nevertheless, attempts have been made to induce GVHD after ABMT in the clinical setting using cyclosporin. These results confirm that acute GVHD is inducible by cyclosporin in the majority of patients, but there is as yet no clear evidence that this confers protection against leukaemic relapse (Jones et al., 1989). Data are conflicting concerning the effect of cyclosporin on relapse potential. After allogeneic BMT, cyclosporin is associated with an increased risk of relapse for both acute leukaemia and CML. In animal experiments, Slavin et al. (1990) have shown the potential of cyclosporin to provoke relapse when administered to successfully transplanted chimeras inoculated with L1210 leukaemia cells. A further approach being investigated is the combination of cyclosporin to induce GVHD followed by IL-2 to expand the autoreactive clone of T lymphocytes. The existence of a potential GVL effect following ABMT therefore remains unclear.

Purging bone marrow and stem cell infusions of malignant cells

There are several areas of uncertainty relating to the nature and re-transplant potential of residual malignant disease in bone marrow or blood.

1 Regrowth potential of infused malignant cells. The transfusion of autologous malignant cells is not necessarily synonymous with relapse of the disease because not all malignant cells have limitless proliferative potential, and host environmental factors may reduce the seeding efficiency further. Animal studies show that the rate of tumour regrowth in a recipient is dose-related and a threshold number of cells must be infused before tumour seeding occurs. Purging methods should focus upon the elimination of clonogenic precursors below the limit of take. Clonogenic assays are available for some leukaemias, lymphomas and solid tumours.

2 The limit of detection of malignant cells in marrow infusions puts constraints upon the evaluation of purging techniques. There are several ways of increasing the detection limit which include the use of clonal assays, and fluorescent activated cell-sorter (FACS) analysis. However, it is not possible even with the best approach to identify cell frequencies of less than 1/10000. The biological implication of such small inocula is not known.

3 While tumour cells represent distinct cell populations from

marrow progenitors, the relationship between leukaemic stem cells and their normal counterparts, for example in AML, is imprecise. Remission marrow from such patients may contain a mixture of residual leukaemia cells, normal stem cells and preleukaemic cells of intermediate malignancy. No purging technique is precise enough to separate true normal stem cells from preleukaemic ones.

4 These considerations aside, there is no incontrovertible clinical evidence that purging reduces the risk of relapse after ABMT. There have been no comparative studies of ABMT with or without purging, and multicentre data for autologous BMT in ALL, lymphoma and neuroblastoma do not demonstrate an advantage for purging. However, one study in AML autografts from multiple European centres indicates an advantage for purging with maphosphamide (but not for other techniques) in first-remission transplants (Gorin et al., 1989). The negative clinical data do not necessarily imply that the purging approach is conceptually at fault. It could be argued, for example, that the failure to demonstrate an effect of purging is because the benefit is obscured by relapse from inadequate high-dose treatment to the patient. Alternatively the technique may be inadequate and malignant cells transfused below the limit of detection are responsible for the relapse. Because of the potential for some relapses to be caused by reinfusion of malignant cells, many transplanters continue to use purging methods in the knowledge that the evidence is lacking.

Purging approaches

The techniques used exploit functional or physical differences between malignant cells and normal stem cells (Table 4.11). They can be divided into immunological and non-immunological techniques.

Immunological techniques

These rely for their specificity upon the presence of antigens on the cell surface of the malignant cell and not on the stem cell. Non-haemopoietic cells such as neuroblastoma cells are ideally removed by such techniques, as are lymphoid malignancies. Alternatively pluripotent stem cells can be purified by positive selection of CD34+ve cells (Lansdorp and Thomas, 1991).

The binding of an antibody to the surface of a malignant cell is not, however, the only consideration. Antibodies may fail to bind to a small population of clonogenic cells; they may dissociate too rapidly from the cell or they may be internalized before they are effective.

Bound antibodies can be used to kill the cell by complement fixation, or by linking the antibody to ricin or other agents as an

Table 4.11 Methods of purging bone marrow (for references see Gee, 1991)

Immunological techniques (positive or negative selection of malignant cells)
Antibody
Antibody + complement
Antibody + ricin A chain
Antibody-coated magnetic beads
LAK cell induction *in vitro*

Chemotherapeutic agents: differential cytoreduction favouring preservation of normal stem cells
Asta-Z
Maphosphamide
4-Hydroperoxycyclophosphamide

Photosensitizing dyes (damages plasma membrane in malignant cells, stem cells spared)
Merocyanin 540 photosensitization

Favouring the survival advantage for normal stem cells
Cryopreservation may selectively reduce leukaemic progenitors
Ten-day culture selects for normal stem cells in CML and possibly AML

LAK, Lymphokine + activated killer; CML, chronic myeloid leukaemia; AML, acute myeloid leukaemia.

immunotoxin (Krolnick *et al.*, 1982). Alternatively the malignant cells can be removed physically using antibody-coated magnetic beads. Many technical difficulties arise with all of these approaches because of the need to achieve high removal efficiency and reproducibility. A novel approach that is currently being explored is the use of IL-2-activated NK cells to purge leukaemia cells by their known cytotoxic effect on leukaemia cells and their progenitors. In rats LAK cells were shown to produce two or three log reductions in lymphoid and myeloid tumour cell lines without compromising normal haemopoietic stem cell function (Long *et al.*, 1990). The technique has not been used in humans.

Non-immunological techniques

Malignant and normal cells differ in their growth and recovery potential under a variety of adverse conditions. It has been suggested that the process of cryopreservation itself favours the survival of normal stem cells and eliminates malignant cells (Douay *et al.*, 1986; Hagenbeek and Martens, 1989). The addition of cytotoxic agents to the bone marrow is widely used as a method of purging leukaemic marrow. Common agents are maphosphamide (Asta-Z; Gorin *et al.*, 1986b; Marchetti-Rossi *et al.*, 1987) and the active cyclophosphamide derivative 4-hydroperoxycyclophosphamide (4-HC) (Körbling *et al.*,

1982; Yeager et al., 1986). Several groups have used long-term marrow culture to select normal stem cells in CML and myelodysplastic syndromes. Remarkably, Ph^1-positive clones can be eliminated in about half of the cultures. Such marrows retransfused into the recipient reconstitute normal haematopoiesis and can remain Ph-negative for long periods (Barnett et al., 1989).

Physical separation methods have also been applied to purging. They include the use of lectins to bind tumour cells, and density gradient separation. The susceptibility of some tumour cells such as neuroblastoma and leukaemias to ultraviolet light forms the basis of an ultraviolet purging technique using the photosensitizing agent merocyanin 540.

Stem cell function after ABMT

Haematological and immunological recovery after ABMT, in contrast to allografts, is typically rapid and complete. Relatively small numbers of stem cells are required for engraftment, and failed engraftment is more related to the quality rather than the quantity of cells infused. In AML, remission marrow or blood cells are used as a source of autologous stem cells. Recovery of platelets may be very delayed in these circumstances. This has been attributed to stem cell functional defects related either to the effect of previous chemotherapy or to the disease process itself.

CURE OF NON-MALIGNANT DISORDERS BY BMT

Bone marrow transplantation can be used to correct metabolic disorders in two distinct ways: replacement of defective bone marrow cell lines by normal donor cells, and replacement of a generalized enzyme deficiency by grafting bone marrow stem cells capable of generating a permanent population of enzyme-competent cells. Other disorders, such as amino acid transport abnormalities, represent a defect occurring in differentiated cells that are not of haemopoietic origin. Bone marrow transplantation cannot be used to correct these abnormalities. Autologous BMT is not at present a relevant form of correction for these disorders, but in future gene therapy will allow retransplantation of autologous, genetically corrected, stem cells.

It is easy to understand how BMT can correct genetic disorders such as thalassaemia major, where the requirement is to ablate defective bone marrow and replace it with that of a normal donor. The mode of correction of metabolic disorders is more involved. Most are examples of lysosomal enzyme defects. Lysosomes contain numerous cytoplasmic enzymes and play a vital role in enzyme transport between

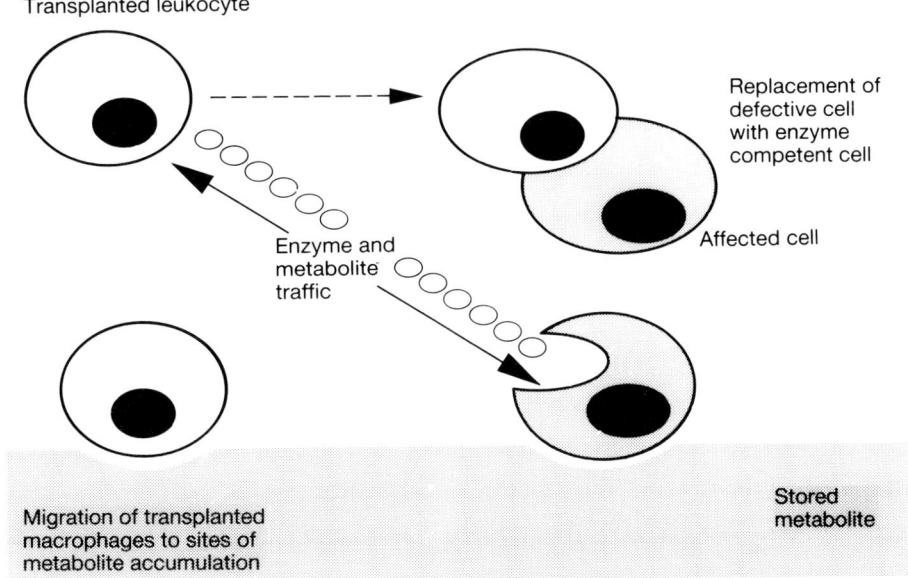

Fig. 4.11 Correction of metabolic disorders by BMT.

cells: they can migrate to the cell membrane and release enzymes into the tissue fluid where they are available to other cells by the process of pinocytosis and lysosome incorporation. Experiments where cell lines from metabolic disorders are co-cultivated with enzyme-competent cells derived from normal individuals have demonstrated exchange of lysosomally packaged enzymes between cells, correcting the abnormality in the defective cell. Three processes responsible for correction of metabolic disorders by BMT can be identified (Barrett and McCarthy, 1990) (Fig. 4.11).

Cell replacement

Massive production of leukocytes by the bone marrow serves as a major source of lysosomal enzymes. Widespread distribution of marrow-derived macrophages and lymphocytes throughout the reticuloendothelial system provides a significant and permanent supply of cells, bringing replacement enzyme into contact with typical sites of accumulation of storage products. These include liver, spleen, lymph nodes, skin and mucous membranes. It is now clear that marrow transplant-derived cells of the monocyte–macrophage line are also precursors to microglia in the central nervous system. This may be an important mechanism for reversing the accumulation of mucopolysaccharide in the brain in conditions such as Hurler's disease.

Enzyme donation

The availability of lysosomal enzymes by exchange between transplanted cell and recipient tissue makes it possible for metabolic correction to occur in extracellular storage material, as well as within cells of the host.

Metabolic gradient

Transplanted cells in an area of storage metabolite will first produce clearance of the metabolite within their immediate vicinity. A concentration gradient is thus established, down which further metabolite will flow. Ultimately metabolic gradients established across the blood–brain barrier may permit the flow of soluble storage metabolite away from areas of high concentration in the brain or other tissues not directly reached by the transplanted cells.

While there is some evidence for these mechanisms, their relative importance in the correction of individual diseases by BMT is not clear.

Conditioning regimens

Many genetic disorders represent conditions where the marrow, while producing defectively functioning cells, proliferates entirely normally. These patients will not have experienced the same degree of normal marrow suppression as leukaemia transplant recipients. It is therefore of particular importance to use conditioning regimens for BMT that not only immunosuppress the recipient but 'make space' for the transplanted stem cells. The implication is that recipient haematopoiesis might persist despite a 100% donor lymphoid engraftment, as is sometimes observed in unpreconditioned SCID recipients of matched sibling marrow. The term 'displacement marrow transplantation' has been used to refer to the combination of a myelotoxic agent (busulphan) with an immunosuppressive agent (cyclophosphamide) as conditioning for genetic disorders (Hobbs, 1986). A precise understanding of what is required is, however, lacking. Marrow transplants for inborn errors other than SCID conditioned with cyclophosphamide immunosuppression alone are usually rejected. Split chimerism (with donor immunity and recipient haemopoiesis) is rare in non-SCID patients and associated with unstable engraftment. It is possible, therefore, that the highly successful busulphan–cyclophosphamide combination simply achieves better immunosuppression than cyclophosphamide alone.

The first inborn errors to be successfully transplanted were infants with SCID. The profound immunodeficiency of these patients made it possible to obtain stable engraftment without any preconditioning, provided a fully HLA-matched sibling donor was used. It was subsequently discovered that not all immune-deficient states would permit engraftment of matched marrow without prior immunosuppression and that even infants with SCID would reject a less than fully compatible bone marrow. Such situations required immunosuppression with cyclophosphamide to achieve stable engraftment. Cyclophosphamide regimens were found to be ineffective in achieving regular graft takes in Wiskott–Aldrich disease, thalassaemia, and neutrophil disorders (Kapoor et al., 1981). This led to the addition of TBI to the regimen. While the combination of TBI and cyclophosphamide did permit engraftment, the mortality from the schedule was found to be unacceptably high. Subsequently, following its introduction as a conditioning regimen in leukaemia patients by Santos, the combination of busulphan and cyclophosphamide (BuCy) was introduced into genetic disease transplant schedules with success (Santos, 1984; Tutschka et al., 1987). More recent studies of conditioning regimens in genetic disorders have concerned selection of the most favourable doses of Cy and Bu – schedules that achieve the highest rate of engraftment with the lowest transplant-related mortality. Lucarelli and colleagues (1985), studying BMT in thalassaemia recipients, carried out trials of conditioning schedules first using TBI and Cy and subsequently with Bu and Cy. Total doses of Bu were varied from 8 to 16 mg/kg. They found that lower doses of Bu did not permit satisfactory engraftment, while high doses were associated with unacceptable mortality from pneumonitis. These results were confirmed from multicentre data on thalassaemia transplants submitted to the IBMTR. The consensus is that a dose of busulphan of 14 mg/kg with cyclophosphamide 200 mg/kg offers the best compromise between graft failure and mortality from pneumonitis (Barrett, 1989).

Patients with Fanconi anaemia represent a special case. Initial attempts to correct the aplastic anaemia by BMT using standard cyclophosphamide schedules resulted in a high mortality from GVHD, complicated by toxic epidermal necrolysis and severe gastrointestinal damage. This complication is presumed to be related to the generalized defect of DNA repair in this condition. Gluckman and coworkers (1984) showed that the skin of Fanconi anaemia patients is extremely sensitive to cyclophosphamide but less so to irradiation. They subsequently obtained successful grafts in Fanconi anaemia by using a dose of cyclophosphamide tailored to the individual patient but usually 10-fold less than the standard dose. Interestingly, this lower dose of cyclophosphamide is not associated with graft rejection, suggesting that the lymphocytes in Fanconi anaemia are also highly sensitive to cyclophosphamide.

Timing of BMT

Many inborn errors present in infancy after an apparently normal birth. Diagnosis of these rare disorders is unlikely to be made by antenatal screening unless a previous child has already been affected. Thus, the condition usually causes clinical problems before BMT can be carried out. Thereafter the disease progresses, causing increasing and irreversible damage to tissue such as the myocardium, central nervous system, peripheral nerves, bones and cartilage. It is crucial, therefore, to carry out BMT before signs of permanent damage are severe. This may mean BMT between 6 months and 1 year of life. Clinical experience indicates that infants under 1 year tolerate BMT more easily than older patients. Thus, early diagnosis and corrective treatment appear to be the best approach.

Metabolic disturbance after BMT

The rapid production by the grafted marrow of previously missing enzyme can lead to metabolic disturbance secondary to rapid degradation of large amounts of stored metabolite. Hypercholesterolaemia occurs after BMT in patients with a cholesterol ester storage defect (Wolman's disease), and patients with osteopetrosis may develop life-threatening hypercalcaemia coincident with engraftment of normal osteoclasts immediately commencing bone remodelling.

Splenomegaly

Splenomegaly is a common feature of storage diseases and haemoglobinopathies. Very large spleens delay marrow engraftment and can cause life-threatening cytopenia in the first 3 months after BMT. Splenectomy before BMT should therefore be considered in patients with very large spleens (Hobbs *et al.*, 1987).

GVHD

The syndrome of secondary disease, a lethal wasting disease in irradiated mice induced by allogeneic but not syngeneic spleen cells, was first described by Barnes and Loutit (1955). Secondary disease, or as it was later called GVHD, was shown to be related to the infusion of allogeneic lymphocytes (Santos and Cole, 1955). A severe form of GVHD was seen in humans in some of the early attempts at BMT between unmatched donor–recipient pairs before the advent of HLA typing.

GVHD is one of the major complications of BMT. It occurs in up to 80% of patients receiving HLA-matched sibling BMT, and is responsible for up to 20% mortality after BMT. Prevention and treatment of GVHD is only partially successful at present because of the inefficiency and lack of specificity of the available treatments. Recently the mechanisms underlying the GVHD process have become better defined and have formed the basis of new treatment approaches.

Clinical features of GVHD

Acute GVHD varies in intensity from a mild self-limiting condition requiring no treatment to a severe and fatal disorder. The first manifestation is usually a rash with or without the accompaniment of fever and influenza-like symptoms. The rash is typically distributed on the extensor surface of the limbs, the face and neck, and the palms and soles. It may be localized to the upper or lower part of the body.

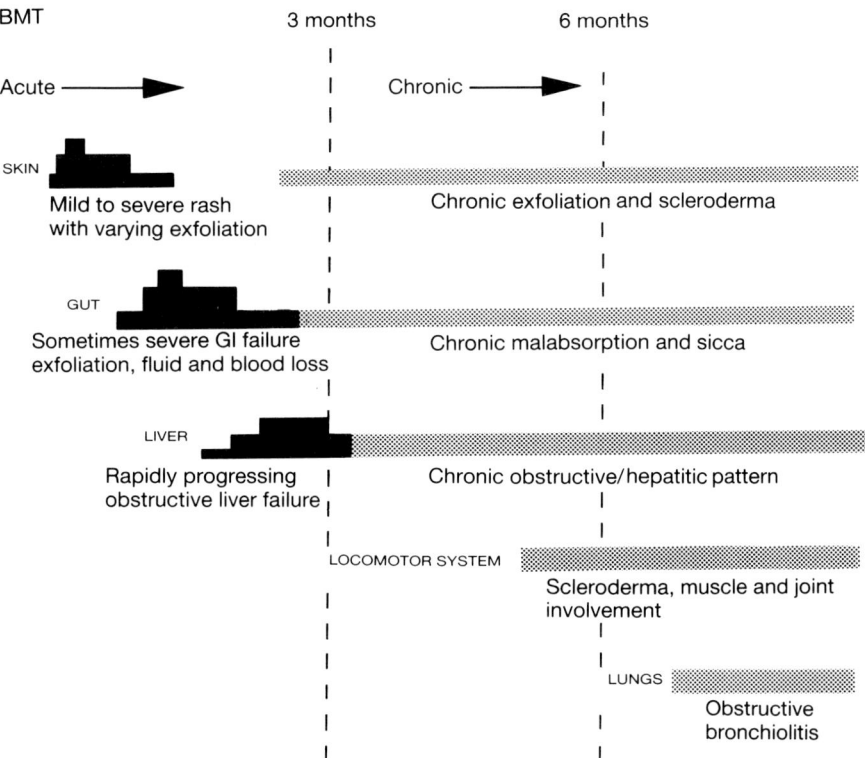

Fig. 4.12 Timecourse of organ involvement in acute and chronic GVHD.

In severe cases the rash spreads to affect most of the body surface, sometimes in progressive waves of extension. The more severe rashes become confluent, and may progress to frank epidermolysis with the formation of bullae. The reaction resolves with exfoliation. If gastro-intestinal (GI) GVHD occurs, it typically follows acute skin GVHD several weeks later. The most frequent manifestation is diarrhoea accompanied by abdominal cramps, nausea and anorexia. The condition may progress to involve the whole of the GI tract with severe fluid and blood loss, and prostration. Barium studies show loss of the normal ridged mucosal pattern and can delineate the extent of the process. Liver GVHD is usually the last to develop – beyond 40 days from BMT, often as a further extension of a continuing GVHD process but sometimes as an isolated manifestation, or after resolution of skin and gastrointestinal GVHD. Pancytopenia and immunological deficiency tend to reflect the severity of the process. Sometimes complete marrow failure occurs, but usually the cytopenia will resolve if the GVHD is controlled. Figure 4.12 and Plate 4.1 (facing p. 148) illustrate the patterns of clinical evolution and pathology of acute GVHD.

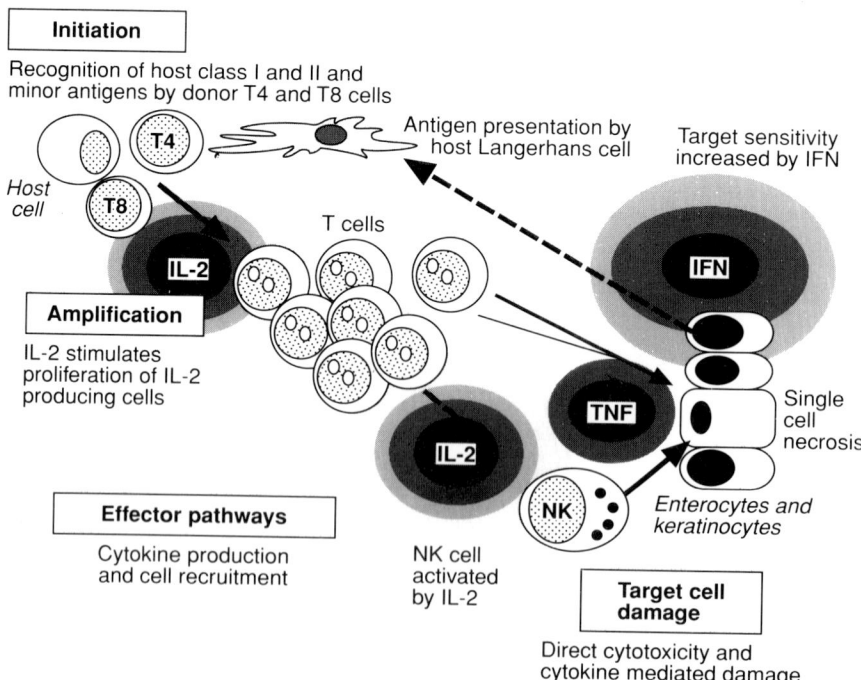

Fig. 4.13 Mechanism of GVHD.

PATHOPHYSIOLOGY OF ACUTE GVHD

Figure 4.13 outlines the stages identified in the development of GVHD.

Initiation

The GVHD process requires the activation of T lymphocytes. Disparity between donor and recipient at either the HLA class I or II loci is a potent stimulus for donor T lymphocytes but minor histocompatibility differences are equally capable of triggering GVHD between HLA-matched siblings (Goulmy et al., 1983). A syndrome histologically indistinguishable from skin GVHD has been described after BMT between identical twins, and also after autologous BMT. This reaction appears to be an autoimmune process. Tutschka et al. (1983) showed that GVHD can readily be induced experimentally in rats receiving syngeneic BMT provided cyclosporin is given following the BMT. The reaction can be blocked by antibodies to MHC class II, suggesting that the process is mediated through CD4 helper cells and may therefore be considered as an autoimmune phenomenon. Cyclosporin induces imbalance in the recovery of helper and suppressor lymphocyte subsets after BMT, and this may provoke an autoimmune reaction.

The most compelling evidence for the central role of T cells in the initiation of GVHD came from the demonstration first in animals (Müller-Ruchholtz et al., 1980) and then in humans (Prentice et al., 1982; Reisner et al., 1983) that T lymphocyte depletion of donor marrow can reduce the frequency and severity of GVHD or even completely abrogate it. Subsequent studies by Cobbold et al. (1986), who transplanted mice with bone marrow and spleen cells selectively depleted of lymphocyte subsets, showed that both helper (Lyt-1) and suppressor (Lyt-2) lymphocytes can initiate GVHD.

Amplification

Activation of donor T lymphocytes without subsequent clonal expansion is unlikely to result in a clinical GVHD syndrome. Interleukin-2 is the central growth factor and activator of T lymphocytes and may play a central role in determining the severity of the reaction. Several studies show that GVHD can be induced after allogeneic transplantation in mice by administration of IL-2. If the marrow transplant is depleted of T lymphocytes, however, IL-2 does not induce GVHD (Malkovsky et al., 1986).

Effector mechanisms

A variety of cells are involved in causing the characteristic tissue damage of the GVHD reaction. Sviland et al. (1989a) measured numbers and characterized the subset of lymphocytes infiltrating the epidermis during the evolution of GVHD reactions. They concluded that there was no particular pattern of cell subset infiltration with both suppressor and helper subsets becoming involved in the histological changes seen. A constant and early occurrence is the detection of enhanced DR antigen expression on the surface of Langerhans cells and neighbouring keratinocytes. Langerhans cells are believed to be involved in antigen presentation. They disappear rapidly from the epidermis during the development of the GVH reaction. Thus the role of macrophages in the effector process is not clear. It is possible that NK cells are implicated in the final effector path of the GVHD reaction. Early reappearance of NK reactivity after BMT is associated with acute GVHD (Dokhelar *et al.*, 1981). Antibodies against cells with NK phenotype in mice can partially block GVHD.

Targets of the GVHD reaction

Although GVHD is a generalized disorder affecting multiple systems, scrutiny of the histological features of the process reveals a reproducible pattern of cell damage in many tissues. The target cells of the GVHD reaction are keratinocytes, epithelial cells of the gastrointestinal mucosa and their embryological outpouchings in the biliary tree and exocrine glands. Curiously, the urothelium is not the site of GVH reactions. In addition the bone marrow is susceptible to GVHD – severe reactions are accompanied by pancytopenia in part due to marrow suppression, and lymphopenia (sometimes with severe immunosuppression) occurs. A common feature of cells susceptible to GVHD damage is their proliferative nature, and the ability to express DR antigens which is enhanced by IFNγ (Basham *et al.*, 1984). There are considerable experimental and clinical data showing that both viral and bacterial infection enhance tissue susceptibility to GVHD. Protective environments have been shown to reduce the incidence and severity of GVHD in aplastic anaemia BMT recipients (Storb *et al.*, 1983). Furthermore there is a relationship between the intensity of the conditioning regimen and GVHD, possibly mediated through the degree of tissue damage caused.

Cytokines in GVHD

The hallmark of the reaction is the appearance of single cell necrosis in the basal layers of the epidermis, the intestinal mucosa or the bile canaliculi. A notable feature is the disparity between the severe disruption of the basal layer of the skin or the submucosa of the GI tract, and the paucity of the lymphocyte infiltrate. The damage is produced by cytokines released locally from relatively few infiltrating cells. Piguet et al. (1987) have shown that TNF is capable of producing GVHD-like changes in the skin, and that GVH reactions are blocked in mice by antibodies to TNF.

The skin explant model has been a useful model for testing the role of different cytokines in GVHD in humans. Additionally, Sviland et al. (1989b) have shown that the supernatant from mixed lymphocyte reactions contains factors that induce features in the basal layer identical to those seen in GVHD. The changes can be reduced by blocking antibodies to TNF but not completely abrogated, indicating that other cytotoxic factors are involved (Cohen, 1988).

Chronic GVHD

Chronic GVHD is defined as GVHD occurring beyond 100 days from BMT. Nevertheless, clinical and histological features typical of chronic GVHD may occur as early as 30 days after BMT in some patients, and overlap between acute and chronic GVHD is not uncommon (see review by Atkinson, 1990b). Chronic GVHD may develop directly from acute GVHD, or following a period of quiescence. Occasionally it occurs without any preceding acute phase. The major pathological feature which characterizes chronic GVHD is an increase in collagen deposition with the development of sclerosis and atrophy of the dermis. Cytotoxic prethymic T suppressor cells are found in patients with chronic GVHD; these may be responsible for tissue damage (Tsoi, 1982). The mechanism underlying this immune dysregulation is incompletely understood. Various autoimmune features occur – autoantibodies to nucleoli (Kier et al., 1990), red cells and platelets, and other tissues have been described. Despite clinical similarities to various autoimmune disorders, such as scleroderma and primary biliary cirrhosis, there are distinct differences in the underlying pathology (Plate 4.2, facing p. 148).

Clinically, the condition has a wider tissue distribution than acute GVHD, often involving the musculoskeletal system and lungs. Much of the pathology results from the widespread deposition of collagen leading to exocrine gland failure (sicca syndrome), fasciitis, dry joints, malabsorption and obstructive bronchiolitis (Beschorner et al., 1978). Chronic liver GVHD can cause cirrhosis. Most patients with chronic GVHD have a mild to moderate disorder with a limited tissue distribution. Occasionally it runs a severe unremitting course, resulting in death from lung or liver failure, or infection. Chronic GVHD is accompanied by an immune dysregulation which leads to the development of autoimmune cytopenias, and immune deficiency. This

Table 4.12 Prevention and treatment of graft-versus-host disease (GVHD)

Prevention
T lymphocyte depletion
    Monoclonal antibodies: Campath-1, anti-CD3, anti-CD5, monoclonals conjugated with ricin, or complement fixing
    Physical methods: countercurrent elutriation, T rosette depletion and soybean lectin-positive stem cell selection
Immunosuppressive agents
    Methotrexate, cyclosporin, ATG, steroids
Combinations of T depletion with immunosuppressives
Combinations of immunosuppressives
    e.g. methotrexate and cyclosporin, methotrexate, ATG and cyclosporin
Protective isolation and gut decontamination
Improved donor selection by predictive tests

Treatment
Immunosuppressives
    High-dose prednisolone, standard-dose prednisolone, ATG, cyclosporin, cyclophosphamide, methotrexate, thalidomide
Monoclonal antilymphocyte antibodies
    Anti CD5-ricin conjugate, anti-CD2 and anti-CD5 combinations, anti-CD25
Anticytokines
    Anti-TNF, pentoxyphyllin
Anticollagen agents (chronic GVHD)
    Penicillamine

ATG, antithymocyte globulin; TNF, tumour necrosis factor.

leads to an increased risk of infection, particularly from encapsulated bacteria such as the pneumococcus.

PREVENTION AND TREATMENT OF GVHD

The methods used to prevent and treat GVHD in clinical BMT and the results obtained are shown in Table 4.12. Prophylactic treatments have largely been developed empirically. However, they can be broadly categorized into:
1 agents that prevent lymphocyte proliferation;
2 *in vitro* or *in vivo* depletion of donor lymphocytes;
3 agents blocking the effector arm of GVHD; and
4 combination treatments.

Agents inhibiting lymphocyte proliferation

Storb *et al.* (1970) attempted to suppress GVHD reactions in dogs undergoing BMT using methotrexate (MTX). These experiments formed the basis for the Seattle MTX schedule which is still in wide use in various modifications of the original schedule. There is no evidence that MTX has any more than a non-specific antiproliferative action on donor lymphocytes. It is therefore the timing of the treatment that is likely to be critical in the inhibition of the developing donor T lymphocyte proliferative response to the host tissues. The early administration of MTX in the first 7 days after the BMT is essential for its anti-GVHD action.

Three studies have compared MTX with no GVHD prophylaxis. Two of them showed that MTX was effective in preventing and reducing the severity of GVHD (Lazarus et al., 1984; Elfenbein et al., 1986; Sullivan et al., 1989b). Cyclophosphamide has also been used with equal effectiveness as an antiproliferative agent (Santos et al., 1987). Nevertheless, severe and lethal GVHD – even between matched donor–recipient sibling pairs – is never completely prevented by cytotoxic agents.

Because of this the introduction of cyclosporin was an important breakthrough (Gluckman et al., 1980; Powles et al., 1980; Tutschka et al., 1983). Cyclosporin blocks the action of IL-2 on lymphocytes, preventing the clonal proliferation in response to a primary challenge. Cyclosporin reduces both the incidence and severity of GVHD. For maximum effectiveness it has to be administered at the time of BMT and continued for at least 3 months thereafter. It is given twice daily (intravenously or orally) in order to maintain immunosuppressive tissue levels. Cyclosporin is the most effective *in vivo* agent for the prevention of GVHD.

Depletion of lymphocytes

T cell depletion

The most effective method of preventing GVHD is the removal of T cells in the donor marrow inoculum. Early attempts using anti-T cell globulins to treat the donor marrow were not successful because of the inefficiency of the technique (Rodt et al., 1981). Reisner et al. (1983) subsequently employed lectins and sheep red cells to select a stem cell-rich T lymphocyte-depleted fraction of bone marrow and demonstrated that efficient T cell removal prevented GVHD in transplants between haplotype-matched parental donors for infants with SCID. Following the development of monoclonal antibodies with T cell specificity it became possible effectively to remove sufficient T cells from the marrow to reduce GVHD in the recipient. Treating the donor marrow with specific mouse monoclonal antibodies against the lymphocyte CD3 receptor (OKT3 antibody), or cocktails of several anti-T cell antibodies achieved a 2 log reduction in T cells which was sufficient almost completely to eliminate GVHD between matched sibling donor—recipient pairs (Filipovitch et al., 1982; Prentice et al., 1982; Mitsuyasu et al., 1986). Mouse monoclonals have the disadvantage of low cytotoxicity with human complement. However, the rat monoclonal Campath-1 developed by Hale and colleagues (1983, 1988) is cytotoxic with human complement and has been used successfully to prevent GVHD by many European BMT teams. Other approaches in current use are ricin-conjugated antibodies and countercurrent elutriation (de Witte et al., 1986).

As T cell depletion became widely adopted, reports of an increased incidence of leukaemic relapse appeared (Apperley et al., 1986; Maraninchi et al., 1987). A further complication was the demonstration of an increased risk of graft rejection or failure occurring even after what was considered an immunoablative dose of TBI (reviewed by Martelli and Aversa, 1991). When the disease-free survival of T-depleted BMTs was compared with BMT using other methods of GVHD prevention, it became increasingly apparent after longer follow-up that there was no survival advantage for T-depleted BMT recipients. Several studies demonstrated that the disadvantages of relapse and graft failure could be, to some extent, reduced by increasing the intensity of the conditioning regimen (Bozdech et al., 1985; Guyotat et al., 1987; Burnett et al., 1988; Prentice et al., 1989). Attention has also focused upon the type of T cell depletion used: 'broad-spectrum' depletion of T and B lymphocytes and NK cells by agents such as Campath-1 is more likely to result in leukaemic relapse (Butturini and Gale, 1990; Hervé, 1991). Highly selective depletion using physical methods such as the soybean lectin approach and countercurrent elutriation appears to have a more favourable outcome (de Witte et al., 1986). Another important consideration is the efficiency of the depletion. Most techniques achieve a 2 log depletion of lymphocytes. Patients receiving larger lymphocyte doses have a high risk of developing GVHD while very efficient depletion increases the risk of graft failure and relapse.

The efficiency of T cell removal from the marrow varies according to the technique used and from one procedure to the next. Attempts have therefore been made to define the optimum number of T cells to infuse. Inefficient T depletion fails to prevent GVHD, while excessive T depletion increases the risk of graft failure (Kernan et al., 1986). As a guideline, the infusion of less than 10^6 lymphocytes per kg recipient weight will effectively prevent GVHD. Several workers have attempted to standardize the number of lymphocytes transfused by carrying out highly efficient T depletion and then adding back a known dose of T cells. There is as yet no clear evidence that this approach is reliable (Poynton, 1988).

In vivo *antibody treatment*

Antilymphocyte globulin has some activity in preventing GVHD but was no more effective than steroids in a randomized trial (Doney et al., 1981). Monoclonal antibodies are still under evaluation. Hervé reported that BB10, an anti-CD25 monoclonal which blocks the IL-2 receptor, reduced the frequency and severity of acute GVHD (Ferrara et al., 1987; Hervé, 1991). In another study, a different antibody delayed but did not reduce the incidence of acute GVHD (Anasetti et al., 1991).

Agents primarily blocking the effector arm of GVHD

Steroids are the most widely used and effective treatment for established acute and chronic GVHD. Prednisolone is commonly used to treat GVHD and has also been shown to have some efficacy in prevention. Steroids act at multiple points in the immune pathway, blocking lymphocyte responsiveness and inhibiting lymphocyte and macrophage function. Response to steroid treatment is rapid, but high doses are required to control severe acute GVHD reactions (Kendra et al., 1981). For no determined reason not all GVHD reactions respond. Steroid responsiveness is the best prognostic indicator for acute GVHD outcome – patients refractory to adequate doses of prednisolone have a mortality of over 80% (Hervé, 1991). Because TNF contributes to the tissue damage in GVHD, attempts to reduce TNF production, by antibodies to TNF or pentoxyphyllin, have been made. Pentoxyphyllin has been shown to have some efficacy in GVHD prevention. Anti-TNF therapy is still under evaluation. The antibiotic ciprofloxacin also has anti-TNF activity but has not been clinically evaluated in this respect.

Combination treatment for prophylaxis

The proven but incomplete efficacy of individual agents in GVHD prevention has led to numerous trials employing combinations of two or three preventive agents. Two approaches in particular appear to show a definite benefit. These are the combination of methylprednisolone, antilymphocyte globulin, and MTX introduced by the Minneapolis group (Ramsay et al., 1982), and the combination of cyclosporin and MTX introduced by the Seattle team (Storb et al., 1985, 1989). Some studies show that the combination of cyclosporin and MTX leads to an increase in relapse (Biggs et al., 1986; Aschan et al., 1991), although this was not confirmed in a recent study (Mrsic et al., 1990). At present, therefore, despite our ability almost completely to abrogate GVHD by T depletion, no prophylactic approach is without its disadvantages, either because of undesirable side-effects, or through inefficiency of the procedure in preventing GVHD. New developments have yet to be translated into improved clinical results (Hervé, 1991). Because of this, the treatment of established GVHD remains an important aspect of clinical BMT.

Combination treatment for established GVHD

The main application of combination treatment of acute GVHD is in patients who are unresponsive to steroids. Agents effective in GVHD prophylaxis such as cyclosporin, MTX and antilymphocyte globulin have been widely used but have low efficacy in this group of patients. Several antilymphocyte monoclonals, such as Campath-1G and anti-CD5, are effective during the period of administration but do not prevent relapse or reduce the ultimate mortality. Anti-TNF has not yet been evaluated in this context.

Prevention and treatment of chronic GVHD

The treatments which prevent acute GvHD also have an impact on the development of chronic GVHD. However, chronic GVHD can occur in patients who have not experienced acute GVHD. Prolonged treatment with cyclosporin is probably beneficial but no studies have examined the relationship of the duration of GVHD prophylaxis on chronic GVHD occurrence.

There is clear evidence that treatment in chronic GVHD is effective in preventing progression (Sullivan et al., 1981, 1988). Many treatments have been used but all are immunosuppressive, and refractoriness occurs in a subgroup of patients who have severe and progressive chronic GVHD. Both cyclosporin and prednisolone are effective. There is no evidence to support the use of azathioprine as an additional agent. The immunosuppressive property of thalidomide has been beneficial in some refractory patients (McCarthy et al., 1989; Vogelsang, 1991). Immunosuppressive treatments for chronic GVHD have the disadvantage of exaggerating further the profound immune defect of the condition. It is therefore essential to give anti-infective prophylaxis. This should include penicillin to reduce the risk of pneumococcal sepsis associated with hyposplenism, co-trimoxazole to prevent pneumocystis infection, and acyclovir either as prophylaxis or as prompt treatment for herpes simplex and varicella-zoster reactivation (Atkinson, 1990b). In chronic GVHD restricted to a particular organ local treatment (e.g. topical steroids) can be helpful.

GRAFT FAILURE

Graft failure manifests itself either as a complete failure of donor haemopoietic recovery, or as a period of haemopoietic recovery followed by a progressive and usually rapid pancytopenia. Failure of haemopoietic reconstitution is sometimes associated with a rejection syndrome characterized by fever, transient splenomegaly, and the presence of large granular lymphocytes in the blood associated with pancytopenia and a hypocellular bone marrow. Although engraftment may be retarded in some recipients, failure of haemopoietic reconstitution at 4 weeks post-transplant constitutes graft failure. Less commonly, patients with established donor haemopoietic recovery develop late graft failure up to 1 year post-transplant. Occasionally patients with aplastic anaemia or congenital disorders regenerate recipient haemopoiesis at the time of the transplant failure. Spontaneous recipient haemopoietic recovery may follow a period of pancytopenia or be undetected except by marker studies demonstrating full recipient haemopoietic recovery. Somewhat remarkably, recipient haemopoiesis is capable of regenerating after high-dose chemotherapy and radiation preparative regimens (Barrett *et al.*, 1989).

Graft failure may be caused by non-immunological factors associated with inadequate transfusion of viable donor cells or an unfavourable recipient environment for haemopoietic engraftment. Rejection by residual recipient immunity is, however, the predominant mechanism responsible for both early and late graft failure and will be discussed in detail below.

Conditions predisposing to graft failure

Clinical BMT experience has identified both donor and host-related factors relating to the risk of marrow graft rejection (Table 4.13).

Host factors

The degree of compatibility between donor and recipient plays a central role in the rejection process. Transplants between identical twins are not rejected except in the special situation of SAA where the failure of about 30% of identical-twin BMTs to take without prior immunosuppression of the recipient suggests a specific process of graft failure associated with aplastic anaemia (Champlin *et al.*, 1984).

The risk of rejection increases with increasing disparity between the donor and the recipient. Minor MHC differences, for example, are responsible for a higher graft failure rate between HLA A, B and DR-matched pairs, but the rejection rate is highest in recipients of haplo-

Table 4.13 Risk factors for graft failure

Recipient-related
Early
    Hostile marrow environment (some aplastic anaemia)
    Residual T lymphocytes
    Circulating inhibitors – drugs, cytokines
    Presensitization to donor
    Splenomegaly

Late
    Competition from host haemopoiesis
    Competition from recovering host lymphopoiesis (mixed chimerism)

Donor-related
Early
    Insufficient stem cells
    Major MHC incompatibility with recipient
    Minor MHC incompatibility with recipient
    T lymphocyte-depleted transplants
    Defective stem cell function (relatives of aplastic patients)
    Stem cell damage from *in vitro* marrow manipulation

Late
    Stem cells with limited self-replication transplanted
    Toxicity to grafted marrow from treatment of GVHD
    Cytomegalovirus infection
    Mixed chimeric state

MHC, Major histocompatibility complex; GVHD, graft-versus-host disease.

identical marrow. Congenital immune deficiency states have helped to elucidate the role of recipient immune function in marrow engraftment. Patients with SCID readily accept transplants from HLA-matched family members but are still capable of rejecting marrow from haplotype-identical parental donors (Fischer *et al.*, 1986). Patients with less severe immune deficiencies such as Wiskott–Aldrich disease are capable of rejecting fully matched sibling bone marrows unless prior immunosuppression is provided. These observations indicate that profound immunosuppression is necessary before even fully matched transplants can be accepted and suggest a role for NK-mediated rejection of bone marrow in T cell-deficient patients. Even after immunosuppressive conditioning it has been shown that CD3+ve lymphocytes with antidonor cytotoxic potential persist (Bordignon *et al.*, 1989) as well as radioresistant NK cells (Yankelevich *et al.*, 1989). Thus MHC restricted and unrestricted recipient immunity appears to play a role in graft rejection. These observations are supported by animal transplant experiments pointing to a role for recipient NK cells as well as helper and suppressor lymphocyte subsets in causing rejection (Cobbold *et al.*, 1986). Clinical transplanters have

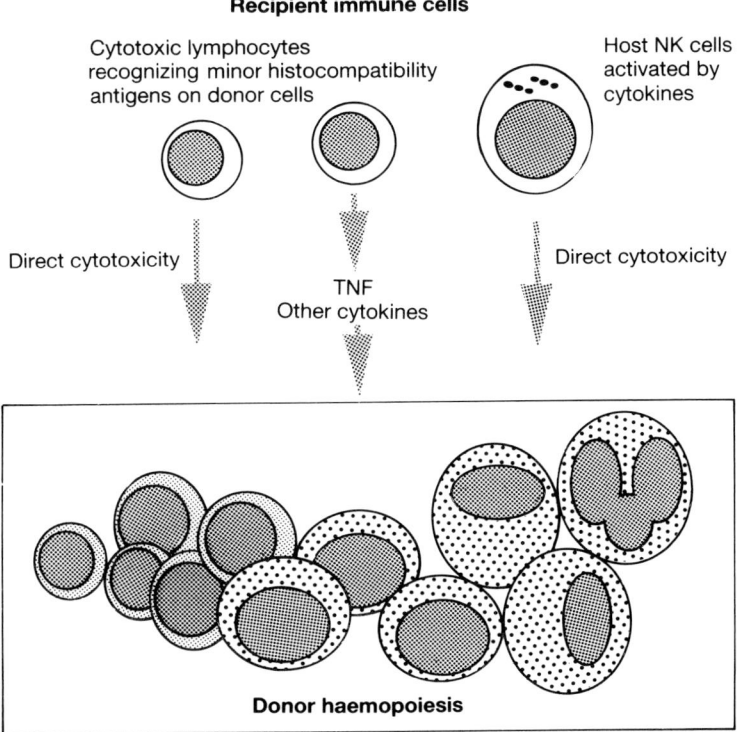

Fig. 4.14 Mechanisms of graft rejection.

had some success in circumventing graft failure in less than fully compatible transplants by augmenting the conditioning schedule with additional radiation (Patterson et al., 1986; Guyotat et al., 1987; Burnett et al., 1988), addition of cytosine arabinoside, antilymphocyte globulin (Bozdech et al., 1985) or monoclonal antilymphocyte antibodies. During graft rejection in humans there is a rise in CD3+ve, CD8+ve lymphocytes, as well as an increase in large granulolymphocytes bearing NK markers. After *in vitro* expansion with IL-2, these cells can be demonstrated to be of recipient origin. Cytotoxic T cell clones derived from patients rejecting donor marrow have been shown to recognize a variety of minor histocompatibility antigens on the donor cells (Goulmy, 1985; Fig. 4.14).

Donor factors

The role of donor T lymphocytes in facilitating graft take has been clearly demonstrated in the increased risk of graft failure incurred by donor marrow T cell depletion from 2 to 25% in matched sibling leukaemia transplants, and from 20 to 50% in closely matched unrelated donor transplants (Martin, 1990). The number of donor marrow cells and haematopoietic progenitors transfused has a bearing on the chance of successful engraftment. However, the relationship between the number of transplanted stem cells and the chance of engraftment remains imprecise, partly because it is not possible to quantitate human pluripotent stem cells directly and partly because any dose relationship between committed progenitors or total nucleated cells is obscured by other factors within the range of cell doses usually transplanted. Increasing the number of donor cells inevitably increases the number of lymphoid cells transfused, thereby providing a protective effect of donor T cells in securing engraftment.

Relationship of graft take to GVHD prevention and chimerism

Gale and Reisner (1986) have proposed that GVHD and graft rejection are mirror images such that the two conditions are mutually incompatible. In this model GVHD represents the successful elimination of residual host immune cells by donor cytotoxic lymphocytes, while engraftment without GVHD is associated with persisting host immune responses, and also host-type haematopoiesis. Such situations may lead to donor–host lymphoid and haematopoietic chimerism, manifest as no take or take, followed by graft failure. The relationship between graft take and the presence of clinical GVHD is not however absolute: there is evidence that cells responsible for graft take are not identical to GVHD-reacting cells, possibly because subsets may recognize host lymphocytes but not host GVHD targets such as epithelial cells (Martin, 1990). Evidence in support of this comes from animal studies using T-depleted allogeneic marrow where donor chimerism can be enhanced by a distinct donor cell population lacking the potential to cause GVHD (Sykes et al., 1988, 1989).

Role of donor lymphocytes

The action of donor lymphocytes in facilitating stem cell engraftment could be mediated through several mechanisms: following the hypothesis that donor T cells and NK cells may be responsible for the immune elimination of 'minimal residual' host immunity (Gale and Reisner, 1986). The lack of a clear reciprocal relationship between GVHD and failure to engraft could be explained by the existence of a degree of specificity of donor lymphocytes for host lymphocytes and not other GVHD targets such as epithelial and endothelial cells. Another possibility is that donor cells exert a 'veto' effect on host antidonor cytotoxic responses. There is experimental evidence for both NK and lymphocytes having a suppressive action on host cytotoxic

T cell function (Fink et al., 1984; Ogasawara et al., 1988; Bosserman et al., 1989). Thirdly, donor lymphocytes may be responsible for the production of cytokines responsible for early engraftment of pluripotent stem cells. It has not been possible however to demonstrate a specific role for GM-CSF in enhancing engraftment (Blazar et al., 1988), and the effects of earlier acting cytokines such as IL-3 (Vallera and Blazar, 1988) and IL-1 have not been studied in rejection models. There is therefore no unequivocal evidence for any of these mechanisms and the interactions between donor and residual host immunity may therefore be complex and variable.

Prevention of graft failure

To a large extent graft failure can be circumvented by adequate immunosuppression of the host. Indeed, with the exception of BMT in SCID disease from HLA-matched family donors and patients with aplastic anaemia transplanted with bone marrow from identical twins, some form of immunosuppression is mandatory. The intensity of the immunosuppressive regimen can be tailored to the perceived risk of rejection. Thus, engraftment is usually achieved with cyclophosphamide and cyclosporin alone in unsensitized patients with aplastic anaemia receiving BMTs from HLA-identical siblings. However, additional irradiation to the lymphatic system is necessary to secure engraftment in sensitized patients or those receiving marrow from matched but unrelated donors. While TBI almost always ensures engraftment in recipients of unmanipulated donor bone marrow, a significant rejection risk is conferred by the use of T lymphocyte-depleted donor marrow. This can be circumvented by increasing the total dose of radiation administered (Patterson et al., 1986; Guyotat et al., 1987; Burnett et al., 1988), addition of cytokine arabinoside or the use of antilymphocyte globulin or monoclonal antibodies (Bozdech et al., 1985; Sondel et al., 1985).

Treatment of graft rejection

Attempts have been made to prevent donor haemopoietic failure by immunosuppression with antilymphocyte globulin, cyclosporin or steroids (Bunjes et al., 1990), or more recently by the use of haemopoietic growth factors (Neumanaitis et al., 1990). Only patients with some residual donor haemopoietic function appear to respond to these treatments and a second transplant is usually the only method of obtaining haemopoietic recovery. Second transplants from an allogeneic donor carry a high risk of treatment failure (Storb et al., 1987).

However, the reinfusion of stored autologous stem cells can be life-saving.

INFECTIONS AFTER BMT

Infections are one of the major causes of morbidity and mortality after BMT. Bacterial, fungal, protozoal and viral agents can cause infectious complications from the time of preparation for the transplant, and persisting for many months afterwards (see Wingard, 1990, for review). The pattern of infection is related to its timing in relation to the transplant: infectious complications can be divided into those occurring in the first month after the BMT during the phase of neutrophil recovery and repair of mucosal surfaces; those occurring in the first 3 months which confer a high mortality, and later infections largely associated with persisting cell-mediated immune deficiency from chronic GVHD.

Variations in susceptibility to infectious complications

The risk of morbidity and mortality from infection is much greater following allogeneic marrow transplantation than after autologous

Table 4.14 Factors contributing to infection after bone marrow transplantation (BMT)

Factor	Bacterial/ fungal	Viral/ protozoal
Haemopoietic recovery		
Neutropenia, monocytopenia	+	−
Defective neutrophil function	+	−
Immunological recovery		
Poor B cell function − low immunoglobulin levels	+	(+)
Defective cell-mediated immunity	+	+
No donor immunity before BMT	−	+
Dysregulation of T helper and suppressors	−	+
Steroids	+	+?
Other immunosuppressives	+	+
Acute GVHD	+	+
Chronic GVHD	+	+
Tissue damage from chemotherapy and radiation		
Mucositis	+	+
Pulmonary damage	−	+
Transfusion of blood products		
HIV, CMV, hepatitis B and C	−	+

GVHD, Graft-versus-host disease; HIV, human immunodeficiency virus; CMV, cytomegalovirus.

BMT or BMT between identical twins. For example, cytomegalovirus infection or reactivation occurs in less than 10% of autograft recipients but in up to 60% of allograft recipients. The implication of this observation is that most of the infectious complications following allogeneic BMT are due to the problems of transplanting a new donor immune system into the recipient. In autografts, the most serious risk of infection comes from delayed haematological reconstitution predisposing to bacterial and fungal infection, while in allografts, mortality from infections relates more to virus reactivation. The risk of infectious complications rises with increasing disparity between donor and recipient. Major contributing factors to infection after allografts are the use of steroids and immunosuppressives after BMT and the development of acute and chronic GVHD. Monoclonals given to enhance engraftment may predispose to infection early after BMT. Anti-LFA-1, in particular, blocks a wide range of immune reactions and is associated with an increased risk of bacterial infection. Table 4.14 summarizes the factors contributing to infection after BMT.

Infections during the early recovery after BMT

The combination of mucositis due to the transplant preparative regimen and the use of MTX, with neutropenia, leads to an increased risk from bacterial infection. Early mortality after BMT due to infection has diminished significantly, largely because of the introduction of highly effective broad-spectrum antibiotic combinations in the last decade. Possibly as a consequence, the pattern of bacterial infectious complications has changed in recent years. Gram-negative infections are largely controllable with oral antibiotic prophylaxis and early introduction of combinations of an aminoglycoside and a penicillin derivative, or monotherapy with agents such as ceftazidime (Pizzo et al., 1986). A persisting problem is the high mortality associated with endotoxic shock. Trials with antiendotoxin and anti-TNF suggest that these agents are promising but less effective once hypotension and renal shut-down have occurred (Bone, 1991).

Gram-positive infections from staphylococci and streptococci of low pathogenicity but broad antibiotic resistance associated with the use of semipermanent intravenous lines have proved difficult to manage because they are often impossible to eradicate once established without removing the intravenous line, and because the vancomycin to which they are usually sensitive is nephrotoxic. *Staphylococcus epidermidis* infecting long-term intravenous cannulae has become the single most frequently encountered pathogen after BMT (Lokich et al., 1985).

Fungal infection facilitated by prolonged neutropenia and the use of

Table 4.15 Antimicrobial treatment of infection after bone marrow transplantation (Hughes *et al.*, 1977; Wingard, 1990)

Bacterial infection	
Gram-positive organisms	Vancomycin, ceftazidime
Gram-negative organisms	Aminoglycosides, broad-spectrum penicillins, ciprofloxacin. Antiendotoxin and anti-TNF monoclonals
Fungal infection	
Candidal mucositis	Topical antifungals, imidazole, antifungals
Aspergillus and invasive fungal infection	Intravenous amphotericin B, liposomal amphotericin
Protozoal infection	
Pneumocystis carinii	Trimethoprim sulphonamide, pentamidine
Toxoplasmosis	Erythromycin sulphonamide
Virus infection	
HSV, VZV,	Acyclovir
CMV	Acyclovir, ganciclovir
Respiratory syncytial virus	Ribavirin

TNF, Tumour necrosis factor; HSV, herpes simplex virus; VZV, varicella-zoster virus; CMV, cytomegalovirus.

steroids remains a continuing therapeutic challenge. *Candida* infections typically spread from a primary site in the oropharynx, and extend down the oesophagus, ultimately disseminating via the portal blood to the liver and blood stream. *Candida* infection can be controlled by topical antifungals, but invasive infection requires systemically absorbed imidazoles, or intravenous amphotericin, to which it responds readily. *Aspergillus* infection originates in the sinuses and pulmonary tree by inhalation of airborne spores. It spreads by destructive local invasion across tissue boundaries and has a high mortality in BMT recipients. Laminar airflow units may offer some protection against infection, as does the use of amphotericin aerosols. Established infection is difficult to diagnose in its early and treatable phase. Because of this, antibiotic policies usually employ intravenous amphotericin as a third-line agent to treat fevers not responding to antibacterial agents as presumed fungal infections. Successful responses are limited by the amount of tissue destruction already incurred, the adverse effect of concurrent steroid use, poor immune recovery, nephrotoxicity of amphotericin, and the relatively poor antifungal activity of amphotericin. There is a need for more effective and less toxic agents which may be partly met by the introduction of new imidazoles, and the use of liposomally packaged amphotericin

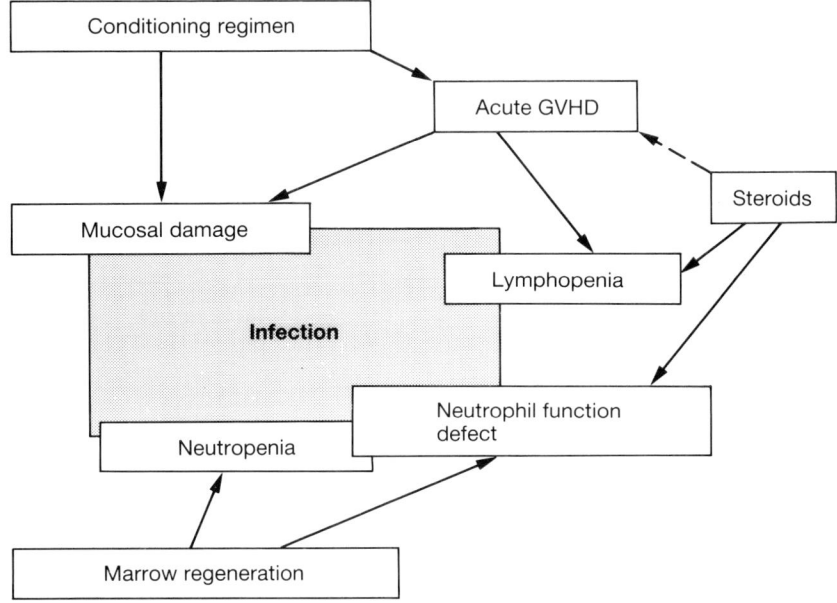

Fig. 4.15 Relationship between acute GVHD, immunosuppressive treatment, and infection after BMT.

(Lopez-Berestein *et al.*, 1989). Table 4.15 summarizes the antimicrobials used in the management of infections following BMT. Figure 4.15 summarizes the relationship between acute GVHD and infection in the early post-graft period.

Late infectious complications

Infections occurring after neutrophil recovery from BMT are related to several factors. Neutrophil function has been found to be defective following BMT. Antibody production, especially IgA, is slow to recover and may remain reduced for some years. Cell-mediated immunity is defective for many months (Atkinson, 1990a), and predisposes particularly to viral infection. The deficient immune response is exacerbated by acute and chronic GVHD and the immunosuppression used for its prevention and treatment. Transmission of hepatitis virus, cytomegalovirus and human immunodeficiency virus (HIV) from blood products is a further cause of infection in the later period following BMT. In the first 3 months after BMT, when immune function is particularly poor, almost any type of infection may occur. As time passes the risk and severity of infection diminishes. However, persisting chronic GVHD is associated with a prolonged risk of infection. A particular feature of chronic GVHD is functional hyposplenism

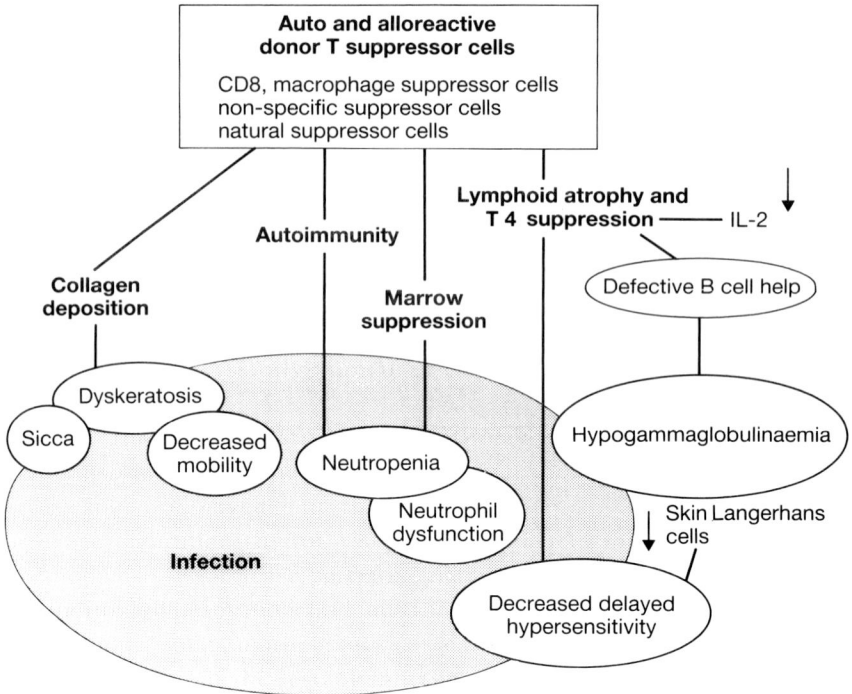

Fig. 4.16 Relationship between chronic GVHD, immune deficiency and infection.

predisposing to life-threatening infection with encapsulated organisms such as pneumococcus and *Haemophilus influenzae* and necessitating continued antibiotic prophylaxis with co-trimoxazole or penicillin in patients with chronic GVHD (Atkinson *et al.*, 1979; Winston *et al.*, 1979). Viral infections in conjunction with GVHD may also facilitate infection by other agents. Protozoal infection by *Pneumocystis carinii* and *Toxoplasma* are uncommon but dangerous infections associated with prolonged immunosuppression. The pathogenesis of late infections and their relationship to chronic GVHD are summarized in Figure 4.16.

Virus infections after BMT

The profound immune suppression and the immune dysregulation associated with GVHD after allogeneic BMT predispose to viral illness due either to new exposure or reactivation of viruses. DNA viruses account for the most frequent and severe problems and in particular cytomegalovirus is responsible directly or indirectly for significant post-transplant mortality (Meyers *et al.*, 1980, 1982). Two components can be identified – the cytopathic effect directly caused by the virus, and host immune factors that cause tissue damage via cytokine and growth factor production, lymphocyte- and macrophage-mediated cytotoxicity, and antibody production. The presence of replicating virus in turn can modify the immune response of the transplanted marrow affecting GVHD and GVL (see below).

Cytomegalovirus infection

Cytomegalovirus is normally acquired by adulthood in over 50% of the population. Bone marrow transplant recipients may already be infected or be infected from prior transfusion of blood products or from the donor marrow. Because of this high prevalence, cytomegalovirus conversion is found in up to 40% of allograft recipients after BMT (Winston and Gale, 1991). The likelihood that this cytomegalovirus reactivation will develop into a clinical syndrome depends upon many factors – the degree to which the immune system has reconstituted normally, and the degree to which target organs like the lungs are damaged by previous conditioning or infection. The main complication associated with cytomegalovirus infection is interstitial pneumonitis. Patients usually develop this condition within the first 4 months after BMT. The syndrome is characterized by increasing dyspnoea, decreased gas diffusion and stiffening of the lungs. Death occurs from respiratory failure. The histopathological appearance is that of a moderate lymphocyte infiltrate, oedema and thickening of the alveolar membrane and proliferation of type II alveolar macrophages which may show cytopathic change and cytomegalovirus inclusion bodies. Viral replication leads to antigen expression and antigen-processing by alveolar macrophages. Such infected cells have been found to cause immune dysregulation inhibiting T lymphocyte proliferation and increasing NK activity. The production of IL-1 and TNFα by infected cells causes damage to the alveolar cells in a manner similar to the effect of GVHD. Release of platelet-derived growth factor leads to pulmonary fibrosis and collagen deposition. Viral damage therefore is probably not a central part of the process. The most effective approach to the problem is to prevent infection in cytomegalovirus-negative recipients, and prevent viral replication in recipients infected either endogenously or by the donor marrow. Administration of cytomegalovirus-negative blood products and the filtering of blood to remove potentially infected lymphocytes can reduce the frequency of infection and pneumonitis in cytomegalovirus-negative individuals. High-dose ganciclovir and high-titre cytomegalovirus immunoglobulin have been shown in one study to reduce the incidence of cytomegalovirus viraemia, and the frequency of interstitial pneumonitis (Schmidt et al., 1991). The treatment of the established infection is unsatisfactory: the only reproducible successes have been with a combination of high-dose intravenous immunoglobulin and ganciclovir. While ganciclovir appears to prevent further viral replication, it may not necessarily halt progression to fatal lung damage, as discussed above. The mechanism of action of high-dose immunoglobulin may be in some way to correct the immune dysregulation. Further attempts to reduce tissue damage by administering antibodies to TNF seem worthwhile.

DNA viruses, GVHD and GVL

Infections with herpes group viruses

Herpes simplex (HSV) and varicella-zoster (VZV) are common problems post-transplant. The risk of developing clinical HSV infection is in the order of 80%, and 30% for VZV presenting either as zoster or disseminated varicella. The incidence of both infections can be reduced by prophylaxis with acyclovir (Wingard, 1990). Several analyses have drawn attention to the association of GVHD with exposure of donor or recipient to the herpes viruses VZV, HSV, Epstein–Barr virus (EBV) and cytomegalovirus. The suggestion that viral antigens expressed in MHC class II antigens can stimulate alloreactivity in HLA-matched responders is supported by the observation that viral antigens stimulate lymphocyte responsiveness in mixed lymphocyte culture (Yasukawa and Zarling, 1984). A multifactorial analysis showed that the risk of severe GVHD was proportional to the overall recipient seropositivity pretransplant for three or four herpes viruses (Gratama *et al.*, 1991). Similarly, donor seropositivity to three or more herpes viruses conferred an increased risk of chronic GVHD (Boström *et al.*, 1989). In another multicentre analysis, donor seropositivity for cytomegalovirus was associated with an increased risk of chronic GVHD (Boström *et al.*, 1990a). There is also a suggestion that patients with positive serology for more than two herpes viruses, in particular recipient cytomegalovirus seropositivity, was associated with a lower risk of relapse (Boström *et al.*, 1991b). If this association is real, it suggests that reactivation of DNA viruses may induce potentially useful cytotoxic T cell or NK responses with antileukaemic activity.

Prevention of infection after BMT

Existing approaches to the prevention of infection after BMT are relatively unsuccessful. Table 4.16 summarizes the available approaches, and outlines some of the future possibilities aimed at improving the speed and quality of immune responses to infection after

Table 4.16 Prevention of infection after bone marrow transplantation (Wingard, 1990; Winston and Gale, 1991)

Bacterial and fungal infection
Topical antimicrobials – skin, mouth, gastrointestinal tract
Systemic antimicrobials – oral or intravenous antibiotics and antifungals
Immunoglobulin infusions
Granulocyte growth factors
Protective isolation
Sterile food

Pneumocystis *infection*
Prophylaxis with co-trimoxazole

Viral infection
Screening blood products
Prophylaxis with acyclovir, ganciclovir
High-titre anticytomegalovirus immunoglobulin

General: future directions
Preventing GVHD without suppressing immune recovery
Accelerating immune recovery –? IL-2, other cytokines
Avoidance of immune dysregulation
Adoptive transfer of immunity – selected donor T cell clones
Reimmunization

GVHD, Graft-versus-host disease; IL-2, interleukin 2.

BMT. Antibacterial, antifungal and antiprotozoal prophylaxis is widely practised to prevent both early neutropenic infection and later infection associated with defective cell-mediated immunity. This approach serves both to prevent the re-emergence of the patient's own bacterial and fungal flora, and to protect against the acquisition of infection from the environment (Karp *et al.*, 1991). The ability to screen blood products for cytomegalovirus, hepatitis B and C, and HIV reduces the risk of exogenously acquired viral infection. Suppression of cytomegalovirus, VZV and HSV reactivation can be achieved with acyclovir (Holland *et al.*, 1990). Ganciclovir is more active than acyclovir against cytomegalovirus, and early studies with this agent both in prophylaxis and treatment of cytomegalovirus pneumonitis are promising (Emanuel *et al.*, 1988; Winston and Gale, 1991).

A much greater impact on the prevention of infection after BMT would be achieved if it were possible to enhance selectively specific immune responses to infective agents after BMT. The use of prophylactic immunoglobulin may confer some benefit in this regard (Sullivan *et al.*, 1990). In the future it may become increasingly possible to transfer specific cell-mediated immunity against viruses with the generation of T lymphocyte clones cytotoxic to virally infected cells. The demonstration by Riddell *et al.* (1991) that cytotoxic

T cell clones with anticytomegalovirus reactivity can be transferred to patients after BMT and persist in the circulation is an important step towards this goal.

NON-HAEMATOLOGICAL COMPLICATIONS AFTER BMT

The morbidity and mortality in the first 3 months following BMT from complications not directly related to haematopoiesis or immunological dysfunction is considerable. Pneumonitis and veno-occlusive disease account for a variable proportion of the 20–30% of post-transplant mortality following allografting (ACIBMTR, 1989) and 10–20% following autologous BMT (Armitage, 1989; Gorin et al., 1989).

Mucositis

Since the gastro-intestinal mucosa is maintained by rapid cell turnover, some degree of immediate damage to the gastro-intestinal tract is inevitable after BMT where cytotoxic chemotherapy or radiation has been used, either in the preparative regimen or after BMT to prevent GVHD. Mucositis affects the whole of the GI tract causing stomatitis, oesophagitis, diarrhoea and intestinal malabsorption. The causes are multifactorial. Post-transplant neutropenia increases the chance of bacterial invasion from the gut into the submucosa, facilitated by the suppressive effect of the preparative regimen on mucosal repair. Herpes simplex virus reactivation is common and contributes significantly to oral mucositis. Acute GVHD causes further damage by targeting the crypt cells responsible for regenerating the mucosa. The severity of acute GVHD of the GI tract is thus partly related to the damage already sustained by these processes. Methotrexate given after BMT to prevent GVHD produces a significant mucositis, compounding pretransplant treatment effects and delaying repair. Treatment is largely supportive with strong analgesics and parenteral feeding until repair occurs in the second week after BMT associated with neutrophil recovery. Prophylactic acyclovir reduces the severity of stomatitis, and topical antifungal and antibacterial agents reduce the problems of secondary infection (Weisdorf et al., 1989).

Interstitial pneumonitis

Interstitial pneumonitis is the single most frequent cause of death in the first 3 months after BMT. The condition is characterized by a mononuclear cell infiltration causing thickening of the alveolar walls from oedema. Acutely the process presents as a respiratory distress

Table 4.17 Aetiology and risk factors for interstitial pneumonitis

Immune dysregulation
Acute and chronic GVHD
Immunosuppression

Infection
Cytomegalovirus
Adenovirus
Pneumocystis carinii
Septicaemia

Radiation and drugs
Radiation to the lung fields
Alkylating agents (busulphan, melphalan, cyclophosphamide)
Cyclosporin toxicity
Prior treatment with radiation and chemotherapy

Exacerbating pulmonary complications
Fluid overload
Cardiac dysfunction
Idiopathic respiratory distress
Pre-existing pneumonia

GVHD, Graft-versus-host disease.

syndrome. Gas exchange is severely impaired, and there is a progressive decrease in lung volume and lung compliance. Death often occurs from hypoxaemia. Patients surviving the acute onset have a high frequency of progression to severe interstitial fibrosis. The process has multiple aetiologies (Table 4.17), and its pathophysiology is poorly understood. Cytomegalovirus infection, irradiation, and GVHD are, however, recurrent associated factors (Torres *et al.*, 1982; Barrett et al., 1983; Weiner *et al.*, 1985; Zaia and Churchill, 1987). Local TNF release by pulmonary macrophages has been implicated in the early phase of the process. This may be associated with a local response to cytomegalovirus infection. However, sepsis and toxicity from cyclosporin causing a capillary leak syndrome may initiate the process (Holler *et al.*, 1988). It is possible that several triggers of interstitial damage lead to a final common path of increasing lung fibrosis.

Interstitial pneumonitis can be partly prevented by measures designed to avoid risk factors. Successful prophylaxis of cytomegalovirus infection would make the largest contribution to interstitial pneumonitis prevention. Fractionated and lower TBI doses are favourable. Prevention of GVHD and prompt treatment of obstructive bronchiolitis caused by chronic GVHD may be beneficial.

Treatment of interstitial pneumonitis is unsatisfactory. Successful elimination of cytomegalovirus by antiviral treatment does not always prevent the progression to lethal interstitial thickening. Monoclonal antibodies to TNF have been proposed as a method of preventing the seemingly irreversible process.

Veno-occlusive disease

Veno-occlusive disease presents usually within 30 days following BMT with increasing hepatomegaly and pain, ascites and jaundice. The process affects the small intrahepatic venules of the portal system. Histologically the liver shows centrilobular congestion, oedema and haemorrhage from disrupted central venules. The condition progresses eventually to a complete fibrosis of the central vein lumina (Berk et al., 1979; McDonald et al., 1984).

The cause is not known. It is related to the use of radiation, high-dose alkylating agents and possibly other agents in the preparative regimen. The risk increases with intensification of the preparative regimen (Kanfer et al., 1987). The process follows damage to the endothelium of the portal venous system. A fall in the level of protein C and antithrombin III may promote platelet adhesion and subsequent endothelial damage from platelet products, and fibrosis due to production of fibroblast growth factor.

The risk of veno-occlusive disease can be reduced by using preparative regimens that are less intensive. Its treatment is equally unsatisfactory. Treatment prophylaxis with heparin may be effective but is hazardous (Bearman et al., 1990). Experimental treatments with prostaglandin E_1 (Ibrahim et al., 1990) and tissue plasminogen activator (Baglin et al., 1990) have had some success but, in the absence of a satisfactory understanding of the factors initiating the disease process, treatments are largely empirical.

Late effects after BMT

Delayed effects of BMT occur from long-term damage to non-haemopoietic tissues by the preparative regimen or of GVHD and immune deficiency after the transplant (see review by Kolb and Bender-Gotze, 1990). Damage to proliferating non-haemopoietic tissues results either in depletion of clonogenic cells, or injury to DNA impairing their postmitotic function and increasing the potential for malignant change. High-dose chemotherapy and radiation and chronic GVHD can damage vascular stroma and lead to fibrosis and organ impairment. Delayed effects can be categorized according to their pathogenesis into effects on proliferating tissues, and effects on non-proliferating cells (Table 4.18).

Radiation damage is schedule- and dose-related. Fractionated

Table 4.18 Delayed complications after bone marrow transplantation

Complication	Cause			
	Irradiation	Chemotherapy	GVHD	Immune suppression
Damage to proliferating tissues				
Growth impairment				
Pituitary failure	+	+	–	–
Gonadal failure				
Retarded or absent puberty	+	+	+	–
Postpubertal ovarian failure	+	+	–	–
Azoospermia	+	+	–	–
Hypothyroidism	+	–	–	–
Haemorrhagic cystitis	–	+	–	–
Chronic skin changes				
Hypotrophy, scleroderma	–	–	+	–
Second malignancy				
Lymphoreticular	–	–	–	+
Solid tumours	+	+	–	–
Damage to non-proliferating tissues				
Pulmonary				
Fibrosis, obstructive bronchiolitis	+	+	+	+
Musculoskeletal				
Osteonecrosis	+	–	–	–
Fasciitis	–	–	+	–
Neurological				
Polyneuropathy, myasthenia	–	–	+	–
Multifocal leukoencephalopathy	–	–	–	+
Ophthalmological				
Cataracts	+	+	–	–
Keratoconjunctivitis	–	–	+	–
Liver				
Cirrhosis, chronic hepatitis	–	–	+	+
Cardiac				
Muscle damage	–	+	–	–
Renal				
Late-onset renal failure	+	+	–	–

GVHD, Graft-versus-host disease.

TBI is less likely to cause cataracts, gonadal failure and pulmonary fibrosis. There are fewer data on the effects of high-dose alkylating agents, but disappointingly the BuCy preparative schedule given to thalassaemic children causes similar impairment of growth as that seen after TBI (Manenti et al., 1989). There is evidence, however, for the potential of some of the damage to repair: ovarian function does return in a small minority of women, and pregnancy has been reported following high-dose chemotherapy BMT preparation. Spermatogenesis may recover after 5 years. The use of chemotherapy-only preparative regimens favours this recovery (Sanders et al., 1983; Milliken et al.,

1990). Cyclophosphamide and anthracyclines specifically affect the heart (Kupari et al., 1990). Other non-cytotoxic agents can be responsible for long-term damage—steroids contribute to cataract formation and bone necrosis, and permanent damage to the VIIIth nerve follows high-dose aminoglycoside administration.

Radiation (Bergstein et al., 1986) and cyclosporin (Atkinson et al., 1983b) are important causes of permanent renal damage. Graft-versus-host disease can lead to severe and permanent damage to the skin, eyes, lungs, GI tract and musculoskeletal system. The prolonged immunosuppression associated with chronic GVHD and immunosuppressive therapy is partly responsible for haemorrhagic cystitis which is provoked by cyclophosphamide and other alkylating agents (Millard, 1981), but which is also associated with reactivation of the BK virus (Rice et al., 1985).

Second malignancies occurring in the first year after BMT include EBV-related lymphomas associated with continued immune deficiency. Long-term survivors of BMT have essentially normal immune function and are not at risk from this type of malignancy. However, the administration of radiation and chemotherapy carries a risk of tumour induction. Surveys carried out on large cohorts of BMT recipients do not yet extend long enough to provide reliable data. The largest survey showed an incidence of 35 second malignancies in 2246 patients (Witherspoon et al., 1989). More than half involved relatively rapid-onset lymphoreticular malignancy, suggesting that the main provocative factor for new malignancy after BMT is prolonged immunodeficiency. Evidence that BMT could be responsible for an increased incidence of later-developing solid tumours is unclear. So far there is no suggestion that this is an important problem (Table 4.19).

Table 4.19 Reported second malignancies after bone marrow transplantation (Witherspoon et al., 1989)

Condition	Number
Patients at risk	2246
Leukaemia and lymphoma	22
Non-Hodgkin's lymphoma	16
Leukaemia	6
Solid tumours	13
Brain tumour	3
Melanoma	3
Hepatocellular carcinoma	1
Squamous cell carcinoma	3
Rectal adenocarcinoma	1

Italics indicate a significant increased incidence compared to the age- and sex-adjusted general population.

REFERENCES

Adams JA, Gordon AA, Jiang YZ et al. (1990) Thrombocytopenia after bone marrow transplantation for leukaemia: changes in megakaryocyte growth and growth promoting activity. *British Journal of Haematology* 75, 195.

Advisory Committee of the International Bone Marrow Transplant Registry (ACIBMTR) (1989) Report from the International Bone Marrow Transplant Registry. *Bone Marrow Transplantation* 4, 221.

Alter BP, Rappeport JM, Hoisman TH et al. (1976) Foetal erythropoiesis following bone marrow transplantation. *Blood* 48, 843.

Anasetti C, Amos D, Beatty P et al. (1989) Effect of HLA compatibility on engraftment of bone marrow transplants in patients with leukaemia and lymphoma. *New England Journal of Medicine* 320, 197.

Anasetti C, Martin PJ, Strob R et al. (1991) Prophylaxis of graft versus host disease by administration of the murine anti-IL-2 receptor antibody 2A3. *Bone Marrow Transplantation* 7, 375.

Apperley JF, Jones L, Hale RG et al. (1986) Bone marrow transplantation for patients with chronic myeloid leukaemia: T cell depletion with Campath-1 reduces the incidence of graft-versus-host disease but may increase the risk of leukaemic relapse. *Bone Marrow Transplantation* 1, 53.

Armitage JO (1989) Bone marrow transplantation in the treatment of patients with lymphoma. *Blood* 73, 1749.

Arnold R, Schmeiser T, Heit W et al. (1986) Haemopoietic reconstitution after bone marrow transplantation. *Experimental Haematology* 14, 271.

Aschan J, Ringden O, Sundberg B et al. (1991) Methotrexate combined with cyclosporin A decreases graft versus host disease but increases leukemic relapse compared to monotherapy. *Bone Marrow Transplantation* 7, 113.

Atkinson K (1990a) Chronic graft-versus-host disease — review. *Bone Marrow Transplantation* 5, 69.

Atkinson K (1990b) Reconstitution of the haemopoietic and immune systems after marrow transplantation. *Bone Marrow Transplantation* 5, 209.

Atkinson K, Storb R, Prentice RL et al. (1979) Analysis of late infections in 89 long term survivors of bone marrow transplantation. *Blood* 53, 720.

Atkinson K, Incefy GS, Storb R et al. (1982) Low serum thymic hormone levels in patients with chronic graft-versus-host disease. *Blood* 53, 1073.

Atkinson K, Luckhurst E, Penny R et al. (1983a) Immunological reconstitution after allogeneic bone marrow transplantation in man. *Transplantation Proceedings* 5, 474.

Atkinson K, Biggs JC, Hayes J et al. (1983b) Cyclosporin A associated nephrotoxicity in the first 100 days after allogeneic bone marrow transplantation: three distinct syndromes. *British Journal of Haematology* 54, 59.

Atkinson K, Norrie S, Chan P (1985) Lack of correlation between nucleated bone marrow cell dose, marrow CFU-GM dose, or marrow CFU-E dose and the rate of HLA identical sibling marrow engraftment. *British Journal of Haematology* 60, 245.

Ault KE, Antin JH, Ginsburg D et al. (1985) Phenotype of recovering lymphoid cell populations after marrow transplantation. *Journal of Experimental Medicine* 161, 1483.

Azogui O, Kalil J, Andersen E et al. (1983) Peripheral blood T-lymphocytes bearing DR antigen after bone marrow transplantation. *Transplantation* 35, 513.

Bach FH, Albertini RJ, Joo P et al. (1968) Bone marrow transplantation in a patient with the Wiskott-Aldrich syndrome. *Lancet* 2, 1364.

Baglin TP, Harper P, Marcus RE (1990) Veno-occlusive disease of the liver complicating ABMT successfully treated with recombinant tissue plasminogen activator (r-TPA). *Bone Marrow Transplantation* 5, 439.

Bagot M, Mary J-Y, Heslan M et al. (1988) The mixed epidermal cell lymphocyte reaction is the most predictive factor of acute graft-versus-host disease in bone marrow graft recipients. *British Journal of Haematology* 70, 403.

Bain B, Vas MR, Lowenstein L (1964) The development of large immature lymphocytes in mixed lymphocyte culture. *Blood* 23, 108.

Barnes DWH, Loutit JF (1955) Spleen protection: the cellular hypothesis. In: Bacq FM (ed.) *Radiobiology Symposium Liege*. Butterworth, London, p. 134.

Barnett MJ, Eaves CJ, Phillips GL et al. (1989) Successful autografting in chronic myeloid leukaemia after maintenance of marrow in culture. *Bone Marrow Transplantation* 4, 345.

Barrett AJ (1989) Bone marrow transplantation, thymus transplantation and thymic factors in the treatment of congenital immune deficiency states. In: Hamblin TJ (ed.) *Immunotherapy of Disease. Immunology and Medicine Series*. Kluwer Academic Publishers, Dordrecht, p. 1.

Barrett AJ (1991) Worldwide bone marrow transplant activity in the last decade. In: Champlin RE, Gale RP (eds) *New Strategies in Bone Marrow Transplantation*. Wiley/Liss, New York, p. 1.

Barrett AJ, McCarthy D (1990) Bone marrow transplantation for genetic disorders. *Blood Reviews* 4, 116.

Barrett AJ, Faille A, Ketels F et al. (1980) Survival of CFU-C in recipient blood after bone marrow transplantation. *Clinical and Laboratory Haematology* 2, 25.

Barrett A, Depledge MH, Powles RL (1983) Interstitial pneumonitis following bone marrow transplantation after low dose rate total body irradiation. *International Journal of Radiation Oncology, Biology and Physics* 9, 1029.

Barrett AJ, Horowitz MM, Gale RP et al. (1989) Marrow transplantation for acute lymphoblastic leukaemia: factors affecting relapse and survival. *Blood* 74, 862.

Basham TY, Nickoloff BJ, Merigan TC et al. (1984) Recombinant gamma interferon induces HLA-DR expression on cultured human keratinocytes.

Journal of Investigative Dermatology 83, 88.

Bearman SI, Hinds MS, Wolford JL et al. (1990) A pilot study of continuous infusion heparin for the prevention of hepatic veno-occlusive disease after bone marrow transplantation. *Bone Marrow Transplantation* 5, 407.

Beatty PG, Clift RA, Mickelson EM et al. (1985) Marrow transplantation from related donors other than HLA-identical siblings. *New England Journal of Medicine* 313, 765.

Beatty PG, Dahlberg S, Michelson EM et al. (1988) Probability of finding HLA matched unrelated marrow donors. *Transplantation* 45, 714.

Beatty PG, Hansen JA, Longton GM et al. (1991) Marrow transplantation from HLA matched unrelated donors for treatment of hematological malignancy. *Transplantation* 51, 443.

Berenson RJ, Andrews RG, Besinger WI et al. (1988) Antigen CD34 marrow cells engraft lethally irradiated baboons. *Journal of Clinical Investigation* 81, 951.

Bergstein J, Andreoli SP, Provisor AJ et al. (1986) Radiation nephritis following total-body irradiation and cyclophosphamide in preparation for bone marrow transplantation. *Transplantation* 41, 63.

Berk PD, Popper H, Krugger GRF et al. (1979) Veno-occlusive disease of the liver after allogeneic bone marrow transplantation. *Annals of Internal Medicine* 90, 158.

Berkman A, Farmer E, Tutschka P et al. (1982) Skin explant culture as a model for cutaneous graft-versus-host disease. *Experimental Hematology* 10 (suppl 12), 33.

Beschorner WE, Saral R, Hutchins GM et al. (1978) Lymphocytic bronchitis associated with graft-versus-host disease. *New England Journal of Medicine* 299, 1030.

Bidwell JL, Bidwell EA, Savage DA et al. (1988) A DNA-RFLP typing system that positively identifies serologically well-defined and ill-defined HLA-DR and DQ alleles including DRw10. *Transplantation* 45, 640.

Biggs JC, Atkinson K, Gillett E et al. (1986) A randomised prospective trial comparing cyclosporine and methotrexate given for prophylaxis of graft versus host disease after bone marrow transplant. *Transplantation Proceedings* 18, 253.

Bjorkman PJ, Saper MA, Samraoui B et al. (1987) Structure of the human class I histocompatibility antigen HLA-A2. *Nature* 329, 506.

Blaise D, Olive D, Stoppa AM et al. (1990) Haematological and immunologic effects of the systemic administration of recombinant interleukin 2 after autologous bone marrow transplantation. *Blood* 76, 1092.

Blazar BR, Widmer MB, Soderling CCB et al. (1988) Augmentation of donor bone marrow engraftment in histoincompatible murine recipients by granulocyte/macrophage colony-stimulating factor. *Blood* 71, 320.

Bone RC (1991) A critical evaluation of new agents for the treatment of sepsis. *Journal of the American Medical Association* 266, 1686.

Bordignon C, Keever CA, Small TN et al. (1989) Graft failure after T-cell-depleted human leukocyte antigen identical marrow transplants for leukemia: II. In vitro analyses of host effector mechanisms. *Blood* 74, 2237.

Bortin MM (1970) A compendium of reported human bone marrow transplants. *Transplantation* 9, 571.

Bortin MM (1987) Factors influencing the risk of acute graft-vs-host disease in man. In: Gale RP, Champlin R (eds) *Progress in Bone Marrow Transplantation*. Alan R Liss, New York, p. 243.

Bortin MM, Rimm AA (1986) Increasing use of bone marrow transplantation. *Transplantation* 42, 229.

Bortin MM, Horowitz MM, Barrett AJ et al. (1992) Changing trends in allogeneic bone marrow transplantation for leukemia in the 1980s. *Journal of the American Medical Association* 262, 607.

Bosserman LD, Murray C, Takvorian T et al. (1989) Mechanisms of graft failure in HLA-matched and HLA-mismatched bone marrow transplant recipients. *Bone Marrow Transplantation* 4, 239.

Boström L, Ringden O, Sunderberg B et al. (1989) Pretransplant herpes virus serology and chronic graft-versus-host disease. *Bone Marrow Transplantation* 4, 547.

Boström L, Ringden O, Jacobsen N et al. (1990a) A European multi-centre study of chronic graft-versus-host disease. *Transplantation* 49, 1100.

Boström L, Ringden O, Jacobsen N, Zwaan F, Nilsson B (1990b) An increased risk of relapse in allogeneic bone marrow recipients seropositive to few herpes viruses. *Bone Marrow Transplantation* 5 (suppl. 2) abstract 46.

Bozdech MJ, Sondel PM, Trigg ME et al. (1985) Transplantation of HLA haploidentical T-cell depleted marrow for leukaemia: addition of cytosine arabinoside to the pretransplant conditioning regimen prevents rejection. *Experimental Haematology* 13, 1201.

Brenner MK, Heslop HE (1991) Graft-versus-leukaemia effects after marrow transplantation in man. In: Proctor SJ (ed.) *Bailliere's Clinical Haematology 4. Minimal Residual Disease in Leukaemia*. Bailliere Tindall, London, p. 727.

Brenner NK, Reittie JE, Grob JP et al. (1986) The contribution of large granular lymphocytes to B-cell activation and differentiation after T-cell depleted allogeneic bone marrow transplantation. *Transplantation* 42, 257.

Brown JH, Jardetzky J, Saper MA et al. (1988) A hypothetical model of the foreign antigen binding sites of class II histocompatibility molecules. *Nature* 332, 845.

Bunjes D, Wiesneth M, Hertenstein B et al. (1990) Graft failure after T-cell depleted bone marrow transplantation: clinical and immunological characteristics and response to immunosuppressive therapy. *Bone Marrow Transplantation* 6, 309.

Burnett AK, Hann IM, Robertson AG et al. (1988) Prevention of graft versus host disease by ex-vivo T cell depletion: reduction in graft failure with augmented total body irradiation. *Leukaemia* 2, 300.

Butturini A, Gale RP (1990) New strategies for T cell

depletion. *Bone Marrow Transplantation* 6, 225.
Butturini A, Bortin MM, Gale RP (1987) Graft-versus-leukaemia following bone marrow transplantation. *Bone Marrow Transplantation* 2, 233.
Cesbron A, Moreau P, Milpied N et al. (1990) Influence of HLA-DP mismatches on primary MLR responses in unrelated HLA-A, B, DR, DQ, Dw identical pairs in allogeneic bone marrow transplantation. *Bone Marrow Transplantation* 6, 337.
Champlin RE, Feig SA, Sparkles RS et al. (1984) Bone marrow transplantation for identical twins in the treatment of aplastic anaemia; implications for the pathogenesis of the disease. *British Journal of Haematology* 56, 455.
Chang J, Morganstern GR, Coutinho LH et al. (1989) The use of bone marrow cells grown in long term culture for autologous bone marrow transplantation in acute myeloid leukaemia: an update. *Bone Marrow Transplantation* 4, 5.
Charak BS, Brynes RK, Groshen S et al. (1990) Bone marrow transplantation with interleukin-2-activated bone marrow followed by interleukin-2 therapy for acute myeloid leukemia in mice. *Blood* 76, 2187.
Cheever MA, Britzmann Thompson D, Klarnet JP et al. (1986) Antigen driven long term cultured T-cells proliferate in vivo, distribute widely, mediate specific tumour therapy, and persist long term as functional memory T-cells. *Journal of Experimental Medicine* 163, 1100.
Cobbold S, Hale G, Waldemann H et al. (1986) Suppressor (T4) and helper (T8) lymphocyte are needed for graft-versus-host disease initiation. *Transplantation* 42, 239.
Cohen J (1988) Cytokines as mediators of graft-versus-host-disease. *Bone Marrow Transplantation* 3, 193.
Cullis JO, Jiang YZ, Schwarer AP et al. (1992) Donor leukocyte infusions for chronic myeloid leukaemia in relapse following allogeneic bone marrow transplantation. *Blood* 79, 1379.
Daar AS, Fuggle SV, Fabre JW et al. (1984) The detailed distribution of HLA-A, B, C antigens in normal human organs. *Transplantation* 38, 287.
Daley GQ, Van Etten RA, Baltimore D (1990) Induction of chronic myelogenous leukemia in mice by the P210 bcr/abl gene of the Philadelphia chromosome. *Science* 247, 824.
de Witte T, Hoogenhout J, de Pauw B et al. (1986) Depletion of donor lymphocytes by counterflow centrifugation successfully prevents acute graft-versus-host disease in matched allogeneic marrow transplantation. *Blood* 67, 1302.
Dick KE, Kamel-Reid S (1991) Animal models of normal and leukaemic human haematopoiesis in immune deficient mice. In: Champlin RK, Gale RP (eds) *New Strategies in Bone Marrow Transplantation*. Wiley/Liss, New York, p. 209.
Dickinson AM, Sviland L, Carey P et al. (1988) Skin explant culture as a model for cutaneous graft-versus-host disease in humans. *Bone Marrow Transplantation* 3, 323.
Dokhelar MC, Wiels J, Lipinski M et al. (1981) Natural killer activity in human bone marrow recipients. Early reappearance of peripheral natural killer activity in graft-versus-host disease. *Bone Marrow Transplantation* 31, 61.
Doney KC, Weiden PL, Storb R et al. (1981) Treatment of GVHD in human marrow graft recipients: a randomised trial comparing antithymocyte globulin and corticosteroids. *American Journal of Hematology* 11, 1.
Douay L, Gorin NC, Mary JY et al. (1986) Recovery of CFU-GM from cryopreserved marrow and in vivo evaluation after autologous bone marrow transplantation are predictive of engraftment. *Experimental Hematology* 14, 358.
Egelund T, Andrews R, Smith FC et al. (1990) Functional studies of immunomagnetically isolated CD34+ cells. *Experimental Hematology* 18, 549.
Elfenbein G, Goedect T, Graham-Pole J et al. (1986) Is prophylaxis against acute graft-versus-host disease necessary if treatment is effective and survival is not impaired? *Journal of the American Society of Clinical Oncology* 5, 643.
Emanuel D, Cunningham I, Jules-Elysee K et al. (1988) Cytomegalovirus pneumonia after bone marrow transplantation successfully treated with the combination of ganciclovir and high-dose intravenous immune globulin. *Annals of Internal Medicine* 109, 777.
Falkenburg JHF, Goselink HM, Van der Harst D et al. (1990) Specific lysis of clonogenic leukaemic cells (CLC) by cytotoxic T lymphocyte (CTL) against minor histocompatibility (mh) antigens: an in vitro model for graft versus leukaemia (GVL). *Experimental Haematology* 18, 682 (abstract).
Fefer A, Cheever MA, Greenberg PD et al. (1982) Treatment of chronic granulocytic leukaemia with chemoradiotherapy and transplantation of marrow from identical twins. *New England Journal of Medicine* 306, 63.
Ferrara J, Marion A, Murphy G et al. (1987) Acute graft-versus-host disease: pathogenesis and prevention with a monoclonal antibody. *Transplantation Proceedings* 19, 2662.
Filipovitch AH, McGlave PB, Ramsay NKC et al. (1982) Pretreatment of donor bone marrow with monoclonal antibody OKT3 for prevention of acute graft-versus-host disease in allogeneic histocompatible bone marrow transplantation. *Lancet* 1, 1266.
Fink PJ, Rammensee J-G, Bevan MJ (1984) Cloned cytolytic T cells can suppress primary cytotoxic responses directed against them. *Journal of Immunology* 133, 1775.
Fischer A, Griscelli C, Blanche S et al. (1986) Prevention of graft failure by an anti-HLA-1 monoclonal antibody in HLA-mismatched bone marrow transplantation, *Lancet* 2, 1058.
Fleischhauer K, Kernan NA, O'Reilly RJ et al. (1990) Bone marrow allograft rejection by T-lymphocytes recognising a single amino acid difference in HLA-B44. *New England Journal of Medicine* 323, 1818.
Foa R, Melone G, Tosti S et al. (1990) Treatment of residual disease in acute leukaemia patients with recombinant interleukin-2 (IL-2): clinical and biological findings. *Bone Marrow Transplantation* 6

(suppl 1), 98.

Gajewski JL, Champlin RE (1991) Enhanced graft-versus-leukaemia effect in patients receiving matched unrelated donor bone marrow transplants. In: Champlin RE, Gale RP (eds) *New Strategies in Bone Marrow Transplantation*. Wiley-Liss, New York, p. 281.

Gale RP (1980) Foetal liver transplantation in man. In: Lucarelli G, Fliedner TM, Gale RP (eds) *Foetal Liver Transplantation: Current Concepts and Future Directions*. Excerpta Medica, Amsterdam, p. 286.

Gale RP, Butturini A (1991) How do bone marrow transplants cure leukaemia? In: Champlin RE, Gale RP (eds) *New Strategies in Bone Marrow Transplantation*. Wiley-Liss, New York, pp. 109–118.

Gale RP, Reisner Y (1986) Graft rejection and graft-versus-host disease: mirror images. *Lancet* 1, 1468.

Gale RP, Horowitz MM, Biggs JC et al. (1989) Transplant or chemotherapy in acute myelogenous leukaemia. *Lancet* 1, 119.

Gatti RA, Meuwissen HJ, Allen HD et al. (1968) Immunological reconstitution of a sex linked lymphopenic immunological deficiency. *Lancet* 2, 1366.

Gee AP (1991) *Bone Marrow Processing and Purging: a Practical Guide*. CRC Press, Boca Raton.

Gething MJ, Sambrook J (1992) Protein folding in the cell. *Nature* 355, 33.

Gluckman E, Devergie A, Arcese W et al. (1980) Cyclosporine A prophylactic treatment of graft-versus-host disease in human allogeneic bone marrow transplants. Preliminary results. *Blut* 41, 182.

Gluckman E, Berger R, Dutreix J (1984) Bone marrow transplantation for Fanconi's anaemia. *Seminars in Hematology* 21, 20.

Gluckman E, Broxmeyer HE, Auerbach AD et al. (1989) Haematological reconstitution in a patient with Fanconi anaemia by means of umbilical cord blood from an HLA identical sibling. *New England Journal of Medicine* 321, 1124.

Goldman JM, Gale RP, Horowitz MM et al. (1988) Bone marrow transplantation for chronic myelogenous leukaemia in chronic phase: increased risk of relapse associated with T-cell depletion. *Annals of Internal Medicine* 108, 806.

Gorin NC, Aegerter P (1986) Autologous bone marrow transplantation for acute leukaemias in remission. Third European survey. *Bone Marrow Transplantation* 1 (suppl 1), 255.

Gorin NC, Hervé P, Aegerter P et al. (1986a) Autologous bone marrow transplantation for acute leukaemia in remission. *British Journal of Haematology* 64, 385.

Gorin N, Donay J, Laporte M et al. (1986b) Autologous bone marrow transplantation using marrow incubated with Asta Z 7557 in adult acute leukaemia. *Blood* 67, 1367.

Gorin NC, Aegerter P, Auvert B for the EBMT (1989) Autologous bone marrow transplantation for acute leukaemia in remission: an analysis of 1322 cases. *Bone Marrow Transplantation* 4 (suppl 2), 3.

Goulmy E (1985) Class I restricted human cytotoxic T lymphocytes directed against minor transplantation antigens and their possible role in organ transplantation. *Progressive Allergy* 36, 44.

Goulmy E, Gratama JW, Blokland E et al. (1983) A minor transplant antigen detected by MHC restricted cytotoxic T lymphocytes during graft-versus-host disease. *Nature* 302, 159.

Goulmy E, Blockland E, Pool J et al. (1986) Correlation between cytotoxic T-cell responses and graft-versus-host disease. *Bone Marrow Transplantation* 1 (suppl 1), 138.

Gratama JW, Sinnige LGF, Weijers TF et al. (1987) Marrow donor immunity to herpes simplex virus: association with acute graft versus host disease. *Experimental Hematology* 15, 735.

Gratama JW, Stijnen T, Weiland HT et al. (1991) Herpes virus immunity and acute graft versus host disease: an update from Leiden. In: Champlin RK, Gale RP (eds) *New Strategies in Bone Marrow Transplantation*. Wiley-Liss, New York, p. 311.

Greaves DR, Frazer P, Vidal MA et al. (1990) A transgenic mouse model of sickle cell disorder. *Nature* 343, 183.

Guyotat D, Dutou L, Erhsam A et al. (1987) Graft rejection after T cell depleted marrow transplantation: role of fractionated irradiation. *British Journal of Haematology* 65, 499.

Hagenbeek A, Martens ACM (1989) Cryopreservation of autologous marrow grafts in acute leukaemia: survival of in vivo clonogenic leukaemic cells and normal haemopoietic stem cells. *Leukaemia* 3, 535.

Hagenbeek A, Lu YL, Ger JA et al. (1991) Minimal residual disease in acute leukaemia: preclinical studies. In: Champlin RE, Gale RP (eds) *New Strategies in Bone Marrow Transplantation*. Wiley-Liss, New York, p. 193.

Hale G, Bright S, Chumbley B et al. (1983) Removal of T-cells from bone marrow for transplantation: a monoclonal antilymphocyte antibody that fixes human complement. *Blood* 62, 873.

Hale G, Cobbold S, Waldmann H (1988) T-cell depletion with Campath-1 in allogeneic bone marrow transplantation. *Transplantation* 45, 753.

Haylock DN, To LB, Dyson PG et al. (1990) Analysis of haemopoietic progenitor cells in recovery phase peripheral blood. *Experimental Haematology* 18, 716.

Heisterkamp N, Jenster G, ten Hoeve J et al. (1990) Acute leukaemia in bcr/abl transgenic mice. *Nature* 344, 251.

Hervé P (1991) Perspectives in the prevention and treatment of graft-versus-host disease. *Bone Marrow Transplantation* 7 (suppl 2), 117.

Higano CS, Brixey M, Bryant EM et al. (1990) Durable complete remission of acute non lymphocytic leukemia with discontinuation of immunosuppression following relapse after allogeneic bone marrow transplantation. A case report of a probable graft versus leukemia effect. *Transplantation* 50, 175.

Hobbs JR (1986) Displacement bone marrow transplantation and immunoprophylaxis to treat some genetic disorders. *Bone Marrow Transplantation* 1, 333.

Hobbs JR, Shaw PJ, Hugh-Jones K et al. (1987) Beneficial effect of pre-transplant splenectomy on displacement bone marrow transplantation for Gaucher's syndrome. *Lancet* 1, 1111.

Holland HK, Wingard JR, Saral R (1990) Viral infections in bone marrow transplantation: clinical presentation, pathogenesis and therapeutic strategies. *Cancer Investigation* 8, 507.

Holler E, Kolb HJ, Hiller E et al. (1988) Microangiopathy after allogeneic BMT: interaction of cellular activation in the course of acute graft-versus-host disease and cyclosporin. *Bone Marrow Transplantation* 3 (suppl 1), 259.

Holmes N (1989) New HLA class 1 molecules. *Immunology Today* 10, 52.

Horowitz MM, Gale R P, Sondel PM et al. (1990) Graft-versus-leukaemia reactions after bone marrow transplantation. *Blood* 75, 555.

Hughes W, Kuhn S, Chaudhary S et al. (1977) Successful chemoprophylaxis for *Pneumocystis carinii* pneumonitis. *New England Journal of Medicine* 279, 1419.

Hurme M, Chandler PR, Hetherington CMJ et al. (1978) Cytotoxic T-cell responses to H-Y: correlation with the rejection of syngeneic male skin grafts. *Experimental Medicine* 147, 768.

Ibrahim A, Pico JL, Ostronoff M et al. (1990) Use of prostaglandin E_1 for the treatment of venoocclusive disease of the liver following autologous bone marrow transplantation. *Bone Marrow Transplantation* 5 (suppl 2), 82.

Ireland RM, Atkinson K, Concannon A et al. (1990) Serum erythropoietin changes in autologous and allogeneic bone marrow transplant patients. *British Journal of Haematology* 76, 128.

Irinondo A, Pastor JM, Hermosa V et al. (1986) Protection against hepatitis B after marrow transplantation. *Annals of Internal Medicine* 105, 293.

Izutsu KT, Sullivan KM, Schubert MM et al. (1983) Disordered salivary immunoglobulin secretion and sodium transport in human chronic graft-versus-host disease. *Transplantation* 35, 441.

Jiang YZ, Kanfer E, Macdonald D et al. (1991a) Graft-versus-leukaemia effect following allogeneic bone marrow transplantation: emergence of cytotoxic T-lymphocytes reacting to host leukaemia cells. *Bone Marrow Transplantation* 8, 253.

Jiang YZ, Macdonald M, Cullis JO et al. (1991b) Is graft-versus-leukaemia effect separable from graft-versus-host reactivity? *Bone Marrow Transplantation* 7 (suppl 2), 26.

Jones RJ, Vogelsang GB, Hess AD (1989) Induction of graft-versus-host disease following autologous bone marrow transplantation. *Lancet* 2, 754.

Juttner CA, To LB, Haylock DM et al. (1985) Circulating autologous stem cells collected in very early recovery from acute non-lymphoblastic leukaemia produce prompt but incomplete haemopoietic recovery after high dose melphalan or supralethal irradiation. *British Journal of Haematology* 61, 739.

Kaminsky E, Sharrock C, Hows J et al. (1988) Frequency analysis of cytotoxic T lymphocyte precursors — possible relevance to HLA-matched unrelated donor bone marrow transplantation. *Bone Marrow Transplantation* 3, 149.

Kanfer EJ, McCarthy DM (1989) Cytoreductive preparation for bone marrow transplantation in leukaemia: to irradiate or not? *British Journal of Haematology* 71, 447.

Kanfer EJ, Buckner CD, Fefer A et al. (1987) Allogeneic and syngeneic marrow transplantation following high-dose dimethylbusulfan, cyclophosphamide and total body irradiation. *Bone Marrow Transplantation* 1, 339.

Kapoor N, Kirkpatrick D, Blaise RM et al. (1981) Reconstitution of normal megakaryocytopoiesis and immunologic functions in Wiskott-Aldrich syndrome by marrow transplantation following myeloablation and immunosuppression with busulfan and cyclophosphamide. *Blood* 57, 692.

Karp JE, Merz WG, Dick JD et al. (1991) Strategies to prevent or control infections after bone marrow transplants. *Bone Marrow Transplantation* 8, 1.

Kendra JR, Barrett AJ, Lucas C et al. (1981) Response of graft versus host disease to high doses of methyl prednisolone. *Clinical and Laboratory Haematology* 3, 19.

Kernan NA, Collins NH, Juliano L et al. (1986) Clonable T lymphocytes in T cell-depleted bone marrow transplants correlate with development of graft-v-host disease. *Blood* 68, 770.

Kessinger A, Armitage JO, Landmark JD et al. (1988) Autologous peripheral hematopoietic stem cells transplantation restores hematopoietic function following marrow ablative therapy. *Blood* 71, 723.

Kier P, Penner E, Bakos S et al. (1990) Autoantibodies in chronic GvHD: high prevalence of antinucleolar antibodies. *Bone Marrow Transplantation* 6, 93.

Klarnet JP, Matis LA, Kern DE et al. (1987) Antigen driven T-cell clones can proliferate in vivo, eradicate disseminated leukaemia, and provide specific immunological memory. *Journal of Immunology* 138, 4012.

Kolb H, Bender-Gotze Ch (1990) Late complications after allogeneic bone marrow transplantation. *Bone Marrow Transplantation* 6, 61.

Kolb HJ, Mittermuller J, Clemm CH et al. (1990) Donor leukocyte transfusions for treatment of recurrent chronic myelogenous leukaemia in marrow transplant patients. *Blood* 76, 2462.

Körbling M, Hess AD, Tutschka PJ et al. (1982) 4-hydroperoxycyclophosphamide: a model for eliminating residual human tumour cells and T-lymphocytes from the bone marrow graft. *British Journal of Haematology* 52, 89.

Körbling M, Dorken B, Ho AD et al. (1986) Autologous transplantation of blood derived haemopoietic stem cells after myeloablative therapy in a patient with Burkitt's lymphoma. *Blood* 67, 529.

Körbling M, Haas R, Knauf W et al. (1990) Therapeutic efficacy of autologous blood stem cell transplantation (ABSCT): the role of cytotoxic/cytokine stem cell mobilisation. *Bone Marrow Transplantation* 5 (suppl 1), 39.

Korngold R, Sprent J (1978) Lethal graft-versus-host disease after bone marrow transplantation across minor histoincompatibility barriers in mice. Prevention by removing mature T-cells from the marrow. *Journal of Experimental Medicine* 148, 1687.

Kourilsky P, Claverie JM (1989) MHC–Antigen interaction: what does the T-cell receptor see? *Advances in Immunology* 45, 107.

Krolnick KA, Uhr JW, Vitetta ES (1982) Selective killing of leukaemia cells by antibody-toxin conjugates: implications for autologous bone marrow transplantation. *Nature* 295, 604.

Kupari M, Volin L, Suokas A et al. (1990) Cardiac involvement in bone marrow transplantation: electrocardiographic changes, arrhythmias, heart failure and autopsy findings. *Bone Marrow Transplantation* 5, 91.

Kurnick NB, Montano A, Gerdes JC et al. (1958) Preliminary observations on the treament of post-irradiation haemopoietic depression in man by the infusion of stored autogenous marrow. *Annals of Internal Medicine* 49, 973.

Lansdorp PM, Thomas TE (1991) Selection of human haemopoietic stem cells. In: Gee AP (ed.) *Bone Marrow Processing and Purging*. CRC Press, Boca Raton, p. 352.

Lazarus HM, Coccia PF, Hertzig RH et al. (1984) Incidence of acute graft-versus-host disease with and without methotrexate prophylaxis in allogeneic bone marrow transplant recipients. *Blood* 64, 215.

Lim SH, Patton WM, Jobson S et al. (1988) Mixed lymphocyte reactions do not predict severity of graft-versus-host disease (GVHD) in HLA-DR compatible sibling bone marrow transplants. *Clinical Pathology* 41, 1155.

Lokich JJ, Bothe A jr, Benotti P et al. (1985) Complications and management of implanted venous access catheters. *Journal of Clinical Oncology* 3, 710.

Long DS, Cramer DV, Harnaha JS et al. (1990) Lymphokine activated killer (LAK) cells purging of leukaemic bone marrow: range of activity against different haematopoietic neoplasms. *Bone Marrow Transplantation* 6, 169.

Lopez-Berestein G, Bodey GP, Fainstein V et al. (1989) Treatment of systemic fungal infections with liposomal amphotericin B. *Archives of Internal Medicine* 149, 2533.

Lorenz E, Uphoff D, Reid TR et al. (1951) Modification of irradiation injury in mice and guinea pigs by bone marrow injections. *Journal of the National Cancer Institute* 12, 197.

Loveland B, Simpson E (1986) The non-MHC transplantation antigens: neither weak nor minor. *Immunology Today* 7, 223.

Lucarelli G, Polchi P, Galimberti M (1985) Marrow transplantation for thalassaemia following busulphan and cyclophosphamide. *Lancet* 1, 1355.

Lucarelli G, Galimberti M, Polchi P et al. (1990) Bone marrow transplantation in patients with thalassemia. *New England Journal of Medicine* 322, 417.

Lum LG (1987) The kinetics of immune reconstitution after human marrow transplantation. *Blood* 69, 369.

McCarthy DM, Kanfer EJ, Barrett AJ (1989) Thalidomide for the therapy of graft-versus-host disease following allogeneic bone marrow transplantation. *Biomedicine and Pharmacotherapy* 43, 693.

McCune JM, Namikawa R, Kaneshima H et al. (1988) The SCID-hu mouse: murine model for the analysis of human haematolymphoid differentiation and function. *Science* 241, 1632.

Macdonald D, Jiang YZ, Swirsky D et al. (1991) Acute myeloid leukaemia relapsing following interleukin-2 treatment expresses the alpha chain of the interleukin-2 receptor. *British Journal of Haematology* 77, 43.

McDonald GB, Sharma P, Matthews DE et al. (1984) Venaocclusive disease of the liver after bone marrow transplantation: diagnosis, incidence and predisposing factors. *Hepatology* 4, 116.

Mackinnon S, Hows JM, Goldman JMG (1990) Induction of in vitro graft versus leukemia activity following bone marrow transplantation for chronic myeloid leukemia. *Blood* 76, 2037.

Malkovsky M, Brenner MK, Hunt R et al. (1986) T-cell depletion of allogeneic bone marrow prevents acceleration of graft-versus-host disease induced by exogenous interleukin-2. *Cellular Immunology* 103, 476.

Manenti F, Galimberti M, Lucarelli G et al. (1989) Growth and endocrine function after bone marrow transplantation for thalassaemia major. In: Buckner CD, Gale RP, Lucarelli G (eds) *Advances and Controversies in Thalassaemia Therapy – Bone Marrow Transplantation and Other Approaches*. Alan R Liss, New York, p. 273.

Maraninchi D, Blaise D, Rio B et al. (1987) Impact of T cell depletion on outcome of allogeneic bone marrow transplantation for standard risk leukaemia. *Lancet* 2, 175.

Maraninchi D, Mawas C, Guyotat D et al. (1988) Selective depletion of marrow T-cytotoxic lymphocytes (CD8) in the prevention of graft-versus-host disease after allogeneic bone marrow transplantation. *Transplantation International* 1, 91.

Marchetti-Rossi M, Centis F, Talevi N et al. (1987) Decontaminating bone marrow with merocyanin 540, mafosphamide or both. In: Dicke K, Spitzer G, Jagannath S (eds) *ABMT Proceedings of the Third International Symposium on Autologous Bone Marrow Transplantation*. University of Texas, MD Anderson Hospital and Tumour Institute, Houston, p. 151.

Marrack P, Kappler J (1988) T-cell can distinguish between allogeneic major histocompatibility complex products on different cell types. *Nature* 332, 840.

Martelli MF, Aversa F (1991) Graft versus-host disease prophylaxis today. *Bone Marrow Transplantation* 7 (suppl 2), 112.

Martin PJ (1990) The role of donor lymphoid cells in allogeneic marrow engraftment. *Bone Marrow Transplantation* 6, 283.

Mathé G, Jammet H, Pendic B et al. (1959) Transfusions et greffes de moelle osseuse homologue chez des humans irradiés a haut dose accidentellement. *Revue Françaises d'Études Cliniques et Biologiques* 4, 226.

Metcalf D, Moore MAS (1971) *Haemopoietic Cells*.

Frontiers of Biology 24. North Holland Press, Amsterdam.

Meyers JD, Flournoy N, Thomas ED (1980) Infection with herpes simplex virus and cell mediated immunity after marrow transplant. *Journal of Infectious Diseases* 142, 338.

Meyers JD, Flournoy N, Thomas ED (1982) Nonbacterial pneumonitis after allogeneic bone marrow transplantation: a review of ten years' experience. *Reviews of Infectious Diseases* 4, 1119.

Millard RJ (1981) Busulphan-induced hemorrhagic cystitis. *Urology* 18, 143.

Milliken S, Powles R, Parikh P et al. (1990) Successful pregnancy after allogeneic transplantation for leukaemia. *Bone Marrow Transplantation* 35, 135.

Mitsuyasu RT, Champlin RE, Gale RP et al. (1986) Treatment of donor bone marrow with monoclonal anti T-cell antibody and complement for the prevention of acute graft-versus-host disease: a prospective randomised double blind trial. *Annals of Internal Medicine* 105, 20.

Mosier DE, Gulizia RJ, Baird SM et al. (1988) Transfer of a functional human immune system to mice with SCID. *Nature* 335, 256.

Mrsic M, Labar B, Bogdanic V et al. (1990) Combination of cyclosporin and methotrexate for prophylaxis of acute graft-versus-host disease after allogeneic bone marrow transplantation for leukaemia. *Bone Marrow Transplantation* 6, 137.

Müller-Ruchholtz W, Wottge H, Müller-Hermelink HK et al. (1980) Restitution potentials of allogeneically or zenageneically grafted lymphocyte-free haemopoietic stem cells. In: Thierfelder S, Rodt H, Kolb HJ (eds) *Immunobiology of Bone Marrow Transplantation*. Springer Verlag, Berlin, p. 153.

Neumanaitis J, Singer JW, Buckner CD et al. (1990) The use of recombinant human granulocytemacrophage colony stimulating factor in graft failure following bone marrow transplantation. *Blood* 76, 245.

Ogasawara M, Iwabuchi K, Good RA et al. (1988) Bone marrow cells from allogeneic bone marrow chimeras inhibit the generation of cytotoxic lymphocyte responses against both donor and recipient cells. *Journal of Immunology* 141, 3306.

Ogawa M (1991) Cellular organisation of the hemopoietic system. *Experimental Haematology* 19, 457a.

OKunewick JP, Kociban DL, Buffo MJ et al. (1987) Graft versus host disease and graft versus leukaemia in experimental systems. In: Baum SJ, Santos GW, Takaku F (eds) *Recent Advances and Future Directions in Bone Marrow Transplantation. Experimental Haematology Today*. Springer Verlag, New York, p. 3.

OKunewick JP, Kociban DL, Machen LL et al. (1990) Effect of CD4 and CD8 T-cell on graft-versusleukaemia. *Experimental Haematology* 18, 652 (abstract).

Patterson J, Prentice HG, Brenner MK et al. (1986) Graft rejection following HLA matched T-lymphocyte depleted bone marrow transplantation. *Blood* 68, 954.

Pegg DE (1966) *Bone Marrow Transplantation*. Lloyd-Luke, London.

Perrault C, Decary F, Brochu S et al. (1990) Minor histocompatibility antigens – a review. *Blood* 76, 1269.

Piguet PF, Grau GE, Allet BE (1987) Tumour necrosis factor/cachectin is an effector of skin and gut lesions of the acute phase of graft-versus-host disease. *Journal of Experimental Medicine* 166, 1280.

Pizzo PA, Hathorn JW, Hiemenz J et al. (1986) A randomized trial comparing ceftazidime alone with combination antibiotic therapy in cancer patients with fever and neutropenia. *New England Journal of Medicine* 315, 552.

Pober JS, Collins T, Gimbrone MA et al. (1983) Lymphocytes recognise human vascular endothelial and dermal fibroblast IA antigens induced by recombinant immune interferon. *Nature* 305, 726.

Powles RL, Clink HM, Spence D et al. (1980) Cyclosporin A to prevent graft-versus-host disease after allogeneic bone marrow transplantation. *Lancet* 1, 327.

Poynton CH (1988) T-cell depletion in bone marrow transplantation. *Bone Marrow Transplantation* 3, 265.

Prentice HG, Blacklock HA, Janossy G et al. (1982) Use of anti-T-cell monoclonal antibody OKT3 to prevent graft-versus-host disease in allogeneic bone marrow transplantation for acute leukaemia. *Lancet* 1, 700.

Prentice HG, Brenner MK, Gottlieb D (1989) T-cell depleted bone marrow transplantation – the way ahead. *Bone Marrow Transplantation* 4, 225.

Ramsay NK, Kersey JH, Robison LL et al. (1982) A randomised study for the prevention of acute graft-versus-host disease. *New England Journal of Medicine* 306, 392.

Rappeport J, Mihn M, Reinherz E et al. (1979) Acute graft-versus-host disease in recipients of bone marrow from identical twin donors. *Lancet* 2, 717.

Rayfield LS, Brent L (1963) Tolerance immunocompetence, and secondary disease in fully allogeneic radiation chimeras. *Transplantation* 36, 183.

Reisner Y, Kapoor N, Kirkpatrick D et al. (1983) Transplantation for severe combined immunodeficiency with HLA-A, B, D, DR incompatible parental marrow cells fractionated by soy bean agglutinin and sheep red blood cells. *Blood* 61, 341.

Reittie JE, Gottlieb DJ, Heslop HE et al. (1989) Endogenously generated activated killer cells circulate after autologous and allogeneic marrow transplantation but not after chemotherapy. *Blood* 73, 1351.

Rice SJ, Bishop J, Apperley J et al. (1985) BK virus as cause of haemorrhagic cystitis after bone marrow transplantation. *Lancet* 2, 844.

Riddell SR, Watanabe KS, Goodrich JM et al. (1991) Reconstitution of CD8+ve cytomegalovirus (CMV)-specific T-cell immunity after bone marrow transplant by adoptive immunotherapy with T-cell clones. *Blood* 78, 77a.

Robertson M (1991) Proteasomes in the pathway. *Nature* 353, 300.

Rodt H, Kolb HJ, Netzel B et al. (1981) Effect of anti-T-cell globulin on graft-versus-host disease in leukaemic patients treated with bone marrow transplantation. *Transplantation Proceedings* 13, 257.

Rooney CM, Wimperis JZ, Brenner MK et al. (1986) Natural killer cell activity following T-cell depleted allogeneic bone marrow transplantation. *British Journal of Haematology* 62, 413.

Sachs H, Sharibi Y, Sykes M (1991) Chimerism and the induction of transplant tolerance. In: Champlin RE, Gale RP (eds) *New Strategies in Bone Marrow Transplantation*. Wiley-Liss, New York, p. 21.

Sallefors B, Olofsson T, Lenhoff S (1991) Granulocyte-macrophage colony stimulating factor (GM-CSF), and granulocyte colony stimulating factor (G-CSF) in serum in bone marrow transplanted patients. *Bone Marrow Transplantation* 8, 191.

Sanders JE, Buckner CD, Leonard JM et al. (1983) Late effects on gonadal function of cyclophosphamide, total body irradiation and marrow transplantation. *Transplantation* 36, 252.

Santos GE, Cole LJ (1955) Effect of donor and host lymphoid and myeloid tissue injections in lethally X-irradiated mice treated with rat bone marrow. *Journal of the National Cancer Institute* 21, 279.

Santos GW (1983) History of bone marrow transplantation. *Clinical Haematology* 12, 611.

Santos GW (1984) Immunosuppression for clinical marrow transplantation. *Seminars in Hematology* 11, 341.

Santos GW, Tutschka PJ, Brookmeyer R et al. (1987) Cyclosporine plus methyl prednisolone versus cyclophosphamide plus methyl prednisolone as prophylaxis for GVHD: a randomised double blind study in patients undergoing bone marrow transplantation. *Clinical Transplantation* 1, 21.

Schmidt GM, Horak D, Niland JC et al. (1991) A randomized, controlled trial of prophylactic ganciclovir for cytomegalovirus pulmonary infection in recipients of allogeneic bone marrow transplants. *New England Journal of Medicine* 324, 1005.

Serota FT, Burkey ED, August CS et al. (1983) Total body irradiation versus fractionated exposure as preparation for bone marrow transplantation in treatment of acute leukaemia and aplastic anaemia. *International Journal of Radiation Oncology, Biology and Physics* 9, 1941.

Sheridan WP, Morstyn G, Wolf M et al. (1989) Granulocyte colony stimulating factor (G-CSF) and neutrophil recovery following high dose chemotherapy and autologous bone marrow transplantation. *Lancet* 2, 891.

Slavin S, Eckerstein A, Weiss L (1988) Adoptive immunotherapy in conjunction with bone marrow transplantation – amplification of natural host defence mechanisms against cancer by recombinant interleukin-2. *Natural Immunity and Cell Growth Regulation* 7, 180.

Slavin S, Ackerstein A, Naparstek E et al. (1990) The graft-versus-leukaemia (GVL) phenomenon: is GVL separable from GVHD? *Bone Marrow Transplantation* 6, 155.

Sondel PM, Bozdech MJ, Trigg ME et al. (1985) Additional immunosuppression allows engraftment following HLA mismatched T-cell depleted bone marrow transplantation for leukaemia. *Transplantation Proceedings* 17, 460.

Sosman JA, Sondel PM (1987) The graft-versus-leukaemia effect following bone marrow transplantation: a review of laboratory and clinical data. *Haematology Reviews* 2, 77.

Sosman JA, Oettel KR, Smith SD et al. (1990) Specific recognition of human leukaemia cells by allogeneic T-cells: II. Evidence for HLA-D restricted determinants on leukaemic cells that are cross reactive with determinants present on unrelated nonleukaemic cells. *Blood* 75, 2005.

Sprent J, Heath W, Korngold R (1991) Protecting mice against lethal graft versus host disease. In: Champlin RE, Gale RP (eds) *New Strategies in Bone Marrow Transplantation*. Wiley-Liss, New York, p. 13.

Storb R, Epstein RB, Graham TC et al. (1970) Methotrexate regimens for control of graft-versus-host disease in dogs with allogeneic marrow grafts. *Transplantation* 9, 240.

Storb R, Thomas ED, Buckner CD et al. (1974) Allogeneic marrow grafting for treatment of aplastic anaemia. *Blood* 43, 157.

Storb R, Prentice RL, Buckner CD et al. (1983) Graft-versus-host disease and survival in patients with aplastic anaemia treated by marrow grafts from HLA-identical siblings: beneficial effects of a protective environment. *New England Journal of Medicine* 308, 302.

Storb R, Deeg HJ, Thomas ED et al. (1985) Marrow transplantation for chronic myelocytic leukaemia: a controlled trial of cyclosporine versus methotrexate for prophylaxis of graft-versus-host disease. *Blood* 66, 698.

Storb R, Weiden PL, Sullivan M et al. (1987) Second marrow transplants in patients with aplastic anaemia rejecting the first graft: use of a conditioning regimen including cyclophosphamide and antilymphocyte globulin. *Blood* 70, 116.

Storb RH, Deeg HJ, Pepe M et al. (1989) Methotrexate and cyclosporine versus cyclosporine alone for prophylaxis of graft-versus-host disease in patients given HLA-identical marrow grafts for leukaemia: long-term follow-up of a controlled trial. *Blood* 73, 1729.

Sullivan KM, Shirlman HM, Storb R et al. (1981) Chronic graft-versus-host disease in 52 patients: adverse natural course and successful treatment with combination immunosuppression. *Blood* 57, 267.

Sullivan KM, Witherspoon RP, Storb RH et al. (1988) Prednisone and azathioprine compared with prednisone and placebo for treatment of chronic graft-versus-host disease: prognostic influence of prolonged thrombocytopenia after allogeneic marrow transplantation. *Blood* 72, 546.

Sullivan KM, Weiden PL, Storb RH et al. (1989a) Influence of acute and chronic graft-versus-host disease on relapse and survival after bone marrow transplantation from HLA-identical siblings as treatment of acute and chronic leukaemia. *Blood* 73, 1720.

Sullivan KM, Storb R, Witherspoon RP et al. (1989b) Deletion of immunosuppressive prophylaxis after marrow transplantation increases hyperacute graft-versus-host disease but does not influence chronic graft-versus-host disease of relapse in patients with advanced leukaemia. *Clinical Transplantation* 3, 511.

Sullivan KM, Kopecky KJ, Jocom J et al. (1990) Immunomodulatory and antimicrobial efficacy of intravenous immunoglobulin in bone marrow transplantation. *New England Journal of Medicine* 323, 705.

Sviland L, Pearson AD, Eastham EJ et al. (1988) Class II antigens expressed by keratinocytes and enterocytes are an early feature of graft-versus-host disease. *Transplantation* 46, 402.

Sviland L, Pearson AD, Green MA et al. (1989a) Expression of MHC class I and II antigens by keratinocytes and enterocytes in graft-versus-host disease. *Bone Marrow Transplantation* 4, 233.

Sviland L, Dickenson AM, Carey P et al. (1989b) An in vitro predictive test for clinical graft-versus-host disease in allogeneic bone marrow transplant recipients. *Bone Marrow Transplantation* 5, 105.

Sykes M, Sheard M, Sachs DH et al. (1988) Effects of T cell depletion in radiation bone marrow chimeras. I. Evidence for a donor cell population which increases allogeneic chimerism and which lacks the potential to produce GVHD. *Journal of Immunology* 141, 2282.

Sykes M, Chester CH, Sundt TM et al. (1989) Effects of T cell depletion in radiation bone marrow chimeras. III. Characterization of allogeneic bone marrow cell populations that increase allogeneic chimerism independently of graft-versus-host disease in mixed marrow recipients. *Journal of Immunology* 143, 3503.

Thein SL, Goldman JM, Galton DG (1981) Acute graft-versus-host disease after autografting for chronic granulocytic leukaemia. *Annals of Internal Medicine* 94, 210.

Thomas ED, Buckner CD, Banaji M et al. (1977) One hundred patients with acute leukemia treated by chemotherapy, total body irradiation and allogenic bone marrow transplant. *Blood* 49, 511.

Till JE, McCulloch EA (1961) Direct measurement of radiation sensitivity of normal mouse bone marrow cells. *Radiation Research* 14, 213.

To LB, Haylock DN, Dyson P et al. (1990) An unusual pattern of haemopoietic reconstitution in patients with acute myeloid leukaemia transplanted with autologous recovery phase peripheral blood. *Bone Marrow Transplantation* 6, 109.

Torres JL, Bross DS, Lam WC et al. (1982) Risk factors in interstitial pneumonitis following allogeneic bone marrow transplantation. *International Journal of Radiation Oncology, Biology and Physics* 8, 1301.

Touraine JL, Philippe N, Betuel N et al. (1981) GVHR and infectious complications in SCID patients treated by bone marrow or foetal liver and thymus transplantation. In: Terrain JL, Gluckman E, Griscelli C (eds) *Bone Marrow Transplantations in Europe* 2, Excerpta Medica, Amsterdam, p. 209.

Travers P, Blondell TL, Sternberg MJE, Bodmer WF (1984) Structural and evolutionary analysis of HLA-D region products. *Nature* 310, 235.

Trowsdale J, Campbell RD (1988) Physical map of a human HLA region. *Immunology Today* 9, 34.

Trowsdale J, Kelly A (1985) The human HLA class II alpha chain gene DZ alpha is distinct from genes in the DP, DQ and DR subregions. *EMBO Journal* 4, 2231.

Truitt RL, Shih CC-Y, LeFever AV (1986) Manipulation of graft-versus-host disease for a graft-versus-leukaemia effect after allogeneic bone marrow transplantation in AKR mice with spontaneous leukaemia/lymphoma. *Bone Marrow Transplantation* 41, 301.

Tsoi MS (1982) Immunological mechanisms of graft-versus-host disease in man. *Transplantation* 33, 459.

Tutschka PJ, Beschorner WE, Hess D et al. (1983) Cyclosporine A to prevent acute graft-versus-host disease. A pilot study in 22 patients receiving allogeneic marrow transplants. *Blood* 61, 318.

Tutschka PJ, Copelan EA, Klein JP (1987) Bone marrow transplantation for leukaemia following a new busulfan and cyclophosphamide regimen. *Blood* 70, 1382.

Vallera DA, Blazar BR (1988) Depressed leukocyte reconstitution and engraftment in murine recipients of T cell-depleted histoincompatible marrow pretreated with interleukin 3. *Transplantation* 46, 616.

Van Bekkum DW, Hagenbeek A (1977) Relevance of the BN leukemia as a model for human acute myeloid leukemia. *Blood Cells* 3, 565.

Van Lochem E, de Gast B, Goulmy E (1992) In vitro dissection of host specific graft-versus-host and graft-versus-leukaemia cytotoxic T-cell activities. *Bone Marrow Transplantation* 10, 181.

Vellodi A, Camba L, McCarthy DM (1992) Bone marrow transplantation for inborn errors of metabolism. In: Treleaven JG, Barrett AJ (eds) *Bone Marrow Transplantation in Practice*. Churchill Livingstone, Edinburgh, p. 161.

Vogelsang GB (1991) Thalidomide treatment of graft-versus-host disease. In: Gale RP, Champlin RE (eds) *New Strategies in Bone Marrow Transplantation*. Wiley-Liss, New York, p. 303.

Vogelsang GB, Hess AD, Berkman AW (1985) An in vitro predictive test for graft-versus-host-disease in patients with genotypic HLA-identical bone marrow transplants. *New England Journal of Medicine* 313, 645.

Volc-Platzer B, Leibel H, Luger T et al. (1985) Human epidermal cells synthesise HLA-DR and alloantigens in vitro upon stimulation with gamma-interferon. *Journal of Investigative Dermatology* 85, 16.

Wagner JE, Santos GW, Noga SJ et al. (1990) Bone marrow graft engineering by counterflow centrifugal elutriation: results of a phase I-II clinical trial. *Blood* 75, 1370.

Wake CT, Long EO, Mach B (1982) Allelic polymorphism and complexity of the genes for HLA-DR beta chains: direct analysis by DNA-DNA hybridization.

Nature 300, 372.

Walker DG (1975) Bone reabsorption restored in osteopetrotic mice by transplants of normal marrow and spleen. *Science* 190, 784.

Weiden PL, Flournoy N, Thomas ED *et al.* (1979) Antileukaemic effects of graft-versus-host disease in human recipients of allogeneic marrow grafts. *New England Journal of Medicine* 300, 1068.

Weiden PL, Sullivan KM, Flournoy N *et al.* (1981) Antileukaemic effect of chronic graft-versus-host disease. Contribution to improved survival after allogeneic marrow transplantation. *New England Journal of Medicine* 304, 1529.

Weiner RS, Bortin MM, Gale RP *et al.* (1985) Risk factors associated with interstitial pneumonitis following allogeneic bone marrow transplantation. *Transplantation Proceedings* 17, 470.

Weisdorf DJ, Bostrom B, Raether D *et al.* (1989) Oropharyngeal mucositis complicating bone marrow transplantation: prognostic factors and the effect of chlorhexidine mouth rinse. *Bone Marrow Transplantation* 4, 89.

Williams SF, Bitran JD, Richards JM *et al.* (1990) Peripheral blood derived stem cell collections for use in autologous transplantation after high dose chemotherapy: an alternative approach. *Bone Marrow Transplantation* 5, 129.

Wimperis JZ, Brenner MK, Prentice HG *et al.* (1986) Transfer of a functioning humoral immune system in transplantation of T lymphocyte depleted bone marrow. *Lancet* 1, 339.

Wingard JR (1990) Advances in the management of infectious complications after bone marrow transplant. *Bone Marrow Transplantation* 6, 439.

Winston DJ, Gale RP (1991) Prevention and treatment of cytomegalovirus infection and disease after bone marrow transplantation in the 1990s. *Bone Marrow Transplantation* 8, 7.

Winston DJ, Schiffman G, Wang DC *et al.* (1979) Pneumococcal infections after human bone marrow transplantation. *Annals of Internal Medicine* 91, 835.

Witherspoon RP, Goehle S, Kretschmer M *et al.* (1986) Regulation of immunoglobulin production after human marrow grafting. The role of helper and suppressor T-cells in acute graft-versus-host disease. *Transplantation* 41, 328.

Witherspoon RP, Fisher LD, Schoch G *et al.* (1989) Secondary cancers after bone marrow transplantation for leukaemia or aplastic anaemia. *New England Journal of Medicine* 321, 784.

Wolf NS, Kone A, Priestly GV (1990) Primitive stem cells obtained with combined Hoechst 33342 and rhodamine 123 sorting: selection and capabilities. *Experimental Haematology* 18, 549.

Yang SY (1989) A standardized method for detection of HLA-A and HLA-B alleles by one-dimensional isoelectric focusing (IEF) gel electrophoresis. In: Dupont B (ed.) *Immunobiology of HLA*. Springer-Verlag, New York, p. 332.

Yankelevich B, Kbobloch C, Nowicki M *et al.* (1989) A novel cell type responsible for marrow graft rejection in mice. *Journal of Immunology* 142, 3423.

Yasukawa M, Zarling J (1984) Human cytotoxic T-cell clones directed against herpes simplex virus-infected cells. 1 lysis restricted by HLA Class II MB and DR antigens. *Journal of Immunology* 133, 422.

Yeager AM, Brennan S, Tiffany C *et al.* (1984) Prolonged survival and remyelination after haematopoietic cell transplantation in the twitcher mouse. *Science* 225, 1052.

Yeager AM, Kaizer H, Santos GW *et al.* (1986) Autologous bone marrow transplantation in patients with acute non-lymphocytic leukemia, using ex-vivo marrow treatment with 4-hydroperoxycyclophosphamide. *New England Journal of Medicine* 315, 141.

Zaia JA, Churchill NA (1987) The biology of human cytomegalovirus infection after marrow transplantation. In: Gale RP, Champlin R (eds) *Progress in Bone Marrow Transplantation*. Alan R Liss, New York, p. 563.

Zeevi A, Duquesnoy RJJ (1985) Specificity of allo-activated human T-lymphocyte clones in secondary proliferation, cell-mediated lympholysis and interleukin-2 release. *Immunogenetics* 12, 17.

Chapter 5
Clinical Application of Haemopoietic Growth Factors

Introduction, 281
  General features of HGF responses *in vivo*, 282
Experimental background, 288
  Preclinical models of growth factor therapy, 288
  Effects of high-level, continuous exposure to HGFs *in vivo*, 289
Principles and practice of HGF therapy, 292
  Administration, 292
  Toxicity, 293
  Contraindications, 294
Clinical HGF therapy, 296
  Treatment of aplastic anaemia with HGFs, 297
  Treatment of neutropenia with HGFs, 299
  Treatment of thrombocytopenia with HGFs, 301

Treatment of anaemia with HGFs, 302
Effects of HGF treatment on neoplastic cell growth, 304
Treatment of myelodysplasia with HGFs, 305
Treatment of acute myeloid leukaemia with HGFs, 307
Treatment of non-myeloid leukaemias with HGFs, 308
Treatment of infections with HGFs, 308
The value of HGFs in chemotherapy, 309
The value of HGFs in bone marrow transplantation, 311
Overview, 314
References, 316

INTRODUCTION

The knowledge that soluble haemopoietic growth factors (HGFs) can stimulate haemopoiesis meant that a clinical role could be considered for them. Several early observations, including the association between tumours producing colony-stimulating factor (CSF) and peripheral granulocytosis (Asano *et al.*, 1977; Sato *et al.*, 1979; Gabrilove *et al.*, 1986), supported the idea that growth factors may be able to reverse neutropenia *in vivo*. Also, patients with graft-versus-host disease (GVHD) following allogeneic bone marrow transplantation have increased levels of CSF in their sera, probably as a result of lymphocyte activation *in vivo* (Singer *et al.*, 1977).

Haemopoietic growth factor therapy was not a clinical reality until recombinant growth factor proteins became widely available. Until then, the tiny amounts of the HGFs that could be purified from culture supernatants and other biological sources did not, generally, provide sufficient material for treating patients. Nevertheless, there were some attempts at therapeutic intervention—for example, treatment of neutropenic patients with CSF derived from human urine (Motoyoshi *et al.*, 1983). The progress made in the molecular cloning of the HGFs was encouraged by a great interest in their potential clinical applications and has been extremely rapid (see Chapter 1).

Recombinant HGFs have been used in the clinic in most of the

Table 5.1 The use of recombinant haemopoietic growth factors in the treatment of haematological disease

Growth factor	Haematological disorders
GM-CSF	Aplastic anaemia; congenital neutropenia; leukocyte adhesion deficiency; myelodysplastic syndromes; acute myeloid leukaemia; infections (AIDS); cytopenias post-chemotherapy; cytopenias post bone marrow transplantation
G-CSF	Aplastic anaemia; congenital neutropenia; glycogen storage disease; idiopathic neutropenia; cyclic neutropenia; myelodysplastic syndromes; acute myeloid leukaemia; cytopenias post-chemotherapy; cytopenias post bone marrow transplantation
IL-3	Aplastic anaemia
M-CSF	Neutropenia; ? fungal infection
Erythropoietin	Aplastic anaemia; anaemia of renal disease; myelodysplastic syndrome; anaemia post-chemotherapy; chronic anaemia associated with cancer; sickle cell anaemia; autologous transfusion
IL-1	Cytopenia post-chemotherapy

GM-CSF, Granulocyte-macrophage colony-stimulating factor; AIDS, acquired immune deficiency syndrome; IL-3, interleukin 3.

situations where cytopenias of one sort or another are important (Table 5.1). They are likely to be most satisfactory when they are used to enhance haematological recovery after myelotoxic treatment or after bone marrow transplantation because this most closely approximates their physiological function, namely, to stimulate rapid cell production in times of emergency (i.e. infection, bleeding etc.). Thus, the HGFs will profoundly affect chemotherapy-induced cytopenia, which is a major contributor to morbidity, mortality and inadequate dosing for therapeutic effectiveness.

Less success could reasonably be foreseen for treating patients with intrinsic marrow failure or abnormal marrow function in whom the target cell populations or the mechanisms for responding to growth factors (receptors; signal transduction pathways; gene expression) might not be intact. None the less, the HGFs have already had a considerable impact on clinical haematology and their precise roles are emerging and becoming more clearly defined.

General features of HGF responses *in vivo*

As we have discussed, the HGFs affect target cells of different lineages and at different levels of development, but they are not as restricted in their actions as they first appeared. Nevertheless, the clinical effects of the HGFs follow experimental predictions remarkably closely. As more is learnt about their combined actions and spectra of target cells *in vivo*, it will become possible to adjust this treatment modality to suit individual circumstances.

GM-CSF

Granulocyte-macrophage (GM) CSF is a pluripoietin which acts throughout the granulomonocytic lineage but influences only the early stages of erythropoiesis (BFU-E) and megakaryopoiesis (Mk-CFC). It seems likely that additional factors (i.e. erythropoietin and thrombopoietin) are required for complete development to mature red cells and platelets.

Overall, the effects of GM-CSF in patients consist of stimulation at the progenitor cell level, increased granulocyte and monocyte production and enhanced neutrophil function. Any effects on platelet, erythrocyte and lymphocyte counts are moderate and may be influenced by the context of the treatment. As a rule, the changes elicited by GM-CSF persist only for as long as it is given and disappear shortly after the treatment is withdrawn.

A reduction in serum cholesterol has been noted following GM-CSF administration (Nimer *et al.*, 1988), which indicates that forms of the GM-CSF molecule, modified in order to isolate this particular activity from its other effects, might be useful in the long-term control of hypercholesterolaemia. This use of HGFs may prove to be safer than other forms of intervention (Oliver, 1991).

G-CSF

Granulocyte CSF is generally thought of as a lineage-restricted HGF which, specifically, stimulates the production of neutrophils to attack the bacteria and other microorganisms responsible for infections. Ogawa and his colleagues have reported that G-CSF also acts on early progenitors but this prediction has not been thoroughly investigated *in vivo*. Intravenous administration of G-CSF results in a dose-dependent increase in circulating mature neutrophils and band forms. Monocyte counts are raised only at high doses and eosinophil and reticulocyte counts are unchanged (Bronchud *et al.*, 1987; Gabrilove *et al.*, 1988; Morstyn *et al.*, 1988; 1989). In addition, Lindemann *et al.* (1989) and Ohsaka *et al.* (1989) have measured increased oxygen radical production and C3bi receptor expression and increased serum levels of enzymes related to granulocyte turnover in recipients of G-CSF. These studies demonstrate that G-CSF is a potent stimulator of neutrophil function *in vivo*.

Based on its actions *in vivo* and *in vitro*, G-CSF might be expected to induce an increase in granulocytes at the expense of earlier progenitor cell pools. Treatment with G-CSF could theoretically lead to stem cell depletion, with obvious implications for bone marrow failure, because the progenitor cells of the G-CFC (i.e. the GM-CFC) have virtually no self-renewal capacity and must be replaced by the proliferative activity of more primitive cells. Duhrsen *et al.* (1988) investigated this aspect by culturing bone marrow cells from G-CSF-treated patients in clonogenic assays. They detected a slight decrease in progenitor cell frequency in marrows from most of the patients but any changes in absolute numbers of progenitor cells cannot be estimated without information about changes in marrow cellularity. In the blood, the numbers of progenitor cells of all lineages increased up to 100-fold after 4 days of G-CSF treatment.

Taking another approach, Lord *et al.* (1989) used tritiated thymidine and autoradiography to investigate myeloid cell kinetics in two haematologically normal patients treated with G-CSF. They calculated that an increase of 3.2 extra cell divisions by myeloid precursor cells could account for the neutrophil response. This increased production occurred at the level of entry into the myeloblast compartment and was considered moderate and unlikely to result in depletion of primitive stem cell populations.

Two studies have reported an effect of G-CSF on BFU-E in humans. In cancer patients, Duhrsen *et al.* (1988) reported increases in circulating BFU-E with corresponding differences in marrow BFU-E and no increases in reticulocytes or haemoglobin. These observations are consistent with premature release of progenitor cells rather than increased production. In myelodysplastic patients, Miles *et al.* (1990) noted reticulocytosis and increased haemoglobin levels in G-CSF-treated patients accompanied by time- and dose-dependent increases in the numbers of circulating BFU-E.

M-CSF

Macrophage CSF (M-CSF or CSF-1) stimulates the development of monocytes and macrophages and enhances the effector functions of mature mononuclear phagocytes *in vitro*. A phase I clinical trial of M-CSF is being conducted in patients with metastatic melanoma. The observed haematological changes include increases in large vacuolated monocytes in the blood and reversible thrombocytopenia (Bajorin *et al.*, 1991). M-CSF also enhances the functions of peripheral blood monocytes *in vivo* and this effect may be beneficial in the treatment of selected infections (Khwaja *et al.*, 1991). Recombinant human M-CSF also reduces plasma cholesterol levels when given to non-human primates, hyperlipidaemic or normal rabbits (Stoudemire and Garnick, 1991), or to patients (Bajorin *et al.*, 1991).

Erythropoietin

Erythropoietin is a major physiological regulator of red blood cell production and is essential for haemoglobin synthesis. In normal individuals, its levels in the serum vary inversely with the oxygen tension and deviations from this relationship can assist in the diagnosis of disorders such as polycythaemia rubra vera and secondary polycythaemia. The CFU-E *in vitro* is the equivalent of the earliest erythropoietin-responsive cell *in vivo*. There is controversial evidence that erythropoietin also stimulates megakaryopoiesis *in vivo* and *in vitro* but higher doses are needed for this effect compared with the doses needed to stimulate erythropoiesis.

Interleukin 3 (IL-3)

Interleukin 3 appears to act on earlier stages of haemopoiesis than the other CSFs (Cannistra *et al.*, 1990). It might, therefore, prove useful in treating cases of bone marrow failure where production of the targets for the later-acting HGFs (GM-CSF, G-CSF, M-CSF and erythropoietin) may be blocked. The early action of IL-3 means that it will probably need to be combined with other growth factors to ensure complete haemopoietic cell development.

The results of phase I and I/II trials have demonstrated that IL-3 is capable of increasing neutrophil, eosinophil, monocyte, reticulocyte and platelet counts (Ganser *et al.*, 1990a,b). These increases were associated with increases in the cell cycle rate of GM-CFC, BFU-E and GEMM-CFC and in marrow cellularity but the concentration of the progenitors was unaltered or slightly decreased (Ottman *et al.*, 1990).

Trilineage haematological responses were seen in patients with preserved bone marrow function and in patients with secondary bone marrow failure but were more marked in the patients with bone marrow failure. Responses to IL-3 differed from responses to GM-CSF and G-CSF in that they were less rapid and of smaller magnitude. The left-shifted myelopoiesis in the marrow and the maintenance of the blood counts following withdrawal of treatment indicate effects on early haemopoietic progenitor cells.

IL-1

Interleukin-1 affects nearly all types of tissue and organ and is involved in increasing host defence mechanisms, especially immunological and haematological responses (see Dinarello, 1991). Phase I/II clinical trials have been initiated to investigate possible myeloprotective effects of IL-1, in combination with 5-fluorouracil, in humans. The patients experienced a significant increase in platelet count and an acute two- to threefold leukocytosis. Increases in cellularity and in the myeloid:erythroid ratio occur in the marrow. In addition, studies have shown that there are elevations in the levels of circulating IL-6 and soluble IL-2 receptor in the blood but no change in tumour necrosis factor α (TNFα), IL-2, GM-CSF or interferon α (IFNα) levels (see Starnes, 1991).

The other interleukins

Recombinant material is available for interleukins 2 and 4–11. The clinical applications of IL-2 will be covered in Chapter 6. The other interleukins have not yet been tested in clinical trials but some of their activities on haemopoietic cells suggest that they may be useful in the future. Interleukin 6 acts on early haemopoietic progenitor cells and IL-1 has been shown to enhance haemopoietic recovery following irradiation in animal models and to protect cells from the effects of exposure to cytotoxic drugs *in vitro*. Interleukin 7 promotes the growth of pre-B cells and of immature T cells and has been suggested to act at the stem cell level to regulate lymphoid differentiation. A role for IL-4 in thrombolysis is indicated by its stimulation of monocytes to produce tissue-type plasminogen activator (Hart *et al.*, 1989). Interleukin 5 stimulates eosinophil production and there are some indications that eosinophils are active against tumour cells since, in several situations, eosinophilia is a favourable prognostic indicator. However, high eosinophil counts can result in tissue damage; patients with hypereosinophilic syndrome are at risk of cardiac damage. Recent evidence indicates that IL-11 may potentiate the effects of IL-3 on megakaryopoiesis (Bruno *et al.*, 1991).

Modified growth factors

We mentioned in Chapter 1 the demonstrations that some of the multiple effects of IL-1β could be ascribed to different structural domains, raising the possibility that selectively active cytokine fragments could be used in therapy, and that modification of the G-CSF molecule can increase its biological activity. Other modifications that may prove of therapeutic value consist of producing hybrid molecules. For example, polyethylene glycol (PEG) has been attached to IL-2 in order to extend its half-life *in vivo*; a fusion protein consisting of GM-CSF and IL-3 has been shown to possess increased receptor-binding affinity and stimulating activity *in vitro* (Curtis *et al.*, 1991); and the fusion product of diphtheria toxin (DAB$_{486}$) and IL-2 produced a therapeutic response in a patient with chronic lymphoblastic leukaemia (CLL) who had not responded to other drugs (LeMaistre *et al.*, 1991).

Agonists and antibodies

In a variety of circumstances, high levels of growth factors and/or target cell responses to them are unfavourable. Ways are now being developed for preventing problems of this nature and include the use of antibodies and other agents that can prevent interactions between growth factors and their cell surface receptors.

High or prolonged production of IL-1 occurs in many diseases and eventually debilitates normal defence functions. Thus, a reduction in IL-1 synthesis or abrogation of its effects becomes a therapeutic target in, for example, rheumatoid arthritis, renal allograft rejection, inflammatory or autoimmune diseases or leukaemia. An IL-1 receptor agonist occurs naturally and is specific for IL-1. It blocks the effects of IL-1 in animals injected with the factor and also prevents shock, sepsis, hypotension and immune complex-induced colitis in model systems. In cultures of leukaemic cells it reduces spontaneous proliferation and the production of endogenous growth factors. Recently, IL-1β has been implicated in the growth advantage enjoyed by chronic myeloid leukaemia (CML) cells and the demonstration that IL-1 receptor agonist suppresses colony formation by CML cells suggests that it might have therapeutic potential (Estrov *et al.*, 1991). Other approaches to blocking IL-1-mediated effects include administration of recombinant soluble receptor (extracellular domain of the transmembrane receptor), which also blocks colony formation in CML (Estrov *et al.*, 1991), and antibodies to the IL-1 receptor (see Dinarello, 1991). Anti-IL-1 and anti-IL-2 receptor antibodies have been tried in the treatment of established GVHD in transplanted patients (Herve *et al.*, 1988, 1990). Also, Blaise *et al.* (1989) used a monoclonal antibody that blocked the IL-2 receptor as prophylaxis for acute GVHD and demonstrated that it did not interfere with engraftment following allogeneic bone marrow transplantation.

Efforts are being made to develop IL-4 agonists for the treatment of excess immunoglobulin E (IgE) production in the hyper-IgE syndrome, in allergic conditions and following bone marrow transplantation. In mice, a combination of anti-IL-4 and anti-IL-4 receptor antibodies completely blocked IgE production but did not affect IgG1 production (Finkelman *et al.*, 1991), supporting its potential usefulness in the treatment of IgE-mediated disorders. Recombinant soluble IL-4 receptor provides another potential therapeutic agent in this context (Jacobs et al., 1991). Agonists to IL-5 may be useful in hypereosinophilia, hypersensitivity diseases and in the treatment of asthma where eosinophils are involved in the formation of lesions on respiratory epithelium. Interleukin 6 agonists may find application in the treatment of Castleman's disease (Yoshizaki et al., 1989). A case of plasma cell leukaemia (myeloma) that responded temporarily to treatment with a monoclonal antil-IL-6 antibody has been reported (Klein et al., 1991).

Interleukin 8 is a neutrophil-activating peptide and agonists or inhibitors could provide new anti-inflammatory agents in, for example, rheumatoid arthritis, idiopathic pulmonary fibrosis and adult respiratory distress syndrome (ARDS) (Bagglioni et al., 1989).

As well as potentially being active in the autocrine stimulation of tumour growth, secretion of growth factors by malignant cells may be involved primarily or secondarily in the pathophysiology of cancer. For example, the production by myeloma of TNF and IL-1 correlates with extensive osteolytic bone disease (Lichtenstein et al., 1989) and it may be possible, therefore, to alleviate this complication by neutralizing the cytokines *in vivo*.

EXPERIMENTAL BACKGROUND

There have been numerous studies of the haematological effects of growth factors administered to laboratory rodents. Clearly, in some respects, the range of studies possible using these species is far wider than the studies that can be undertaken using non-human primates and humans. In other respects, studies in animals are limited because, for example, side-effects that need to be communicated verbally cannot be evaluated.

Preclinical models of growth factor therapy

It is beyond the scope of this text to describe in detail all of the preclinical models of human disease and treatment that have been used to evaluate the clinical potential of the HGFs. They have been tested using laboratory rodents, hamsters, dogs and non-human primates. In the majority of cases, administration of the HGFs at clinically relevant doses has not produced unexpected effects on blood counts, progenitor cell numbers or mature cell function.

Studies have explored the roles of the HGFs in the management of bone marrow transplant recipients using models for allogeneic transplantation (Atkinson et al., 1991), for T cell-depleted histincompatible transplantation (Blazar et al., 1988), for autologous bone marrow transplantation (Monroy et al., 1987) and for transplantation of stem cells induced to circulate in the peripheral blood (Craddock et al., 1990; Molineux et al., 1990). Similarly, their effectiveness in enhancing haematological recovery following treatment with myelotoxic drugs or radiation has been investigated (Neta and Oppenheim, 1988; Moreb et al., 1990; Waddick et al., 1991) and the idea that pretreatment with growth factors *in vitro* can enhance subsequent graft performance *in vivo* has been tested in mice by Tavassoli and colleagues (1991).

The *in vivo* effects of the HGFs on the development of leukaemic cell populations have been tested. There are indications from this work that GM-CSF may, in some types of leukaemia, cause terminal differentiation and loss of tumorigenicity (Jiminez and Yunis, 1988) and that B cell leukaemias do not respond to GM-CSF or to GM-CSF plus IL-3 (Fabian et al., 1988).

Certain genetically determined deficiency disorders in experimental animals provide further opportunities for testing the HGFs. Canine cyclic neutropenia in grey collie dogs is one such condition. It is an autosomal recessive disorder characterized by peaks and troughs in the neutrophil count that occur with a periodicity of 14 days. Treatment of the dogs with recombinant human G-CSF caused a marked leukocytosis and prevented two predicted episodes of neutropenia (Lothrop et al., 1988). Recombinant IL-3 had no effect and GM-CSF, whilst increasing the neutrophil count, did not prevent cyclic blood cell production (Hammond et al., 1990). Anaemic W/W^v and Sl/Sl^d mice have been used to test the effects of erythropoietin. Cynshi et al. (1990) found that W/W^v anaemia, which is the result of a stem cell defect, responded to erythropoietin but Sl/Sl^d anaemia, due to a defect on the haemopoietic microenvironment, did not. The product of the Steel (Sl) locus is a factor that is often referred to as 'stem cell factor' (see Chapter 1) and repeated subcutaneous injection of the stem cell factor into Sl/Sl^d mice results in marked increases in white blood cell count and platelets (Zsebo et al., 1990). It has also been administered to baboons, rats and mice (Andrews et al., 1990; Rosen et al., 1990; Molineux et al., 1991; Ulich et al., 1991), with some differences in response between the species.

Effects of high-level, continuous exposure to HGFs *in vivo*

The genetic disorders considered above are deficiency disorders and have been informative in establishing the effects of low HGF levels *in vivo*. However, the effects of high levels are of real clinical concern in the context of administering pharmacological amounts of biologically active recombinant protein. The most realistic model involves the long-term administration of HGFs to experimental animals. This did not result in any major adverse effects, although there was evidence of osteoclast activation and marked remodelling of bone in animals treated with GM-CSF, G-CSF or erythropoietin (Lee et al., 1991). This aspect has been approached also using the transfer and expression *in vivo* of the HGF genes in transgenic mice. Alternatively, bone marrow cells or factor-dependent haemopoietic cell lines have been infected with retroviruses incorporating the HGF gene.

To study the long-term effects of whole-body exposure to high levels of GM-CSF, Lang et al. (1987) produced transgenic mice carrying the murine GM-CSF gene. These mice developed increased (80 × normal) levels of GM-CSF in the urine, peritoneal cavity and eye. Pathological changes associated with these increased GM-CSF levels consisted of accumulations of macrophages in the lens, retina and striated muscle. Surprisingly, there was little change in the cellularity of the blood, marrow or lymph nodes and the haemopoietic tissue responded normally to GM-CSF *in vitro* by forming colonies. The relevance of these findings to HGF therapy is uncertain because the transgene was expressed in ocular, muscle and peritoneal cells but not in the bone marrow. However, the serious consequences of prolonged, high-level exposure to GM-CSF are evident and all of the mice died prematurely.

Even higher levels of GM-CSF than those observed in transgenic mice have been achieved by transplanting lethally irradiated mice with bone marrow cells infected with recombinant GM-CSF-containing retroviruses (Johnson et al., 1989). The mice were afflicted by a fatal disease associated with large numbers of circulating, infiltrating neutrophils, macrophages and eosinophils. There was a massive expansion of granulocyte and macrophage populations in the peripheral blood, spleen and peritoneal cavity but decreased cellularity in the marrow. However, this decrease in marrow cellularity resulted from reductions in number of lymphoid and erythroid cells and the absolute numbers of neutrophils and eosinophils were, in fact, increased. There was also extensive infiltration of the liver and lungs and some infiltration of the heart, skeletal muscle and eyes of some mice. Haemopoietic tissue from the mice secreted GM-CSF *in vitro* and haemopoietic progenitor cells produced growth factor-independent colonies in semisolid cultures. In spite of these abnormalities, the numbers of GM-CFC in the femoral marrow were lower than in control animals and transplantation of bone marrow cells into new recipients did not result in any haematological disorder. This demonstrates that chronic exposure of normal cells to high levels of GM-CSF is not sufficient to induce leukaemia.

To examine further the events that take place in cells that have been manipulated to produce the growth factor to which they normally respond, thereby constructing an autocrine loop, factor-dependent myeloid cell lines have been infected with retroviral constructs containing the GM-CSF gene (Lang et al., 1985; Laker et al., 1987). The autonomous growth pattern of the infected cells showed that they secreted GM-CSF and, in some experiments, the cells were tumorigenic upon transplantation *in vivo*.

Mice transplanted with retrovirus-infected stem and progenitor cells expressing the IL-3 gene develop a myeloproliferative disorder with excessive proliferation and accumulation of mature, functional haemopoietic cells plus splenomegaly and hepatomegaly caused by myeloid cell infiltration. In spite of the amplification in stem and progenitor cell number, there was no discernible alteration in the self-renewal capacity of the progenitor cells or their ability to complete apparently normal cellular maturation. The mice died of the myelo-proliferative syndrome about 5 weeks after the transplant but the disease was not transmitted to mice transplanted with cells from the infected animals or with mast cell lines derived from their tissues. In contrast, injection of IL-3-infected factor-dependent FDCP-1 cells did lead to tumour formation *in vivo*, showing that, whereas high levels of IL-3 do not transform normal cells, FDCP-1 cells readily become malignant (Chang et al., 1989a; Wong et al., 1989).

Mice transplanted with cells expressing the G-CSF gene did not suffer severe tissue damage and no tumours developed in the recipients (Chang et al., 1989b). The mice did not die prematurely and none of them developed myeloid leukaemia, which confirms that overstimulation, by itself, is not sufficient for leukaemic transformation. Animals expressing the human erythropoietin transgene are polycythaemic, with increased numbers of erythroid precursors in their haemopoietic tissue and high levels of erythropoietin in their sera (Semenza et al., 1989).

The dramatic effects of high-level production of haemopoietic growth factors by transplanted cells do not seem to affect the self-renewal capacity of the spleen colony-forming cells (CFU-S) in mice. Chang and Johnson (1991) transplanted marrow expressing the IL-3, GM-CSF or G-CSF genes to obtain spleen colonies in lethally irradiated recipients. The spleen colonies were then dissected out and analysed for secondary CFU-S (the products of self-renewal) by re-transplantation, and for differential cell morphology (the products of differentiation). In no case did high levels of the haemopoietic growth factors alter the self-renewal probability or differential cell production of virus-positive CFU-S.

Many of the *in vivo* effects of the HGFs and other cytokines are probably not yet known and experimental expression of the genes *in vivo* can be used to reveal some of their unknown activities. This was illustrated recently by a study done by Metcalf and Gearing (1989) on the effects of leukaemia inhibitory factor (LIF). They transplanted mice with factor-dependent FDCP-1 cells that had been retrovirally infected with the LIF gene. The mice rapidly (17–20 days later) developed a fatal syndrome involving cachexia, formation of new bone, calcification of muscle tissue, pancreatitis, atrophy of the thymus and abnormalities of the adrenal cortex, ovaries and tests.

PRINCIPLES AND PRACTICE OF HGF THERAPY

Administration

Information about the most effective way of administering the HGFs in different circumstances is limited because of the different routes and schedules that have been used in the studies reported so far. Other differences that make it very difficult to compare results from different trials include the use of glycosylated versus non-glycosylated recombinant proteins and doses calculated according to ideal body weight, actual body weight or surface area. Nevertheless, some principles are beginning to emerge.

It is generally thought that it is necessary to maintain constant high levels of the HGFs *in vivo* in order to obtain a clinically useful response. However, dose–response relationships *in vivo* are likely to be complex and, as a result of the multiple actions of growth factors, a high dose need not necessarily produce the desired response. This point was made by Kurzrock *et al.* (1991) who found that some patients treated with high doses of GM-CSF responded by producing eosinophils rather than neutrophils. When their dose of GM-CSF was reduced, these patients produced larger numbers of neutrophils without any increase in their eosinophilia.

Continuous infusions are demonstrably more effective than intravenous bolus injections (Steward *et al.*, 1988). Also, the subcutaneous route is superior to intravenous bolus injection, presumably because the active factor is dispersed more slowly than if it is introduced directly into the blood stream. In some studies, this route has been more effective than continuous infusion (Morstyn *et al.*, 1988) but in others it has been the same (Aglietta *et al.*, 1990). In the case of IL-1, the subcutaneous route is associated with fewer side-effects (see Dinarello, 1991). To a certain extent, the choice of route depends on practical factors such as venous access and patient compliance. Continuous subcutaneous infusion has the advantage that patients can remain at home without the need for daily injections. In addition, new ways of maintaining constant levels of HGFs *in vivo* are being developed. In mice, Tani et al. (1989) have developed a method for the sustained delivery of G-CSF by subcutaneous implants of diffusion chambers containing fibroblasts expressing the transfected human G-CSF gene. Other possibilities include the use of 'organoids' consisting of genetically engineered endothelial cells supported by Gore-Tex fibres (Thompson et al., 1989) or transfusion of lymphocytes retrovirally infected with growth factor genes (Kantoff et al., 1986).

Studies using glycosylated and non-glycosylated recombinant GM-CSF have indicated that glycosylation reduces its specific activity (see Chapter 1). In the case of erythropoietin, however, glycosylation increases its survival in the circulation (Spivak and Hogans, 1989).

Toxicity

The HGFs have generally been well-tolerated in phase I and I/II trials in concentrations at which biological activity can be expected or has been observed. Particular toxicities include the severe pericarditis and dyspnoea, ascribed to a 'capillary leak syndrome' that occurs in 80% of patients treated with the maximum tolerated dose (60 µg/kg per day) of GM-CSF (Steward et al., 1989). At the higher clinical dose levels (32 µg/kg per day), there have been marked weight gain, generalized oedema and acute renal failure (Brandt et al., 1988) and pericarditis can be dose-limiting at doses as low as 15 µg/kg per day (Lieschke et al., 1989).

About 15–30 minutes after injection of a bolus of GM-CSF, there is a reproducible acute leukopenia associated with increased expression of a cell adhesion molecule on neutrophils and monocytes and transient sequestration of cells in the lungs. This effect suggests that GM-CSF may not be suitable for treating patients with underlying pulmonary disease (Devereaux et al., 1987; Phillips et al., 1989). Also, GM-CSF can play a role in activating antigen-presenting cells which, in patients with pre-existing autoantibodies, can activate autoaggressive T cell clones (Hoekman et al., 1991). Similarly, it can aggravate seropositive arthritis (Hazenberg et al., 1989). In spite of these documented toxicities, the results of a phase III trial revealed no differences between the treatment and placebo groups (Rabinowe et al., 1991).

No significant toxicities have been observed for G-CSF or IL-3 (Morstyn et al., 1988, 1989; Ganser et al., 1990a,b) although an acute leukopenia follows G-CSF treatment as well as GM-CSF treatment (Morstyn et al., 1988). Macrophage-CSF reduced the platelet count but had no effect on neutrophils, monocytes or lymphocytes (Nemunaitis et al., 1991b). Hypertension and an increased incidence of thrombotic episodes may result from erythropoietin-induced increases in haematocrit and alterations in vasculature (Anagnostou et al., 1990), although no hypertensive, convulsive or thrombotic events were observed during a trial of erythropoietin in normal healthy volunteers (McMahon et al., 1990).

Administration of IL-1 caused fever and chills in most patients and was accompanied in many by tachycardia, headache and flu-like symptoms. Significant cardiac and renal toxicities are seen occasionally at the maximum tolerated dose (see Dinarello, 1991; Starnes, 1991). Crown et al. (1991) reported that hypotension was dose-limiting at the highest dose they tested.

Contraindications

The systemic administration of the HGFs means that any cells that are exposed to them and are capable of responding will have the opportunity to do so. There has been a considerable amount of concern and debate about the possible undesirable effects that could result from these responses. For example, GM-CSF activates mature neu-

Table 5.2 Stimulatory effects of growth factors on malignant cells in acute myeloid leukaemia

Growth factor	System	References
IL-3	Clonogenic	Delwel et al., 1987; Miyauchi et al., 1987; Vellenga et al., 1987a; Saeland et al., 1988
	Suspension	Miyauchi et al., 1987; Vellenga et al., 1987a; Lowenberg et al., 1988; Saeland et al., 1988
GM-CSF	Clonogenic	Hoang et al., 1986; Begley et al., 1987; Delwel et al., 1987; Miyauchi et al., 1987; Vellenga et al., 1987a,b
	Suspension	Hoang et al., 1986; Miyauchi et al., 1987; Vellenga et al., 1987a; Lowenberg et al., 1988
G-CSF	Clonogenic	Begley et al., 1987; Delwel et al., 1987; Kelleher et al., 1987; Miyauchi et al., 1987; Vellenga et al., 1987a,b
	Suspension	Kelleher et al., 1987; Miyauchi et al., 1987; Vellenga et al., 1987a; Lowenberg et al., 1988
M-CSF	Suspension	Lowenberg et al., 1988; Miyauchi et al., 1988
SCF	Clonogenic	Wang et al., 1991
	Suspension	Wang et al., 1991
IL-2	Suspension	Carron and Cawley, 1989

IL-3, Interleukin 3; GM-CSF, granulocyte-macrophage colony-stimulating factor; SCF, stem cell factor.

trophils which leads to the release of activated oxygen radicals and of many potentially damaging proteolytic enzymes (Klausmann et al., 1988). These agents are known to play a part in ARDS, emphysema, coagulation defects, arthritis and inflammation.

Myeloid leukaemia cells express growth factor receptors and potentially can respond to the HGFs proposed for therapeutic use. Moreover, autocrine stimulation of proliferation is one mechanism for the expansion of leukaemic cell populations. Many studies of the responses of leukaemic cells to HGFs have been performed *in vitro* using clonogenic and suspension culture systems (Table 5.2). In general, these studies have shown responses by acute myeloid leukaemia (AML) cells to one or several HGFs; a lack of cellular maturation in response to HGFs and a poor correlation between HGF responsiveness and French–American–British (FAB) classification subtype. However, a specific association has been noted between *in vitro* responses to G-CSF and AML cells with translocations involving the q12q21 region of chromosome 17. This association is particularly characteristic of acute promyelocytic leukaemia (APL) with the pathognomonic t(15;17) translocation (Pebusque et al., 1988). In lymphoid leukaemias, T-lineage acute lymphoblastic leukaemia (ALL), B-lineage ALL and CLL cells express IL-7 receptors and respond to IL-7 (Dibirdik et al., 1991; Digel et al., 1991) which may contraindicate any clinical use of IL-7 in these disorders. Similarly, the demonstration that anti-IL-6 monoclonal antibody can suppress myeloma cell proliferation *in vivo* might indicate that IL-6 should not be used in the treatment of myeloma patients (Klein et al., 1991).

Haemopoietic growth factors may also stimulate the preleukaemic clone in patients with one of the myelodysplastic syndromes (MDS). The proportion of blast cells in the marrow of MDS patients has been seen to increase during treatment with GM-CSF and this effect was particularly noticeable in patients with a higher (>14%) blast cell count prior to treatment (Ganser et al., 1989). Also, *in vitro* experiments have demonstrated that GM-CSF increases the size of the blast cell population in long-term cultures of MDS marrow (Marley et al., 1990). These observations indicate that HGF therapy alone might be inappropriate in the management of MDS, although a combination of growth factors with the capacity to induce differentiation or selective cytotoxic drugs might overcome the problem of increased 'preleukaemic' cell proliferation.

There is a known association between treatment with chemotherapy and the development of a second malignancy. Also, following chemotherapy, tumour recurrence can originate in a very small population of residual tumour cells. Several recent reports have indicated that HGFs can affect the proliferation of a variety of non-haemopoietic malignant cell types, suggesting that HGF therapy has the potential to accelerate tumour regrowth. Dedhar et al. (1988) showed that GM-CSF stimulated several tumour cell lines in vitro but that these cells only responded to doses that were 10–20-fold greater than the doses required to stimulate proliferation of GM-CFC. In another study, Berdel et al. (1989) found that three adenocarcinoma cell lines responded to IL-3, GM-CSF and G-CSF and high-affinity GM-CSF receptors have been demonstrated in small cell lung carcinoma cell lines (Baldwin et al., 1989). In contrast, Nemunaitis and Singer (1989) were unable to demonstrate proliferation by glioblastoma, leiomyosarcoma, bladder cancer, small cell lung cancer, hepatoma, lung adenocarcinoma, melanoma or breast cancer cell lines to GM-CSF but did find that IL-1 stimulated the leiomyosarcoma cell line. Primary melanoma cells apparently express low-affinity GM-CSF receptors that bind GM-CSF but do not transduce a signal across the cell membrane (Baldwin et al., 1991).

Several non-haemopoietic types of normal cells express HGF receptors and can respond to them. The study by Dedhar et al. (1988) referred to above also showed that fibroblast precursors in normal bone marrow respond to GM-CSF. Bussolino et al. (1989) studied the effect of GM-CSF and G-CSF on human endothelial cells in culture and found that they responded by migrating and proliferating and that c-*fos* messenger (m)RNA was induced following exposure to these HGFs. High-affinity binding sites for GM-CSF and G-CSF were identified on the endothelial cells and the effects of the HGFs were abolished by neutralizing antibodies. Similarly, erythropoietin has mitogenic and chemotactic effects on endothelial cells, which might be relevant to the vascular complications that can occur in erythropoietin-treated patients (Anagnostou et al., 1990).

The information summarized in this section suggests that a variety of normal and malignant cells can respond to HGFs and may cause complications in HGF-treated patients. However, the implications for clinical practice have yet to be assessed and issues concerning the affinities of receptors on malignant cells and the status of the signal transduction mechanisms required to bring about a proliferative response have not been fully addressed.

CLINICAL HGF THERAPY

The preceding sections have indicated the potential benefits and possible hazards in the use of the HGFs to treat haematological diseases and insufficiencies. This section is concerned with the clinical experience of applying them to specific conditions and circumstances.

Treatment of aplastic anaemia with HGFs

Patients with aplastic anaemia have complete trilineage bone marrow failure marked by bone marrow hypocellularity, fatty changes in the marrow stroma and peripheral pancytopenia. The peripheral blood counts and bone marrow cellularity have been used to construct a classification for very severe, severe and non-severe disease. Clearly, bone marrow replacement is required in severe cases and bone marrow transplantation is an obvious therapeutic option if a human leukocyte antigen (HLA) identical sibling donor is available. Indeed, it is the treatment of choice for patients who are younger than 45–50 years (see Hows, 1991).

Treatment with HGFs presents another possible means of improving peripheral counts in aplastic patients and could be used either as a primary treatment or in combination with bone marrow transplantation or immunosuppression. Since it is important to treat severely aplastic patients early, one potential benefit of HGF therapy might be to combat infection and other complications whilst an appropriate HLA-compatible donor is being sought. This would have the advantage, over supportive transfusions, that there would be no danger of alloimmunization through multiple blood donations that could later compromise engraftment, and no requirement for cytomegalovirus (CMV) negative blood products for seronegative patients who have seronegative donors.

Clearly, a response to HGFs in aplastic anaemia depends on the presence of the corresponding target cells in the bone marrow and, in fact, combinations of several growth factors may prove necessary to support the full development of mature circulating red cells, white cells and platelets. The existence of residual early progenitor cells that potentially provide HGF targets has been demonstrated in aplastic anaemia using the long-term bone marrow culture system (Gibson and Gordon-Smith, 1990). Marrow from some aplastic patients produced a wave of GM-CFC in this culture system which demonstrates the presence of earlier (pre-GM-CFC) progenitors.

Other difficulties with the use of HGF therapy in aplastic anaemia include the high levels of endogenous activity that have been measured in the sera of aplastic patients. High levels of G-CSF have been documented (Watari et al., 1989) and it is likely that the levels of all HGFs are elevated in response to bone marrow failure and peripheral cytopenia. This might be expected to reduce the efficiency of exogenously supplied HGFs in the treatment of aplastic anaemia. Finally, the beneficial effects of the HGFs could be counteracted or prevented by the inhibitory action of an immunological pathomechanism or the presence of a damaged or hostile haemopoietic microenvironment. The existence, in some patients, of the first problem is suggested by the success of immunosuppressive therapy in some cases; the existence of the second problem is not, in general, supported by the success of bone marrow transplantation in many cases. Overall, the limiting factor in the response of aplastic anaemia to HGF treatment appears to be the amount of residual haemopoiesis, i.e. the availability of target cells to respond.

Clinical experience using GM-CSF to treat aplastic anaemia has shown that the haematological response is related to the white cell count prior to intervention and to the severity of the disease. For example, two patients with agranulocytosis (Champlin et al., 1988) and four with very severe aplastic anaemia (Nissen et al., 1988) failed to respond whilst responses were achieved in relatively less severe cases. The lineage-related responses also vary from study to study. Six of 14 patients investigated by Vadhan-Raj et al. (1988b) sustained multilineage responses and three of them became independent of red cell and platelet transfusions. Champlin et al. (1989) reported results from 11 evaluable aplastic patients treated with GM-CSF, 10 of whom responded with substantial increments in blood granulocytes, eosinophils and monocytes with myeloid and eosinophilic hyperplasia of the bone marrow. A response at the progenitor cell level was seen in an increase in GM-CFC numbers and, again, responses were related to the white cell count before treatment. Responses to GM-CSF have been maintained by continuous infusion for 2 months (Champlin et al., 1989) but, almost invariably, blood counts fall to pretreatment values once therapy is discontinued and there is no long-lasting benefit.

Recently, it has been shown that treatment of refractory patients with GM-CSF increased B cells and T cells and that natural killer (NK) cell activity was unaffected. However, proliferative responses to phytohaemagglutinin, *Candida* antigen and tetanus toxoid were unchanged (Faisal et al., 1990). The mechanism responsible for these GM-CSF-induced changes is not defined and their implications in terms of resistance to infection are not established.

Granulocyte CSF can be expected to increase the neutrophil count in more than 80% of patients with aplastic anaemia. The results of a study by Kojima et al. (1991) suggest that this response will be valuable in managing patients with fungal or bacterial infections, will reduce mortality and prolong survival. This could allow patients to survive, for example, the period between diagnosis and bone marrow engraftment or a response to immunosuppression.

Interleukin 3 has recently been administered to patients with aplastic anaemia in a phase I/II trial (Ganser et al., 1990a). Platelet responses with reduced transfusion requirements were rare and, in most patients, transfusion requirements were unchanged. Similarly, red cell transfusion requirements were not altered. In some, there was an increase in marrow cellularity but this did not produce substantial increases in leukocyte count, although neutrophil counts did show some increase in about half of the patients.

Treatment of neutropenia with HGFs

A variety of neutropenic disorders have been treated with GM-CSF and G-CSF. These disorders differ in their aetiology and the level at which neutrophil production and function is defective and, accordingly, responses have also been varied. The examples listed below indicate some of the situations in which HGF therapy might be useful in the treatment of neutropenia and where it might be anticipated to fail. In addition, there may be some cases of neutropenia in which the cells lack the appropriate receptors or intracellular signal transduction pathways may be defective. However, such patients, if they exist, have not been identified. The treatment with HGFs of neutropenia as a consequence of treatment is covered in the sections on chemotherapy and bone marrow transplantation.

Congenital neutropenia

Welte et al. (1990) found that G-CSF was effective in the treatment of congenital neutropenia with maturation arrest at the promyelocyte stage and that G-CSF was superior to GM-CSF. Initially, five patients were treated with GM-CSF but only one of them experienced an absolute increase in neutrophil count. Subsequent treatment with G-CSF produced a neutrophil response in all five that was sustained during maintenance therapy and associated with an improvement or absence of infections. Presumably, this requirement for G-CSF indicates that it is needed to complete neutrophil development in these patients and this is consistent with the known action of G-CSF in the later stages of granulocyte formation. However, responses to administered G-CSF in these patients do not necessarily reflect an *in vivo* deficiency in G-CSF synthesis since monocytes from patients who respond clinically to G-CSF are capable of releasing biologically active G-CSF *in vitro* (Pietsch et al., 1991) and increased G-CSF levels can be measured in their serum (Mempel et al., 1991). Thus, the patients are unable to respond to endogenous G-CSF but can respond to administered G-CSF.

In Kostmann's syndrome (congenital agranulocytosis), G-CSF treatment increased neutrophil counts from less than 500 per μl to over 1000 per μl and improved maturation of the myeloid series to polymorphonuclear neutrophils occurred in the bone marrow. There was a delay of 8–9 days after administration before a response was seen in the peripheral blood, which suggests that the G-CSF was acting on early progenitor cells in these patients. The response was maintained by subcutaneous G-CSF treatment for up to 13 months with resolution of existing infections, a reduction in new infections and a reduced requirement for antibiotics (Bonilla et al., 1989). The Pelger–Huët anomaly is transmitted as an autosomal dominant trait and consists of a defect in nuclear lobulation in neutrophils and eosinophils. Morphologically, neutrophils respond to G-CSF *in vitro* by forming lobed nuclei but eosinophils do not respond to G-CSF or IL-5 (Teshima et al., 1991). These observations suggest that G-CSF may have a role in the management of Pelger–Huët anomaly which can be shown to result in neutrophil dysfunction (Park et al., 1977; Repo et al., 1979; Teshima et al., 1991). It may already have been beneficial in G-CSF-treated leukaemic, myelodysplastic and cancer patients with acquired morphological features of this condition.

Vadhan-Raj et al. (1990) treated a 13-year-old patient with GM-CSF to overcome a neutrophilic maturation defect and obtained responses by eosinophilic and monocytic lineages but not by neutrophils. This patient may have corresponded to the patients described by Kurzrock et al. (1991) who benefited, in terms of their neutrophil response, from a greatly reduced dose of GM-CSF (see above).

Recently, Wang et al. (1991) treated a patient with an inherited metabolic disorder, glycogen storage disease. Daily treatment with G-CSF for a period of 18 months reduced the severity and frequency of infections, eliminated mouth ulcers and greatly improved the quality of the patient's life. In leukocyte adhesion deficiency (LAD), the neutrophils are functionally deficient because they do not express integrin cell adhesion molecules at sufficiently high levels. *In vitro*, adhesion by LAD neutrophils is improved by treatment with GM-CSF and, *in vivo*, GM-CSF increased phagocyte margination and improved neutrophil phagocytosis and killing (Yong et al., 1991).

Idiopathic neutropenia

Treatment with G-CSF accomplished normalization of the absolute neutrophil count and improved neutrophil function, which removed the necessity for prophylactic antibiotics to prevent infection. This, of course, has the supplementary advantage of reducing the risk of antibiotic-resistant infections emerging. Treatment was continued for more than 6 months, during which time the neutrophil and monocyte counts oscillated in phase and there was evidence of cycling in the eosinophil, platelet and lymphocyte counts. The bone marrow changes were moderate but the number of GM-CFC fell on treatment. This, together with the cycling in the peripheral counts, could be a reflection of a reduced marrow reserve (Jakubowski et al., 1989).

Cyclic neutropenia

Granulocyte-CSF was effective in the treatment of cyclic neutropenia and reduced considerably the symptoms and signs of the illness (Hammond et al., 1989). Although the cycling persisted, the periodicity decreased and the number of days of severe neutropenia fell. In this study, treatment was maintained for more than 40 months without clinical side-effects. Studies of progenitor cells *in vitro* revealed an acute increase in circulating GM-CFC, and a lesser increase in circulating BFU-E after G-CSF treatment and there are indications that the progenitor populations in the marrow are increased as well. These acute changes followed each administration of G-CSF during a chronic course of therapy (Migliaccio et al., 1990).

Immune-mediated neutropenia

Granulocytopenia was corrected by GM-CSF treatment in Felty's syndrome (neutropenia plus splenomegaly and rheumatoid arthritis) but this caused a flare-up of the arthritis that was attributed to increased production of IL-6 (Hazenberg et al., 1989).

Certain patients suffer neutropenia or agranulocytosis associated with a T lymphocytosis and, in some cases, the lymphocytes or their soluble products have been shown to inhibit haemopoiesis *in vitro*. Such a pathophysiology could potentially interfere with any beneficial effects of HGF treatment. This seemed to be the case when a patient with agranulocytosis associated with a Tγ lymphocytosis failed to produce neutrophils in response to GM-CSF and his serum prevented autologous colony formation and the release of growth factors by his cells *in vitro* (Thomssen et al., 1989).

Treatment of thrombocytopenia with HGFs

Thrombocytopenia remains a serious problem in clinical management but recombinant HGFs for the megakaryocyte lineage are not yet available. The multilineage growth factors, IL-3 and GM-CSF, may be hoped to have some stimulatory effect on platelet production. Preliminary evidence from phase I/II trials indicates that platelet responses to IL-3 are found in patients with preserved bone marrow function and, more obviously, in patients with secondary bone marrow failure (Ganser et al., 1990a,b). Responses by megakaryocytic cells to GM-CSF have also been seen in haematologically normal patients

(Aglietta et al., 1991) and platelet responses to IL-1 have been documented in patients treated with 5-fluorouracil (see Starnes, 1991). In rhesus monkeys, sequential administration of IL-3 and IL-1 is a more effective stimulant of platelet production, maturation and release than either agent used alone (Monroy et al., 1991). There are indications from in vivo and in vitro experiments that erythropoietin has a genuine stimulatory effect on megakaryopoiesis (Berridge et al., 1988) as well as on erythropoiesis but clinical confirmation is not available. Interleukin 6 has megakaryopoiesis-stimulating activities and its effectiveness has been demonstrated in primates (Asano et al., 1990; Stahl et al., 1991), although IL-6-induced platelet production differs morphologically from physiologically accelerated platelet production and they should not be considered to be comparable processes. To date, the clinical potential of IL-6 has not been evaluated in humans. Similarly, effects of IL-11 on megakaryopoiesis have been indicated but not tested (Bruno et al., 1991).

Treatment of anaemia with HGFs

Erythropoietin was first used to treat anaemia in patients with renal disease but it is now being investigated for use in other anaemias associated with chronic non-malignant disease (Means et al., 1989), with haemopoietic disorders (e.g. MDS) or with treatment (e.g. chemotherapy) and in a variety of other clinical situations (Abels and Rudnick, 1991).

Erythropoietin is an effective treatment for anaemia in end-stage renal failure and the majority of patients achieve a rise in haematocrit and increases in transferrin uptake and reticulocyte counts. In general, transfusion requirements are reduced and it may be necessary to adjust the dose of erythropoietin to stabilize the haematocrit and avoid hypertension (Winearls et al., 1986; Eschbach et al., 1987). Some investigators (Winearls et al., 1986; Zins et al., 1986) have not observed the changes in white cell and platelet counts that have been seen by others (Bommer et al., 1987). These, in combination with the raised haematocrit, could potentially exacerbate the risk of thrombotic episodes in some patients.

Prolonged treatment with recombinant human erythropoietin (150–300 u/kg three times weekly) of patients with transfusion-dependent anaemia in end-stage renal disease first increases the number of CFU-E (4.2-fold), BFU-E (3.4-fold), GM-CFC (1.9-fold) and Mk-CFC (2-fold) compared with their respective concentrations in pretreatment marrows. These numerical changes were accompanied by a doubling of the percentage of cells in S-phase of the cell cycle measured by the thymidine suicide technique (Dessypris et al., 1988).

After several months of erythropoietin treatment, there is a fall in BFU-E numbers in the marrow to about 25% of pretreatment values but no decrease in circulating BFU-E. It has been suggested that this reduction in BFU-E numbers can be explained by failure to replace the lost progenitors from the stem cell compartment (Reid et al., 1988).

Erythropoietin has recently been used to treat patients with chronic anaemia associated with cancer (Ludwig et al., 1990; Miller et al., 1990) and to avoid chemotherapy-induced anaemia (Oster et al., 1990). The cancer patients had inappropriately low levels of erythropoietin in relation to their haemoglobin levels and treatment with erythropoietin improved the haemoglobin levels, corrected the anaemia and restored BFU-E numbers in the bone marrow and peripheral blood. Chronic anaemia is also associated with chronic infections and inflammatory conditions and the levels of erythropoietin in the serum are generally lower than would be expected for the haemoglobin levels in these patients. This suggests that erythropoietin might be useful in the anaemia of chronic disease and it has been tested in human immunodeficiency virus (HIV) infected patients (acquired immune deficiency syndrome; AIDS) and in rheumatoid arthritis. In clinical trials of erythropoietin in AIDS, patients with a serum erythropoietin level below 500 mu/ml responded to the treatment but those with higher erythropoietin levels did not, presumably because other factors were involved in the pathogenesis of the anaemia and blunted the response to endogenous and administered erythropoietin (Fischl et al., 1990; Abels and Rudnick, 1991). In rheumatoid arthritis, it has been reported that erythropoietin corrects the anaemia but this required higher doses than those needed to correct the same degree of anaemia in chronic renal failure (Pincus et al., 1990).

In sickle cell anaemia, erythropoietin might be expected to increase haemoglobin F (HbF) production, which would be beneficial because HbF inhibits the polymerization of deoxyhaemoglobin S. Although the anticipated effect was seen in one study of erythropoietin treatment (Al-Khatti et al., 1988), it was not seen in another, when no measurable benefit could be found (Goldberg et al., 1990). Experimental evidence from homozygous β-thalassaemic mice, which resemble human β-thalassaemia intermedia, suggests that erythropoietin treatment might modulate the globin chain imbalance in favour of β chain synthesis, increase the red cell mass and reduce erythrocyte abnormalities (Leroy-Viard et al., 1991). In a preliminary trial of erythropoietin treatment in patients with β-thalassaemia intermedia, there were elevations in haemoglobin concentration, haematocrit and red cell count but no changes in the α/β globin chain synthetic ratio or in HbF synthesis (Rachmilewitz et al., 1991).

Anaemia in premature infants is common and requires multiple blood transfusions. It may be caused by inadequate erythropoiesis, excessive phlebotomy for monitoring purposes or a low level of erythropoietin production by the kidney at this stage of development. It does not occur because of low numbers of erythroid progenitor cells (see Abels and Rudnick, 1991). The results of clinical trials suggest that erythropoietin treatment reduces transfusion requirements in infants with low requirements for phlebotomy (Halpern et al., 1990; Abels and Rudnick, 1991).

Finally, erythropoietin can be used to increase the numbers of units of blood that can be obtained from patients undergoing elective surgery so that it can be stored and used later for autologous transfusion. This procedure avoids the risks that accompany the use of blood transfusions from multiple donors (Goodnough, 1990). Its use in the perisurgical setting, to reduce the numbers of transfusions required by hastening red cell recovery, is under evaluation (Abels and Rudnick, 1991) and it has been used as an alternative to blood transfusion in a Jehovah's Witness (Rothstein et al., 1990). Erythropoietin may also provide a useful alternative to transfusion in patients with antibodies against potenial donors' cells. Its use in the treatment of other haematological disorders is discussed in the relevant sections.

Effects of HGF treatment on neoplastic cell growth

The expression of HGF receptors by a wide variety of malignant cell types, referred to earlier in this chapter, has led to concern that treatment with growth factors could stimulate tumour cell proliferation. So far, these fears have remained largely unfounded. However, a few instances of apparently increased malignant cell growth associated with HGF treatment have been reported.

First, several patients with myelodysplasia have experienced increases in blast cell count whilst on treatment and, in some, chemotherapy has been required (Hoelzer et al., 1988; Ganser et al., 1989b). Second, there was some evidence for increased tumour cell proliferation in two lymphoma patients treated with IL-3 but no obvious acceleration of tumour growth in patients with non-haematological malignancies (Ganser et al., 1990b).

Against this pessimistic view, administration of GM-CSF to cancer patients increased the numbers and function (secretion of TNFα and IFN and antibody-dependent cytotoxicity) of monocytes and increased primed superoxide release by neutrophils (Kaplan et al., 1989; Wing et al., 1989). An effect of GM-CSF on lymphocyte activation has been indicated by increases in lymphocyte counts, soluble IL-2 receptor levels and soluble CD8 levels (Ho et al., 1990). Also, G-CSF in vivo induces neutrophils to express high-affinity receptors for IgG (FcγR1;

CD64), which enables neutrophils to kill extracellular targets, and neutrophils from G-CSF-treated cancer patients have an increased capacity for antibody-dependent cellular cytotoxicity (Repp et al., 1991). These observations suggest that G-CSF and GM-CSF might, in selected circumstances, improve host defences against tumour cells and could explain the observation made by Steward et al. (1989) that metastatic disease stabilized or even regressed on GM-CSF therapy.

Treatment of myelodysplasia with HGFs

Patients with one or another of the MDS have been treated with GM-CSF or G-CSF. The MDS belong to a group of disorders characterized by progressive bone marrow failure associated with anaemia, neutropenia and thrombocytopenia. Cytopenia is the cause of death in many cases but AML develops in a proportion of them. Myelodysplasia is also known as preleukaemia for this reason.

Even in the early stages of the disease, haemopoiesis in MDS is clonal and in vitro data have indicated that myeloid progenitors in the abnormal clone are hyporesponsive to growth factors. The neutrophil defect can be overcome in culture by exposing the cells to high GM-CSF concentrations but erythroid, megakaryocytic and mixed-lineage colony numbers are not improved (Carlo-Stella et al., 1989; Mayani et al., 1989). Correction of neutropenia by GM-CSF therapy might therefore be anticipated, but not correction of anaemia and thrombocytopenia, which may require a combination of different HGFs. It is relevant that the production of factors stimulating pluripotent colony-forming cells in vitro is not impaired in MDS (Merchav et al., 1987), whereas megakaryocyte colony-stimulating activity is defective (Giessler et al., 1987).

A dose-dependent increase in leukocyte count has been seen in some patients treated with recombinant human GM-CSF (Vadhan-Raj et al., 1987, 1989a; Antin et al., 1988, 1990; Hoelzer et al., 1988; Ganser et al., 1989b). The earlier study reported by Vadhan-Raj et al. (1987) indicated that, in addition to marked increases in leukocyte count, there were considerable increases in red cell and platelet production, to the extent that two previously transfusion-dependent patients did not require red cell and platelet support for 20–27 weeks of follow-up. However, further investigation revealed that responses on this scale were limited to a minority (1/8) of MDS patients (Vadhan-Raj et al., 1989). The other studies have shown very little, if any, effect on reticulocytes and platelets. Treatment with GM-CSF may increase or decrease marrow fibrosis in patients with this complication, although an increase does not preclude a haematological response (Antin et al., 1990).

Several patients, particularly those with higher blast cell counts in the marrow at the beginning of treatment, have developed increases in blast cell concentration and, in some cases, low-dose cytotoxic chemotherapy with cytosine arabinoside has become necessary (Hoelzer et al., 1988; Ganser et al., 1989b). In response to the unwanted effects of GM-CSF on the blast cell populations, Estey et al. (1991) evaluated the effects of low-dose subcutaneous treatment, starting at 5 µg/m^2 and escalating in patients who did not show a haematological response. However, increases in blasts and reductions in platelets were still seen. Ganser and colleagues (1991) evaluated the effects of GM-CSF and IL-3 on clonal and non-clonal haemopoiesis using restriction fragment length polymorphisms (RFLPs) of the phosphoglycerate kinase and hypoxanthine phosphoribosyl transferase genes (see Chapter 2) in combination with karyotyping. Results varied from patient to patient and ranged from persistence of monoclonality to totally non-clonal cell populations in the peripheral blood. In contrast to these cases, a patient with therapy-related MDS who was studied by Vadhan-Raj et al. (1989b) remained in polyclonal, cytogenetically normal remission for nearly a year after GM-CSF treatment. These observations show that GM-CSF treatment elicits a variety of responses in MDS patients and occasionally stimulates non-clonal haemopoiesis.

Treatment of MDS patients with escalating doses of G-CSF results in dose-related increases in neutrophil count in most cases but the counts fall to baseline levels once the treatment is stopped (Negrin et al., 1989). Prolonged treatment with G-CSF is needed if the counts are to be maintained and maintenance therapy can produce responses lasting from 3 to 16 months with attendant reductions in bacterial infections and decreased red cell transfusion requirements. Myeloid maturation indices in the marrow improved in responding patients but 3/18 converted to acute myeloid leukaemia whilst on treatment. The persistence of cytogenetic abnormalities during the clinical response suggested that G-CSF might have induced maturation of the abnormal clone and, in one case, this maturation-inducing effect was confirmed by RFLP analysis of X-linked genes (Negrin et al., 1990).

Erythropoietin has been used to treat MDS patients in an attempt to alleviate their anaemia but only a few patients respond with an increase in haematocrit. An increase in marrow erythropoiesis has been seen morphologically, suggesting that ineffective red cell production is stimulated, but no change in BFU-E or CFU-E numbers in the blood or bone marrow has been reported. It is still possible that erythropoietin will be useful in a subgroup of patients and ways of identifying them are needed (Hirashima et al., 1989; Bowen et al., 1991; Schouten et al., 1991).

Treatment of acute myeloid leukaemia with HGFs

Haemopoietic growth factors have not been widely used in the treatment of AML. Whilst they might be expected to improve normal haematological recovery they may, as we have discussed, also stimulate the growth of the leukaemic cell population. Cautious administration of GM-CSF after completion of induction chemotherapy failed to have any beneficial effect on infections, complete remission rate or neutrophil recovery. Neither was there any detectable increase in the regrowth of the leukaemic cells (Estey et al., 1990). Relapsed or elderly (over 65 years old) patients have been given GM-CSF after chemotherapy to ameliorate neutropenia, with the result that the complete remission rate was increased and the early death rate was reduced. Marked regrowth of leukaemic cells occurred in two of the 30 patients but, in one of them, did not seem to be associated with the GM-CSF therapy; in the other the reappearance of the leukaemia was reversible (Buchner et al., 1991).

Treatment with G-CSF following remission-induction chemotherapy for leukaemia enhanced neutrophil recovery. There was no consistent effect on the blast cell count and it is difficult to attribute any increases or decreases in blast cells to the administration of G-CSF (Teshima et al., 1989). There has been one prospective randomized trial in patients with relapsed or refractory leukaemia and the results indicated that neutrophil recovery was improved, infections were reduced and there was no evidence of leukaemic cell stimulation (Ohno et al., 1990).

Granulocyte CSF has been used as treatment in a patient with hypoplastic AML who was not sufficiently fit to receive high-dose chemotherapy. The patient entered complete remission, possibly as a result of a differentiation-inducing effect of the G-CSF, with neutrophilia followed by a stable neutrophil count and normal cell differentiation (Toki et al., 1989). Another patient who did not achieve remission on chemotherapy and developed septicaemia and ARDS was treated with high-dose methylprednisolone and G-CSF. His illness resolved and he entered a complete remission (Sugawara et al., 1991). Thus, G-CSF might be a useful therapeutic option in hypoplastic AML, for which there is no known cure, and in patients who do not enter remission on chemotherapy and are too sick to receive further cytoreductive treatment. However, in view of the information about the response of AML blasts to G-CSF, this approach should perhaps be reserved for patients for whom there is no reasonable alternative.

Exposure to GM-CSF increases the drug sensitivity of AML cells (Cannistra et al., 1989) and it has been suggested that a strategy could be developed involving combinations of growth factors and cell cycle-active drugs. The success of this approach would depend on the drug sensitivity of normal haemopoietic cells not being increased to the same extent as that of the leukaemic cells. *In vivo* recruitment of leukaemic cells into drug-sensitive phases of the cell cycle has been demonstrated in AML patients treated with GM-CSF 24–48 hours before chemotherapy and GM-CSF given to the same patients after cytotoxic chemotherapy enhanced recovery of the neutrophil count. The combined treatment produced complete aplasia 14 days after chemotherapy, and two patients died from fungal infection during this period, but the remission rate for the group (18 patients) was 83% (Bettelheim *et al.*, 1991).

Treatment of non-myeloid leukaemias with HGFs

Glaspy *et al.* (1988) treated hairy cell leukaemia patients with IFN plus G-CSF with the result that neutrophil recovery from the myelosuppressive effects of the IFN occurred within 2–4 weeks instead of 2–3 months. Erythropoietin has been used to treat anaemia in patients with myeloma and responses have been seen in those with lower basal serum erythropoietin levels (Ludwig *et al.*, 1990).

Treatment of infections with HGFs

Infection is a major cause of death in cancer patients and the incidence of bacterial and fungal infections is a function of the duration and severity of neutropenia (Gerson *et al.*,1984; Pizzo, 1984). Neutropenia is also associated with most forms of cancer therapy and follows bone marrow transplantation. Improvement of the neutrophil count using HGFs would be of tremendous benefit to these groups of patients and has indeed proved effective in combating infections. Also, treatment with GM-CSF can enable cytopenic patients to undergo procedures such as dental surgery (Vadhan-Raj *et al.*, 1989b) which would otherwise be dangerous.

The demonstration that neutrophil migration is reduced during GM-CSF administration (Peters *et al.*, 1988) means that neutrophils might not localize properly to areas of infection in GM-CSF-treated patients. However, neutrophil localization to a site of invasive fungal infection has been shown in a patient given the xanthine derivative pentoxyfylline in addition to GM-CSF (Montgomery *et al.*, 1991). In this case, the pentoxyfylline may have prevented the GM-CSF-mediated inhibition of neutrophil migration and adhesion. Recent results from a phase I trial of M-CSF suggest that this factor also may have a role in the treatment of fungal infections (Nemunaitis *et al.*, 1991b).

Since GM-CSF can activate macrophages, it is conceivable that it might restrict viral infection in these cells. This concept has been applied to HIV infection in particular, although there are conflicting reports on the effect of GM-CSF on the replication and expression of HIV *in vitro* (Hammer *et al.*, 1986; Folks *et al.*, 1987). Also, in some studies of AIDS patients treated with GM-CSF, monitoring for HIV p24 antigen levels in plasma and culturing peripheral blood mononuclear cells for production of the virus produced no firm evidence for either suppression or enhancement in the presence of GM-CSF *in vivo* (Mitsuyasu *et al.*, 1988). In other studies, significant increases in circulating p24 antigen have been found in response to GM-CSF (Pluda *et al.*, 1990). Results of an *in vitro* study on infected normal stem cells suggest that GM-CSF and IL-3 can enhance virus production but that G-CSF does not (Kitano *et al.*, 1991).

Intravenous or subcutaneous administration of GM-CSF to patients with AIDS or AIDS-related complex achieved dose-related increments in leukocyte counts, most of which were neutrophils. However, they fell to pretreatment levels when the infusions were stopped. There was little effect on the numbers of monocytes or lymphocytes or on the ratio of helper:suppressor T cells and no alterations in red cells or platelets (Groopman *et al.*, 1987; Mitsuyasu *et al.*, 1988). In combination with the thymidine analogue AZT (otherwise known as zidovudine or azidothymidine), GM-CSF reduced the myelotoxicity associated with the treatment and apparently enhanced its antiviral activity (Pluda *et al.*, 1990). Also, the combined effects of G-CSF and erythropoietin decreased neutropenia and anaemia with no apparent effect of HIV expression on the therapeutic efficiency of AZT (Miles *et al.*, 1991).

The role of HGF therapy in the management of AIDS patients remains to be established but the increase in leukocyte count can be expected to allow treatment with myelotoxic antibiotics or antiviral agents and to decrease morbidity and mortality due to opportunistic infections. The beneficial effects of HGF therapy on infections associated with various neutropenias have been described earlier in this chapter and its role in the management of neutropenias following chemotherapy and bone marrow transplantation is discussed in the next two sections.

The value of HGFs in chemotherapy

Myelotoxicity is the most important dose–limiting factor in chemotherapy and often prevents patients from receiving clinically effective antitumour treatment. It is in this area that HGF therapy has found one of its most significant applications and its value is now well-

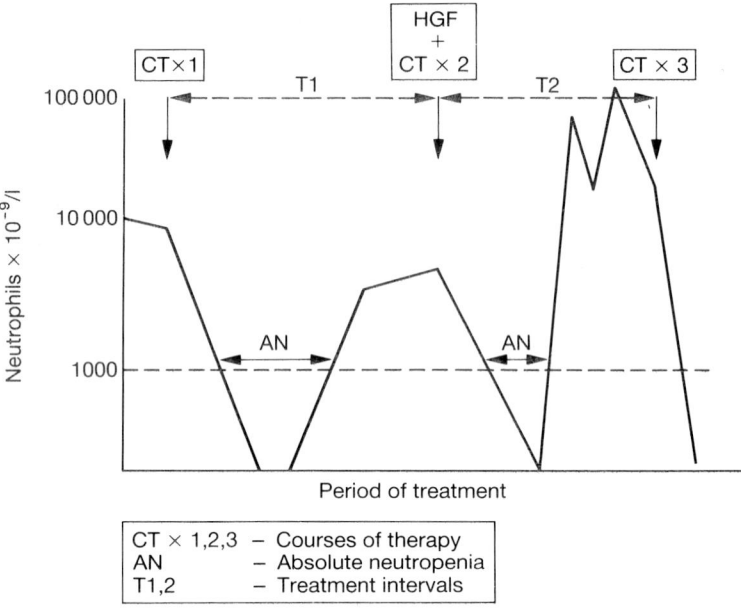

Fig. 5.1 Effect of growth factors on neutrophil recovery and timing of chemotherapy.

established. Favourable results have been obtained using GM-CSF and G-CSF and, in general terms, they reduce the duration and degree of neutropenia following chemotherapy and, consequently, the risks of infection. As a result, the time period between courses of chemotherapy can be reduced so that patients can receive more chemotherapy in a given time. These improvements can be expected to improve the efficiency of cancer chemotherapy. It is not yet clear, however, if treatment with different drugs requires the same or different growth factor therapy to improve haematological recovery. Experiments in mice indicate that the required HGFs may depend on the type of chemotherapy (Mizushima et al., 1990) and this is likely to correspond to the level of damage in the haemopoietic system.

By treating patients with alternating courses of chemotherapy with and chemotherapy without HGFs they can act as their own controls and the effects of the HGFs can be evaluated internally (Fig. 5.1). In this way, GM-CSF was shown to result in less suppression of neutrophil and platelet counts in patients with soft tissue sarcomas (Antman et al., 1988). In patients with myeloma treated with high-dose melphalan, GM-CSF hastens haematological recovery in younger patients who have received relatively little therapy, presumably because they have sufficient marrow reserve to respond to the treatment (Barlogie et al., 1990).

Bronchud et al. (1987) demonstrated that G-CSF treatment resulted in faster and greater neutrophil recovery after chemotherapy and, in addition to improvements in granulocyte counts, Morstyn et al. (1988, 1989) noted increases in monocytes, lymphocytes and immature myeloid cells in cancer patients who were given G-CSF and melphalan. The major effect on the marrow was an increase in the proportion of early myeloid cells, particularly promyelocytes and myelocytes, and a decrease in the proportion of mature myeloid cells. Also, G-CSF administration reduced the severity of oral mucositis in patients treated with a combination of methotrexate, vinblastine, doxorubicin and cisplatin (Gabrilove et al., 1988).

A phase I trial of IL-1β, alone or in combination with myelosuppressive doses of 5-fluorouracil, has been conducted in patients with gastrointestinal cancer (Crown et al., 1991). Although there were fewer days of neutropenia following 5-fluorouracil plus IL-1β than following 5-fluorouracil alone, this difference did not achieve statistical significance.

The value of HGFs in bone marrow transplantation

In autologous or allogeneic bone marrow transplantation, the intended outcome of HGF therapy is to reduce the period of severe neutropenia immediately postgraft and decrease morbidity and mortality resulting from opportunistic infections. In the context of bone marrow transplantation, it is relevant that plasma collected from marrow recipients regularly stimulates proliferation of GM-CFC and Mk-CFC with peak activities 7-21 days after marrow infusion. Erythroid burst-promoting activity is occasionally found and stimulators of GEMM-CFC are rare. Values usually return to pretransplant levels by the 30th day in patients with prompt engraftment but remain higher in patients with delayed engraftment (Messner, 1988).

The influence of HGFs on postgraft reconstitution in recipients of allogeneic marrow does not appear to have been as widely studied as it has been in recipients of autologous marrow. One study has shown that G-CSF accelerates neutrophil and monocyte recovery with no effect on platelets and reticulocytes (Teshima et al., 1989). In another study, human urinary CSF reduced the time taken for neutrophil recovery in patients treated by allogeneic bone marrow transplantation (Masaoka et al., 1988). Nemunaitis et al. (1991a) have reported a phase I/II trial of recombinant GM-CSF given daily to recipients of allogeneic bone marrow grafts. The patients received two different types of GVHD prophylaxis, with and without methotrexate which is myelotoxic. Those patients whose treatment did not include methotrexate, compared with those whose treatment did include methotrexate, had faster neutrophil recovery, fewer febrile days, a shorter period of hospitalization and no increase in GVHD. Erythropoietin has been used to alleviate anaemia in a patient treated for CML by ABO-incompatible bone marrow transplantation (Heyll et al., 1991). The use of erythropoietin after allogeneic bone marrow transplantation is further indicated by the inappropriately low erythropoietin levels seen in allogeneic transplant recipients (Beguin et al., 1991).

Recombinant human GM-CSF has been given to patients with breast cancer or malignant melanoma following aggressive chemotherapy and autologous bone marrow rescue (Brandt et al., 1988). The nadir in the white cell count was reduced and myeloid recovery was accelerated. There was no effect on the platelet count and the neutrophil count fell on withdrawal of GM-CSF therapy. Nevertheless, even transient elevations in the neutrophil count can help to combat infections and a reduction in the duration of neutropenia can shorten the period of hospitalization for transplanted patients (Appelbaum et al., 1988; Nemunaitis et al., 1988). In lymphoma patients given GM-CSF after autologous marrow, studies on progenitor populations showed reductions in the levels of GM-CFC and BFU-E in the blood and marrow 60–90 days after treatment, which may have resulted from mature cell production at the expense of progenitor cell expansion (Lazarus et al., 1991).

It has become clear that the growth factors used clinically do not abolish the early phase of absolute neutropenia (neutrophils less than $100/mm^3$) after marrow transplantation (Fig. 5.2). It is at this stage

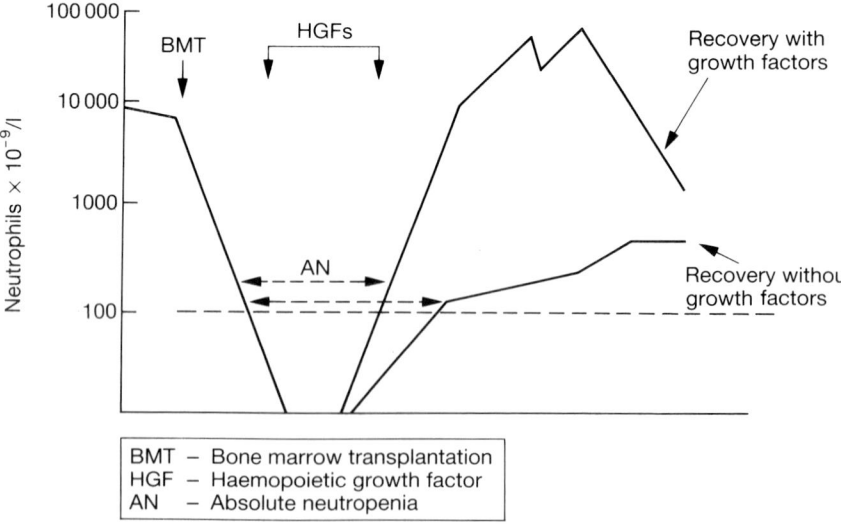

Fig. 5.2 Influence of growth factors on absolute neutropenia and neutrophil recovery following bone marrow transplantation.

that most fatal complications become established and other measures are required to solve the problem. Suggestions include the *in vitro* incubation of marrow with growth factors to raise the numbers of granulocyte precursors prior to infusion (Dicke *et al.*, 1991).

Treatment with growth factors offers a potential alternative to supportive care or a second transplant in patients whose grafts have failed. Using this approach with GM-CSF, Nemunaitis *et al.* (1990) obtained increases in neutrophil numbers and function with consequent reductions in infection and increased survival. Importantly, there was no evidence for an increase in leukaemic relapse rate and no exacerbation of GVHD in patients initially treated with allogeneic marrow. Similarly, 50% of patients with markedly delayed (more than 55 days) engraftment after autologous bone marrow transplantation benefit from treatment with GM-CSF (Brandwein *et al.*, 1991). Even more striking are indications that treatment with GM-CSF may entirely replace the need for autologous transplantation following high-dose BEAM (carmustine, etoposide, cytosine arabinoside, melphalan) therapy for non-Hodgkin's lymphoma (Láporte *et al.*, 1991). This strategy was used because blood and bone marrow involvement precluded autografting and may offer an alternative in some cases. However, one possible disadvantage of this approach is that the recovering stem cells would have been exposed to the full impact of the chemotherapy, rather than being harvested for autografting and hence protected, and this extra damage may manifest itself as an increase in secondary treatment-related leukaemias.

In patients given autografts purged (see Chapter 6) of ALL cells using 4-hydroperoxycyclophosphamide, which depletes the marrow of colony-forming progenitor cells, the response to GM-CSF was related to the numbers of residual GM-CFC infused (Blazar *et al.*, 1989). This emphasizes the necessity of providing target cell populations for responses to growth factors. Similarly, in cases of graft failure, patients who originally received chemically purged autografts failed to respond to GM-CSF, whereas recipients of unpurged marrow or marrow purged using monoclonal antibodies did respond (Nemunaitis *et al.*, 1990).

Several phase III clinical trials of GM-CSF treatment following autologous bone marrow transplantation for lymphoma have now been completed (see Rabinowe *et al.*, 1991). Neutrophil recovery was hastened in the treatment arm, although the time taken for the first neutrophil to appear was no shorter. Benefits included a reduction in infections and use of antibiotics and the recipients of GM-CSF were able to leave hospital more rapidly than recipients of placebo. The effect on platelet recovery seen in phase I/II trials was not confirmed in the phase III trial and the toxicities observed were essentially the same in the treatment and placebo groups.

There are fewer reports of the use of G-CSF in autologous transplantation (see Rabinowe et al., 1991, for references). In these studies there is an apparent increase in neutrophil recovery with reduction in fever and infection but no effect on platelet recovery.

Another application of GM-CSF and G-CSF exploits their capacity, alone or in combination with chemotherapy, to expand the pool of circulating progenitors. These cells can be harvested by leukapheresis and used as an autograft to rescue patients from chemotherapy-induced cytopenias (Socinski et al., 1988; Gianni et al., 1989, 1990; Davis and Morstyn, 1991). This manoeuvre can result in complete haematological recovery and it has been shown in an animal model that the circulating progenitor cells include long-term marrow-repopulating cells (Molineaux et al., 1990). In humans, the GM-CSF-induced circulating cells include CD34-positive, CD33-negative cells, which indicates that primitive cells are present (Siena et al., 1989).

OVERVIEW

The clinical benefits of HGF therapy are listed in Table 5.3. The HGFs GM-CSF and G-CSF are now firmly established in the clinical management of the neutropenic complications of cancer treatment and bone marrow transplantation. Erythropoietin has a longer history of effectiveness in the treatment of anaemia and its applications have now extended beyond the management of the anaemia of renal disease. Macrophage CSF has only recently been tested using the recombinant protein in phase I studies. In general, at least for short-term administration and at the doses used clinically, toxicity problems have been remarkable for their absence, as might be expected for biological agents of this type.

None the less, many questions remain regarding the further use of the HGFs and relate to definition of dose–response relationships *in vivo*, the choice of the most appropriate factor in different cytopenic situations and the inability of the HGFs to eliminate the early total neutropenia following bone marrow transplantation and high-dose

Table 5.3 Clinical benefits of haemopoietic growth factor therapy

Amelioration of neutropenia and infection
Improvements in chemotherapy
  Prevention of dose reduction
  Increased frequency of chemotherapy cycles
  Dose intensification
Treatment of bone marrow failure
Improved recovery after bone marrow transplantation
Mobilization of stem cells into peripheral blood for harvesting and autografting
Possible alternative to autografting

chemotherapy. Little information is available concerning the effects of prolonged administration, although it is clear from animal experiments that exposure to high HGF doses *in vivo* does not, by itself, precipitate leukaemic transformation. It is equally clear from experiments using transgenic mice and transplantation of cells expressing growth factor genes that severe toxicities can be produced in these artificial systems (see earlier in this chapter). However, the toxicities are seen only when the HGF levels are very high and the localization of the HGFs is not physiologically controlled. Perhaps this is a consequence of the use of recombinant growth factors which may not be susceptible to the 'damping' mechanisms, such as binding to extracellular matrix or to carrier molecules, described in Chapter 1. There is little evidence to suggest that the prolonged use of growth factors in chronic disorders can lead to eventual stem cell exhaustion but this possibility has not been tested thoroughly and should not be discounted at present. It is noteworthy that the use of HGFs (GM-CSF, G-CSF and erythropoietin) to sustain high levels of haemopoietic activity for 3 weeks in mice led to increased osteoclast numbers, enlargement of the medullary cavity and a reduction in bone thickness (Lee *et al.*, 1991). This finding may be relevant to the bone pain experienced by many patients treated with HGFs and bone modulation could be a possible deleterious effect of long-term clinical administration.

The role of the HGFs in the therapy of myeloid leukaemia is rather uncertain. Several of the HGF genes and their receptors are proto-oncogenes and the autocrine production of growth factors has been implicated as one step in the pathogenesis of AML. Furthermore, HGF receptor expression and responsiveness have been demonstrated *in vitro* for AML cells and for a wide variety of other malignant cell types. No serious problems have arisen from the (limited) clinical use of HGFs in AML or in patients with solid tumours in terms of stimulating neoplastic cell proliferation but the increased blast cell count in some myelodysplastic patients gives cause for concern.

So far, the great majority of the reported clinical trials have been unrandomized and uncontrolled and some of the available information remains anecdotal. Randomized trials are now in progress to confirm the clinical observations and benefits in large groups of unselected patients. It is unlikely that single-agent therapy will produce the maximum effect. The realization that combinations of growth factors can act synergistically *in vitro* has led to a limited number of *in vivo* experiments and phase I trials of more than one factor given simultaneously (Donahue *et al.*, 1988; Giessler *et al.*, 1990). It can be anticipated that the next generation of clinical trials will address the complicated questions of synergistic activities and the most effective dosing, sequencing and timing of administration.

REFERENCES

Abels RI, Rudnick SA (1991) Erythropoietin: evolving clinical applications. *Experimental Hematology* 19, 842.

Aglietta M, Monzeglio C, Piacibello W et al. (1990) GM-CSF: intravenous versus subcutaneous treatment. *Leukemia* 4, 523.

Aglietta M, Monzeglio C, Sanavio F et al. (1991) In vivo effect of human granulocyte-macrophage colony-stimulating factor on megakaryocytopoiesis. *Blood* 77, 1991.

Al-Khatti A, Umemura T, Clow J et al. (1988) Erythropoietin stimulates F-reticulocyte formation in sickle cell anaemia. *Transactions of the Association of American Physicians* 101, 54.

Anagnostou A, Lee ES, Kessiman N, Levinson R, Steiner M (1990) Erythropoietin has a mitogenic and a positive chemotactic effect on endothelial cells. *Proceedings of the National Academy of Sciences of the USA* 87, 5978.

Andrews RG, Bartelmez SH, Egrie JE, Bernstein ID, Zsebo KM (1990) Recombinant human stem cell factor (RHSCF) stimulates in vitro and in vivo hematopoiesis in baboons. *Blood* 76, 130a.

Antin JH, Smith BR, Holmes W, Rosenthal DS (1988) Phase I/II study of recombinant human granulocyte-macrophage colony-stimulating factor in aplastic anemia and myelodysplastic syndrome. *Blood* 72, 705.

Antin JH, Weinberg DS, Rosenthal DS (1990) Variable effect of recombinant human granulocyte-macrophage colony-stimulating factor on bone marrow fibrosis in patients with myelodysplasia. *Experimental Hematology* 18, 266.

Appelbaum FR, Nemunaitis J, Singer J (1988) Recombinant human granulocyte-macrophage colony-stimulating factor (rhGM-CSF) following autologous marrow transplantation in man. *Proceedings of the American Society of Clinical Oncology* 7, 231.

Asano S, Urabe A, Okabe T et al. (1977) Demonstration of granulopoietic factor(s) in the plasma of nude mice transplanted with human lung cancer and in the tumour tissue. *Blood* 49, 845.

Asano S, Okano A, Ozawa K et al. (1990) In vivo effects of recombinant interleukin-6 in primates: stimulated production of platelets. *Blood* 75, 1602.

Atkinson K, Matias C, Guiffre A et al. (1991) In vivo administration of granulocyte colony-stimulating factor (GM-CSF), granulocyte-macrophage CSF, interleukin-1 (IL-1) and IL-4, alone and in combination, after allogeneic murine hematopoietic stem cell transplantation. *Blood* 77, 1376.

Bagglioni M, Walz A, Kunkel SL (1989) Neutrophil-activating peptide-1/interleukin 8, a novel cytokine that activates neutrophils. *Journal of Clinical Investigation* 84, 1045.

Bajorin DF, Cheung N-KV, Houghton AN (1991) Macrophage colony-stimulating factor: biological effects and potential applications for cancer therapy. *Seminars in Hematology* 28, 42.

Baldwin GC, Gasson JC, Kaufman SE et al. (1989) Nonhematopoietic tumor cells express functional CSF receptors. *Blood* 73, 1033.

Baldwin GC, Golde DW, Widhopf GF, Economou J, Gasson JC (1991) Identification and characterisation of low-affinity granulocyte-macrophage colony-stimulating factor receptor on primary and cultured human melanoma cells. *Blood* 78, 609.

Barlogie B, Jagannath S, Dixon DO et al. (1990) High-dose melphalan and granulocyte-macrophage colony-stimulating factor for refractory multiple myeloma. *Blood* 76, 677.

Begley CG, Metcalf D, Nicola NA (1987) Purified colony stimulating factors (G-CSF and GM-CSF) induce differentiation in human HL60 leukemic cells with suppression of clonogenicity. *International Journal of Cancer* 39, 99.

Beguin Y, Glemons GK, Oris R, Fillet G (1991) Circulating erythropoietin levels after bone marrow transplantation: inappropriate response to anemia in allogeneic transplants. *Blood* 77, 868.

Berdel WE, Danhauser-Riedl S, Steinhauser G, Winton EF (1989) Various human hematopoietic growth factors (interleukin-3, GM-CSF, G-CSF) stimulate clonal growth of nonhematopoietic tumor cells. *Blood* 73, 80.

Berridge MV, Fraser JK, Carter JM, Lin F-K (1988) Effects of recombinant erythropoietin on megakaryocytes and on platelet production in the rat. *Blood* 72, 970.

Bettelheim P, Valent P, Andreef M et al. (1991) Recombinant human granulocyte-macrophage colony-stimulating factor in combination with standard induction chemotherapy in de novo acute myeloid leukemia. *Blood* 77, 700.

Blaise D, Maraninchi D, Mawas C et al. (1989) Prevention of acute graft-versus-host disease by monoclonal antibody to interleukin-2 receptor. *Lancet* ii, 1333.

Blazar BR, Widmer MB, Soderling CCB, Gillis S, Vallera DA (1988) Enhanced survival but reduced engraftment in murine recipients of recombinant granulocyte/macrophage colony-stimulating factor following transplantation of T-cell depleted histoincompatible bone marrow. *Blood* 72, 1148.

Blazar BR, Kersey JH, McGlave PB et al. (1989) In vivo administration of recombinant human granulocyte/macrophage colony-stimulating factor in acute lymphoblastic leukaemia patients receiving purged autografts. *Blood* 73, 849.

Bommer J, Muller-Buhl E, Ritz E, Eifert J (1987) Recombinant human erythropoietin in anaemic patients on haemodialysis. *Lancet* i, 392.

Bonilla MA, Gillio AP, Ruggeiro M et al. (1989) Effects of recombinant human granulocyte colony-stimulating factor on neutropenia in patients with congenital agranulocytosis. *New England Journal of Medicine* 320, 1574.

Bowen D, Culligan D, Jacobs A (1991) The treatment of anaemia in the myelodysplastic syndromes with recombinant human erythropoietin. *British Journal of Haematology* 77, 419.

Brandt SJ, Peters WP, Atwater SK et al. (1988) Effect of recombinant human granulocyte-macrophage colony-stimulating factor on hematopoietic reconstitution after high-dose chemotherapy and autologous bone marrow transplantation. *New England Journal of Medicine* 318, 869.

Brandwein JM, Nayar R, Baker MA et al. (1991) GM-CSF therapy for delayed engraftment after autologous bone marrow transplantation. *Experimental Hematology* 19, 191.

Bronchud MH, Scarffe JA, Thatcher N et al. (1987) A phase I/II study of recombinant granulocyte colony-stimulating factor in patients receiving intensive chemotherapy for small cell lung cancer. *British Journal of Cancer* 56, 809.

Bruno E, Briddell RA, Cooper RJ, Hoffman R (1991) Effects of recombinant interleukin-II on human megakaryocyte progenitor cells. *Experimental Hematology* 19, 378.

Buchner T, Hiddemann W, Koenigsmann M et al. (1991) Recombinant human granulocyte-macrophage colony-stimulating factor after chemotherapy in elderly patients with acute leukemia or after relapse. *Blood* 78, 1190.

Bussolino F, Wang JM, Defillippi P et al. (1989) Granulocyte and granulocyte-macrophage-colony stimulating factors induce endothelial cells to migrate and proliferate. *Nature* 337, 471.

Cannistra SA, Groshek P, Griffin JD (1989) Granulocyte-macrophage colony-stimulating factor enhances the cytotoxic effects of cytosine arabinoside in acute myeloblastic leukemia and in the myeloid blast crisis phase of chronic myeloid leukemia. *Leukemia* 3, 328.

Cannistra SA, Koenigsman M, DiCarlo J, Groshek P, Griffin JD (1990) Differentiation-associated expression of two functionally distinct classes of granulocyte-macrophage colony-stimulating factor receptors by human myeloid cells. *Journal of Biological Chemistry* 265, 12656.

Carlo-Stella C, Cazzola M, Bergamaschi G et al. (1989) Growth of human hematopoietic colonies from patients with myelodysplastic syndromes in response to recombinant human granulocyte-macrophage colony-stimulating factor. *Leukemia* 3, 363.

Carron JA, Cawley JC (1989) IL-2 and myelopoiesis: IL-2 induces blast cell proliferation in some cases of acute myeloid leukaemia. *British Journal of Haematology* 73, 168.

Champlin RE, Nimer SD, Oette D, Golde DW (1988) Granulocyte-macrophage colony-stimulating factor (GM-CSF) treatment for aplastic anemia (AA) or agranulocytosis. *Experimental Hematology* 16, 519a.

Champlin RE, Nimer SD, Ireland P, Oette DH, Golde DW (1989) Treatment of refractory aplastic anemia with recombinant granulocyte-macrophage colony-stimulating factor. *Blood* 73, 694.

Chang JM, Johnson GR (1991) Effects on spleen colony-forming unit self-renewal after retroviral-mediated gene transfer of multi-colony-stimulating factor, granulocyte-macrophage colony-stimulating factor and granulocyte colony-stimulating factor. *Experimental Hematology* 19, 602.

Chang JM, Metcalf D, Lang RA, Gonda TJ, Johnson GR (1989a) Nonneoplastic hematopoietic myeloproliferative syndrome induced by dysregulated multi-CSF (IL-3) expression. *Blood* 73, 1487.

Chang JM, Metcalf D, Gonda TJ, Johnson GR (1989b) Long-term exposure to retrovirally expressed granulocyte colony-stimulating factor induces a nonneoplastic granulocyte and progenitor cell hyperplasia without tissue damage in mice. *Journal of Clinical Investigation* 84, 1488.

Craddock CF, Apperley JF, Corbo M, Gordon MY (1990) Long term reconstituting capacity of circulating murine stem cells mobilised by cyclophosphamide. *Experimental Hematology* 18, 24a.

Crown J, Jakubowski A, Kemeny M et al. (1991) A phase I trial of recombinant interleukin-1β alone and in combination with myelosuppressive doses of 5-fluorouracil in patients with gastrointestinal cancer. *Blood* 78, 1420.

Curtis BM, Williams DE, Broxmeyer HE et al. (1991) Enhanced hematopoietic activity of a human granulocyte/macrophage colony-stimulating factor – interleukin 3 fusion protein. *Proceedings of the National Academy of Sciences of the USA* 88, 5809.

Cynshi O, Satoh K, Higuchi M, Imai N, Kawaguchi T, Hirashima K (1990) Effects of recombinant human erythropoietin on anaemic W/Wv and Sl/Sld mice. *British Journal of Haematology* 75, 319.

Davis I, Morstyn G (1991) The role of granulocyte colony-stimulating factor in cancer chemotherapy. *Seminars in Hematology* 28, 25.

Dedhar S, Gaboury L, Galloway P, Eaves C (1988) Human granulocyte-macrophage colony-stimulating factor is a growth factor active on a variety of cell types of nonhemopoietic origin. *Proceedings of the National Academy of Sciences of the USA* 85, 9253.

Delwel R, Dorssers L, Tour I, Wagenaker G, Lorrenberg B (1987) Human recombinant multilineage colony stimulating factor (interleukin 3): stimulator of acute myelocytic leukemia progenitor cells in vitro. *Blood* 70, 333.

Dessypris EN, Graber SE, Krantz SB, Stone WJ (1988) Effects of recombinant erythropoietin on the concentration and cycling status of human marrow hematopoietic progenitor cells in vivo. *Blood* 72, 2060.

Devereaux S, Linch DC, Campos Costa D, Spittle MF, Jellife AM (1987) Transient leukopenia induced by granulocyte-macrophage colony-stimulating factor. *Lancet* ii, 1523.

Dibirdik I, Langlie M-C, Ledbetter J et al. (1991) Engagement of interleukin-7 receptor stimulates tyrosine phosphorylation, phosphinositide turnover and clonal proliferation of human T-lineage acute lymphoblastic leukaemia cells. *Blood* 78, 564.

Dicke KA, Jackson J, Murphy B (1991) The use of hematopoietic growth factors in autologous marrow transplantation. *Experimental Hematology* 19, 416a.

Digel W, Schmid M, Heil G, Conrad P, Gillis S, Porzsolt F (1991) Human interleukin-7 induces proliferation of neoplastic cells from chronic lymphocytic leukemia and acute leukemias. *Blood* 78, 753.

Dinarello CA (1991) Interleukin-1 and interleukin-1 antagonism. *Blood* 77, 1627.

Donahue RE, Seehra J, Metzger M et al. (1988) Human IL-3 and GM-CSF act synergistically in stimulating hematopoiesis in primates. *Science* 241, 1820.

Duhrsen U, Villeval J-L, Boyd J, Kannourakis G, Morstyn G, Metcalf D (1988) Effects of recombinant human granulocyte colony-stimulating factor on hematopoietic progenitor cells in cancer patients. *Blood* 72, 2074.

Eschbach JW, Egrie JC, Downing MR, Browne JK, Adamson JW (1987) Correction of the anemia of end-stage renal disease with recombinant human erythropoietin. *New England Journal of Medicine* 316, 73.

Estey EH, Dixon D, Kantarjian HM et al. (1990) Treatment of poor-prognosis, newly diagnosed acute myeloid leukemia with ara-C and recombinant human granulocyte-macrophage colony-stimulating factor. *Blood* 75, 1766.

Estey EH, Kurzrock R, Talpaz M et al. (1991) Effects of low doses of recombinant human granulocyte-macrophage colony-stimulating factor (GM-CSF) in patients with myelodysplastic syndromes. *British Journal of Haematology* 77, 291.

Estrov Z, Kurzrock R, Wetzler M et al. (1991) Suppression of chronic myelogenous leukemia colony growth by interleukin-1 (IL-1) receptor agonist and soluble IL-1 receptors: a novel application for inhibitors of IL-1 activity. *Blood* 78, 1476.

Fabian I, Kletter Y, Slavin S (1988) Therapeutic potential of recombinant granulocyte-macrophage colony-stimulating factor and interleukin-3 in murine B-cell leukemia. *Blood* 72, 913.

Faisal M, Cumberland W, Champlin R, Fahey JL (1990) Effect of recombinant human granulocyte-macrophage colony-stimulating factor administration on the lymphocyte subsets of patients with refractory aplastic anemia. *Blood* 76, 1580.

Finkelman FD, Urban JF, Beckmann MP, Schooley KA, Holmes JM, Katona IM (1991) Regulation of murine in vivo IgG and IgE responses by a monoclonal anti IL-4 receptor antibody. *International Immunology* 3, 599.

Fischl M, Galpin J, Levine J et al. (1990) Recombinant human erythropoietin for patients with AIDS treated with zidovudine. *New England Journal of Medicine* 322, 1488.

Folks TM, Justment J, Kinter A, Dinarello CA, Fauci AS (1987) Cytokine-induced expression of HIV-1 in a chronically infected promonocyte cell line. *Science* 238, 800.

Gabrilove JL, Welte K, Harris P et al. (1986) Pluripoietin α: a second human hematopoietic colony-stimulating factor produced by the human bladder carcinoma cell line 5637. *Proceedings of the National Academy of Sciences of the USA* 83, 2478.

Gabrilove JL, Jakubowski A, Scher H et al. (1988) Effect of granulocyte colony-stimulating factor on neutropenia and associated morbidity due to chemotherapy for transitional-cell carcinoma of the urothelium. *New England Journal of Medicine* 318, 1414.

Ganser A, Lindemann A, Ottman OG et al. (1989a) Effect of recombinant interleukin-3 in vivo – a phase I trial. *Experimental Hematology* 17, 484.

Ganser A, Volkers B, Greher J et al. (1989b) Recombinant human granulocyte-macrophage colony-stimulating factor in patients with myelodysplastic syndromes – a phase I/II trial. *Blood* 73, 31.

Ganser A, Lindemann A, Siepelt G et al. (1990a) Effects of recombinant human interleukin-3 in aplastic anemia. *Blood* 76, 1287.

Ganser A, Lindemann A, Siefelt G et al. (1990b) Effects of recombinant human interleukin-3 in patients with normal hematopoiesis and in patients with bone marrow failure. *Blood* 76, 666.

Ganser A, Janssen JWG, Ottman OG et al. (1991) In vivo effects of granulocyte-macrophage colony-stimulating factor and interleukin-3 on clonal and non-clonal cell populations in patients with clonal hematopoietic disorders. *Leukemia* 5, 487.

Gerson SC, Talbot GH, Hurwitz S, Strom BL, Lusk EJ, Casileth PA (1984) Prolonged granulocytopenia: the major risk factor for invasive pulmonary aspergillosis in patients with acute leukemia. *Annals of Internal Medicine* 100, 345.

Gianni AM, Bregni M, Stern AC et al. (1989) Granulocyte-macrophage colony-stimulating factor to harvest circulating haemopoietic stem cells for autotransplantation. *Lancet* ii, 580.

Gianni AM, Tarella C, Siena S et al. (1990) Durable and complete hematopoietic reconstitution after autografting of rhGM-CSF exposed peripheral blood progenitor cells. *Bone Marrow Transplantation* 6, 143.

Gibson FM, Gordon-Smith EC (1990) Long term culture of aplastic anaemia bone marrow. *British Journal of Haematology* 75, 421.

Giessler D, Thaler J, Konwalinka G, Peschel C (1987) Progressive preleukaemia presenting as amegakaryocytic thrombocytopenic purpura: association of the 5q-syndrome with a decreased megakaryocytic colony formation and a defective production of meg-CSF. *Leukemia Research* 11, 731.

Giessler K, Valent P, Mayer P et al. (1990) Recombinant human interleukin-3 expands the pool of circulating hematopoietic progenitor cells in primates – synergism with recombinant granulocyte-macrophage colony-stimulating factor. *Blood* 75, 2305.

Glaspy JA, Baldwin GC, Robertson PA et al. (1988) Therapy for neutropenia in hairy cell leukemia with recombinant human granulocyte colony-stimulating factor. *Annals of Internal Medicine* 109, 789.

Goldberg MA, Brugnara C, Dover GJ, Schapira L, Charache S, Bunn F (1990) Treatment of sickle cell anaemia with hydroxyurea and erythropoietin. *New England Journal of Medicine* 323, 366.

Groopman JE, Mitsuyasu RT, Deleo MJ, Oette DH, Golde DW (1987) Effect of recombinant human granulocyte-macrophage colony-stimulating factor on myelopoiesis in the acquired immunodeficiency syndrome. *New England Journal of Medicine* 317, 593.

Halpern D, Wakker P, Lacourt G et al. (1990) Effects of recombinant human erythropoietin in infants with the anemia of prematurity: a pilot study. *Journal of Pediatrics* 116, 779.

Hammer SM, Gillis JM, Groopmen JE, Rose RM (1986) In vitro modification of human immunodeficiency virus infection by granulocyte-macrophage colony-stimulating factor and γ interferon. *Proceedings of* the National Academy of Sciences of the USA 83, 8734.

Hammond WP, Price TH, Souza LM, Dale DC (1989) Treatment of cyclic neutropenia with granulocyte colony-stimulating factor. New England Journal of Medicine 320, 1306.

Hammond WP, Boone TC, Donahue RE, Souza LM, Dale DC (1990) A comparison of treatment of canine cyclic hematopoiesis with recombinant human granulocyte-macrophage colony-stimulating factor (GM-CSF), G-CSF, interleukin-3 and canine G-CSF. Blood 76, 523.

Hart PH, Burgess DR, Vitti GF, Hamilton JA (1989) Interleukin-4 stimulates human monocytes to produce tissue-type plasminogen activator. Blood 74, 1222.

Hazenberg BPC, Van Leeuwen MA, Van Rijswijk MH, Stern AC, Vellenga E (1989) Correction of granulocytopenia in Felty's syndrome by granulocyte-macrophage colony-stimulating factor. Simultaneous induction of IL-6 and flare-up of the arthritis. Blood 74, 2769.

Herrmann F, Schulz G, Lindemann A et al. (1988) Yeast expressed granulocyte-macrophage colony-stimulating factor in cancer patients: a phase Ib clinical study. Behring Institute Mitteilungen 83, 107.

Herve P, Wijdenes J, Bergerat JP, Milpied N, Gaud C, Bordigoni P (1988) Treatment of acute graft-versus-host disease with monoclonal antibody to IL-2 receptor. Lancet ii, 1072.

Herve P, Wijdenes J, Bergerat JP et al. (1990) Treatment of corticosteroid resistant acute graft-versus-host disease by in vivo administration of anti-interleukin-2 receptor monoclonal antibody (B-B10). Blood 75, 1017.

Heyll A, Aul C, Runde V, Arning M, Schneider W, Wernet P (1991) Treatment of pure red cell aplasia after major ABO-incompatible bone marrow transplantation with recombinant erythropoietin. Blood 77, 906.

Hirashima K, Bessho M, Susaki L, Miyazawa K, Nagashima M (1989) Improvement of anemia by intravenous injection of recombinant erythropoietin in patients with myelodysplastic syndrome and aplastic anemia. Experimental Hematology 17, 385.

Ho AD, Haas R, Wulf G et al. (1990) Activation of lymphocytes induced by recombinant human granulocyte-macrophage colony-stimulating factor in patients with malignant lymphoma. Blood 75, 203.

Hoang T, Nara N, Wong G, Minden MD, McCulloch EA (1986) Effects of recombinant GM-CSF on the blast cells of acute myeloblastic leukemia. Blood 68, 313.

Hoekman K, Von Blomberg-Van Der Flier BME, Wagstaff J, Drexhage HA, Pinedo HM (1991) Reversible thyroid dysfunction during treatment with GM-CSF. Lancet 338, 541.

Hoelzer D, Ganser A, Volkers B, Greher J, Walther F (1988) In vitro and in vivo action of recombinant human GM-CSF (rhGM-CSF) in patients with myelodysplastic syndromes. Blood Cells 14, 551.

Hows JM (1991) Severe aplastic anaemia: the patient without an HLA-identical sibling. British Journal of Haematology 77, 1.

Jacobs CA, Lynch DH, Roux ER et al. (1991) Characterisation and pharmacokinetic parameters of recombinant soluble interleukin-4 receptor. Blood 77, 2396.

Jakubowski A, Souza L, Kelly F et al. (1989) Effects of human granulocyte colony-stimulating factor in a patient with idiopathic neutropenia. New England Journal of Medicine 320, 38.

Jiminez JJ, Yunis AA (1988) Treatment with monocyte-derived partially purified GM-CSF but not G-CSF aborts the development of transplanted chloroleukemia in rats. Blood 72, 1077.

Johnson GR, Gonda TJ, Metcalf D, Hariharan IK, Cory S (1989) A lethal myeloproliferative syndrome in mice transplanted with bone marrow cells infected with a retrovirus expressing granulocyte-macrophage colony-stimulating factor. EMBO Journal 8, 441.

Kantoff PW, Kohn DB, Mitsuya H et al. (1986) Correction of adenosine deaminase deficiency in cultured human T and B lymphocytes by retrovirus-mediated gene transfer. Proceedings of the National Academy of Sciences of the USA 83, 6563.

Kaplan SS, Basford RE, Wing EJ, Shadduck RK (1989) The effect of recombinant human granulocyte macrophage colony-stimulating factor on neutrophil activation in patients with refractory carcinoma. Blood 73, 636.

Kelleher C, Miyauchi J, Wong G, Clarke S, Minden MD, McCulloch EA (1987) Synergism between recombinant growth factor, GM-CSF and G-CSF, acting on the blast cells of acute myeloblastic leukemia. Blood 69, 1498.

Khwaja A, Johnson B, Addison IE et al. (1991) In vivo effects of macrophage colony-stimulating factor on human monocyte function. British Journal of Haematology 77, 25.

Kitano K, Abboud CN, Ryan DH, Quan SG, Baldwin GC, Golde DW (1991) Macrophage-active colony-stimulating factors enhance immunodeficiency virus type 1 infection in bone marrow stem cells. Blood 77, 1699.

Klausmann M, Pfluger KH, Krumweih D, Seiler FR, Havemann K (1988) Modulations of functions of granulocytes by recombinant human GM-CSF and possible complications of GM-CSF therapy. Leukemia Research (suppl), 63.

Klein B, Wijdenes Z, Zhang XG et al. (1991) Murine anti-interleukin-6 monoclonal antibody therapy for a patient with plasma cell leukemia. Blood 78, 1198.

Kojima S, Fukuda M, Miyajima Y, Matsuyama T, Horibe K (1991) Treatment of aplastic anemia in children with recombinant human granulocyte colony-stimulating factor. Blood 77, 937.

Kurzrock R, Talpaz M, Gomez JA et al. (1991) Differential dose-related haematological effects of GM-CSF in pancytopenia: evidence supporting the advantage of low- over high-dose administration in selected patients. British Journal of Haematology 78, 352.

Laker C, Stocking C, Bergholz U, Ness N, Delamarter JF, Ostertag W (1987) Autocrine stimulation after transfer of the granulocyte/macrophage colony-stimulating factor gene and autonomous growth are distinct but interdependent steps in the oncogenic pathway. *Proceedings of the National Academy of Sciences of the USA* 84, 8458.

Lang RA, Metcalf D, Gough NM, Dunn AR, Gonda TJ (1985) Expression of hemopoietic growth factor cDNA in a factor-dependent cell line results in autonomous growth and tumorigenicity. *Cell* 43, 531.

Lang RA, Metcalf D, Cuthbertson RA et al. (1987) Transgenic mice expressing a hemopoietic growth factor gene (GM-CSF) develop accumulations of macrophages, blindness, and a fatal syndrome of tissue damage. *Cell* 51, 675.

Laporte JP, Fouillard L, Douayl et al. (1991) GM-CSF instead of autologous bone marrow transplantation after BEAM regimen. *Lancet* 338, 601.

Lazarus HM, Andersen J, Chen MG et al. (1991) Recombinant granulocyte-macrophage colony-stimulating factor after autologous bone marrow transplantation for relapsed non-Hodgkin's lymphoma: blood and bone marrow progenitor growth studies. A phase II Eastern Cooperative Oncology Group Trial. *Blood* 78, 830.

Lee MY, Fukunaga R, Lee TJ, Lottsfelt JL, Nagata S (1991) Bone modulation in sustained hematopoietic stimulation in mice. *Blood* 77, 2135.

LeMaistre CF, Rosenblum MG, Reuben JM et al. (1991) Therapeutic effects of genetically engineered toxin (DAB_{486}Il-2) in patients with chronic lymphocytic leukemia. *Lancet* 337, 1124.

Leroy-Viard K, Rouyer-Fessard P, Beuzard Y (1991) Improvement of mouse β-thalassemia by recombinant human erythropoietin. *Blood* 78, 1596.

Lichtenstein A, Berenson J, Norman D, Chang MP, Canile A (1989) Production of cytokines by bone marrow cells obtained from patients with multiple myeloma. *Blood* 74, 1266.

Lieschke G, Cebon J, Morstyn G (1989) Characterization of the clinical effects after the first dose of bacterially synthesized recombinant human granulocyte-macrophage colony-stimulating factor. *Blood* 74, 2634.

Lindemann A, Herrmann F, Oster W et al. (1989) Hematologic effects of recombinant human granulocyte colony-stimulating factor in patients with malignancy. *Blood* 74, 2644.

Lord BI, Bronchud MH, Owens S et al. (1989) The kinetics of human granulopoiesis following treatment with granulocyte colony-stimulating factor in vivo. *Proceedings of the National Academy of Sciences of the USA* 86, 9499.

Lothrop CD, Warren DJ, Souza LM, Jones JB, Moore MAS (1988) Correction of canine cyclic hematopoiesis with recombinant human granulocyte colony stimulating factor. *Blood* 72, 1234.

Lowenberg B, Salen M, Delwel R (1988) Effects of recombinant multi CSF, GM-CSF and M-CSF on the proliferation and maturation of human AML in vitro. *Blood Cells* 14, 539.

Ludwig H, Fritz E, Kotzmann H, Gisslinger H, Barnas U (1990) Erythropoietin treatment of anemia associated with multiple myeloma. *New England Journal of Medicine* 322, 1693.

McMahon FG, Vargas R, Ryan M, Jain AK, Perry B, Smith IL (1990) Pharmacokinetics and effects of recombinant human erythropoietin after intravenous and subcutaneous injections in healthy volunteers. *Blood* 76, 1718.

Marley SB, Russell NH, Reilly IAG (1990) GM-CSF stimulates blast cell proliferation in long-term culture of bone marrow from patients with myelodysplasia. *Leukemia and Lymphoma* 2, 29.

Masaoka T, Motoyoshi K, Takaku F et al. (1988) Administration of human urinary colony stimulating factor after bone marrow transplantation. *Bone Marrow Transplantation* 3, 121.

Mayani H, Baines P, Bowen DT, Jacobs A (1989) In vitro growth of myeloid and erythroid progenitor cells from myelodysplastic patients in response to recombinant human granulocyte-macrophage colony-stimulating activity. *Leukemia* 3, 29.

Means RT, Olsen NJ, Krantz SB et al. (1989) Treatment of the anaemia of rheumatoid arthritis with recombinant erythropoietin: clinical and in vitro studies. *Arthritis and Rheumatism* 32, 368.

Mempel K, Pietsch T, Menzel T, Ziedler C, Welte K (1991) Increased serum levels of granulocyte colony-stimulating factor in patients with severe congenital neutropenia. *Blood* 77, 1919.

Merchav S, Nagler A, Sahar E, Tatarsky I (1987) Production of human pluripotent progenitor cell colony stimulating activity (CFU-GEMM.CSA) in patients with myelodysplastic syndromes. *Leukemia Research* 11, 273.

Messner HA (1988) Growth factors in bone marrow transplant recipients. *Blood Cells* 14, 385.

Metcalf D, Gearing DP (1989) Fatal syndrome in mice engrafted with cells producing high levels of the leukemia inhibitory factor. *Proceedings of the National Academy of Sciences of the USA* 86, 5948.

Migliaccio AR, Migliaccio G, Dale DC, Hammond WP (1990) Hematopoietic progenitors in cyclic neutropenia: effect of granulocyte colony-stimulating factor in vivo. *Blood* 75, 1951.

Miles SA, Mitsuyasu RT, Lee K et al. (1990) Recombinant human granulocyte colony-stimulating factor increases circulating burst-forming unit-erythron and red blood cell production in patients with severe human immunodeficiency virus infection. *Blood* 75, 2137.

Miles SA, Miltsuyasu RT, Moreno J et al. (1991) Combined therapy with recombinant colony-stimulating factor and erythropoietin decreases hematologic toxcity from zidovudine. *Blood* 77, 2109.

Miller CB, Jones RJ, Piantadosi S, Abeloff MD, Spivak JI (1990) Decreased erythropoietin response in patients with the anemia of cancer. *New England Journal of Medicine* 322, 1689.

Mitsuyasu R, Deleo M, Miles SA, Levine J, Oette D, Golde D (1988) Chronic dose subcutaneous (sc) administration of recombinant GM-CSF in patients with HIV-related neutropenia. In: *IV International Conference on AIDS* Stockholm, p. 3517a.

Miyauchi J, Kelleher CA, Wong GG et al. (1988) The effects of combinations of the recombinant growth factors GM-CSF, G-CSF, IL-3 and CSF-1 on leukemic blast cells in suppression culture. *Leukemia* 2, 382.

Miyauchi J, Kelleher CA, Yang Y et al. (1987) The effects of three recombinant growth factors, IL-3, GM-CSF and G-CSF on the blast cells of acute myeloblastic leukemia maintained in short-term suspension culture. Blood 70, 657.

Mizushima Y, Morikage T, Yano S (1990) Differences in in vitro proliferative responses to granulocyte colony-stimulating factor and interleukin 2 of bone marrow from mice treated with chemotherapeutic drugs. Cancer Research 50, 1847.

Molineux G, Pojda Z, Hampson IN, Lord BI, Dexter TM (1990) Transplantation potential of peripheral blood stem cells induced by granulocyte colony-stimulating factor. Blood 76, 2153.

Molineux G, Migdalska A, Smitzkowski M, Zsebo K, Dexter TM (1991) The effects on hematopoiesis of recombinant stem cell factor (ligand for c-kit) administered in vivo to mice either alone or in combination with granulocyte colony-stimulating factor. Blood 78, 961.

Monroy RL, Skelly RR, Macvittie TJ et al. (1987) The effect of recombinant GM-CSF on the recovery of monkeys transplanted with autologous bone marrow. Blood 70, 1696.

Monroy RL, Davis TA, Donahue RE, Macvittie TJ (1991) In vivo stimulation of platelet production in a primate model using IL-1 and IL-3. Experimental Hematology 19, 629.

Montgomery B, Bianco JA, Jacobsen A, Singer JW (1991) Localization of transfused neutrophils to site of infection during treatment with recombinant human granulocyte-macrophage colony-stimulating factor and pentoxypylline. Blood 78, 533.

Moreb J, Zucali JR, Rueth S (1990) The effects of tumor necrosis factor α on early human hematopoietic cells treated with 4-hydroperoxycyclophosphamide. Blood 76, 681.

Morstyn G, Campbell L, Souza LM et al. (1988) Effect of granulocyte colony-stimulating factor on neutropenia induced by cytotoxic chemotherapy. Lancet 1, 667.

Morstyn G, Campbell L, Lieschke G et al. (1989) Treatment of chemotherapy-induced neutropenia by subcutaneously administered granulocyte colony-stimulating factor with optimization of dose and duration of therapy. Journal of Clinical Oncology 7, 1554.

Motoyoshi K, Takaku F, Miura Y (1983) High serum colony-stimulating activity of leukocytopenic patients after intravenous infusion of human urinary colony-stimulating factor. Blood 62, 685.

Negrin RS, Haeuber DH, Nagler A et al. (1989) Treatment of myelodysplastic syndromes with recombinant human granulocyte colony-stimulating factor. A phase I/II trial. Annals of Internal Medicine 110, 976.

Negrin RS, Haeuber DH, Nagler A et al. (1990) Maintenance treatment of patients with myelodysplastic syndrome using recombinant human granulocyte colony-stimulating factor. Blood 76, 36.

Nemunaitis J, Singer JW (1989) The effect of recombinant human granulocyte-macrophage-colony stimulating factor (rhGM-CSF) and recombinant human interleukin-1 (rhIL-1) on proliferation of human tumor cell lines. The Cancer Journal 2, 369.

Nemunaitis J, Singer JW, Buckner CD et al. (1988) Use of recombinant human granulocyte-macrophage-colony-stimulating factor in autologous marrow transplantation for lymphoid malignancies. Blood 72, 834.

Nemunaitis J, Singer JW, Buckner CD et al. (1990) Use of recombinant human granulocyte-macrophage colony-stimulating factor in graft failure after bone marrow transplantation. Blood 76, 245.

Nemunaitis J, Buckner CD, Appelbaum FR et al. (1991a) Phase I/II trial of recombinant human granulocyte-macrophage colony-stimulating factor following allogeneic bone marrow transplantation. Blood 77, 2065.

Nemunaitis J, Meyers JD, Buckner CD et al. (1991b) Phase I trial of recombinant human macrophage colony-stimulating factor in patients with invasive fungal infections. Blood 78, 907.

Neta R, Oppenheim JJ (1988) Cytokines in therapy of radiation injury. Blood 72, 1093.

Nimer SD, Champlin RE, Golde DW (1988) Serum cholesterol-lowering activity of granulocyte-macrophage colony-stimulating factor. Journal of the American Medical Association 260, 3297.

Nissen C, Tichelli A, Gratwohl A et al. (1988) Failure of recombinant human granulocyte-macrophage colony-stimulating factor in aplastic anemia patients with very severe neutropenia. Blood 72, 2045.

Ohno R, Tomonaga M, Kobayashi T et al. (1990) Effect of granulocyte colony-stimulating factor after intensive induction therapy in relapsed or refractory acute leukemia. New England Journal of Medicine 323, 871.

Ohsaka A, Kitagawa S, Sakamoto S et al. (1989) In vivo activation of human neutrophil functions by administration of recombinant human granulocyte colony-stimulating factor in patients with malignant lymphoma. Blood 74, 2743.

Oliver MF (1991) Might treatment of hypercholesterolaemia increase non-cardiac mortality? Lancet 337, 1529.

Oster W, Herrmann F, Cicco A et al. (1990) Erythropoietin prevents chemotherapy-induced anaemia. Blut 60, 88.

Ottman OG, Ganser A, Seipelt G, Eder M, Hoelzer D (1990) Effects of recombinant human interleukin-3 on human hematopoietic progenitor and precursor cells in vivo. Blood 76, 1494.

Park BH, Dolen J, Snyder B (1977) Defective chemotactic migration of polymorphonuclear leukocytes in Pelger-Huet anomaly. Proceedings of the Society of Experimental and Biological Medicine 155, 51.

Pebusque M-J, Lafage M, Lopez M, Mannoni P (1988) Preferential response of the acute myeloid leukemias with translocation involving chromosome 17 to human recombinant colony-stimulating factor. Blood 72, 257.

Peters WP, Stuart A, Affronti ML, Kim CS, Coleman RE (1988) Neutrophil migration is defective during recombinant human granulocyte-macrophage colony-stimulating factor infusion after autologous bone marrow transplantation in humans. Blood 72, 1310.

Phillips N, Jacobs S, Stoller R, Earle M, Przepiorka D,

Shadduck RK (1989) Effect of recombinant human granulocyte-macrophage colony-stimulating factor on myelopoiesis in patients with refractory metastatic carcinoma. *Blood* 74, 26.

Pietsch T, Buhrer G, Mempel K et al. (1991) Blood mono-nuclear cells from patients with severe congenital neutropenia are capable of producing granulocyte colony stimulating factor. *Blood* 77, 1234.

Pincus T, Olsen W, Russell I et al. (1990) Multicenter study of recombinant human erythropoietin in correction of anemia in rheumatoid arthritis. *American Journal of Medicine* 89, 161.

Pizzo PA (1984) Granulocytopenia and cancer therapy: past problems, current solutions, future challenges. *Cancer* 54, 2649.

Pluda JM, Yarchoan R, Smith PD et al. (1990) Subcutaneous recombinant granulocyte-macrophage colony-stimulating factor used as a single agent and in an alternating regimen with azidothymidine in leukopenic patients with severe human immunodeficiency virus infection. *Blood* 76, 463.

Pollack MN (1988) Recombinant GM-CSF in myelosuppression of chemotherapy. *New England Journal of Medicine* 320, 253.

Rabinowe SN, Nemunaitis J, Armitage J, Nadler LM (1991) The impact of myeloid growth factors on engraftment following autologous bone marrow transplantation for malignant lymphoma. *Seminars in Hematology* 28, 6.

Rachmilewtz EA, Goldfarb A, Dover G (1991) Administration of erythropoietin to patients with β-thalassemia intermedia: a preliminary trial. *Blood* 78, 1145.

Reid CDL, Fidler J, Oliver DO, Cotes PM, Pippard MJ, Winearls CG (1988) Erythroid progenitor cell kinetics in chronic haemodialysis patients responding to treatment with recombinant human erythropoietin. *British Journal of Haematology* 70, 375.

Repo H, Vuopio P, Leirisalo M, Jansson SE, Kosunen TU (1979) Impaired neutrophil chemotaxis in Pelger-Huet anomaly. *Clinical and Experimental Immunology* 36, 326.

Repp R, Valerius Th, Sendler A et al. (1991) Neutrophils express the high affinity receptor for IgG (FcRγ1, CD64) after in vivo application of recombinant human granulocyte colony-stimulating factor. *Blood* 78, 885.

Rosen BA, Catchatourian R, Egrie JE et al. (1990) The in vivo effects of recombinant human stem cell factor (rh-SCF) on hematopoiesis in nonhuman primates. *Blood* 76, 163a.

Rothstein P, Roye D, Verdisco R, Stern L (1990) Preoperative use of erythropoietin in an adolescent Jehovah's Witness. *Anesthesiology* 75, 568.

Sailand S, Caux C, Favre C et al. (1988) Effects of recombinant human interleukin-3 on CD34 enriched normal hematopoietic progenitor cells and on myeloblastic leukemia cells. *Blood* 72, 1580.

Sato N, Asano S, Ueyama Y et al. (1979) Granulocytosis and colony-stimulating activity (CSA) produced by human squamous cell carcinoma. *Cancer* 43, 605.

Schouten HC, Vellenga E, Van Rhenen DJ, De Wolf JTM, Coppens PJW, Blijham GH (1991) Recombinant human erythropoietin in patients with myelodysplastic syndromes. *Leukemia* 5, 432.

Semenza GL, Traystman MD, Gearhart JD, Antonarakis SE (1989) Polycythaemia in transgenic mice expressing the human erythropoietin gene. *Proceedings of the National Academy of Sciences of the USA* 86, 2301.

Siena S, Bregni M, Brando B, Ravagnani F, Bonnadonna G, Gianni AM (1989) Circulation of CD34-positive haemopoietic stem cells in the peripheral blood of high-dose cyclophosphamide-treated patients: enhancement by intravenous recombinant GM-CSF. *Blood* 74, 1905.

Singer JW, James MC, Thomas ED (1977) Serum colony-stimulating factor: a marker for graft-versus-host disease in humans. In: Baum SJ, Ledney GD (eds) *Experimental Hematology Today*. Springer-Verlag, New York, p. 221.

Socinski MA, Cannista SA, Elias A, Antman KH, Schnipper L, Griffin JD (1988) Granulocyte-macrophage colony-stimulating factor expands the circulating haemopoietic progenitor cell compartment in man. *Lancet* i, 1194.

Spivak JL, Hogans BB (1989) The in vivo metabolism of recombinant human erythropoietin in the rat. *Blood* 73, 90.

Stahl CP, Zucker-Franklin D, Evatt BL, Winton EF (1991) Effects of human interleukin-6 on megakaryocyte development and thrombopoiesis in primates. *Blood* 78, 1467.

Starnes HF (1991) Biological effects and possible clinical applications of interleukin 1. *Seminars in Hematology* 28, 34.

Steward WP, Scarffe JE, Austen R, Crowther D, Loynds P (1988) Phase I study of recombinant DNA granulocyte-macrophage colony-stimulating factor (rGM-CSF). *Proceedings of the American Society of Clinical Oncology* 7, 614.

Steward WP, Scarffe JH, Austin R et al. (1989) Recombinant human granulocyte macrophage colony-stimulating factor (rhGM-CSF) given as daily short infusions – a phase I dose-toxicity study. *British Journal of Cancer* 59, 142.

Stoudemire JB, Garnick MB (1991) Effects of recombinant human macrophage colony-stimulating factor on plasma cholesterol levels. *Blood* 77, 750.

Sugawara T, Sato A, Shishido T et al. (1991) Complete remission in acute myeloid leukaemia after treatment with recombinant human granulocyte colony-stimulating factor and high dose intravenous methylprednisolone. *British Journal of Haematology* 77, 561.

Tani K, Ozawa K, Ogura H et al. (1989) Implantation of fibroblasts transfected with human granulocyte colony-stimulating factor cDNA into mice as a model of cytokine-supplement gene therapy. *Blood* 74, 1274.

Tavassoli M, Konno M, Shiota Y, Omoto E, Minguell JJ, Zanjani ED (1991) Enhancement of grafting efficiency of transplanted marrow cells by pre-incubation with interleukin-3 and granulocyte-macrophage colony-stimulating factor. *Blood* 77, 1599.

Teshima H, Ishikawa J, Kitayama H et al. (1989) Clinical effects of recombinant human granulocyte colony-stimulating factor in leukemia patients: a phase I/II study. *Experimental Hematology* 17, 853.

Teshima H, Shibuya T, Harada M et al. (1991) Effects of G-CSF, GM-CSF and IL-5 on nuclear segmentation of neutrophils and eosinophils in congenital or acquired Pelger-Huet anomaly. *Experimental Hematology* 19, 322.

Thompson JA, Haudenschild CC, Anderson KD, Dipietro JM, Anderson WF, Macaig T (1989) Heparin-binding growth factor-1 induces the formation of organoid neovascular structures in vivo. *Proceedings of the National Academy of Sciences of the USA* 86, 7928.

Thomssen C, Nissen C, Gratwohl A, Tichelli A, Stern A (1989) Agranulocytosis associated with T-gamma-lymphocytosis: no improvement of peripheral blood granulocyte counts with human-recombinant granulocyte-macrophage colony-stimulating factor (GM-CSF). *British Journal of Haematology* 71, 157.

Toki H, Matsutomo S, Okabe K-I, Shimokawa T (1989) Remission in hypoplastic acute myeloid leukaemia induced by granulocyte colony-stimulating factor. *Lancet* i, 1389.

Ulich TR, Del Castillo J, Yi ES et al. (1991) Hematopoietic effect of stem cell factor in vivo and in vitro in rodents. *Blood* 75, 645.

Vadhan-Raj S, Keating M, Lemaistre A et al. (1987) Effects of recombinant human granulocyte-macrophage colony-stimulating factor in patients with myelodysplastic syndrome. *New England Journal of Medicine* 317, 1545.

Vadhan-Raj S, Buescher S, Lemaistre A et al. (1988a) Stimulation of hematopoiesis in patients with bone marrow failure and in patients with malignancy by recombinant human granulocyte-macrophage colony-stimulating factor. *Blood* 72, 134.

Vadhan-Raj S, Buescher S, Lemaistre A et al. (1988b) Effects of recombinant human granulocyte-macrophage colony-stimulating factor in patients with aplastic anemia. *Experimental Hematology* 16, 519a.

Vadhan-Raj S, Hittelman WN, Ventura C, Buescher S, Keating MJ, Gutterman JU (1989a) Granulocyte-macrophage colony-stimulating factor and myelodysplastic syndromes. *New England Journal of Medicine* 319, 51.

Vadhan-Raj S, Broxmeyer HE, Spitzer G et al. (1989b) Stimulation of nonclonal hematopoiesis and suppression of the neoplastic clone with recombinant human granulocyte-macrophage colony-stimulating factor in a patient with therapy-related myelodysplastic syndrome. *Blood* 74, 1491.

Vadhan-Raj S, Jeha SS, Buescher S et al. (1990) Stimulation of myelopoiesis in a patient with congenital neutropenia: biology and nature of response to recombinant human granulocyte-macrophage colony-stimulating factor. *Blood* 75, 858.

Vellenga E, Ostapovicz D, O'Rourke B, Griffin JD (1987a) Effects of recombinant IL-3, GM-CSF and G-CSF on proliferation of leukemic clonogenic cells in short-term and long-term culture. *Leukemia* 1, 584.

Vellenga E, Young DC, Wagner K, Wiper D, Ostapovicz D, Griffin JD (1987b) The effects of GM-CSF and G-CSF in promoting growth of clonogenic cells in acute myeloblastic leukemia. *Blood* 69, 1771.

Waddick KG, Song CW, Souza L, Uckun FM (1991) Comparative analysis of the in vivo radioprotective effects of recombinant granulocyte colony-stimulating factor (G-CSF), recombinant granulocyte-macrophage CSF and their combination. *Blood* 77, 2364.

Wang C, Koistinen P, Yang GS et al. (1991) Mast cell growth factor, a ligand for the receptor encoded by c-kit, affects the growth in culture of the blast cells of acute myeloblastic leukemia. *Leukemia* 5, 493.

Wang WC, Crist WM, Ihle JN, Arnold BA, Keating JP (1991) Granulocyte colony-stimulating factor corrects the neutropenia associated with glycogen storage disease type 1b. *Leukemia* 5, 347.

Watari K, Asano S, Shirafuji N et al. (1989) Serum granulocyte colony-stimulating factor levels in healthy volunteers and patients with various disorders as estimated by enzyme immunoassay. *Blood* 73, 117.

Welte K, Zeidler C, Reiter A et al. (1990) Differential effects of granulocyte-macrophage colony-stimulating factor in children with severe congenital neutropenia. *Blood* 75, 1056.

Winearls CG, Pippard MJ, Downing MR, Oliver DO, Reid C, Cotes PM (1986) Effect of human erythropoietin derived from recombinant DNA on the anaemia of patients maintained by chronic haemodialysis. *Lancet* ii, 1175.

Wing EJ, Magee DM, Whiteside TL, Kaplan SS, Shadduck RK (1989) Recombinant human granulocyte/macrophage colony-stimulating factor enhances monocyte toxicity and secretion of tumor necrosis factor α and interferon in cancer patients. *Blood* 73, 636.

Wong PC, Chung S-W, Dunbar CA, Bodine DM, Ruscetti S, Nienhuis AW (1989) Retrovirus-mediated transfer and expression of the interleukin-3 gene in mouse hematopoietic cells result in a myeloproliferative disorder. *Molecular and Cellular Biology* 9, 798.

Yong K, Addison IE, Johnson B, Webster ADB, Lynch DC (1991) Role of leukocyte integrins in phagocyte responses to granulocyte-macrophage colony-stimulating factor (GM-CSF): in vitro and in vivo studies on leukocyte adhesion deficiency neutrophils. *British Journal of Haematology* 77, 150.

Yoshizaki K, Matsuda T, Nishimoto N et al. (1989) Pathogenic significance of interleukin-6 (IL-6/BSF-2) in Castleman's disease. *Blood* 74, 1360.

Zins B, Drueke T, Zingraff J et al. (1986) Erythropoietin treatment in anaemic patients on haemodialysis. *Lancet* ii, 1329.

Zsebo KM, Williams DA, Geissler EN et al. (1990) Stem cell factor is encoded at the Sl locus of the mouse and is the ligand for the c-kit tyrosine kinase receptor. *Cell* 63, 213.

Chapter 6
Immunotherapy

Historical introduction, 324
Tumour immunobiology, 326
   Relationship between the immune system and haematological malignancies, 326
   Experimental methods for the study of immune interactions with haematological malignancies, 329
   Tumour cells as targets for immune attack, 336
   Immune responses against haematological malignancies, 348
   NK and LAK cells, 349
   Lymphocytes expressing the $\alpha\beta$ receptor, 353

$\gamma\delta$ T cells, 354
Other cells, 354
Immunotherapy, 355
   Cytokines and interleukins, 355
   Interferons, 358
   Clinical applications of interferons, 361
   IL-2, 367
   TNF, 379
   IL-4, 382
   IL-6, 382
   M-CSF, 382
   Tumour-specific immune cells, 383
   Antibodies, 387
   Future developments, 393
References, 395

HISTORICAL INTRODUCTION

The concept that immune cells could be stimulated to kill malignant cells originated in the work of Metchnikoff who described phagocytosis (Metchnikoff, 1899), and Ehrlich (1906) who proposed at the turn of the 20th century that cellular defence systems might also regulate the proliferation of cancer. A few years later several experimenters showed that tumours transplanted from one animal to another were rejected. It was not until after 1940, however, that these observations were related to syngeneic animal systems (Gross, 1943; Sikora and Lennox, 1982). Several themes dominated early thinking on immunity and cancer: the idea that antibodies could be raised against specific cancer antigens led to a largely unrewarding search for tumour-specific antigens. Another approach was the use of stimulators of the immune system non-specifically to boost cellular immunity against cancer. This culminated in the trials started in the 1960s using Calmette-Guérin bacillus (BCG), *Corynebacterium parvum* extract and autologous leukaemia cells to maintain remission in acute leukaemias (Mathé et al., 1969). In the absence of controlled trials conclusively demonstrating a therapeutic benefit from immunotherapy, interest waned, coincident with improved results from chemotherapy in childhood acute lymphoblastic leukaemia (ALL), and developments in the application of bone marrow transplantation (BMT) to leukaemia.

The idea that the immune system could have a significant impact in human cancers gained support from several clinical observations:
1 Some tumours and their metastases have a low but well-documented tendency to regress spontaneously, and some malignancies have a long latency before relapse (Everson, 1964).

2   Lymphocytes infiltrate tumours.
3   Congenital immune deficiency states have an increased incidence of lymphoreticular malignancy (Kersey et al., 1953).

These observations supported the concept proposed by Burnet (1970) that spontaneous tumour formation in healthy individuals was prevented from progression to disease by 'immune surveillance'. There was however little direct evidence for the idea, apart from a possible role of the immune system in the development of lymphomas (Schwartz, 1975) and the later demonstration that the proliferation of B cell malignancies associated with the Epstein–Barr virus are under T cell regulation. B cell malignancies evolving under conditions of immunosuppression undergo dramatic regression when immune competence is restored (Thomas et al., 1990; Ziegler, 1991). This reinforced the view that immune regulation of at least some haematological malignancies might be possible. The revolution in immunological understanding that accompanied the mapping of lymphocyte ontogeny and differentiation in the 1960s, and later the description of the major histocompatibility complex (MHC) class I and II antigens, paved the way for a more detailed understanding of immunological interactions with malignant cells that facilitated attempts to manipulate the immune system to control cancer, and in particular haematological malignancies.

The possibility that T lymphocytes might react against *autologous* tumour targets rested heavily upon attempts to demonstrate specific tumour antigens. In the 1970s the characterization of the surface phenotype of normal and leukaemic cells led to a brief period of optimism that therapeutic antibodies could be raised against unique leukaemia antigens. Despite extensive research it became apparent that tumour antigens were expressed exceptionally in some malignancies such as melanoma, and more typically represented antigens present in smaller quantities on normal cells, either at a particular phase of development – for example the common (c)ALL antigen (Greaves et al., 1980) – or expressed only during embryonic development, for example carcinoembryonic antigen and α-fetoprotein. The use of monoclonal antibodies to detect specific leukaemic antigens in humans was equally unsuccessful.

The development of BMT led to interest in the potential of *alloreactive* lymphocytes to exert antitumour reactivity: the realization that graft-versus-host disease (GVHD) was an immunological phenomenon mediated by donor lymphocytes led Barnes and Loutit (1957), and later Mathé to suggest that the reaction might include a potentially useful antileukaemia reactivity (Mathé et al., 1965). The term graft versus leukaemia (GVL) was introduced to describe this effect. It has been only recently, however, that this concept has gained general acceptance as an important mechanism in the curative potential of BMT.

New impetus to the idea that cellular immune processes might be involved in the regulation of malignant cell growth came from the identification of cells with 'natural' killer (NK) activity (i.e. not requiring prior sensitization) by Herbermann (reviewed in Herbermann and Bellanti, 1985). It was demonstrated that NK cells could kill syngeneic tumours (Haller et al., 1977), leukaemia cell lines and fresh autologous tumour cells, and the finding that they could be activated further by interferon α (IFNα) and interleukin 2 (IL-2; Riccardi et al., 1982; Hercend et al., 1986; Lotzova et al., 1989) was the rationale for the preliminary clinical trials using IL-2 and lymphokine activated killer (LAK) cells to treat end-stage malignancies carried out by Rosenberg et al. (1985).

In the last decade the biotechnological revolution has made monoclonal antibodies, recombinant growth factors and cytokines available for clinical experimentation. With these powerful and specific biologically active molecules it has been possible to return to the previously abandoned therapeutic strategies of antibody treatment and immunostimulation with a much greater possibility of success. This chapter describes recent developments in our understanding of immune reactions against malignant cells, and the treatment applications arising from them.

TUMOUR IMMUNOBIOLOGY

Relationship between the immune system and haematological malignancies

Because of their similarity to normal counterparts, malignant myeloid and lymphoid cells remain sensitive to some of the processes of normal haematological and lymphoid regulation by cells and cytokines of the immune system. In this respect, the immune response to haematological malignancies differs from immune responses to tumours arising from other tissues. There is some evidence that both NK cells and T lymphocytes play a part in the regulation of normal haemopoiesis (Hansson and Beran, 1982; O'Brien et al., 1983; Wisniewski et al., 1985; Harada et al., 1986; Vinci et al., 1987, 1988; Voogt et al., 1989). Several lines of evidence indicate that both NK cells and T lymphocytes also prevent the spontaneous development of lymphoreticular malignancy (Table 6.1).

Animals deficient in NK cells (e.g. beige mice), or functioning T lymphocytes (e.g. SCID mice) have an increased risk of developing lymphoreticular malignancies, while animals such as the Syrian

Table 6.1 Immune defects and lymphoreticular malignancies in animals and humans

Examples	Defect	Malignancy
INHERITED STATES		
Animals		
Beige mice	NK cells	Myeloid leukaemias
SCID/SCID mice	T cells	Lymphomas
Humans		
SCID syndromes	T lymphocytes	Lymphomas, leukaemias
Wiskott–Aldrich disease	Immune adhesion (CD43 deficiency)	Lymphomas and myeloid leukaemia
Chédiak–Higashi disease	NK defect	Myeloid leukaemia
Fanconi anaemia	DNA repair, NK function defect	Myelodysplasia and myeloid leukaemia
Bloom's syndrome	Lymphocyte DNA repair	Lymphoma and lymphocytic leukaemia
Purtillo's syndrome	X-linked specific EBV handling defect	EBV lymphomas
ACQUIRED STATES		
Immunosuppression for organ transplantation	T lymphocyte defects	EBV lymphomas
HIV disease	T lymphocyte defects	B cell lymphomas
Radiation and cancer chemotherapy	Stem cell damage, ?NK and T cell suppression	Myeloid leukaemias
Cause unknown	Depressed NK function at diagnosis	AML, CML, myeloproliferative disorders

NK, Natural killer; SCID, severe combined immune deficiency; EBV, Epstein–Barr virus; HIV, human immunodeficiency virus; AML, acute myeloid leukaemia; CML, chronic myeloid leukaemia.

hamster and mouse strains which exhibit high NK activity, have a low incidence of spontaneous malignancy (Haddada et al., 1982). Congenital immune deficiency states in humans are associated with a predisposition to develop B cell lymphomas and some conditions (e.g. Wiskott–Aldrich disease, and the NK deficiency of Chédiak–Higashi disease) also confer a high risk of developing myeloid malignancy (Gatti and Good, 1971). Low NK function is a common feature of acute leukaemias and myeloproliferative disorders as well as Fanconi anaemia (which confers a predisposition to develop myeloid leukaemia; Alter, 1987; Froom et al., 1987). Finally, acute leukaemias and myeloproliferative syndromes usually have depressed NK function at

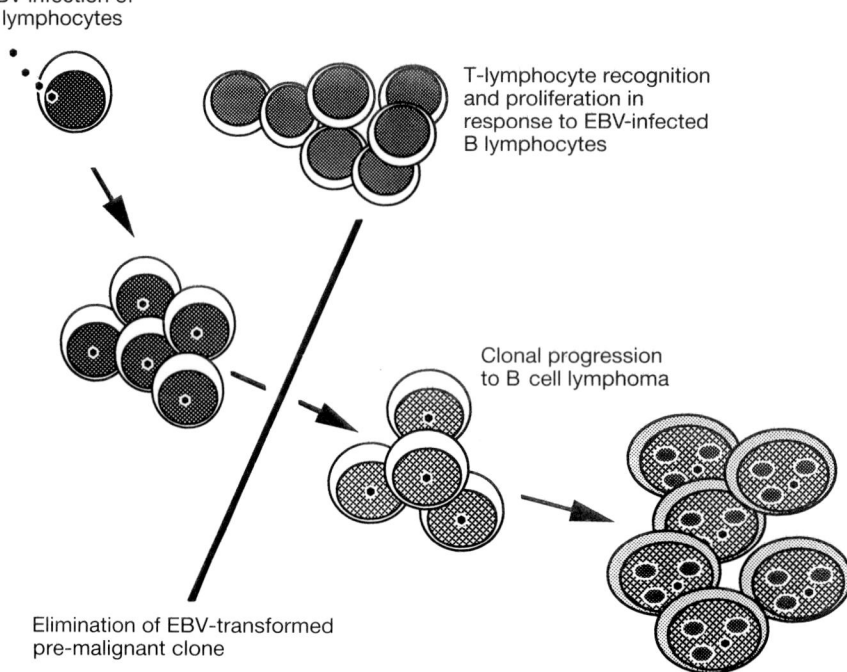

Fig. 6.1 Effect of T cell immune competence on EBV induced B cell malignancy. EBV binds to receptors in the nasopharynx and infects B lymphocytes stimulating proliferation and inducing immortalization of stimulated clones by activation of BCL-2 genes. This may be facilitated by IL-10 production induced in EBV-infected B cells which enhances B cell viability and inhibits T and NK cell function. Normal T lymphocyte function eliminates B cell clonal expansion by recognition of viral antigens presented by B cells. Unregulated proliferation of EBV-infected B cells permits stepwise malignant transformation to high-grade B lymphoma. Reintroduction of T cell control can block the further proliferation of such tumours.

presentation (Jiang et al., 1990). These observations suggest that defective NK activity in particular may contribute to the development of myeloid malignancies.

Malignancies associated with acquired immune deficiency from T cell defects occur after organ transplantation, and in association with human immunodeficiency virus (HIV) infection. T cell deficiency is specially linked to B lymphocyte malignancy arising in Epstein–Barr virus (EBV)-transformed cells. T lymphocytes play a central role in the elimination of virally infected cells (Fig. 6.1). In the normal immune state T lymphocytes eliminate EBV-infected B cell clones early after primary infection by the virus. T cell deficiency induced by treatment (reviewed by Sullivan, 1988), in association with endemic malaria infection (Geser et al., 1983), HIV infection (Kalter et al., 1985), or the rare X-linked lymphoproliferative syndrome (Purtillo et al., 1982) permits continued proliferation of B cell lines with a propensity to evolve into a high-grade lymphoma. The role of T cells in regulating growth of such tumours is demonstrated by the dramatic regression of lymphomas associated with organ transplantation when immunotherapy is discontinued (Thomas *et al.*, 1990). During the course of an EBV infection in healthy individuals, cytotoxic T lymphocytes recognizing EBV antigenic determinants on the surface of the infected B cell eliminate proliferating infected cells. Whether T lymphocytes are also involved in the immune surveillance of haematological malignancy not associated with virus infection is not known.

Experimental methods for the study of immune interactions with haematological malignancies

The interaction of immune cells with their targets can be considered under three headings:
1 Recognition by the responder cell of surface adhesion molecules and antigens on the malignant cell.
2 Amplification of the immune response by clonal proliferation of the stimulated lymphocyte.
3 Effector responses of the activated immune cell resulting either in the lysis or growth inhibition of the target cell.

Unlike T lymphocytes, NK cells are competent to kill certain cell types without prior clonal expansion so that processes (1) and (3) happen almost simultaneously. Interactions between lymphocytes and their targets may be cytotoxic (NK and LAK cells and cytotoxic T cells) or cytokine and growth factor-releasing. Immune recognition is measured by proliferative responses. The frequency of the precursor lymphocytes exhibiting a particular response can also be measured by a limiting dilution assay. Effector function is measured by detecting cytotoxicity or cytokine release in the presence of the target cells.

Proliferative assays

The response of lymphocytes to stimulation by allogeneic cells was developed first as an organ transplant compatibility test in the form of the mixed-lymphocyte reaction (Bain *et al.*, 1964). Other cells such as keratinocytes (Bagot *et al.*, 1986) and leukaemia or lymphoma cells can be used as stimulators to measure tissue-specific responses of alloreactive and autologous lymphocytes. The response is assessed by pulsing a 4–5-day culture with tritiated thymidine 18 hours before harvesting the cells and counting the radioactivity taken up by the proliferating cells in a β counter (Masucci *et al.*, 1980).

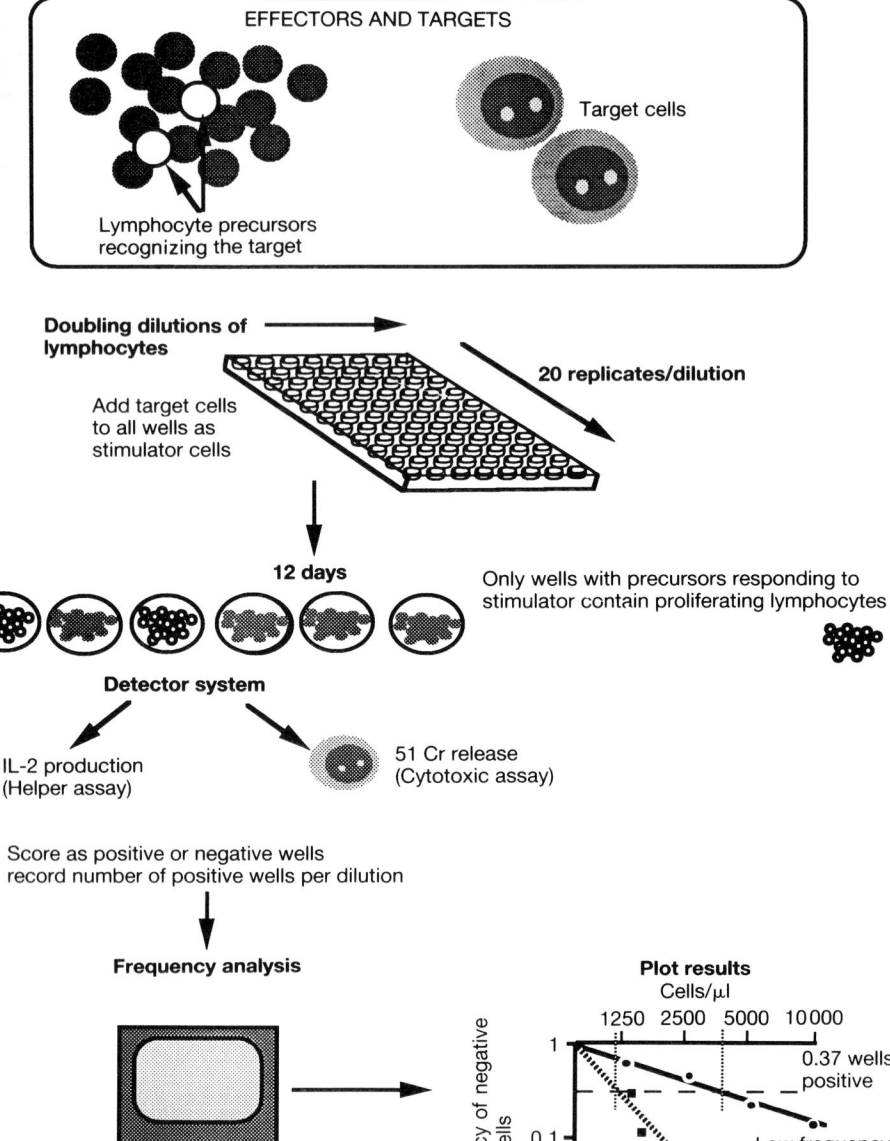

Fig. 6.2 Limiting dilution technique for CTLP and HTLP assay.

Limiting dilution assays and measurements of T cell cytotoxicity (Fig. 6.2)

Because only a very small part of the T cell repertoire responds to the stimulator, the proliferative assay may not detect responses where the responding cell is present at a very low frequency in the circulation. To detect such cells a more sensitive approach is to use a limiting dilution assay for cytotoxic T lymphocyte precursors (CTLps) or helper cell precursors (HTLps; Sharrock et al., 1990). Lymphocytes are diluted out in multiples of 20 wells where they are exposed to the stimulator cells. The cultures are expanded with the help of a low concentration of IL-2 and can be restimulated with the original cells after 6–10 days if necessary. After 12 days the CTLps are assayed by measuring release of radioactive chromium from labelled stimulator cells (now acting as targets). HTLps are detected by measuring IL-2 or IFNγ production by the responding cells. Interleukin 2 production can be conveniently measured by adding an IL-2-sensitive cell line and measuring the uptake of tritiated thymidine after a further 48 hours. The responder frequency is measured by using limiting dilution. Repeated dilutions diminish the concentration of responding cells to a point where only a single responding precursor is likely to be present in each well. Since the chance of any well being positive or negative at that particular dilution obeys the laws of a Poisson distribution, it is possible to calculate the precursor cell frequency by measuring positive wells at different dilutions and plotting the results. The dilution where 33% of the wells would score positive represents the single cell per well dilution from which the precursor frequency can be calculated.

Cytotoxicity assays

The end-result of cytotoxicity by T cells, NK cells, macrophages and antibody-dependent cytotoxic cells is the same – the delivery of a lethal hit, and the subsequent degeneration and lysis of the target cell. Chromium release assays form the basis of NK cell, LAK cell, and cytotoxic T cell assays (Masucci et al., 1980; Grimm et al., 1983). Radiolabelled chromium salts are readily taken up by many cells. Once internalized, the chromium binds to intracellular membranes and is only released by cell lysis. The percentage of radioactivity detected in the supernatant measured in a γ counter is proportional to the amount of lysis produced. To measure NK and LAK function, and make valid comparisons between individuals, standard cell lines are used. The K562 leukaemia cell line is the standard NK cell target, and the (NK-resistant) Daudi Burkitt's lymphoma cell line is used as a LAK cell target. However, any cell that takes up and retains radioactive chromium salts can serve as target for cytotoxicity tests, including leukaemia or lymphoma cells from individual patients. The cytotoxicity exerted *in vitro* by NK and LAK cells depends on the ratio of effector cells to sensitive targets. The cytotoxicity measured therefore depends on the effector:target (E:T) ratio. Assays are carried

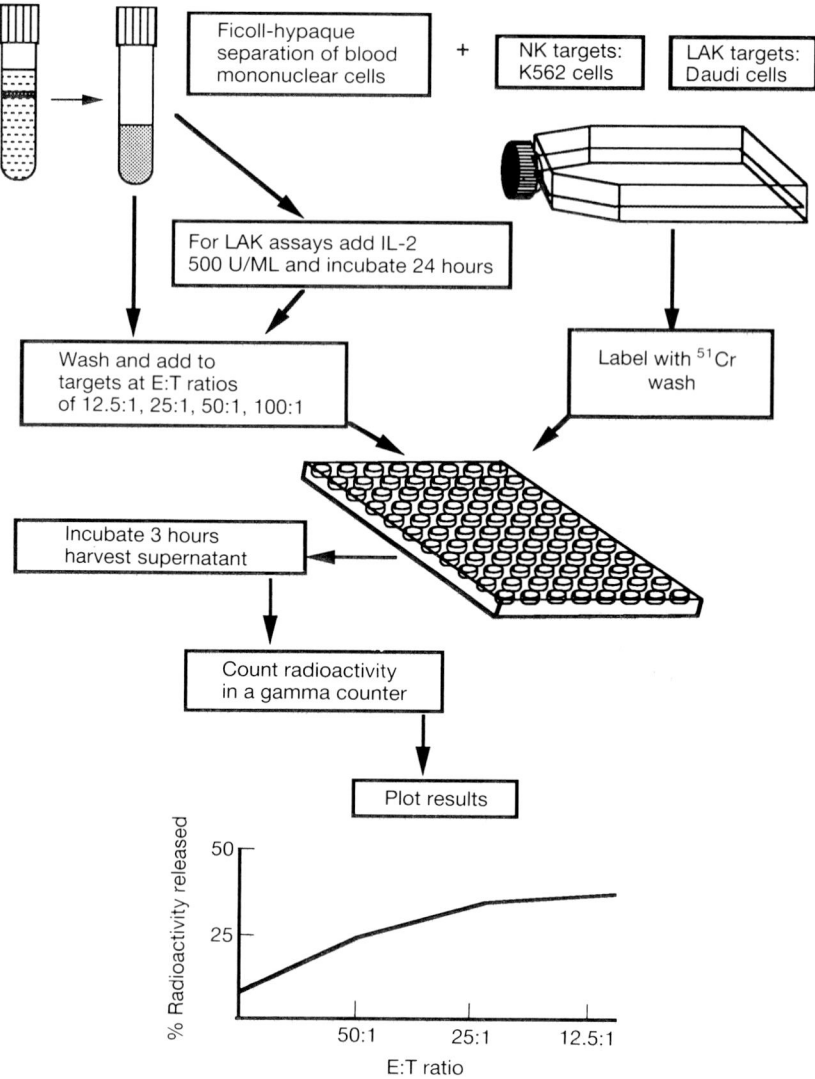

Fig. 6.3 Natural killer and LAK cell assays.

out at different E:T ratios and the results expressed as cytotoxicity for a given E:T ratio or in lytic units. The effector cell dose–response relationship should be a straight line (Fig. 6.3). Factors which critically affect the results are the time between blood collection and NK assay – NK activity falls off rapidly – and the incubation time with the targets – NK cells recycle and can exert cytotoxicity against more than one target.

Natural killer activity is sensitive to the effects of cytokines: IFNα enhances cytotoxicity, as does IL-2 which confers LAK activity on NK cells. Because IL-2 is a proliferative stimulus to T lymphocytes and

NK progenitors, as well as an activator of NK cells and T cells, the population of cells with LAK activity is heterogeneous, and will vary with increasing duration of cell exposure to IL-2. Exposure of less than 6 hours will result largely in the activation of NK cells with the CD56 surface phenotype. Incubation for longer than 24 hours generates an increasing number of LAK cells of mixed phenotype, the majority being CD56+ and the remainder being CD3+ cytotoxic T-lymphocytes. Thus the conditions of the assay determine the results obtained to a great extent.

Alternatives to radiolabelled target assays

A limitation of ^{51}chromium (^{51}Cr) release assays in general is their questionable biological relevance to the regulation of malignant cell proliferation *in vivo*. ^{51}Cr labels end-cells and proliferating cells alike, and if the predominant target cell population is a non-proliferating end-cell, the effect on the more biologically relevant progenitor cells will not be measured (Fig. 6.4). Assays detecting an inhibitory effect on malignant cell proliferation are therefore more likely to reflect an *in vivo* antitumour effect than ^{51}Cr release methods.

Proliferative assays can be applied to leukaemia and lymphoma cell

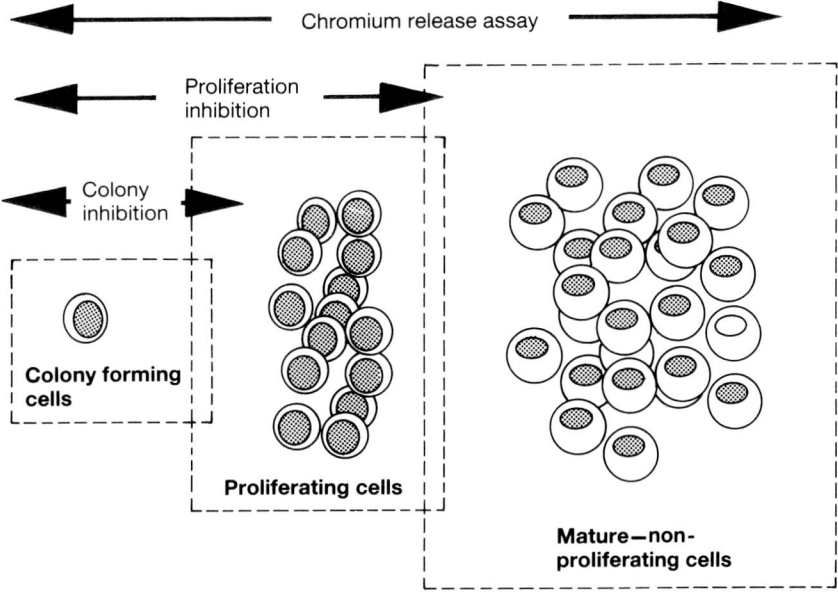

Fig. 6.4 Target cells detected by different cytotoxicity assays. Assays which detect immune interactions with small numbers of leukaemia and lymphoma progenitor cells are more likely to be biologically relevant than assays that detect immune interactions with mature and non-dividing cells.

lines, and to fresh leukaemia and lymphoma cells. However, there are no standardized approaches.

Another technique applicable to progenitor cells which form colonies in culture are colony inhibition assays (for example, as used by Mackinnon et al., 1990; Gibson et al., 1991). Their advantage is that it is possible to determine immune interactions at a very early level of normal or malignant cell differentiation. However the technique is fraught with difficulties. T cells and NK cells have complicated interactions with normal haematopoietic progenitors, cell–cell contact may lead to cell lysis, but the responding lymphocytes may also produce haemopoietic growth factors counteracting the inhibitory effect on colony growth. Normal controls are required to validate specific inhibition of malignant cells. Preincubation of cytotoxic cells with targets allows cell contact and direct lysis, while direct plating of colony-forming cells and responding lymphocytes measures the influence of cytokines and growth factors.

In vivo *techniques*

There are many well-characterized animal leukaemia and lymphoma models, some of which have been used to evaluate the interaction of immune processes with tumour growth. The techniques used are listed in Table 6.2. With an established leukaemia cell line it is possible to determine a direct relationship between the number of malignant cells injected and the survival of the animal. The approach has been used to evaluate both autologous and allogeneic responses to transplanted leukaemia and lymphoma. Irradiated recipients are given donor marrow stem cells with increasing doses of leukaemia cells. The effect of immune cells or cytokines on prolongation of survival can then be determined. Such models have been used to explore the GVL effect, and the use of IL-2 as an immune stimulator in both autologous and allogeneic settings (see also Chapter 4).

The relevance of these rather artificial models to human haematological malignancies has been questioned. There are problems both with the nature of the malignant cells and the type of immune response generated. A major drawback is the fact that cell lines which are well-characterized and stable in their behaviour bear little resemblance to *de novo* leukaemias and lymphomas. Virus-induced malignancies in animals can stimulate significant immune responses in the host by the expression of viral neoantigens. They are not reliable models of immunotherapy for the majority of human haematological malignancies many are not virus-induced. A further problem is that animal bone marrow and tumour transplantation models do not accurately reflect the usual situation in humans where human leukocyte

Table 6.2 *In vivo* models of haematological malignancy used to evaluate immunotherapy

Name	Application
Spontaneous leukaemia BN rat leukaemia Radiation-induced AML in mice (Hagenbeek *et al.*, 1991)	Models with close similarity to natural haematological malignancies–models for GVL and BMT
Leukaemia and lymphoma cell lines EL4, L1210, BCL1 (Slavin *et al.*, 1990)	Immunogenic malignancies. Used as models for GVL and to test the effect of IL-2 on tumour growth
SCID mice transplanted with human cells Daudi cell line, leukaemia, lymphoma (McCune *et al.*, 1988; Kamel-Reid *et al.*, 1989; Malkovska *et al.*, 1992)	Models for *in vivo* function of human immune cells reacting to human haematological malignancies
Athymic nude mice Lymphoma (Phillips *et al.*, 1989)	Models for solid tumour haemopoietic malignancies
Transgenic leukaemia in mice bcr/abl gene inserts p210 (Daley *et al.*, 1990) p190 (Heisterkamp *et al.*, 1990)	Potential models for identifying specific immune recognition of leukaemia antigens

BN, Brown Norway; AML, acute myeloid leukaemia; GVL, graft versus leukaemia; BMT, bone marrow transplantation; IL-2, interleukin 2.

antigen (HLA) matched sibling donors are the source of marrow and immune cells. Since laboratory animals are highly inbred, transplants between animals of the same strain are essentially syngeneic. To produce allograft effects a frequently used approach is to crossbreed two mouse strains to obtain F1 hybrid offspring that are used as recipients of bone marrow from their haplotype-matched parents. Alloimmune antileukaemia or antilymphoma effects from the donor marrow and immune cells in such mouse models mediated by MHC class differences are unlikely to be the same as the GVL effects mediated through minor histocompatibility antigen differences in human matched sibling marrow transplants.

Some of these limitations can be overcome by the severe combined immune deficiency (SCID) hu mouse model. These immune-deficient mice can be transplanted with human cells and used as tumour models (McCune *et al.*, 1988). Recently, human lymphoma cells have been established as tumours in SCID mice to investigate the ability of alloreactive T cell clones to control lymphoma and leukaemia growth

(Kamel-Reid et al., 1989; Phillips et al., 1989). Transplanted human leukaemias and lymphomas may change their nature, becoming easier to establish as a cell line, by losing surface adhesion molecules and undergoing further malignant evolution. Nevertheless the system offers the possibility of evaluating the effects of MHC- and non-MHC-restricted immune processes on the proliferation and spread of human leukaemias and lymphomas in vivo (Malkovska et al., 1992).

Clinical studies

Immune monitoring of experimental immunotherapy treatments involves the quantitation of lymphocyte subsets. A suitable antibody panel would include the following markers: T lymphocytes (CD3), helper cytotoxic T cells (CD4), cytotoxic suppressor T cells (CD8), NK cells (CD16, CD56) and lymphocyte activation markers (CD25 and DR).

In addition, NK and LAK cell function can be monitored, and circulating cytokines (e.g. IL-1, IL-2, IFNα, IFNγ, tumour necrosis factor (TNF) and haematopoietic growth factors) can be assayed by an enzyme-linked immunosorbent assay (ELISA) technique. Although alterations in immune parameters in association with particular immunotherapy treatments are becoming well-characterized, caution should be applied in relating tumour responses directly to these blood changes since they may not reflect more relevant local changes at the site of the malignancy.

Tumour cells as targets for immune attack

The immune response to malignant cells in general, and haematological malignancies in particular, depends upon the recognition of the cell as a target by the immune system and the efficiency of the immune response in preventing malignant cell proliferation. Furthermore, effective immune suppression of lymphohaemopoietic malignancies probably requires the recognition of the progenitor cells rather than the more mature cells in the malignant hierarchy.

Target structures on malignant cells

The repertoire of surface molecules involved in tumour cell recognition by autologous and allogeneic lymphocytes is very wide. Table 6.3 lists a range of surface adhesion molecules, antigenic structures and receptors that may either initiate immune responses or render the cell carrying the structure susceptible to attack by the immune system. They can be classified as non-specific adhesion molecules which

Table 6.3 Target structures on malignant lymphoid and haemopoietic cells

Surface adhesion molecules
ICAM-1
LFA-1
LFA-3
NK ligand (? transferrin receptor)

Receptors
Immune system structures: CD4, CD8, Fc
Cytokine receptors IL-1, IL-2, IL-4, IL-6, TNF, TGFβ, IFNα and IFNγ
Haematopoietic growth factor receptors: GM-CSF, G-CSF, M-CSF, IL-3

Surface antigens
MHC class I presented peptide antigens
MHC class II presented peptide antigens
Superantigens (heat shock proteins)
Other membrane antigens binding to antibodies

ICAM, intracellular adhesion molecule; NK, Natural killer; IL-1, interleukin 1; TNF, tumour necrosis factor; TGFβ, transforming growth factor β; IFN, interferon; GM-CSF, granulocyte-macrophage colony-stimulating factor; MHC, major histocompatibility complex; LFA, leukocyte fixation antigen.

Table 6.4 Adhesion molecules of the immune system and other leukocytes

	Distribution	Ligand (where known)
Immunoglobulin superfamily		
CD2	All T cells	LFA-3
CD3γ, CD3δ	T helper	MHC, other
CD4	T cell monocytes	MHC II
CD8α, CD8β	T suppressor	MHC I
LFA-3	Leukocytes	CD2
CD54 (ICAM-1) (ICAM-2)	and many other cells	LFA-1
Integrins		
CD11a/CD18 LFA-1	T cells, NK cells	ICAM-1 and 2
CD61 GpIIb/IIIa	Platelets and megakaryocytes	Fibrinogen
CD45 (leukocyte common antigen)	All leukocytes	

For explanation of abbreviations *see* footnote to Table 6.3.

permit effector cells to bind to their targets and include as yet poorly defined target structures recognized by NK cells, antigens presented by MHC molecules to T lymphocytes, and membrane antigens against which antibodies are directed.

Adhesion molecules of the immune system

Adhesion molecules represent several molecular families which are widely distributed on many cells (Table 6.4). These cell adhesion molecules enhance the efficiency of specific receptor-dependent lymphocyte–accessory cell and lymphocyte–target cell interactions (Springer et al., 1987; Makgoba et al., 1989). They are also important in leukocyte–endothelial cell interaction and lymphocyte recirculation (Hughes et al., 1990). Of these, the adhesion molecule pairs, LFA-1–ICAM-1 and CD2–LFA-3 have been studied in greatest detail.

Characteristics of adhesion molecules

LFA-1 is a member of a distinct, large and functionally important family of adhesion molecules known as the integrins. LFA-1, like all integrins, is a heterodimer of two non-covalently associated transmembrane proteins which comprise a unique α chain (CD11a) and a β chain (CD18; Larson, 1985; Kishimoto et al., 1987). LFA-1 is expressed by all leukocytes with the exception of resting macrophages. There are 15 000–40 000 LFA-1 surface sites on each peripheral blood lymphocyte, with more abundant expression on T than B cells, and increased expression on T lymphoblasts and activated T cells. LFA-1 is present on up to 50% of bone marrow cells. It is first seen within the myeloid lineage at the late myeloblast stage and is absent or poorly expressed on myeloid and erythroid progenitor cells. It is absent from non-haematopoietic cells (Kurzinger et al., 1981; Campana et al., 1986).

ICAM-1 was shown to be one of the ligands for LFA-1 on the basis of monoclonal antibody inhibition of LFA-1-dependent adhesion, and by studies with purified protein. ICAM-1 is an integral membrane glycoprotein with five immunoglobulin-like domains. It is widely distributed on cells of both haemopoietic and non-haemopoietic origin. ICAM-1 is expressed on most vascular endothelial cells, tissue macrophages, dendritic cells, thymic and mucosal epithelial cells, and it is strongly expressed in inflammatory tissues. Its expression on peripheral blood cells is low, but it is present at high levels on activated T cells and NK cells, EBV-transformed B cells, early haemopoietic progenitors and some cell lines of T cell and myeloid lineage (Dustin et al., 1986; Arkin et al., 1991). Among the adhesion molecules, ICAM-1 is the most variable in its expression. It is induced on many cell types in response to activation, differentiation, inflammatory lymphokines or lymphocyte transformation and is upregulated by IFNγ, TNF and IL-1 (Dustin et al., 1986, 1988; Nickoloff, 1988; Nickoloff and Griffiths, 1989), but not IL-2 (Morhenn et al., 1989).

CD2 is a glycoprotein uniquely expressed on all T lymphocytes and thymocytes. It has been identified as the sheep erythrocyte receptor. Recently, a soluble material has been isolated from T cells that binds to CD2 on resting T cells and induces their activation, and it is also known that anti-CD2 antibodies can induce T cell activation. These findings suggest that CD2 may play a role in an alternative pathway of activation distinct from that mediated through the antigen-receptor heterodimer (Howard et al., 1981). The CD2 molecule has been shown to be a receptor for LFA-3.

LFA-3 is a protein expressed on most peripheral blood cells including erythrocytes, endothelial, epithelial, and connective tissue cells in most organs (Krensky et al., 1983). LFA-3 has two alternative forms anchoring into the membrane. One is in the form of a conventional transmembrane stretch of hydrophobic amino acids and the other is in a phosphatidylinositol linked form (Dustin et al., 1987).

Interaction of lymphocytes with their targets

The process of lymphocyte interaction with the target cell can be divided into three components:
1 contact and binding via non-specific adhesion molecule systems;
2 recognition by the lymphocyte receptor of a specific target cell structure;
3 activation, which may be a proliferative signal or the triggering of cytokine production and cytotoxicity.

It is not always possible, however, to assign specific roles for surface molecules to these specific functions (Springer et al., 1987).

Non-specific adhesion is an early step in the engagement between T cells and other cells, and thus is critical in immune surveillance against tumours or virus-infected cells. Lymphoma cells often express very low levels of LFA-1, LFA-3 and ICAM-1, and are frequently resistant to lysis by specific cytotoxic T lymphocytes. Susceptibility increases during culture as adhesion molecule expression increases (Billaud et al., 1990; Maio et al., 1990). Therefore, lower expression of adhesion molecules on tumour cells appears to be one of the mechanisms by which tumour cells evade immune surveillance (Webb and Gerrard, 1990).

Non-specific adhesion between cells is the initiating event in T cell recognition. The LFA-1/ICAM-1 and CD2/LFA-3 molecules play a critical role in establishing this non-specific binding between a T cell and its potential stimulator or target cell (Krensky et al., 1983; van Kooyk et al., 1989). It is believed that adhesion molecule-mediated cell–cell contacts are able firstly, to overcome the mutual repulsion between cells; secondly, to permit a contact time during which membrane diffusion brings the T cell receptor (TCR) into contact with antigen presented in low density by MHCs on the opposing cell, and thirdly, to allow effector cells efficiently to deliver lethal agents to target cells (Makgoba et al., 1989). Monoclonal antibodies to LFA-1 inhibit CTL-mediated lysis of allogeneic, virus-infected, and hapten-modified targets (Pierres *et al.*, 1982). They also inhibit NK cell-mediated cytotoxicity and antibody-dependent cytotoxic cells (ADCC; Kohl *et al.*, 1984), and helper T cell proliferation in response to soluble antigens, viruses, alloantigens and mitogens. Thus, LFA-1 is a key mediator of many immune functions (Figdor *et al.*, 1990). Patients with the autosomally recessive inherited disease leucocyte adhesion deficiency (LAD) have a SCID syndrome, characterized by recurrent life-threatening bacterial and fungal infections, progressive periodontitis, and failure to form pus. Granulocytes, monocytes and lymphocytes display profound defects, both *in vivo* and *in vitro*, in adherence-dependent immune functions (Anderson *et al.*, 1985). LFA-1 antibody had been used to prevent graft rejection (Fischer *et al.*, 1986). Since ICAM-1 is an important ligand for LFA-1, it is involved in many of the functions of LFA-1. As ICAM-1 expression on many cells can be induced and augmented by cytokines and inflammatory responses (Dustin *et al.*, 1986; Nickoloff, 1988), it is also by itself a fundamental factor for many immunological reactions and lysis of certain target cells. It has been shown that there is a correlation between T cell infiltration and ICAM-1 expression in biopsies from GVHD, cutaneous T cell lymphoma and carcinoma (Vogetseder *et al.*, 1989; Weetman *et al.*, 1989).

LFA-3 binding to CD2 is important in either triggering T cell activation or providing a partial activation signal in certain circumstances (Hunig *et al.*, 1987; Bierer *et al.*, 1988), since CD2 molecules can serve as an alternative pathway of T-cell activation (Meuer *et al.*, 1989). T lymphocyte activation can occur only if a sufficient number of TCRs become occupied with specific antigen. Moreover, TCR occupancy resulting in TCR aggregation is a necessary but not a sufficient condition for activation, particularly when the antigen concentration is limiting. Thus, co-stimuli from other molecular interactions are required for induction of proliferation, or effector functions such as lymphokine secretion or granule release. Facilitating signals can be provided by the same molecular pathways that are critical to adhesion (Mueller *et al.*, 1989), such as the CD2/LFA-3 pathway.

The three types of activation triggers used by lymphocytes distinguish functionally between MHC-restricted, MHC-non-restricted, and ADCCs (Fig. 6.5). Non-MHC-restricted responses of NK cells require a specific glycophorin-like structure on the target cell, rendering it susceptible to attack. This NK receptor has not been characterized. Activation of T cells requires the interaction of the specific αβ or γδ TCR with MHC molecules on the target. T8 lymphocytes interact with antigens presented by MHC class I molecules, while T4 lymphocytes interact with MHC class II presented antigens. These responses are MHC-restricted in that only antigens presented by MHC

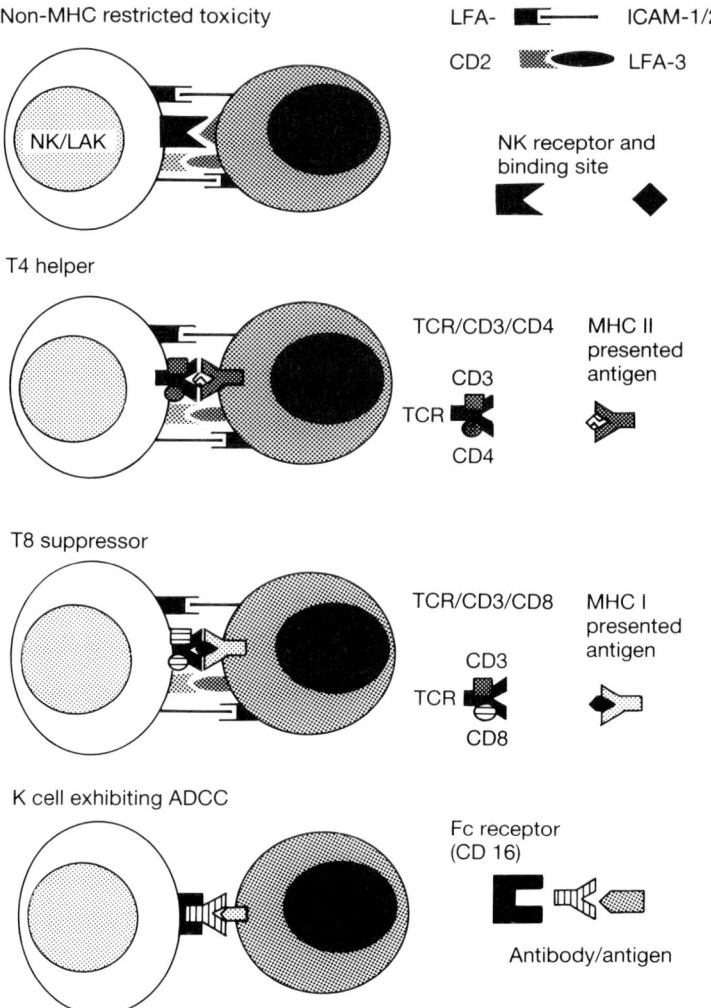

Fig. 6.5 Binding sites for cytotoxicity by different immune reacting cells.

molecules identical to the responder will trigger activation. There is a strict relationship between MHC molecule expression and the interacting lymphocyte type: NK cells interact with cells which do not express MHC molecules, while most T cells require the presence of MHC molecules on the target for activation.

A wide spectrum of protein and sugar residues on the cell surface initiate antibody responses. Antibodies binding to target cells facilitate cytotoxic damage by ADCC. Natural killer cells, B cells, and macrophages which use their Fc receptor to bind to the antibody are all capable of antibody-dependent cytotoxicity. Fc receptor binding activates the cell, rendering it cytotoxic to the target.

Tumour antigens

The search for tumour-specific antigens (TSAs) using antibodies has been largely unrewarding. Despite many years of work it has to be said in summary that investigators have failed to identify antigens on tumour cells that are truly tumour-specific. A number of tumour-associated antigens have been characterized which are either oncofetal antigens (such as the carcinoembryonic antigen) or alloantigens. Alloantibodies generated against tumours in animal systems have not always shown tumour cytotoxicity, and have sometimes enhanced the tumour growth by a protective blocking effect (Manson, 1991). Attention has been directed to the investigation of T lymphocyte responses to antigens presented in the context of MHC molecules (Vose and Bonnard, 1982). MHC-restricted antigens include not only normal inherited major (Phillips *et al.*, 1985), and minor histocompatibility antigens which may be restricted to individual cell types (Marrack and Kappler, 1988) such as mutated *ras* oncogene proteins (Jung and Schluesener, 1991) or the BCR/ABL fusion peptide derived from the Philadelphia chromosome translocation in chronic myeloid leukaemia (CML; Barrett and Jiang, 1992), but possibly also truly tumour-specific antigens (Brenner and Heslop, 1991).

Antigen presentation

Only antigens presented by MHC molecules are seen by T cells. Major histocompatibility complex molecules are therefore central to the fundamental T cell processes of self-recognition and antigen response. It is important to realize that there is a constant traffic of antigen incorporation into MHC molecules, and that surface MHC molecules are usually occupied by antigens. In this way MHC-expressing cells present both internal cytoplasmic (self-antigens) and externally derived antigens for the scrutiny of T cells. Self-antigen recognition results in clonal deletion of potentially autoreactive T cells during the development of the immune system. The pathways of internal processing of antigens by cells and their presentation at the cell surface by MHC molecules are becoming increasingly well-characterized (see reviews by Gerlier and Rabourdin-Combe, 1989; and Harding *et al.*, 1988). There are two main pathways: endogenous antigen-processing via class I MHC molecules, and exogenous antigen-processing via class II molecules (Long, 1989; Lotteau *et al.*, 1991; Rudensky *et al.*, 1991; Fig. 6.6). Endogenous antigens derived from internal cell proteins include membrane protein sequences and many other as yet uncharacterized peptides (Madden *et al.*, 1991). The process of protein turnover in the cytoplasm is believed to be carried out by large grouped enzyme

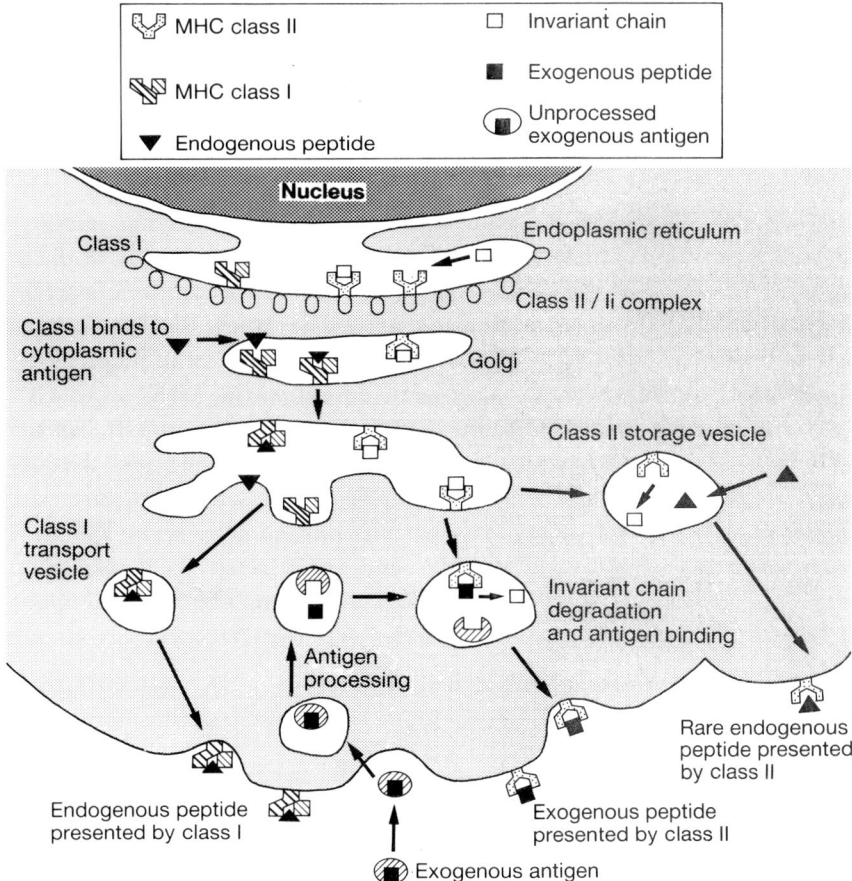

Fig. 6.6 MHC class I and II pathways for internal and exogenous antigen presentation.

structures called proteasomes (Robertson, 1991). They are coded for by two loci RING 10 and 12 situated in the class II region of the sixth chromosome. The peptides produced by this internal degradation are transported across the membrane of the Golgi apparatus by an adenosine triphosphate (ATP) activated membrane transport protein (ATP-binding cassette or ABC) closely similar to the membrane pump responsible for multiple drug resistance. The ABC genes are also located in the ring complex. In the Golgi peptides bind to the variable α chain class I molecule where they are trimmed by proteases to peptides, typically 9 amino acids in length. The peptide-bound variable chain binds to the invariant β_2-microglobulin chain to form the class I heterodimer. Assembled class I molecules are stable only in the presence of the peptide, which ensures that only peptide-occupying MHC molecules reach the cell surface. The class I molecules reach the cell surface in a post-Golgi vacuole, and are constantly recycled.

Antigens exogenous to the cell, such as viral and bacterial proteins, are pinocytosed and fuse with lysosomal vacuoles where they are digested into short peptides (Germain, 1991; Germain and Hendrix, 1991). Lysosomal vacuoles fuse with other vacuoles containing unassembled class II molecules blocked from taking up internal cytoplasmic peptides by the presence of an invariant chain (Long, 1989; Lotteau et al., 1991). The digestion of the invariant chain by lysosomal enzymes facilitates the assembly of the two variable chains of the class II molecule, incorporating the exogenous peptide into the antigen-presenting groove between the two α-helices of the class II molecule (Rudensky et al., 1991). Long peptides are further trimmed once they have been bound to the MHC groove to molecules of less than 15 amino acids in length. Recently it has been confirmed that antigens presented by the HLA DR4 class II molecule include exogenously derived peptides, but somewhat surprisingly, up to 25% of the molecules also incorporate self-peptides from the cell membrane and from the invariant chain itself. This incorporation of membrane proteins in class II molecules may be an important mechanism for the presentation of virally determined membrane proteins.

Immunological implications of antigen presentation

The peptide products of antigens derived from micro-organisms, parasites, viruses, allogeneic cells and antigens present in serum are mainly processed through the class II pathway. Macrophages and B lymphocytes are mainly responsible for exogenous antigen-processing but any cell expressing class II (HLA-DR) such as endothelial cells can function in the same manner. The T4 lymphocyte response to class II-presented antigens involves helper activity with production of IL-2 and other cytokines mediating activation of B lymphocytes and NK cells. A subset of T4 lymphocytes is capable of direct cytotoxicity. Whether this pathway of antigen presentation is important in responses to tumours is not known. It is possible, for example, that malignancies associated with oncogenic viruses might present viral antigens in this way.

Endogenous antigens largely represent normal products of protein turnover and degradation within the cell. Their presentation through class I molecules to CD8+ve lymphocytes permits self-recognition during development of the immune system. Neoantigens formed after this time from virus-determined proteins, and conceivably also from malignant cells, will be recognized as foreign and excite a cytotoxic T lymphocyte response against the antigen-presenting cell (Rees et al., 1989). Almost nothing is known about the variety and distribution of self-peptides. A few are recognized as minor histocompatibility

Table 6.5 Characteristics of minor histocompatibility antigens

Structure
Peptides presented as antigens by MHC class I or II molecules

Genetics
Hundreds of loci throughout genome. Low polymorphism

Specificity
Y chromosome (H-Y) antigen
Tissue-restricted
Viral
Oncogene products
Tumour-specific

Immune function
Physiological
   Antigens recognized as self during lymphocyte ontogeny
Pathological
   Involved in autoimmune disease
Role in BMT
   GVHD
   Rejection
   GVL

MHC, Major histocompatibility complex; BMT, bone marrow transplantation; GVHD, graft-versus-host disease; GVL, graft-versus-leukaemia.

antigens. In the mouse over 200 minor antigens have been described. They include transplantation antigens, Y chromosome-determined antigens, and retrovirally encoded antigens (Janeway, 1991). Even less is known about the extent of the minor histocompatibility system in humans (reviewed by Perrault et al., 1990). Table 6.5 lists the characteristics of the minor histocompatibility antigen system. In particular it should be noted that some minor antigens may be tissue-specific. Thus, immune responses by donor T cells after BMT may recognize only myeloid antigens including those present on leukaemia cells. Such a selective response could be harnessed to provide a GVL response without a GVH reaction (see Chapter 4).

An important question, therefore, is whether there is any evidence for specific tumour antigens behaving as minor histocompatibility antigens, and if they may consequently be recognized by the host's immune system. There is evidence that some solid tumours may be antigenic to autoreacting T lymphocytes. The studies by Rosenberg et al. (1988a) show the presence of tumour-infiltrating lymphocytes (TILs) with specificity against the malignant cells. This response can be blocked by antibodies to HLA-DR. The nature of the antigens stimulating such MHC-restricted responses remains largely unknown. In melanoma Hersey et al. (1988) demonstrated that the patient's own

Table 6.6 Candidate antigens specific for leukaemia and lymphoma

Disease	Chromosome	Gene	Candidate antigen	Possible mode of presentation
CML	t9;22	b2a2 b3a2	p210 fusion peptide	MHC
ALL	t9;22	e1a2	p190 fusion peptide	"
AML M3	t15;17	myl	Retinoic acid receptor Fusion peptide	" "
AML	t8;21	?	?	"
MDS	variable	ras	ras mutated oncogene peptide	"
B lymphoma	14	Heavy chain	Idiotypic immunoglobulin	Membrane
HTLV-I lymphoma		Viral genes	Viral proteins	"
EBV lymphomas		Viral genes	Viral proteins	"
Daudi cell line	6	hsp and others	Heat shock proteins	"

CML, Chronic myeloid leukaemia; MHC, major histocompatibility complex; ALL, acute lymphoblastic leukaemia; AML, acute myeloid leukaemia; MDS, myelodysplastic syndrome; HTLV, human T lymphotropic virus I; EBV, Epstein–Barr virus.

T cells made a proliferative response to a particular melanoma peptide which was presented on the cell surface by class I molecules. Recently Jung and Schluesener (1991) showed that T cell clones could be generated against a single-point mutation in a cell line bearing a mutated *ras* gene. The specificity was such that only the mutated oncogene peptide product was recognized by the T cell clone.

All previous investigations of surface antigens on haematological malignancies have shown them to be differentiation antigens represented by a subpopulation of normal cells (e.g. the common ALL antigen CD10). Candidate antigen molecules that might be presented by MHC class I or II molecules do however exist (Brenner and Heslop, 1991; Table 6.6). They include viral antigens, B cell idiotypic immunoglobulins, fusion proteins derived from disease-specific chromosome translocations, and mutated oncogenes. Figure 6.7 illustrates a hypothetical pathway whereby a novel leukaemia-specific fusion protein such as that coded by the BCR/ABL gene specific for CML is degraded into small peptides and presented as a leukaemia-specific antigen at the cell surface within a class I molecule. The presence of such leukaemia-specific neoantigens within MHC molecules has not so far been demonstrated.

While autoreactive responses to malignant cells would require the presence of truly leukaemia-specific antigens for recognition by the patient's own immune system, the possibility exists that tissue-

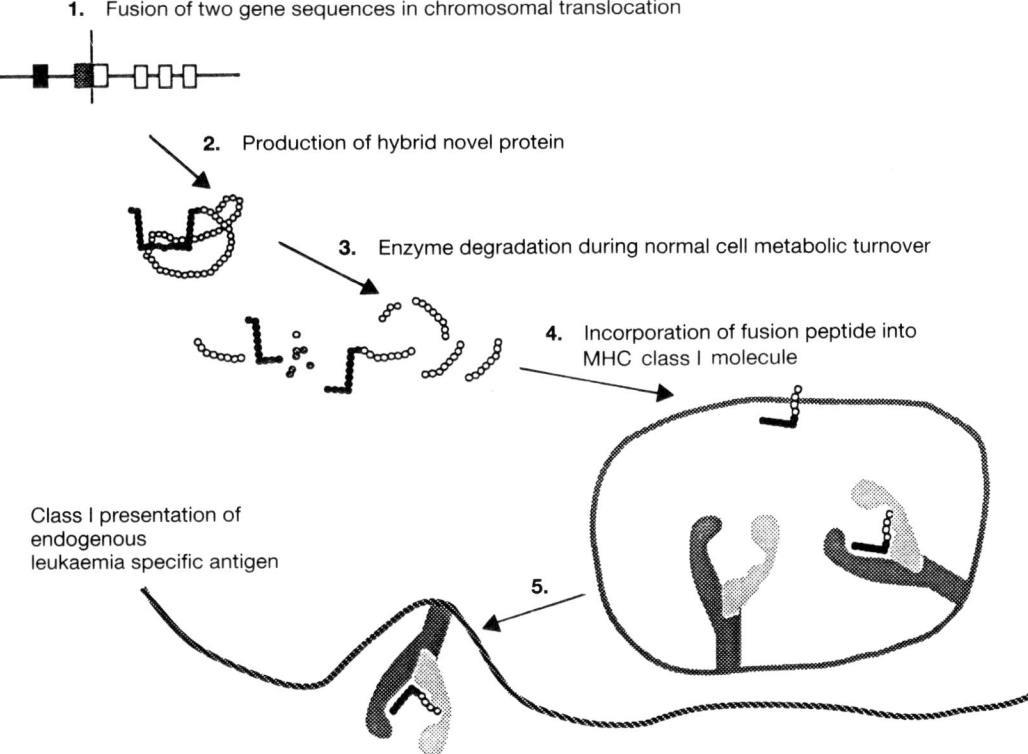

Fig. 6.7 Hypothetical model of leukaemia antigen processing and presentation.

specific alloreactive T cell responses could be important in the GVL response of allogeneic BMTs. Myeloid leukaemia cells, for example, may express minor histocompatibility surface antigens common to both the normal and the malignant cells of that individual, recognized as foreign by the donor and rendering them susceptible to immune control by the grafted T cells.

Superantigens are a class of antigen derived from a variety of bacterial, viral and cellular origins. They may form part of the mechanism whereby heat-damaged cells are eliminated from the body. These antigens can initiate a cytotoxic response from a wide subclass of γ/δ CD3+ve T cells in an MHC-unrestricted fashion. The Daudi lymphoma cell line routinely expresses a heat-shock protein superantigen on the cell membrane and cytotoxic T lymphocyte clones can readily be raised against the cell line (Fisch *et al.*, 1990a,b). Unfortunately lymphoma cells in general do not usually express heat shock protein superantigens and little is known about the possible significance of superantigens in the immune response to haematological malignancy.

Variations in susceptibility of malignant cells as targets

A wide number of factors determine the susceptibility of malignant targets to immune attack.

Lack of adhesion molecules. Leukaemia and lymphoma cells may escape cytotoxic lysis by reduced expression of adhesion molecules.

It is well-recognized, for example, that cell lines vary in their sensitivity to lysis by NK cells. The K562 cell line (derived from a patient with CML) and fresh autologous leukaemia cells are NK-sensitive, while lymphoma cell lines such as the Daudi line, fresh lymphoma cells, and myeloma cells are characteristically resistant to NK cells but more susceptible to cytotoxicity by LAK cells.

Failure of MHC molecule expression. This appears to be a relatively common abnormality of malignant cells in general. Some lymphoma cells may evade recognition in this way (Swan *et al.*, 1991).

Various cytokines affect the expression of adhesion molecules. Thus IFNγ can up-regulate ICAM-1 expression and render the target cell more susceptible to lysis. Many cells only express their DR antigens when activated by other cytokines. Target cell susceptibility to cytotoxic damage is therefore variable and modifiable by the presence of cytokines.

Antigens recognized by antibodies. Susceptibility to antibody-mediated cell damage of malignant cells may vary according to how much the surface antigen is expressed. Antibody attachment may cause up- or down-regulation of particular antigen expression, and cells may become immune from attack either by non-expression of antigen or shedding of antigen from the cell surface when bound to the antibody.

In vivo many other factors may determine how effective the immune response is to the malignancy. Little is known about the ability of lymphocytes to home to the tumour and reach potential sanctuary areas such as the central nervous system. A rapidly proliferating malignancy may outstrip the ability of the immune system to contain it. Alternatively, leukaemic progenitor cells may escape from immune regulation because they lack target structures found only on more mature cells in the leukaemic hierarchy. Large amounts of circulating soluble antigen will neutralize circulating antibody.

Immune responses against haematological malignancies

Figure 6.8 summarizes the repertoire of cellular and humoral immune responses against malignant cells, with particular emphasis on

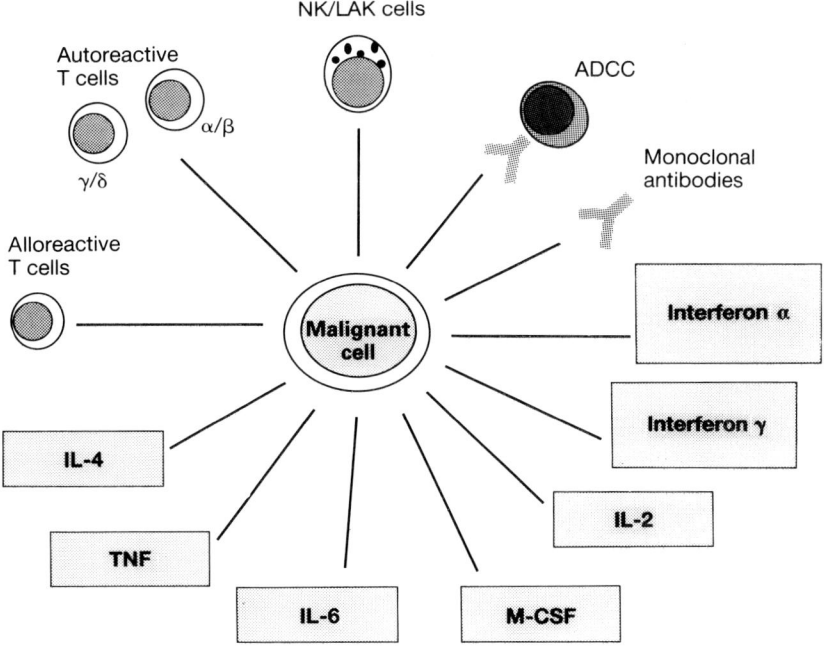

Fig. 6.8 Cellular and humeral approaches to immunotherapy. (Interactions between cytokines, interleukins and cellular immunity not shown.)

reactions of potential use in the treatment of haematological malignancies. Responding cells may exert direct antitumour cytotoxicity, or affect malignant cells indirectly by producing cytokines which regulate growth and differentiation of malignant cells, or activate other cytotoxic cells. MHC-unrestricted responses include those of NK and LAK cells, and of non-specific effectors rendered specific by the presence of antibody (ADCC). As discussed above, MHC-specific T cell responses are important in their potential for antimalignant cell reactivity. *In vivo* the integrated response to the malignancy may involve synergy between cytokines, MHC-restricted, and unrestricted effector cells.

NK and LAK cells

About 10–15% of the circulating lymphocytes are NK cells. They appear morphologically as large granular lymphocytes. Functionally they are distinguished by their ability to lyse certain cells without prior sensitization, hence the term 'natural killer'. There has been

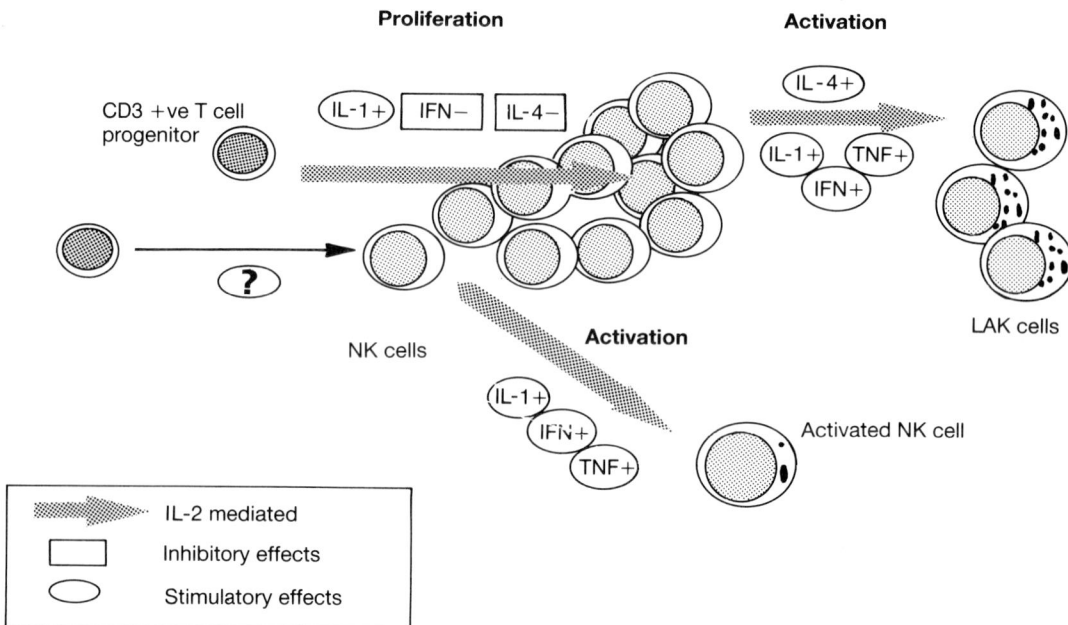

Fig. 6.9 Cytokine regulation of NK and LAK cell growth and activation. IL-2 is the main factor necessary for NK and LAK cell production and function. IL-4 has an inhibitory effect on new NK cell production but enhances activity of preformed IL-2 stimulated cells. LAK cells include activated classical NK cells and a mixed population of CD3 positive derived from IL-2 stimulated proliferation.

confusion over the phenotype of cells expressing NK activity because this function is possessed by two cell subsets – the classical NK cell which is CD3−ve, CD56+ve, CD16+ve, and T cells which are CD3+ CD56+ CD11+ and sometimes CD7+ve, CD4, CD8−ve T cells. The CD56 antigen is related to NCAM, a neural cell adhesion molecule. It is the common denominator for all leukocytes with NK activity, responsible for NK adhesion to the target cell. The target structure on NK-susceptible cells may be the transferrin receptor (Newman et al., 1984). The progenitor to the NK cell is not known. In culture IL-2 rapidly activates mature NK cells, and also induces new NK production both from classical NK and CD3+ve progenitors. IFNα and β, IL-4, IL-1 and TNF are also involved in the activation and proliferation of NK cells and LAK cells (Fig. 6.9). Activation of these cells increases their cytotoxic potential so that they become able to kill a wide range of targets which are resistant to lysis not exposed to IL-2 cells. Cytotoxic cells induced by IL-2 are termed LAK cells. The classical target for measuring NK activity is the K562 cell line. Its important characteristic is that it does not possess MHC antigens and therefore is not a target for MHC-restricted cytotoxicity. Cell lines show an inverse relationship between sensitivity to NK lysis and MHC expression and it has been suggested that MHC molecules directly inhibit NK cytolysis. In contrast, LAK cells kill a wider range of targets irrespective of whether or not they express MHC.

Cytotoxicity by granular lymphocytes

Natural killer cells kill by producing a battery of potent molecules, the most important being locally acting perforins, NK cytotoxic factor, serine proteases and esterases. Natural killer cells have the ability to carry out multiple hits upon many cells in this way (Bonauida and Wright, 1986). They also produce distantly acting cytokines and growth factors, in particular IL-1 (Scala *et al.*, 1984), IL-2 granulocyte-macrophage colony-stimulating factor (GM-CSF), B cell growth factors, TNFα (Peters *et al.*, 1986) and IFNγ and α. Interferons directly enhance NK cytotoxicity, and indirectly increase the cytotoxic response by producing IL-2, which stimulates proliferation and activation of more NK cells.

The presence of cytoplasmic granules in lymphocytes, whether of the T cell or NK cell subset, is the morphological hallmark of their

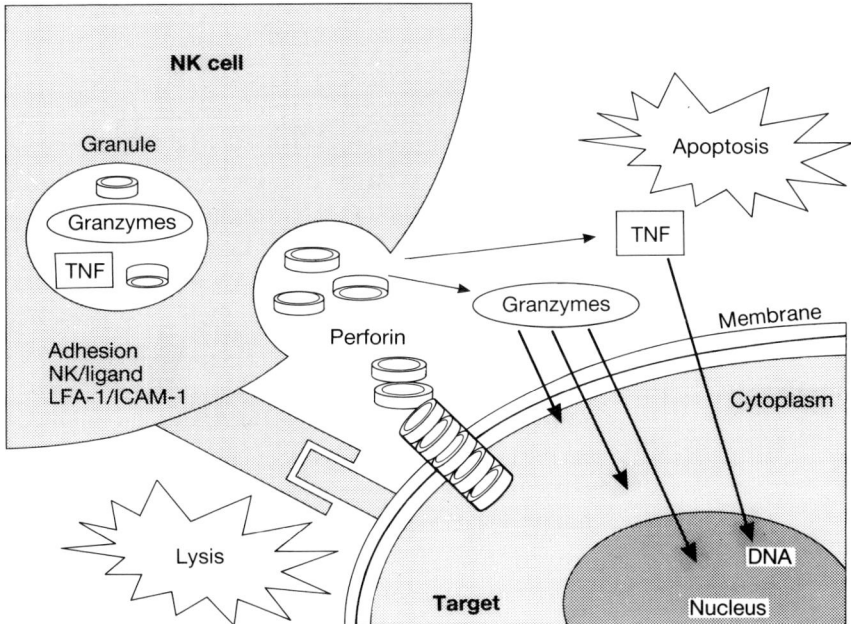

Fig. 6.10 Cytotoxicity of NK cells and LAK cells. After adhesion to the target cell (not shown) granule release results in the assembly of perforin which is a tubular polymer that breaks through the cell wall and induces lysis. Granule enzymes damage the cell membrane, cytoplasmic organelles and fragment DNA. Combined with TNF they induce apoptosis – programmed cell death.

cytotoxicity. The granules contain a package of enzymes (granzymes) including proteases and cathepsin-G, leukalexin (a molecule identical or closely similar to TNFα), and perforin (Litchfield et al., 1988; Shinkai et al., 1988; Lowrey et al., 1989). Perforin is a microtubular structure in a sulphated proteoglycan matrix with close similarity to the ninth complement component. After activation of the cell by binding and triggering through the MHC molecule or the NK target antigen, perforin is released. The lipophilic region of the molecule inserts into the cell membrane, causing the cell to leak fluid and electrolytes through the tubule. In addition granzymes and leukalexin pass into the cell, interfering with many aspects of cytoplasmic and nuclear function-activating cellular endonucleases to cause delayed cell death by DNA degradation (apoptosis; Fig. 6.10).

Role of NK cells in tumour regulation

The rate of spontaneous haematological malignancy varies between strains of mice and particular inbred strains show a high risk of spontaneous leukaemia or lymphoma (Kiessling et al., 1975; Stutman et al., 1978; Herberman and Ortaldo, 1981). Low NK activity appears to be responsible for the high rate of lymphoreticular malignancies observed in the giant lysosomal anomaly which characterizes the Chédiak–Higashi disease in humans and several animals. It may be relevant that NK cell function is reduced in patients presenting with acute leukaemia, myeloproliferative disorders and in Fanconi anaemia (which has an increased risk of developing myeloid and other malignancies; Froom et al., 1987). Whether the low NK function is intrinsically related to the origin of the malignancy or whether it is a secondary phenomenon is not possible to establish however. *In vitro* NK cells are cytotoxic to some leukaemia cell lines, and can be activated by IFN and IL-2 to show greatly enhanced cytotoxicity to a wide range of lymphoid and myeloid leukaemia and lymphoma cell lines (Nunn et al., 1977; Kiessling et al., 1984; Fierro et al., 1988; Lotzova et al., 1989). Of potential clinical significance is the observation that activated NK cells exhibit cytotoxicity against autologous leukaemia targets and leukaemia colony-forming cells. There is evidence that NK cells can also play an active role in suppressing established haematological malignancies *in vivo* (Herberman et al., 1975; Stutman, 1982). For example, Slavin et al. (1990) showed that NK cell activation by IL-2 after syngeneic marrow transplantation can eliminate the experimental EL-4 leukaemia. There is thus a body of evidence that NK cells have a potential role in regulating the emergence of haematological malignancy, and therefore may exert a controlling influence on relapse of treated disease. Furthermore, the ability to activate such cells with cytokines opens up the possibility of manipulating the immune environment to prevent relapse of leukaemia and lymphoma reduced to a residual disease state by chemotherapy.

Lymphocytes expressing the αβ receptor

Major histocompatibility complex (MHC)-restricted immune processes use both T4 and T8 lymphocytes for the full response. The interaction between the specific CD4+ helper cell and MHC class II-bearing antigen-presenting cell results in the release of helper cytokines, which is the crucial event in the induction of the immune response. In particular, IL-2 production by T4+ cells is the main engine for amplifying the cell-mediated immune response. T8+ lymphocytes recognize endogenously presented antigens and play an important role in regulating and suppressing immune responses. They therefore act in an opposing fashion to T4+ cells. The balance between helper and suppressor function prevents autoimmune reactions, and regulates the duration of cell-mediated immune responses. However, the full picture is more complicated than this. For example, some CD4+ T cells are directly cytotoxic.

The relative importance of T4+ and T8+ lymphocyte responses to haematological malignancies has not been determined. Since endogenous rather than exogenous antigen presentation by malignant cells is the more likely recognition mechanism, it seems likely that T8+ cells are particularly involved in the cytotoxic response. Cytokines produced by T helper cells, while not directly cytotoxic, might affect the immune response to tumour cells indirectly by stimulating and recruiting other cytotoxic cells by IL-2 and IFNγ production, or by producing IFNs, which up-regulate the expression of MHC molecules on the surface of the malignant cell, rendering it more antigenic.

The activation of cytotoxic T cells results in cytolysis and death of the target cell, and also in release of cytokines, the most important being 'lymphotoxin' or TNFβ, which induces apoptosis and also inhibits proliferation of many haematological malignancies (Munker and Koeffler, 1987).

Evidence for MHC-restricted antitumour responses

The most powerful evidence that allogeneic responses of MHC-restricted immune responses form an effective antitumour mechanism is the demonstration of the GVL response occurring after marrow transplantation. Minor antigenic differences between recipient and donor may be responsible for the effect (see tumour antigen section, above). The evidence for an autologous response against haematological malignancies is tenuous, but has been shown to occur in some solid tumours. For example, tumour-specific T cells have been successfully generated using purified melanoma antigens incubated with antigen-presenting EBV-transformed B lymphocytes and autologous T cell responders (Hersey et al., 1988). These T cell clones expanded with IL-2, were found to have cytotoxic activity against other melanomas and melanoma cell lines. These promising developments have not yet been repeated in haematological malignancies (Mukherji and MacAlister, 1983; Herin et al., 1987; Mukherji et al., 1989).

γδ T cells

Recently, a T lymphocyte subset expressing the so-called γδ TCR has been identified. The physiological role of these T cells is unknown. These potent cytotoxic cells lyse a variety of different tumour cell lines as well as virus-infected cells in an MHC-unrestricted manner. The epithelial tropism of γδ cells led to the hypothesis that they are involved in monitoring the integrity of epithelial surfaces (Brandtzaeg et al., 1989), and it has been suggested that they participate in host immune surveillance against tumours and infection (Brenner et al., 1987; Fisch et al., 1990a). The repertoires of variable gene segments for the γ and δ genes appear to be much more limited than those of the α and β genes (Takihara et al., 1989). Consequently the diversity of ligands that can be recognized by the γδ TCR may also be more limited. Unlike the αβ T cells, γδ cells may not be suited to recognize highly polymorphic foreign antigens. They may instead detect and eliminate transformed or infected autologous cells expressing stress proteins or altered MHC antigens distinct from the classical class I and class II molecules (Bluestone and Matis, 1989). The identification of the target structures for γδ T cells will help to predict the role, if any, of these cytotoxic cells in antitumour immunity.

Other cells

Antibodies can, in particular circumstances, bind killer cells to their targets. Antibodies coating a target cell expose their Fc immunoglobulin regions, allowing a variety of cytotoxic cells possessing Fc receptors (Leu 11 positive cells), to bind and activate cytotoxic mechanisms. These include some B cells (K cells), macrophages and neutrophil and eosinophil granulocytes. Cytotoxicity is exerted at antibody densities far below that required for complement activation. Such cytotoxicity is rendered specific by virtue of the particular antigen recognized by the antibody. K cells can kill tumour cell lines resistant to NK cells.

Macrophages may play a role in the response to solid tumours and activated macrophages can kill a number of tumour cell lines. Macrophages are cytotoxic either by their phagocytic potential, in which internalized cells are destroyed by lysozymal contents, or by the release of cytotoxic factors and other cytokines. There is little evidence that they are important in direct cytotoxicity of haematological malignancies. They are however potent sources of cytokines such as IFN and TNF and may therefore play an indirect role in immune responses to leukaemias and lymphomas (Andreesen *et al.*, 1988; reviewed by Malkovska and Sondel, 1990).

IMMUNOTHERAPY

Immunotherapy involves either stimulating antitumour immunity by the host cells through *in vitro* manipulation of host cells, or their *in vivo* modification by the administration of cytokines. Alternatively, the immune response may be created by the transfer of antitumour immune cells from other individuals to the host by lymphocyte infusion or marrow transplantation.

Immunotherapy against haematological malignancies is still largely in its infancy. The recombinant cytokines IFNα and γ, and IL-2 have been evaluated fairly widely in the treatment of leukaemias and lymphomas. Bone marrow transplantation is widely practised but the mechanisms involved in the GVL response are poorly understood. Treatment with autologous or allogeneic LAK cells, and T lymphocytes outside the context of BMT (adoptive immunotherapy) is still at a very preliminary stage of evaluation. A relatively new and promising field is the development of monoclonal antibodies with antitumour activity. The following section describes the use of cytokines, immune cells and antibodies in the treatment of haematological malignancies.

Cytokines and interleukins

The last decade has seen the discovery and characterization of a large number of potent molecules which have a wide range of activity on the immune response and on haemopoiesis, as well as diverse activities on other tissues. The first of this type of biological response modifier to be described were the IFNs. Subsequently it became customary to call such agents interleukins to emphasize their production by leukocytes and interaction with other leukocytes. Several other factors such as TNF and transforming growth factor β (TGFβ) could also arguably be termed interleukins. Most of these molecules have been characterized, their DNA sequences cloned, and their chromosome location identified. Many have been synthesized by recombinant gene technology. Their corresponding receptor structure is also known in

Table 6.7 Interleukins (ILs) and other biological response modifiers

Name	Main action
IL-1	Acute-phase response, regulator of early events in haematopoiesis, widely acting
IL-2	Main growth factor for T and NK cells, adjuvant for B cells. Activates NK, LAK and T cells
IL-3	Pluripoietin for haematopoietic cells
IL-4	Regulator of T and B cell development, antagonist of IFNγ
IL-5	Eosinophil growth factor
IL-6	B cell growth factor, megakaryocyte growth factor
IL-7	Early B cell growth factor
IL-8	Neutrophil chemotactic factor
IL-9	Leukaemia inhibitory factor
IL-10	Cytokine synthesis inhibitory factor. Promotes Th^1 helper cell function (delayed hypersensitivity), increases antigen presentation
TGFβ	Diverse regulator of immune function
TNF	Major immune response modifier, IL-1-like activity
IFNα	Antiproliferative, antiviral, MHC up-regulation
IFNγ	Potent immune regulator, less antiproliferative, MHC class II up-regulation

NK, Natural killer; LAK, lymphokine activated killer; IFN, interferon; TGFβ, transforming growth factor β; TNF, tumour necrosis factor; MHC, major histocompatibility complex.

Table 6.8 Diversity of actions and interactions of cytokines

Biological activity	Interactions with other cytokines
Proliferation stimulus	Enhancement
Maturation factor	Inhibition/antagonism
Cell survival factor	Modulation
Activation of cell function	
Modulation of surface adhesion molecules	
Regulation of receptors for other growth factors	
Induction of protein synthesis	
Induction or inhibition of apoptosis	

some cases. Table 6.7 lists the first 10 interleukins described, and some other important biological response modifiers that have been well-characterized. Their potential role in immunotherapy of malignant disease is indicated.

It is important to appreciate the wide range of activities exerted by lymphokines and other factors on both normal and malignant cells.

Table 6.8 lists the spectrum of activities that should be considered when evaluating the possible impact of cytokines used in treatment. Cytokines can affect tumour growth and spread through several mechanisms:
1 Direct antiproliferative effect (e.g. IFNα).
2 Enhancement of specific or non-specific antitumour immune responses (e.g. IL-2 induction of LAK cells, TIL cells or ADCC).
3 Increased tumour cell sensitivity to cytotoxic cells (e.g. IFNs).
4 Direct cytotoxicity (e.g. TNF).
5 Impairment of tumour vasculature (IL-2, TNFα, IL-6).
6 Effect on malignant cell motility and adhesion (IL-6, IFN).

Investigation into the *in vitro* and *in vivo* activities of interleukins and cytokines is revealing an increasingly complex interrelationship between the actions of the various factors. It is almost impossible to predict the end-result of administering a particular cytokine *in vivo* because of the complexity of the interactions that any one factor produces. The network of cytokines interacts in a number of ways (Table 6.8):

Table 6.9 Potential therapeutic and harmful effects of cytokines

Immune system
Stimulation, e.g. IL-2, IFN
   Cytotoxicity
   Autoimmunity
   GVHD
   Helper activity
   Antibody production

Inhibition, e.g. TNF, IL-4
   Antibody production
   Cytotoxicity

Non-haemopoietic tissues
Fibrosis-GM-CSF
Respiratory distress syndrome – TNF

Malignant cells
Growth inhibition – IFN
Growth induction – TNF, GM-CSF, IL-2, others
Maturation induction – IFN
Cell death – TNF

Haemopoiesis
Marrow suppression – IFN
Neutropenia – IL-2
Thrombocytopenia – IL-2
Leukocytosis – haemopoietic growth factors
Thrombocytosis – IL-6

IL-2, Interleukin 2; IFN, interferon; GVHD, graft-versus-host disease; TNF, tumour necrosis factor; GM-CSF, granulocyte-macrophage colony-stimulating factor.

1 Secondary cytokine release, e.g. the release of myeloid growth factors by IL-2-stimulated lymphocytes.
2 Modulation of the effect of other cytokines on immune reacting cells causing enhancement or suppression of their effect, e.g.
3 Changing the expression of target structures on the surface of cells, making them more or less susceptible to cytotoxic effects from other mechanisms, e.g. the up-regulation of class I by IFNα makes such cells more susceptible to lysis by NK cells.
4 Alteration of cell mobility may cause accumulation of activated cells with local enhancement of their activity.

This close network of interactions implies that even though it is possible to administer pure recombinant factors in treatment, the outcome *in vivo* will be less specific. The administration of IL-2 for example will bring about substantial endogenous production of IFN, TNF, and IL-5. *In vitro* the effects of cytokines can be easier to predict and control. The diversity of potentially therapeutic or harmful actions of cytokines is summarized in Table 6.9.

Interferons

Isaacs and Lindenmann (1957) discovered that embryonic chick cells exposed to inactivated influenza virus secreted a substance that interfered with replication of the live virus in other cells. They called this factor interferon (Lindenmann *et al.*, 1957). In the 1960s it became apparent that IFN-like substances were produced by several cell types. These IFNs were termed IFNα, or leukocyte IFN secreted by lymphocytes in response to viruses, IFNβ produced by fibroblasts, and IFNγ (or immune interferon) produced by cells in response to T cell mitogens or specific antigens. It became clear that the IFN family had a range of actions extending beyond their antiviral properties (Baron *et al.*, 1982). Interferons fall into two main subcategories: type I includes α and β. These two IFNs have closely located genes (Shows *et al.*, 1982). They are acid-stable and share the same receptor. Interferon γ is termed type II IFN. The molecule is acid-labile, has a specific receptor, and is encoded by a gene distant from the type I region (Branca and Baglioni, 1981). Their properties are summarized in Table 6.10.

Interferon α

The binding of IFNα to the surface receptor triggers signal transduction with the production of an intermediate molecule that activates a number of genes (IFNα-stimulated genes or ISGs). The promoters of such genes contain an IFN-sensitive enhancer sequence called the IFNα-stimulated response element (ISRE). Several intermediate mol-

Table 6.10 The interferons (IFNs)

Nature and origin
IFNα, IFNβ 23 genes on chromosome 9; large family of similar 18–20 kDa glycoproteins; produced by a wide variety of cells
IFNγ 20–25 kDa; no sequence homology with IFNα and IFNβ; two genes on chromosome 12

Receptor
IFNα and IFNβ present on many cell types
IFNγ different receptor; high-affinity single chain glycoprotein

MHC expression
IFNα enhances class I; inhibits class II; induced by IFNγ
IFNγ enhances class II expression

Interactions with other cytokines
IFNγ antagonizes IL-4

Action on immune system
IFNα activates NK, macrophages, cytotoxic T cells; inhibits IFNγ-induced class II expression; inhibits IgE production
IFNγ augments IL-2 receptor expression on T cells; late-acting B cell growth and differentiation factor; induces class switching IgG ↑ IgE ↓ ; antagonizes IL-4; NK recruitment from NK precursors; widens spectrum of cell types lysed

Action on haemopoiesis
IFNα suppression of haemopoietic cell proliferation
IFNγ suppression of haemopoiesis in aplastic anaemia – and other situations?

Action on tumours
IFNα, IFNβ antiviral action
IFNβ antiproliferative action
IFNα, IFNγ immune activation mainly via NK cells and MHC class I and II up-regulation

MHC, Major histocompatibility complex; IL-4, interleukin 4; NK, natural killer; IgE, immunoglobulin E.

ecules may be involved in the generation of ISG-targeted factors (ISGF) which migrate from the cytosol to the nucleus, bind with and activate the ISG (Veals et al., 1991). Activation of ISG results in a positive feedback with the stimulation of IFNα-production, and the production of a protein kinase which inactivates an enzyme needed for ribosome assembly, and a 2′–5′ oligoadenylate synthetase which leads to degradation of viral DNA (Fig. 6.11) (Lebleu et al., 1976; Shulman and Revel, 1980).

It was initially thought that IFN exerted all its effects through its antiviral properties. Early studies showed that IFNα and β inhibited growth of viral-induced leukaemias in mice leading to prolonged survival. However, it was subsequently discovered that IFN had an

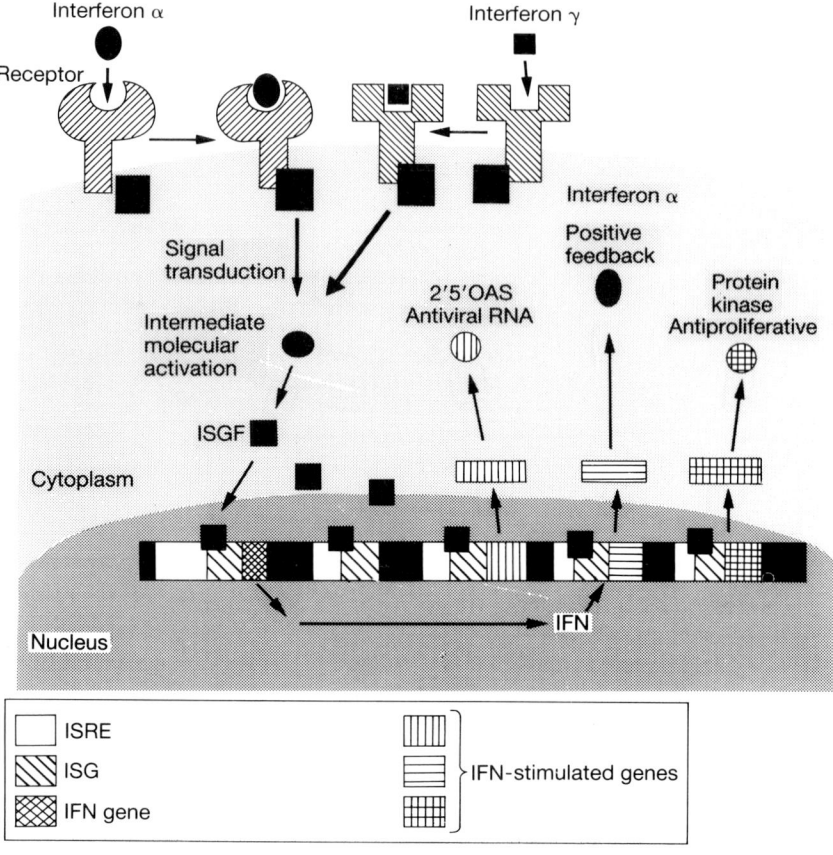

Fig. 6.11 Mode of action of IFNα and γ. Interferon α and γ have different receptors but trigger intermediate systems leading to the production of ISGFs which cross the nuclear membrane and bind to ISRE stimulating production of a variety of factors involved in proliferation and RNA synthesis of the cell and of viruses. Interferon also stimulates the production of more IFNα. ISGF, interferon-stimulated gene targeted factors; ISG, interferon-stimulated genes; ISRE, interferon-stimulated response element; PK, protein kinase; OAS, 2' 5'oligoadenylate synthetase.

effect on non-virally-induced transplantable tumours. Interferon given to immune-competent mice was found to have a protective effect against proliferation of the injected IFN-resistant L1210 mouse lymphoma cell line, but this effect was absent in athymic (nu/nu mice) and SCID mice, or mice treated with antibodies to helper or suppressor T lymphocytes. A similar protective effect of IFNα against Friend erythroleukaemia virus has been found (Gresser, 1991). The actions of type I and II IFNs overlap; however, IFNα has a more potent antiproliferative effect and IFNγ has a more extensive immune stimulatory action. Interferon α and γ both activate NK cells, pre-NK cells, and macrophages and increase antibody-dependent cellular cytotoxicity. They increase MHC expression on a wide variety of

Table 6.11 Haematological disorders treated by interferon α

Lymphoproliferative disorders	
Hairly cell leukaemia	Primary treatment
B cell lymphoma (low-grade)	Adjuvant with chemotherapy
CLL	
Myeloma	Remission/plateau maintenance
Myeloid disorders	
AML	(Remission prolongation)
CML	Reduction in Ph$^+$ clone
MRV	
ET	Myelosuppression
MDS	Maturation induction

CLL, Chronic lymphoblastic leukaemia; AML, acute myeloid leukaemia; CML, chronic myeloid leukaemia; PV, polycythaemia vera; ET, essential thrombocythaemia; MDS, myelodysplastic syndrome.

cells, and may also increase tumour antigen expression (Collins et al., 1984). The direct effects of IFNs on normal and malignant haemopoietic cells are varied. Interferons have an antiproliferative action on EBV-transformed B lymphoblastoid cell lines. Committed normal haemopoietic progenitors burst forming units-erythoid (BFU-E), and granulocyte-monocyte colony forming units (CFU-GM) are also inhibited, IFNα administration causes modest and reversible cytopenias. Interferons suppress oncogene activation, exert a direct antiproliferative action and a direct cytolytic effect on some cell types. Malignant cells differ in their sensitivity to IFNs. In general, haematological malignancies are sensitive to IFN whereas solid tumours with few exceptions are insensitive to any regulatory effects (Fleischmann et al., 1984; reviewed by Borden and Ball, 1981).

Clinical applications of interferons

Interferons have been evaluated in the treatment of most haematological malignancies (Table 6.11). Generally the approach to treatment has been empirical but based on the possibility that therapeutic effects might be achieved in one of three ways (Fig. 6.12) – and via the antiproliferative action; by activating natural immunity; and by an antiviral action on malignancies putatively associated with an oncogenic virus. Interferon α has emerged as a highly effective agent in the treatment of hairy cell leukaemia, and may have a place in the control of several other lymphoid and myeloid marrow disorders described below. The main therapeutic action of IFNα in haematological malignancies is a direct inhibition of proliferation. Interferon is most effective on slowly cycling malignant cells when the tumour burden is low. With the important exception of hairy cell leukaemia,

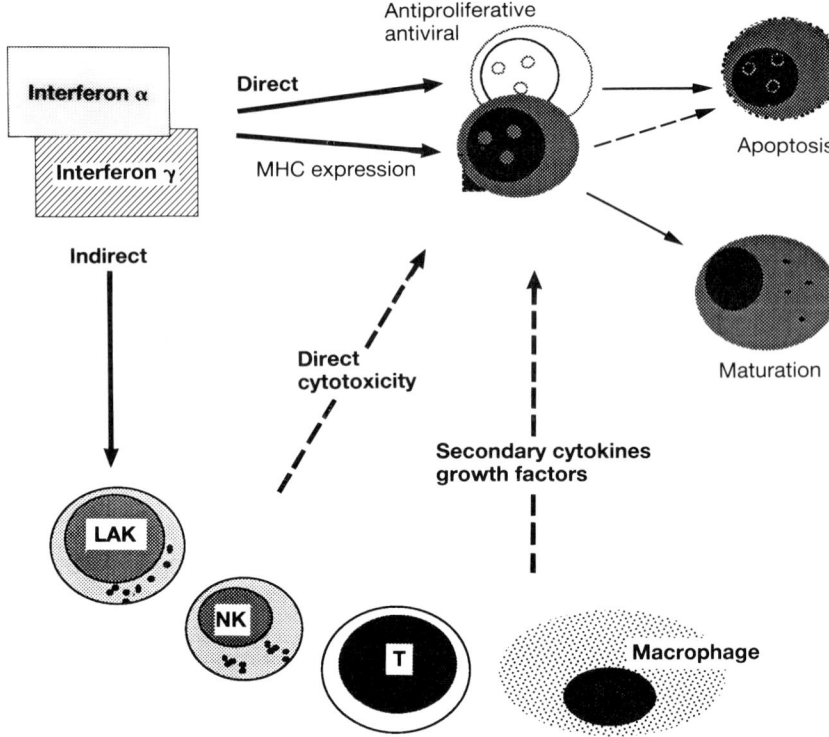

Fig. 6.12 Therapeutic mechanisms of the interferons in haematolological malignancies.

where IFN is effective as a single agent, clinical experience in haematological malignancies indicates that IFNs act best in combination with other cytokines or chemotherapeutic agents.

Of the IFNs, the best evaluated clinically is IFNα which was initially obtained from lymphoblastoid cell lines and latterly as a recombinant product. Interferon α was the first of the cytokines to be evaluated clinically in the 1970s. Early studies in end-stage malignant disease established safe dose ranges and side-effects, but did not demonstrate any important therapeutic benefit (Spiegel, 1985). Interferon is usually administered by intramuscular injection daily or an alternate days for prolonged periods. Side-effects are worse in the first few weeks of treatment. They include influenza-like symptoms, nausea, headache and fever occurring within hours of injection and persisting for about 6 hours. These side-effects are dose-related and it may be possible to continue administration of IFN at a lower dose in intolerant individuals. Some unusual long-term effects of IFN have been described – these include alopecia, depression, and a degenerative encephalopathy affecting the frontal lobes in particular. Antibody formation to recombinant IFN appears to be schedule-related – the highest rates of antibody formation occur in patients given intermittent IFN. Antibodies decrease the biological efficacy of IFN either by increasing clearance or by neutralizing behaviour (Steis et al., 1988).

Hairy cell leukaemia

The demonstration by Quesada and his colleagues (Quesada et al., 1984) that patients with hairy cell leukaemia responded dramatically to lymphoblastoid IFNα was the first clear evidence for a useful therapeutic role of IFNs in haematological malignancies. The results have since been confirmed and the effect of IFN further characterized in numerous trials which show that both the recombinant and cell line-derived IFNα are equally effective. In contrast, IFNγ does not show a therapeutic effect, although IFNβ has been shown to be effective in a patient resistant to IFNα. Sufficient experience with IFN in hairy cell leukaemia has now accrued so that it is possible to come to a consensus view of its place in treatment and the optimum treatment approach.

Response to IFN occurs in over 90% of patients. More rapid and complete responses can be achieved with higher doses, but potential benefits may be offset by severity of the side-effects. Responses are characterized by a fall in circulating hairy cells, a decrease in spleen size and a reduction in bone marrow hairy cell numbers. Complete remissions, as characterized by the elimination of recognizable hairy cells from the marrow, are rare. Nevertheless the reduction in tumour burden is usually associated with complete recovery of bone marrow function. This haemopoietic response may be attributed to the reduced production of inhibitory cytokines by hairy cells.

Treatment with IFN is typically continued for periods of 6–12 months. When treatment is stopped, relapse of hairy cell leukaemia with worsening bone marrow function usually ensues. However, the disease remains responsive to further treatment. The definition of the optimum treatment time and the best approach to maintenance is an area of continuing study. There is a general consensus however that true resistance to IFN does not occur. Some patients develop neutralizing antibodies to IFN (as demonstrated by *in vitro* viral replication assays) after long-term treatment. Surprisingly, however, many of these patients still respond clinically to continued treatment.

Because IFN is so effective in controlling hairy cell leukaemia many investigators advocate its use as first-line therapy. Several studies demonstrate that even patients with a large tumour burden with massive splenomegaly respond well. An alternative approach is to reserve IFN for patients who do not respond or who relapse after

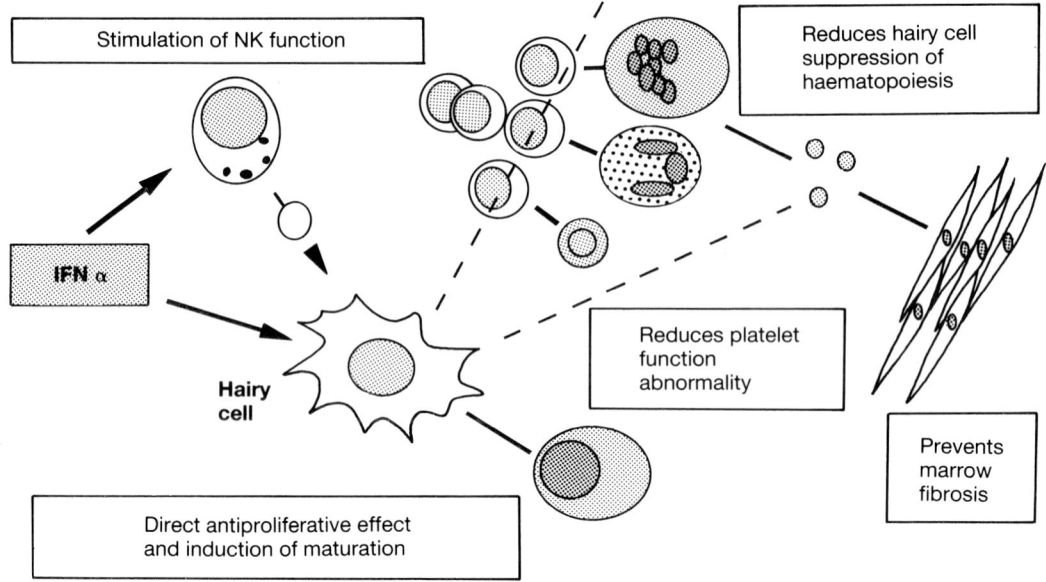

Fig. 6.13 Mode of action of IFNα in hairy cell leukaemia.

splenectomy. Interferon is equally active in these more advanced cases. There remains a small group of patients who fail to respond or who have incomplete responses to treatment. Such patients have been successfully treated with 2-deoxycoformycin (pentostatin), which inhibits adenosine deaminase activity in hairy cells.

Mode of action of IFN in hairy cell leukaemia. The clinical benefit of IFN treatment in hairy cell leukaemia is related to a specific interaction of IFNα with the hairy cell. Although IFN treatment increases NK activity, NK-mediated cytoreduction does not appear to play a role in the response. Hairy cells have been found to bear greatly increased numbers of type I receptors for IFN, suggesting that they may have increased sensitivity to a direct effect of IFNα, which induces RNA synthesis and differentiation in hairy cell leukaemia, while reducing the expression of CD23.

Interferon treatment has also been shown to improve the α granule defect in platelets caused by cytokines released from hairy cells. This in turn may play a role in reducing the marrow fibrosis secondary to the release of platelet-derived fibroblast-stimulating factors produced by premature platelet degranulation in the marrow. The suppression of haematopoiesis by hairy cell leukaemia cytokines is also reversed by IFN treatment, as demonstrated by the reduction in serum-mediated inhibition of CFU-GM characteristic of untreated hairy cell leukamia (Fig. 6.13).

Multiple myeloma

In a study by Mandelli *et al.* (1988) patients who had achieved a complete or partial response to initial chemotherapy were randomized to receive IFNα. By 23 months, five of 26 evaluable IFN-treated patients had relapsed compared with 14/31 controls. The trial was stopped when a significant advantage for relapse and survival was observed in the IFN-treated group. Subsequent follow-up has confirmed the initial observation that IFN prolonged the plateau phase of response (Mandelli *et al.*, 1990). Other studies have explored the use of IFNα as single therapy or in combination with chemotherapy to induce responses in myeloma. These trials demonstrate an antiproliferative action of IFNα. Higher dose regimens are required to achieve responses when IFN is used in this way, and many of the studies report dose-limiting toxicity. There is some evidence that IFNα acts synergistically with other agents such as melphalan and cyclophosphamide but not steroids (Harley, *et al.*, 1979; Cooper *et al.*, 1986).

Other lymphoproliferative disorders

Interferon has been used both in the initial treatment and maintenance treatment of B cell disorders such as non-Hodgkin's lymphoma and chronic lymphoblastic leukaemia (CLL), and in T cell disorders such as mycosis fungoides. The results are in general poor and do not compare with the quality of response seen in myeloma and hairy cell leukaemia. The best responses occur in low-grade non-Hodgkin's lymphomas where IFN is used as an adjunct to chemotherapy or is given following successful debulking by prior treatment (Malkovska *et al.*, 1989).

CML

In 1983, Talpaz and others demonstrated that lymphoblastoid IFNα given to patients in the chronic phase of CML could control the chronic phase by suppressing the leukocyte count (reviewed in Talpaz *et al.*, 1988). They also showed that IFN reduced the percentage of marrow metaphases bearing the Ph^1 chromosome in some patients. Occasional patients become Ph^1 chromosome-negative. Subsequent studies confirmed these findings and showed that the reduction of the leukaemic clone is dose-dependent, more effective in conditions of low tumour burden, and when initial control has been achieved with standard chemotherapy. The bone marrow can retain a normal karyotype for many months after stopping treatment but eventually relapses to a Ph^1 positive state. There is therefore a suggestion that

IFNα may have a selective antiproliferative action against leukaemic cells. However even in patients with a normal karyotype, the presence of the BCR/ABL fusion gene of the Ph^1 chromosome remains detectable, suggesting that IFNα suppresses but does not cure the leukaemia (Hughes et al., 1991). Follow-up is still too short to determine with confidence whether IFN is capable of delaying transformation to the acute terminal phase.

The mechanism of action of IFN in CML is not known. The available data suggest that NK activation does not play a regulatory role and that IFN has a suppressive action on late progenitors (Galvani, 1989; Galvani and Cawley, 1989). Recent work indicates that IFNα in some way reverses the defective adhesiveness of CML progenitors to stromal cells in suspension marrow cultures, and may thus normalize their growth factor dependence on stromal cells (Dowding et al., 1991).

Other myeloproliferative disorders

The antiproliferative effect of IFN on haemopoiesis has led to several studies of IFN in the control of excessive red cell, platelet and leukocyte production in essential thrombocythaemia (ET), polycythaemia vera (PV), and myelofibrosis (MF). Results from a trial in 30 patients (Gisslinger et al., 1989), and smaller studies (May et al., 1989; Tichelli, 1989; Silver, 1990) show that myeloproliferative disorders respond readily to IFNα with a fall in red cell, platelet and leukocyte counts. It is not known whether the myelosuppression is a direct antiproliferative effect, or if it is mediated by NK cells. A recent study indicates that in myeloproliferative disorders, monocytes produce aberrant growth factors responsible for the formation of 'spontaneous' (erythropoietin-independent) erythrocyte colonies which are a feature of ET, PV and MF (Shabbad et al., 1990). It not known whether IFNα modifies this aberrant growth factor production. An important and unanswered question is whether IFNs have any effect upon the natural evolution of myeloproliferative disorders. There is as yet no evidence that IFNα reduces the tendency to increasing marrow fibrosis, and nothing to suggest that there is a return to normal haematopoiesis with treatment. It is therefore unclear whether IFNα offers any therapeutic advantage over conventional chemotherapy with hydroxyurea. There is no evidence as yet that IFNα changes the clinical course of these very slowly evolving disorders – very long controlled studies will be required to show whether IFN has a beneficial effect in myeloproliferative disorders over and above myelosuppression. It can, however, be argued that IFN treatment avoids exposure to potentially leukaemogenic agents such as busulphan or possibly hydroxyurea. Interferon α has been used in MF in an attempt to reduce fibrosis and improve haematopoiesis, but with only occasional modest benefit seen in the small numbers of patients treated (Seewann *et al.*, 1988).

Myelodysplastic syndromes

Interferon has been evaluated in myelodysplastic syndromes with the aim of inducing maturation in the dysplastic myeloid series leading to an increase in numbers and improvement in function of granulocytes, red cells and platelets (Editorial, 1987). The results with IFNα treatment are largely disappointing: troublesome side-effects are common and only a proportion of patients show a measurable response in terms of increase in blood counts (Gisslinger *et al.*, 1990). Occasional patients show more favourable responses such as the disappearance of clones with an abnormal karyotype (Blok *et al.*, 1988). There is no conclusive evidence that IFNα has any clinically useful effect in MDS, but in a recent study of 31 patients with myelodysplastic syndrome IFNγ was shown to produce a dose-related haematological improvement with 27% responding to low-dose and 60% responding to high-dose IFNγ. Disease progression and survival were superior in the high-dose treatment group, but the high-dose regimen was associated with toxic side-effects, and the overall outcome was poor. The results suggest a place for IFNγ in combination with other maturation inducers in myelodysplastic syndromes (Maiolo *et al.*, 1990).

Acute myeloblastic leukaemia

Interferon has been used both during remission-induction and as a maintenance agent. There are few data to support its use as an adjunct to chemotherapy in inducing remission, and trials are under way to determine whether IFN has any effect on prolonging remission.

IL-2

Interferon 2 is a 170 kDa glycoprotein. It is produced almost entirely by activated T lymphocytes, and has been manufactured from lymphoblastoid cell lines. The IL-2 gene complex is situated on chromosome 9. The gene sequence has been established for human and murine IL-2 and has been found to be highly conserved. The IL-2 gene has been cloned and inserted via retroviral sequences into *Escherichia coli*. Several recombinant human IL-2 products are available for clinical trial.

Table 6.12 Interleukin-2

Nature and origin
15 kDa glycoprotein produced by T helper cells

Receptors
Two: high- and low-affinity (see Fig. 6.14)

Cytokine release
TNF
IFNγ
IL-3
IL-4
IL-5
IL-6
GM-CSF

Action on immune system
T cell growth factor
B cell growth factor
NK/LAK precursor proliferation
NK activation
B cell activation
Macrophage activation

Action on haemopoiesis
See Figure 6.16

Antitumour action
See Table 6.13 and Figure 6.15

TNF, Tumour necrosis factor; IFNγ, interferon γ; IL-3, interleukin 3; GM-CSF, granulocyte-macrophage colony-stimulating factor; NK, natural killer; LAK, lymphokine activated killer.

The IL-2 receptor

The IL-2 receptor is a heterodimer consisting of a 70 kDa β chain with a transmembrane component, and a 55 kDa α chain (Tsudo et al., 1989). The complex of IL-2 with the two components is necessary for cell activation. The β chain has a higher affinity than the α chain, but both chains are needed for efficient signal transduction. Figure 6.14 shows the relationship of the IL-2 molecule with its receptor.

Action of IL-2 (Table 6.12)

Interleukin 2 has a diverse range of activities (reviewed by Malkovsky and Sondel, 1987). It has a proliferative and maturational effect on T cells, B cells, NK cells, LAK precursors, and activates NK and LAK function (Grimm et al., 1982; Robertson and Ritz, 1990), MHC-restricted T cell responses (Smith, 1988), B cell (Jung et al., 1984), and monocyte function (Malkovsky et al., 1987). Interleukin 2 also

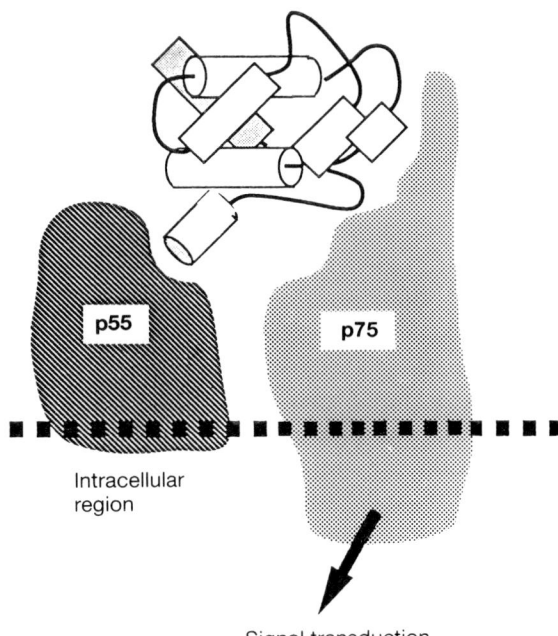

Fig. 6.14 Interleukin 2 and its receptor.

induces a range of further effects through secondary cytokine release. It thus has a powerful effect on both MHC-restricted and unrestricted immune responses.

Interleukin 2 also affects haemopoiesis largely through secondary cytokine production. Interleukin 2-stimulated T cells produce the group of haemopoietic growth factors located on chromosome 5q: IL-3, GM-CSF, IL-5 and IL-6 (Enokihara et al., 1989; Jablons et al., 1989; Neimeyer et al., 1989; Macdonald et al., 1990a). Interleukin 2 also stimulates T cells, macrophages and NK/LAK cells to produce inhibitors and regulators of myelopoiesis such as TNF and IFNγ (Reem and Yeh, 1984; Selby et al., 1987; Murphy et al., 1988; Heslop et al., 1989b). The overall haemopoietic effect of secondary cytokine production depends on the balance between the production of growth-inhibiting and stimulating cytokines. Interleukin 2 may also affect the haematopoietic microenvironment: it inhibits marrow fibroblast proliferation in vitro, interfering with the formation of the adherent stromal layer necessary to support haematopoiesis in suspension culture (Macdonald et al., 1990b). It can directly enhance the proliferation of the granulocyte-erythrocyte-megakaryocyte-macrophage progenitor (CFU-GEMM) which express the p55 (non-signal-transducing) IL-2 receptor (Michalevicz et al., 1988). Other haemopoietic stem cells have not been shown to carry the IL-2 receptor, and IL-2 does not directly stimulate committed progenitors (Burdach and Levitt, 1987; Burdach et al., 1987; Macdonald et al., 1991).

Animal tumours and IL-2

Several animal models have shown the therapeutic potential of IL-2 in the treatment of haematological malignancies: IL-2 infusion with or without LAK cells produces potent antitumour effects in mice (Greenberg, 1986; Thompson et al., 1986). Intraperitoneal administration of IL-2 exhibits a biphasic tumour response in mice bearing a transplantable lymphoma. High doses exert an antitumour effect via LAK cells while a low-dose effect (which was not observed in nude mice) was ascribed to an anti-tumour effect of T cells (Talmadge et al., 1987). Interleukin 2 enhances the survival of mice receiving syngeneic transplants accompanied by a transplantable lymphoma. It promotes the GVL effect in experimental allograft models and exerts a protective effect against relapse from the experimental transplantable EL4 leukaemia in situations where the transplant has been rendered tolerant to the host (Slavin et al., 1990; Sachs et al., 1991). Interleukin 2 enhances the incidence and severity of GVHD in recipients of non-T cell-depleted bone marrow (Malkovsky et al., 1986). However, in a mouse leukaemia model, incubation of non-T-depleted marrow with IL-2 pretransplant, followed by IL-2 infusion, resulted in the highest cure rates without lethal GVHD (Charak et al., 1990).

Effect of IL-2 on leukaemias and lymphoma cells

Interleukin 2 may have direct effects on the malignant clone leading to a favourable induction of maturation, or an unfavourable proliferative stimulus to malignant cells. However, most leukaemias are not stimulated to proliferate *in vitro* (Foa et al., 1990a). Indirectly it may have an inhibitory effect on tumour cell proliferation by its immunostimulatory action on T cells, NK and LAK cells and their secondary cytokine release. The action of IL-2 on myeloid malignancies is likely to differ from its effect on lymphoid malignancies since the latter group includes cells whose normal counterparts have proliferative responses to IL-2. Most *in vitro* experimentation has focused upon the cytotoxic action of LAK cells which lyse an extensive repertoire of leukaemia and lymphoma cell lines. However, there is evidence that in some patients autologous LAK activity is defective (Foa et al., 1990b). The possible role of IL-2 in stimulating autologous T cells equivalent to TIL cells (Rosenberg et al., 1988a) exhibiting MHC-restricted cytotoxic responses to haematological malignancies has not yet been adequately explored.

Acute leukaemias and CML. Extensive *in vitro* studies support an antileukaemic action of IL-2, through a cytotoxic effect of LAK cells on leukaemia blasts and their progenitors (Oshimi *et al.*, 1986; Adler *et al.*, 1988; Lotzova *et al.*, 1989). When incubated in suspension culture with IL-2, leukaemia cell growth of AML, ALL and CML cells is either unaffected or inhibited. Similarly, in semisolid assays IL-2 has either no effect or inhibits AML and CML clonogenic cells (Visani *et al.*, 1987; Heslop *et al.*, 1989a). Low cytotoxic activity of peripheral blood lymphocytes (PBL) against blasts is seen at presentation in myeloid leukaemias but, by culture *in vitro* with IL-2, cells expressing CD16, and CD56 increase and can lyse autologous leukaemic blasts (Lotzova *et al.*, 1989; Savary and Lotzova, 1990). Following chemotherapy or autologous BMT in patients with ALL or AML, LAK cells cytotoxic to leukaemic cell lines, autologous and allogeneic blasts and leukaemic clonogenic cells are generated (Gottieb *et al.*, 1989b; Lista *et al.*, 1989). *In vivo*, the production of secondary cytokines by IL-2 may exert an important regulatory effect. Both IFNγ and TNF are inhibitory to leukaemic cell growth. In addition, IFNγ increases the sensitivity of certain tumour cells to LAK cell lysis. Tumour necrosis factor is cytotoxic to certain tumour cells and acts synergistically with IL-2 to generate LAK cells (Winkelhake *et al.*, 1987; Heslop *et al.*, 1989a, 1989b; Stotter *et al.*, 1989). There is, however, a risk that IL-2 or induced secondary cytokines could stimulate leukaemia cell proliferation. Many haematological malignancies express the β chain of the IL-2 receptor (Rosolen *et al.*, 1989), but only rarely do they express both α and β chains necessary for an efficient IL-2 proliferative response. A small proportion of cases of AML which express the p55 portion of the IL-2 receptor exhibit blast cell proliferation in the presence of IL-2 (Armitage *et al.*, 1986; Allouche *et al.*, 1989; Carron and Cawley, 1989; Hoshino *et al.*, 1990; Macdonald *et al.*, 1991). The *in vivo* significance of this is not clear.

Lymphoid malignancies. The greater activity against malignant lymphoid cell lines of NK cells induced by IL-2 to become LAK cells suggests the possible therapeutic use of IL-2 in B cell malignancies. Lymphokine activated killer cell cytotoxicity and differentiating activity have been demonstrated against CLL cells (Malkovska *et al.*, 1987) and lymphoma cells, but myeloma cells appear to be relatively resistant to the cytotoxic effect of LAK cells (Bianchi *et al.*, 1990). Some B-ALL exhibit the p55 and the p75 IL-2 receptors and IL-2 has both a clonogenic-stimulating as well as a maturation-inducing action. Both T and B lymphomas, CLL, T-ALL and c-ALL often express both the p55 and the p75 receptor (Barnet *et al.*, 1990). The potential cytotoxic action of stimulated immune cells may therefore be offset

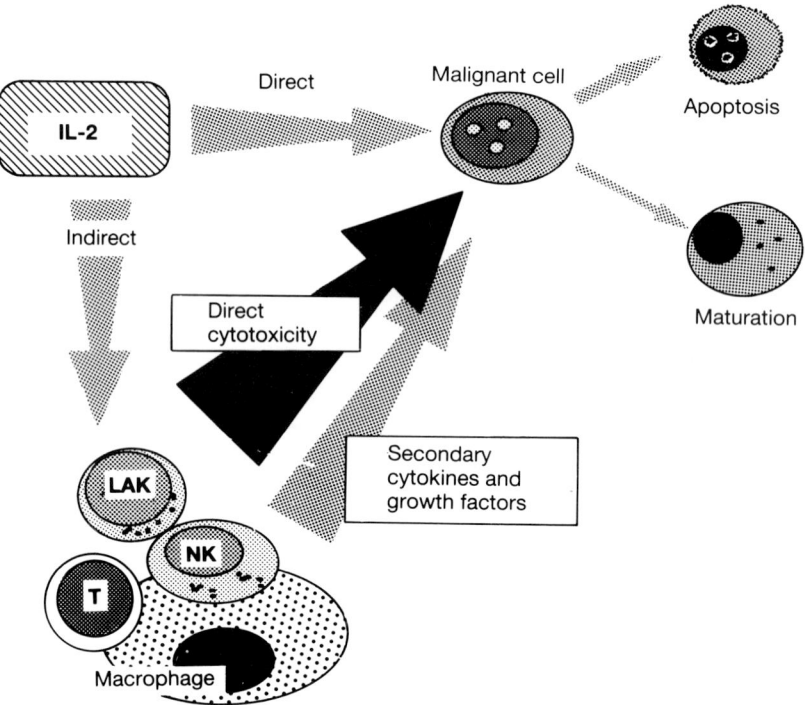

Fig. 6.15 Potential mechanisms of IL-2 in the treatment of haematological malignancy.

by a direct stimulatory action of IL-2 on the lymphoid malignancy (Kaufmann *et al.*, 1987; Malkovska *et al.*, 1987; Rosolen *et al.*, 1989). In addition, TNF acts as a growth stimulator *in vitro* for B cell malignancies (Cordingly *et al.*, 1988).

Clinical trials of IL-2

The rationale for the use of IL-2 in the treatment of haematological malignancies and other neoplasms is based largely upon its immunostimulatory properties. Figure 6.15 and Table 6.13 illustrate the mechanisms of action of IL-2 that could potentially be used in treatment, and its possible disadvantages. Interleukin 2 derived from the Jurkatt cell line was evaluated first in 1980. Subsequently, recombinant IL-2 was cloned and manufactured in sufficient quantity to evaluate its therapeutic activity and toxicity in phase I trials. Detailed evaluations of dose and schedule were carried out by Rosenberg in end-stage cancer patients. Phase I studies demonstrated that the toxicity of both rh IL-2 and the Jurkatt cell line-derived IL-2 was severe (Rosenberg *et al.*, 1987). The most dangerous complication is a capillary leak

Table 6.13 The potential and limitations of interleukin 2 (IL-2) treatment in haematological malignancies

Antitumour strategy	Disadvantages
Stimulating MHC non-restricted LAK cell immunity	Non-specific, role of LAK cells in immunotherapy not defined
Stimulating MHC restricted immune response to tumour	Specific T cell responses to haematological malignancies not well characterized
Generating antiproliferative cytokines, e.g. TNF, IFNγ	Non-specific, toxic side-effects
Induction of maturation in B and T cell malignancies	May also stimulate malignant cell proliferation
Promoting normal haematopoiesis Increase in circulating stem cells for collection and reinfusion	Other less toxic agents are as effective
Stimulation of granulopoiesis (G-CSF)	*In vivo* IL-2 causes only modest neutrophilia and induces cytopenia during infusion

MHC, Major histocompatibility complex; LAK, lymphokine activated killer; TNF, tumour necrosis factor; IFNγ, interferon γ, G-CSF, granulocyte colony-stimulating factor.

syndrome associated with reduced gas transfer and respiratory distress (Gottlieb *et al.*, 1989a). Hypotension occurs due to increased vascular permeability.

Management is complicated by the difficulty of maintaining blood pressure with colloids, while at the same time avoiding decreasing gas transfer resulting from pulmonary oedema. The effects are partly mediated through secondary cytokine release. There is an acute-phase reaction, presumably due to the release of IL-1. It is sometimes difficult to distinguish between bacterial sepsis and IL-2 side-effects. Because of this, some studies have used prophylactic antibiotic treatment throughout the period of IL-2 treatment. Fever, tachycardia, and hypotension are almost always encountered. Toxic erythema is common. Other less frequent side-effects are severe mental depression and alopecia. Patients given high doses of IL-2 in experimental protocols require intensive care. Toxic effects can, however, be avoided since they are dose rate-related and are rapidly reversed by stopping the IL-2 infusion. Since safe administration of IL-2 is a prerequisite for its general application in the management of patients with malignancies, more recent trials have used continuous infusion of lower doses of IL-2, or subcutaneously administered IL-2 to avoid life-threatening complications. It is not yet resolved whether the administration of lower doses of IL-2 is accompanied by as effective stimulation of the immune system, nor whether antimalignant activity is dose- or route-dependent. These considerations are important since animal tumour responses to IL-2 are dependent on both the dose and the treatment duration.

IL-2 and haemopoiesis

Interleukin 2 has its greatest immediate effect on the peripheral blood when given intravenously, by bolus infusion of doses in the region of 18×10^6 World Health Organization units. Similar but less extreme effects are seen during continuous intravenous infusion. Within 24 hours patients may develop thrombocytopenia, lymphopenia and neutrophilia. Anaemia develops during repeated courses of IL-2 administration (Ettinghauser *et al.*, 1987; Richards, 1989). The cytopenia in patients who have received intensive chemotherapy to induce remission in acute leukaemia might be expected to be enhanced by

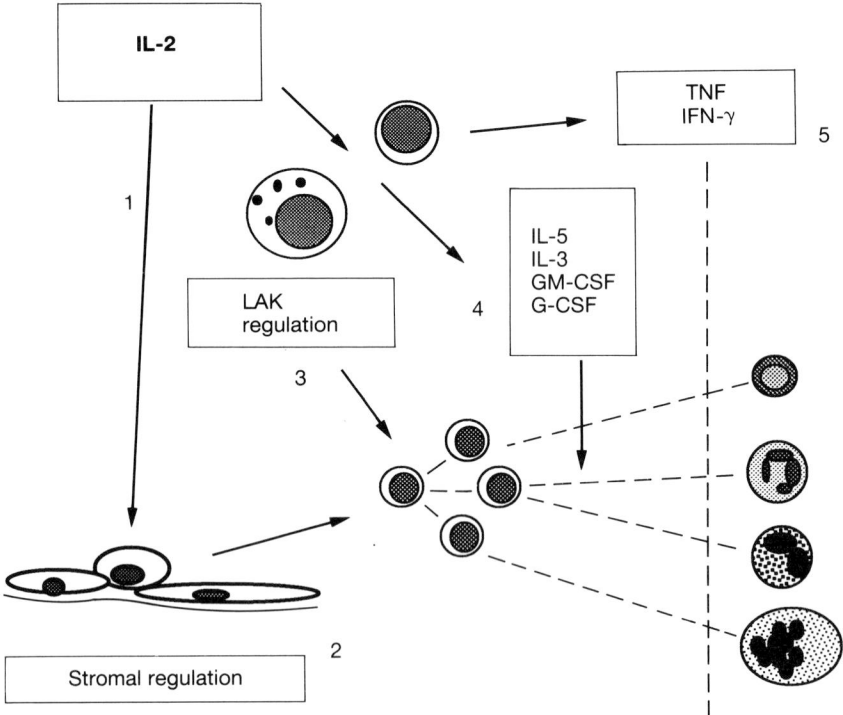

Fig. 6.16 Interactions of IL-2 with haemopoiesis. (1) Direct effect on stroma formation; (2) indirect suppression of haemopoiesis via defective stroma; (3) regulation of progenitor cells by LAK cells and NK cells; (4) production of haemopoietic growth factors; (5) production of cytokines with a negative effect on haemopoiesis.

poor stem cell function. However, in a study in patients with AML in remission, similar degrees of cytopenia to that described in patients with solid tumours receiving IL-2 were seen (Macdonald et al., 1990c). Eosinophilia is a later effect maximal after stopping IL-2 infusion and persisting for 2–3 weeks. There is no distinct pattern to the effect of IL-2 on circulating neutrophils: some studies report no change, and others a slight neutrophilia (Macdonald et al., 1990a, 1990c; Heslop et al., 1991). Interleukin 2 infusion interferes with neutrophil function causing a neutrophil chemotactic defect. This may partly explain the increased incidence of bacterial infection seen during infusion, despite near normal neutrophil numbers (Klempner et al., 1990). Interleukin 2 infusion causes an immediate fall in circulating haemopoietic progenitor cells, followed by a dramatic increase on cessation of treatment. This rise of circulating haemopoietic progenitor cells includes pluripotent stem cells and is large enough to make feasible peripheral blood autografts using haemopoietic progenitor cells collected post IL-2 infusion (Schaafsma et al., 1990). Figure 6.16 summarizes the immediate and delayed haematological effects of IL-2.

Changes in lymphocyte subsets and lymphocyte function

The initial fall in the lymphocyte count during IL-2 infusion is followed by a rebound lymphocytosis which may be very marked (in the order of $10-20 \times 100/l$; Lotze et al., 1985). Figure 6.17 illustrates the typical changes in blood cells seen during and after IL-2 infusion. The increase affects all lymphocyte subsets proportionally: the rise in absolute numbers of T helper, T cytotoxic/suppressor, and NK cells does not alter the ratios of CD4+ to CD8+ cells nor the relative frequency of NK/LAK cells. However, the proportion and absolute number of activated T cells as measured by DR surface antigen expression is greatly increased (Macdonald et al., 1991). Numerous studies demonstrate that NK function is enhanced, and LAK cell activity is induced by IL-2 infusion. Cytotoxicity to autologous leukaemia targets is enhanced (Gottlieb et al., 1989b). The degree of lymphocytosis achieved varies according to the type of patient treated – patients who have been less heavily treated with chemotherapy may achieve lymphocytoses in the order of $20 \times 10^9/l$, while in a trial of IL-2 in patients in remission Macdonald and colleagues (1991) reported only modest lymphcytoses in the order of $6 \times 10^9/l$. Several investigators have reported increases in activated cytotoxic lymphocytes of the NK/LAK phenotype, and have demonstrated increased cytotoxicity against the K562 NK target, as well as against NK-resistant, LAK cell-sensitive targets such as the Daudi B cell line and autologous leukaemia or lymphoma targets (Gottlieb et al., 1989b). There is no evidence however that IL-2 causes selective expansion of LAK cells over and above the increase in other subsets, or how much the lymphocytosis represents a true increase in lymphocyte numbers, or how much it represents a compartmental shift. Whether the degree of lymphocytosis parallels an antitumour effect is also not certain. The demonstration that IL-2 also activates a subpopulation of cytotoxic lymphocytes with restricted specificity against the autologous tumour raises the possibility that the therapeutic effect of IL-2 may relate more closely to the activation of this special subclass of cells (Fisher et al., 1989; Rosenberg et al., 1988a).

IL-2 in the treatment of lymphoma

A number of patients with non-Hodgkin's lymphoma have been treated with high-dose IL-2/LAK therapy, and although these patients generally had advanced and resistant disease, a minority responded, one patient having a complete remission and four patients a partial remission from 20 treated patients. In the treatment of non-Hodgkin's lymphoma, it seems that high-dose IL-2/LAK is currently the most successful, as regimes using IL-2 only or IL-2 with IFNα produced no significant response in small groups of patients with non-Hodgkin's lymphoma or low-grade B cell malignancies (Janson et al., 1989; Kolitz et al., 1990; Malkovska and Sondel, 1990). This observation may be modified by studies on patients with less advanced and heavily treated disease. Current trials are investigating the use of ABMT followed by continuous low-dose infusion of IL-2. This regimen avoids significant toxicity, and generates an increase in circulating NK cells able to lyse tumour cells, with minimal T cell proliferation. The results of this type of protocol are awaited (Allison et al., 1989; Soiffer et al., 1990).

IL-2 in the treatment of leukaemia

As acute leukaemia was not one of the diseases treated in initial clinical trials of high-dose IL-2 with or without LAK cells, only a very few patients with acute leukaemia have received IL-2, and the published trials have a short follow-up. Trials in acute myeloid leukaemia (AML) have employed IL-2 only without LAK cells. In a study of 16 patients with relapsed or refractory AML, complete remission, or a significant reduction in blast cells of 3–4-month duration was seen in five patients (Foa et al., 1989). This suggests that patients in remission from AML with minimal residual disease may be the best candidates for IL-2 treatment, as in theory the highest ratios of effector to target cells would be achieved at this stage. Unfortunately the hypothesis was not borne out in a trial of IL-2 as maintenance for

AML in first remission, where no survival advantage was demonstrated for a group of nine patients (Macdonald et al., 1991). As noted previously, many leukaemic cells retain the growth responsiveness to cytokines that is a feature of their normal counterparts. It is of concern that in a proportion of cases leukaemic blasts express either or both chains of the IL-2 receptor (see above). Additionally, Carron and Cawley (1989) noted proliferation of some monocytic leukaemias *in vitro* in response to IL-2. However, a correlation between receptor expression and leukaemic relapse induced by treatment with IL-2 has not been confirmed.

IL-2 in autologous BMT

The therapeutic use of IL-2 following ABMT has not been clearly evaluated. Theoretically, IL-2 could be used to control minimal residual disease following intensive cytoreduction and autologous BMT. It might enhance the prominent early recovery of NK/LAK cells after autologous marrow infusion (Higuchi et al., 1989; Reittie et al., 1989). IL-2 can be safely administered early after ABMT. It can be shown to enhance the generation of potentially antileukaemic cytokines (IFNγ and TNF) as well as cells with cytoxicity against leukaemic cells (Gottlieb et al., 1989b; Heslop et al., 1989a; Higuchi et al., 1989). The effect on disease-free survival of this type of protocol on survival is awaited (Blaise et al., 1990).

IL-2 in allogeneic BMT

Following marrow transplantation there is a rise in non-specific cytotoxic cells of the NK class as well as an increase in non-MHC-restricted cytotoxic helper T cells (Stotter et al., 1989). Interleukin 2 could therefore be used to expand further the cells responsible for the early re-emergence of non-restricted cytotoxicity.

One limitation of giving IL-2 following non-T-depleted BMT is the risk of inducing fatal GVHD. In mice, IL-2 induces GVHD in recipients of non-T cell-depleted BMT but GVHD was not enhanced in T-depleted recipients (Malkovsky et al., 1986). Trials of IL-2 after T-depleted allogeneic BMT would therefore be justifiable.

Interleukin 2 has a potential role in stimulation of the immune system following BMT and could be used to rescue the GVL response in BMT selectively depleted of GVHD reacting cells (Butturini and Gale, 1990). After BMT for CML, circulating lymphocytes generate LAK cells in the presence of IL-2 with activity against pretransplant CML cells. This activity is mediated by CD16, and CD56 positive cells and can be generated from peripheral blood post T-depleted BMT

(Mackinnon et al., 1990). It is of relevance that the risk of leukaemic relapse was greatest in patients who did not develop lytic activity against host leukaemia, in post-transplant (donor-derived) lymphocytes (Hauch et al., 1990). The main concern before further trials of IL-2 are carried out is that severe GVHD could result from IL-2 treatment. Clinical trials using IL-2 post-BMT are largely limited to autologous BMT and T cell-depleted BMT. Only three patients have been reported and in none of these did overwhelming GVHD develop (Favrot et al., 1989).

Improving the therapeutic index of IL-2

Several clinical trials have investigated different treatment approaches designed to reduce toxicity while retaining an effective antitumour action.

Low-dose IL-2 with LAK cells. West et al. (1987) treated 40 patients with various end-stage malignancies with continuous infusion of IL-2 over 5 days. Major toxicity was avoided and dose reduction was employed if side-effects were considered dangerous. The results in 24 patients with renal cell carcinoma and 22 patients with melanoma compare favourably with those achieved by Rosenberg et al. (1988b) using high dose IL-2 and LAK cells. Similar responses have been achieved in other studies.

Subcutaneous low-dose IL-2. Several reports demonstrate that low-dose subcutaneous IL-2 given by continuous pump infusion was well-tolerated outside the hospital setting and was associated with tumour responses (Whitehead et al., 1990; Stein et al., 1991).

IL-2 and chemotherapy. In mice, cyclophosphamide can exert synergy with IL-2 but not LAK cells. A trial of IL-2 with cyclophosphamide in melanoma produced 6/24 responses but the results are unevaluable in the absence of a non-cyclophosphamide control group (Mitchell et al., 1988).

IL-2 and cytokines. The targets of IL-2-stimulated cytotoxic cells may be rendered more susceptible to cytolysis by factors that increase their expression of MHC class I, necessary for interaction with cytotoxic T cells. Interferon α enhances the susceptibility of target cell lysis in this way. Animal experiments demonstrate synergy between IL-2 and IFN (Rosenberg et al., 1988b) and IL-2 and TNF (McIntosh et al., 1988).

IL-2 and antibodies. Interleukin 2-mediated cytotoxicity can be enhanced *in vitro* by antitumour antibody, which converts LAK cells bearing the Fc receptor into antibody-dependent cytotoxic cells, thereby rendering them specific to cells coated with antibody (Lotze et al., 1987; Shiloni et al., 1987; Dearman et al., 1988).

Future developments

Currently the role of IL-2 in haematopoietic malignancies remains unclear, though studies in the areas outlined above may clarify the situation. Many unanswered questions remain, including the basic questions of how best to administer IL-2, by which route and for how long. These considerations are hampered by the lack of reliable ways of monitoring its efficacy. The synergy of IL-2 with other cytokines such as the IFNs, IL-4 (Nagler et al., 1988) and TNF have yet to be evaluated. Of particular interest in the future is the possibility of using IL-2 to increase the GVL effect following either autologous or allogeneic BMT. A novel modality of IL-2 treatment currently being investigated is the combination of IL-2 with a toxin. These molecules may provide novel therapies for some of the haematopoietic malignancies such as T cell lymphoma, and adult T cell leukaemia/lymphoma which can be induced to, or may constitutively express the IL-2 receptor (Walz et al., 1989). Finally, despite the high purity of the IL-2 now available for clinical use, its effects *in vivo* are toxic and nonspecific. The future for IL-2 may therefore lie more in its property as an *in vitro* growth factor for the production of immune cells with specific and possibly enhanced toxicity for haematological malignancies. Such cells cloned *in vitro* could be used in large numbers on repeated occasions to exert a cell-mediated antitumour effect.

TNF

Tumour necrosis factor α and lymphotoxin (TNFβ) are similar but distinct products of T lymphocyte and NK cell activation. Tumour necrosis factor was first identified as a factor causing necrosis of tumours and cachexia (reviewed by Brenner, 1988). It has a very wide action, being involved in inflammation and toxic shock, immunoregulation, stimulation of angiogenesis and inhibition of growth of many normal cells and tumours.

Tumour necrosis factors represent a family of molecules with wide-ranging effects. Its characteristics are shown in Table 6.14. Tumour necrosis factor α and β are important in cytotoxicity. Tumour necrosis factor β is a 19 kDa glycoprotein which exerts cytostatic and cytotoxic effects against a variety of normal and malignant cells. Its action is enhanced by IFNγ. Tumour necrosis factor causes DNA damage by activating endonucleases. It exerts a wide range of effects by the

Table 6.14 Tumour necrosis factor (TNF)

Origin and nature
TNFα 17 kDa (cachexin) and TNFβ 25 kDa (lymphotoxin) are closely similar glycoproteins produced on chromosome 16 by macrophages and T cells. Released by endotoxin, IFNα, TNF, IL-1

Receptor
Same receptor for TNFα and β. Single 55 kDa, sharing homology with nerve growth factor

Cytokine release
IL-1, IL-6, TGFβ, M-CSF, GM-CSF, PDGF, TNF, prostaglandin release, acute-phase protein release

Action on immune system
Central role in tissue destruction in association with acute-phase reactions
Leukostasis via ICAM activation
Activates T cells up-regulating IL-2 receptor expression
Increases phagocytosis by neutrophils
Activates eosinophils

Action on haemopoiesis
Inhibits erythroid colony (BFU-E) and granulocyte-monocyte (CFU-GM) growth

Action on tumours
Immune stimulation
Cytotoxic to some haematological malignancies, inducing apoptosis (see Fig. 6.10)
A growth factor for some B cell malignancies

IFN, Interferon; IL-1, interleukin 1; TGFβ, transforming growth factor β; M-CSF, macrophage colony-stimulating factor; GM-CSF, granulocyte-macrophage colony-stimulating factor; PDGF, platelet-derived growth factor; ICAM, intracellular adhesion molecule.

activation of other cells: it induces cytotoxic T lymphocytes (CTLs) and releases IL-2, IFNs and colony-stimulating factors from other lymphocytes. Macrophages and neutrophils are powerfully activated by TNF. Class I antigen expression is also enhanced. Tumour necrosis factor therefore has an important modulating effect both in the immune response but also to the susceptibility of target cells of the immune reaction. It is a growth factor for some human diploid cell lines and tumour cell lines, synergizing with insulin, platelet-derived growth factor and epidermal growth factor. The response of the cell to TNF depends upon whether protein synthesis is active or suppressed: TNF is cytotoxic to cells when protein synthesis is inhibited. The mechanism is unclear. Tumour necrosis factor is cytostatic and cytotoxic against a variety of malignant cells. While TNF is cytostatic to myeloid leukaemias, it is paradoxically a growth factor in B-CLL and hairy cell leukaemia. *In vivo*, it plays a role in toxic shock and its local release is implicated in acute respiratory distress syndrome, and veno-occlusive disease.

Table 6.15 Interleukin-4 (IL-4)

Origin
20 kDa glycoprotein mainly produced by a T helper lymphocyte subset

Receptor
140 kDa high affinity. Same receptor superfamily as IL-2
Present on B cells, haemopoietic cells, fibroblasts, endothelial cells

Interactions with other cytokines
Antagonist to interferons and some actions of IL-2
Inhibits M-CSF

Interactions with other receptors
Up-regulates class II
Induces VCAM expression on endothelial cells
Up-regulates IL-2 receptor on B and T cells

Action on B cells
Growth and maturation factor for pre-B cells
Inhibits differentiation of later B cells
Class switching IgE ↑ IgG ↓ IgM ↓
Up-regulates IL-4 receptor

Action on T cells
Stimulates T cell growth

Haemopoiesis
Promotes CFU-GM and BFU-E growth
Stimulates megakaryopoiesis
Inhibits macrophage colony growth (suppresses M-CSF)

Action on tumours
Increases tumour killing by up-regulation of receptors and activation of macrophages

M-CSF, macrophage colony-stimulating factor; IgG, immunoglobulin G; VCAM, vascular cell adhesion molecule; CFU-GM, granulocyte-monocyte colony forming units; BFU-E, erythroid burst forming units.

Clinical studies

The observation that TNF makes some experimental tumours regress has led to several preliminary trials of TNF in end-stage malignant disease. In phase I trials worldwide, recombinant human TNF only rarely produces regressions to less than 50% of the tumour bulk (Malkovska and Sondel, 1990). There have been no trials of TNF in haematological malignancies. Tumour necrosis factor administration alone does not appear to be a useful immunotherapeutic agent since it suppressess NK activity. It may find a place as an adjuvant to other cytokines.

IL-4

Interleukin 4 was first described as B cell-stimulating factor but is best regarded as a wide-ranging growth factor and regulator of B cells, T cells, and haemopoietic cells. It is a 20 kDa glycoprotein produced mainly by T cells and some B cells. Its main characteristics are shown in Table 6.15.

Interleukin 4 has complicated actions on B cells. It promotes differentiation of pre-B cells, and is involved in class switching to IgG1. It inhibits the differentiation of earlier B cells. It synergizes with IL-2, stimulating the growth of helper T cell lines (Fernandez-Botran et al., 1986). It can also substitute for IL-2 to allow post-thymic T cell differentiation in IL-2-deficient mice. However, in mice where the IL-2 gene has been deleted it does not alone permit clonal amplification following T cell activation (Schorle et al., 1991). It has been shown to be a potent regulator of IL-2 activation and NK cell proliferation (Nagler et al., 1988). Interleukin 4 mediates the induction of LAK cells and enhances their effect on tumour targets (Mule et al., 1987). It further increases immune responsiveness by increasing class II expression. In other actions, however, it is an antagonist of IFN-γ. Recombinant human IL-4 has been manufactured and the way is therefore open for clinical trials of IL-4, probably used in combination with other cytokines.

IL-6

Receptors for IL-6 are expressed on activated T cells, B cells, fibroblasts, endothelial cells and monocyte/macrophages. It has therefore been implicated in local regulation of immune responses to infection. Interleukin 6 has a very wide range of actions (Table 6.16).

Interleukin-6 is of potential interest in immunotherapy because together with IL-2, IL-4, and IFNγ, it serves as a differentiation factor for the development of cytotoxic T cells from immature thymocytes (Wong and Clark, 1988). Together with IL-2, IL-6 synergizes to augment perforin gene expression and enhances the cytotoxic potential of human T cells (Smythe et al., 1990). Interleukin 6 is a late-acting B cell growth factor, and is also involved in the stimulation of pluripotent haemopoietic progenitors and megakaryocytopoiesis and can enhance haematological recovery after marrow transplantation (Okano et al., 1988).

M-CSF

Macrophage-stimulating factor (CSF-1) is a glycoprotein dimer of

Table 6.16 Interleukin 6 (IL-6)

Nature and origin
21–28 kDa glycoprotein, made by macrophages and a wide variety of cells
Production stimulated by IL-1, IL-2, TNF and haemopoietic growth factors

Receptors
Two: low- and high-affinity Ig superfamily; present on many cell types

Action on the immune system
Involved with IL-1 in the acute-phase response
Terminal differentiation of B cells – stimulates Ig production and specific antibody responses
Enhances T cell response to alloantigens via up-regulation of the IL-2 receptor
Enhances response of T cells to IL-4

Action on haemopoiesis
Stimulates megakaryopoiesis
Synergy with other growth factors in stimulating entry into G_1 of the cell cycle, mainly affecting pluripotent stem cell proliferation

Other actions
Increases mesangial proliferation of renal glomeruli
Stimulates nerve growth factor production
Stimulates hypothalamus, causing pyrexia

Action on tumours
Growth factor for myeloma cells
Potential adjuvant with other immune-stimulatory cytokines

TNF, Tumour necrosis factor; Ig, immunoglobulin.

29 kDa. It stimulates growth and differentiation of monocyte-macrophages and is also a potent macrophage activator (Table 6.17). Recombinant M-CSF has been evaluated in phase I trials and may have a role in increasing cytotoxic responses to tumours. It has not been used in the immunotherapeutic setting in haematological malignancies.

Tumour-specific immune cells

LAK cells

LAK cells can be prepared from lymphocytes obtained by leukapheresis and incubated for 48–72 hours with IL-2 in gas-permeable collection bags. Autologous LAK cells can be safely reinfused without any reaction. Such LAK cell preparations contain activated T lymphocytes as well as activated NK cells. They can be shown to possess enhanced cytotoxic activity against the recipient's leukaemia. Since most studies combine LAK cell infusions with IL-2 treatment it is not

Table 6.17 Macrophage colony-stimulating factor (CSF-1)

Nature and origin
70–90 kDa glycoprotein produced by macrophages and lymphocytes

Receptor
c-*fms* proto-oncogene on macrophages and other cells

Cytokine release
TNF
G/GM-CSF
IL-1
IFN
Thromboplastin antecedent
Prostaglandins
Thromboplastins

Action on immune system
Stimulation of intracellular killing by macrophages

Action on haemopoiesis
Monocyte-macrophage production from earlier progenitor

Action on tumours
Increases tumour cell lysis by macrophages

Other actions
Placental trophoblast regulation

TNF, Tumour necrosis factor; GM-CSF, granulocyte-macrophage colony-stimulating factor; IL-1, interleukin 1; IFN, interferon.

possible to determine the therapeutic impact of the addition of LAK cells generated *in vitro* to the *in vivo* LAK cell induction by IL-2. A recent trial has investigated the use of LAK cell infusions and IL-2 during remission-induction of AML (Boughton *et al.*, 1991). It was possible to administer LAK cells and IL-2 without major toxicity, and this regimen induced a skin rash clinically and histologically identical to GVHD.

There is as yet no evidence that treatments augmenting LAK cell production confer an antileukaemia effect.

Tumour-specific lymphocytes

Adoptive immunotherapy with tumour-specific T cells has been studied extensively in several animal experimental systems, including the murine FBL leukaemia model (Greenberg *et al.*, 1989) and the AKR/Gross immune leukaemia model (Green *et al.*, 1979). It appears that the adoptive transfer of tumour-sensitized lymphocytes effectively mediates the regression of a variety of established syngeneic tumours. In animal models, T cell therapy shows dose-responsiveness with higher T cell numbers inducing longer survival times and greater percentages of cures. It is therefore probable that larger numbers of effector cells will also be required to treat human tumours. Studies aimed at defining the principles and developing techniques for isolating and propagating tumour-reactive lymphocytes from tumour-bearing hosts are in progress (reviewed by Greenberg, 1991).

The precise mechanisms of tumour elimination *in vivo* are also being investigated. For example, the complete eradication of the retrovirus-induced syngeneic FBL leukaemia requires that transfected cells proliferate in the host and mediate the antitumour effect for at least 30 days. Interestingly, both cytolytic CD8+ T cells and non-cytolytic CD4+ T cells can promote leukaemia eradication in this model. The antitumour activity of the helper cells apparently results from lymphokine secretion that activates macrophages to kill tumours. The antitumour effects of CTL populations which do not secrete sufficient amounts of cytokines could be enhanced by simultaneous administration of IL-2 (Greenberg *et al.*, 1989). By analogy, it might be predicted that successful immunotherapy of human tumours with T cells may be complex and require administration of different T cell-promoting cytokines.

Further studies on human autologous and allogeneic antitumour T cell responses should determine if any of the above approaches are feasible in the clinical setting.

In search of human tumour antigens eliciting a specific immune response, several groups of investigators have obtained CTL generated by B cell lymphomas (reviewed by Anichi *et al.*, 1987). Alloreactive CTLs which lysed leukaemic lymphoblasts but not normal lymphocytes from the same patient have also been generated (Sosman *et al.*, 1990). Both CD8+ and CD4+ CTLs appear to be capable of tumour cell lysis in different systems. Improved culture techniques and availability of recombinant cytokines have facilitated the generation and expansion of stable tumour-specific CTL clones and raised the possibility of using such clones for adoptive immunotherapy (Miescher *et al.*, 1987; Hersey *et al.*, 1988; Topalian *et al.*, 1988). They also represent an important tool for studying tumour-specific antigens. Attempts to identify the molecular structure of these antigens with monoclonal antibodies have been largely unsuccessful. This is not surprising, since tumour antigens which are recognized by tumour-specific T cells are not intact integrated membrane glycoproteins. New approaches to antigen detection involve the transfection of target cells with different protein genes and testing the transfectants for their ability to stimulate specific CTL clones.

TILs

Rosenberg showed that T cells obtained from the vicinity of tumour metastases represented clones of T cells with specific reactivity against the tumour (Rosenberg *et al.*, 1988a,b). They could be expanded *in vitro* in the presence of the tumour cells and IL-2 and showed proliferative and cytotoxic responses to the tumour. These TILs were more easily derived from patients with melanoma than with other tumours.

GVL reactions

The GVL response and its relationship to the GVHD reaction has been considered extensively in Chapter 4. In this section is discussed only the application of alloreactive T cells outside the context of marrow transplantation (reviewed by Sosman and Sondel, 1987).

The concept of using alloreacting lymphocytes to eliminate leukaemic cells *in vivo* is an attractive one. Cytotoxic donor lymphocytes chosen to recognize major or minor histocompatibility antigen differences on the surface of the leukaemic cell could theoretically be used to eliminate minimal residual disease (Zarling *et al.*, 1978). However, the approach has many shortcomings:

1 Infused MHC-incompatible lymphocytes have only a brief survival in the recipient.
2 The potential of such lymphocytes to home to the leukaemia targets may be limited by their tendency to sequester in the lung capillaries.
3 Engraftment of alloreactive lymphocytes in an immunosuppressed recipient can lead to fatal GVHD. Study of transfusion-related GVHD shows that the donor and the recipient usually share at least one MHC class I or II antigen and usually the whole haplotype. It therefore seems likely that haplotype-indentical siblings would in practice be a useful source of alloreactive cells with the capacity to engraft and exert an allograft effect (Anderson and Weinstein, 1990).

Recent studies suggest that leukaemia-specific human CTL may be generated from peripheral lymphocytes obtained from normal HLA-identical marrow donors (Sosman *et al.*, 1989; Falkenburg *et al.*, 1990). These allogeneic CTL did not lyse the patients' remission lymphocytes but their precise target structures remain to be defined. A potential therapeutic use of such T cells from allogeneic sources would be to bypass the problem of generating and obtaining large numbers of functional leukaemia-reactive lymphocytes from leukaemia patients on chemotherapy.

Antibodies

The idea of using antibodies to treat cancers has its origins in the ideas of Ehrlich who sought for 'the magic bullet seeking out the enemy' (Ehrlich, 1906), and Metchnikoff who prepared an antiserum against lymphoid cells (Metchnikoff, 1899). While hopes that specific antisera could be used to treat malignancies were never fulfilled, the development of antilymphocyte globulin as an immunosuppressive agent gave an opportunity to test it in the treatment of T cell lymphomas. Responses occurred but were transient, and the immunosuppressive action of the antilymphoctyte globulin caused lethal infectious complications (Barrett et al., 1976). The introduction of the technique to make monoclonal antibodies by Kohler and Milstein (1975) heralded a new wave of enthusiasm for the use of antibodies in treatment of haematological malignancies (reviewed by Larner, 1989). Compared with solid tumour tissues, the antigen systems of leukocytes are well-characterized, making haematological malignancies good subjects for experimental antibody treatment studies. The advantage of monoclonal antibodies is their reproducibility and specificity, and the ability to manufacture large quantities for clinical use. Nevertheless, these rodent cell-derived monoclonal antibodies still have major shortcomings as therapeutic agents. The following section describes the characteristics of monoclonals, their advantages and disadvantages, and approaches being used to improve their therapeutic efficacy and widen their therapeutic application. (For a description of antibody structure see Chapter 3.)

Modes of action of monoclonal antibodies

Most monoclonals, such as those which have been used to treat lymphomas, are directed against tumour-associated rather than tumour-specific antigens. An exception to this are the anti-idiotypic antibodies raised against unique variable sequences of monoclonal surface immunoglobulins from B lymphomas and myeloma (Stevenson and Stevenson, 1975).

Several mechanisms may be involved in the antitumour effect of monoclonal antibodies.

Complement fixation. The triggering of the complement cascade by antibody-binding, and a configurational change at the hinge region of the antibody, results in the activation of the ninth component which perforates the cell membrane causing lysis (see Male et al., 1991 for review). In order to lyse cells a sufficiently high antibody density is needed to fix complement. Mouse monoclonals are much less able to bind human complement, and as a consequence exhibit little lytic activity against human cells. They can, however, be rendered lytic to human cells in the presence of rabbit complement. Rat monoclonals fix human complement more efficiently, and the rat immunoglobulin M (IgM) monoclonal Campath-1 is lytic to human lymphocytes in the presence of human complement.

ADCC. Antibody-dependent cellular cytotoxicity depends upon the recognition of mouse Fc by human Fc receptors on monocytes, B cells and NK cells. Mouse IgG2 antibodies can stimulate ADCC but IgG1 and IgG2b do not. There is also some question about the ability of macrophages to cooperate in ADCC reactions with mouse monoclonals.

Cooperation with the reticuloendothelial system. In vivo, non-lytic antibodies binding to circulating cells should enhance cell removal and elimination by the reticuloendothelial system through ADCC. While studies of radioantibody-labelled lymphoma cells demonstrate the clearance of injected cells by the reticuloendothelial system, the ultimate fate of such sequestered cells cannot be ascertained.

Other effects. The administration of an antibody from another species induces a polyclonal response which includes the production of anti-idiotypic antibodies against the variable portion of the monoclonal. In some individuals a cascade of anti-anti-idiotypic antibodies may be generated (Schroff *et al.*, 1985). Some of these third-generation antibodies have specificity for the original antigen. It is possible that an antitumour effect could be prolonged by this transfer of immunological memory for the original antigen. Antibodies with specificity for growth factor or cytokine receptors may have special modes of action on the growth of the malignant cell. Blocking the receptor may inhibit growth, but paradoxically may act as a counterfeit trigger for proliferation: antilymphocyte globulin is mitogenic in low doses but antibodies to the IL-2 receptor are highly efficient at preventing IL-2-driven proliferation.

Limitations to the therapeutic use of monoclonals

The property of high purity and specificity of monoclonals is not sufficient on its own to render them immediately useful in treatment of haematological malignancies. The limited cooperation of mouse monoclonals with the human immune system across a species barrier has already been mentioned. In addition, the behaviour of the malignant cell itself places limitations on the effectiveness of the antibody, and *in vivo* monoclonals may have only limited access to the malignant cells.

Tumour cell escape. Efficient antibody binding and function depend upon a relatively high density of surface antigen, and there are many ways in which the cell may evade antibody binding and subsequent damage: antigen expression may be variable from cell to cell and may be absent on progenitor cells which can therefore escape damage. Some antigens are only expressed at particular times in the cell cycle. *In vivo*, soluble antigen shed into the circulation may neutralize the antibody before it reaches the malignant cell. Tissue-specific antibodies may similarly bind to sites other than the malignancy itself. Some cells may escape damage by shedding the antigen–antibody complexes. Rapid internalization of the bound antibody in the capping process may prevent complement and ADCC-mediated damage. Lastly lymphoma cells have been found to change their idiotype during antibody treatment (Gordon *et al.*, 1984; Meeker *et al.*, 1985).

Deficiencies in the monoclonal antibody. Monoclonals from rodents cooperate only partially with the human immune system, thus reducing their potential for recruitment of important cytotoxic mechanisms. Antibodies raised in other species induce neutralizing antibodies within 2 weeks with subsequent rapid clearance and inactivation of further antibody administrations. The half-life of mouse monoclonals is considerably shorter than the equivalent human immunoglobulin subtype. However, some patients may be sufficiently immunosuppressed that the clearance of circulating antibody is prolonged.

Access to the tumour. While IgM antibodies are more efficient at complement-directed lysis, they are too large to exit from the circulation and will not therefore reach extravascular compartments. Because of their wide tissue distribution IgG monoclonals are much more likely to be effective *in vivo*. Antibodies will have greatest efficiency against small numbers of well-dispersed cells. Cells in the centre of a tumour mass may be poorly vascularized and could escape from encountering the antibody. Certain sites, such as the central nervous system, act as sanctuary sites for leukaemias and lymphomas. Effective treatment of central nervous system disease would therefore require intrathecally injected antibody.

Overcoming the problems with artificial antibody constructs

Some of these shortcomings have been overcome by the production of artificially modified 'designer' antibodies (Fig. 6.17).

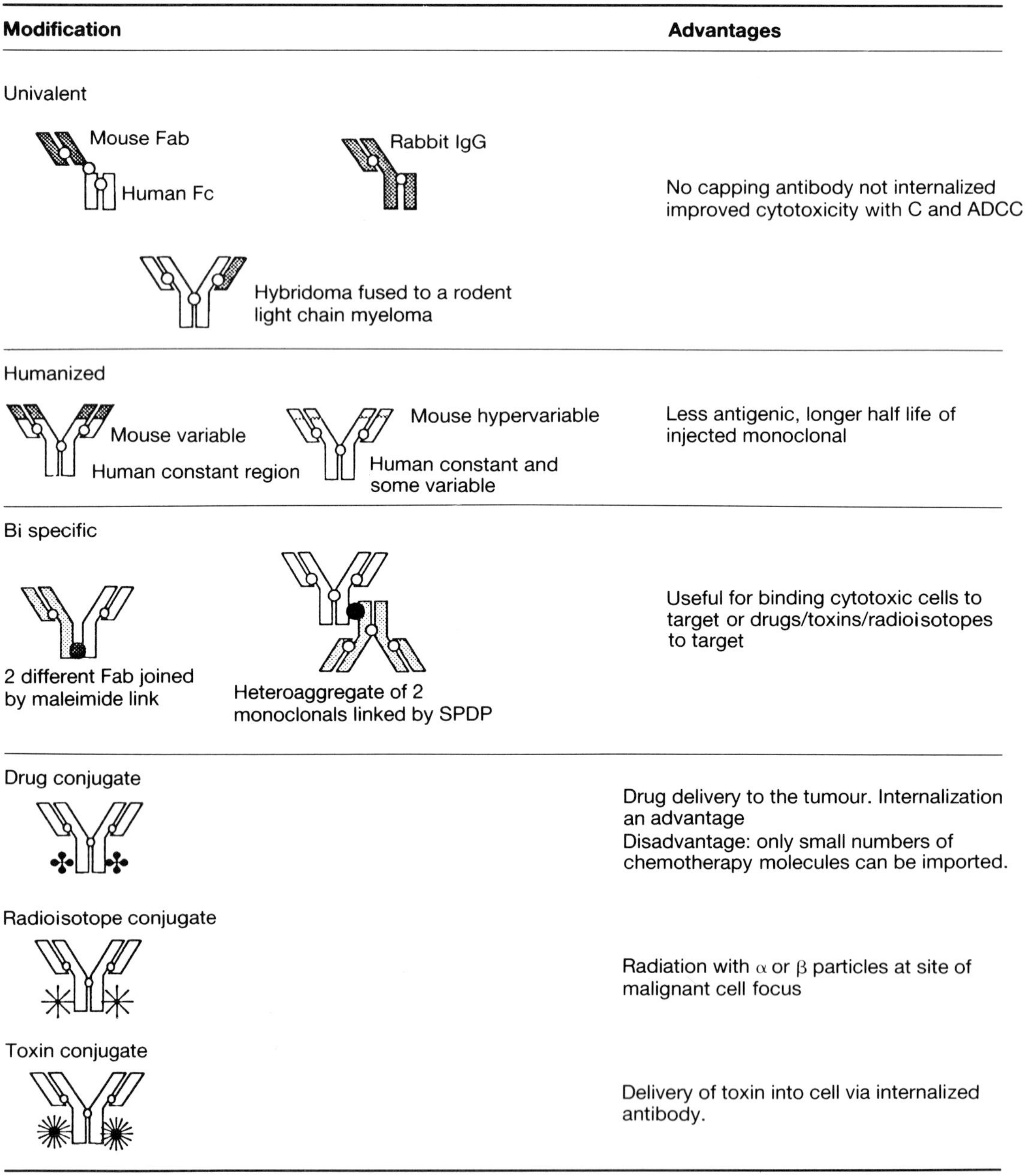

Modification	Advantages
Univalent Mouse Fab / Human Fc Rabbit IgG Hybridoma fused to a rodent light chain myeloma	No capping antibody not internalized improved cytotoxicity with C and ADCC
Humanized Mouse variable / Human constant region Mouse hypervariable / Human constant and some variable	Less antigenic, longer half life of injected monoclonal
Bi specific 2 different Fab joined by maleimide link Heteroaggregate of 2 monoclonals linked by SPDP	Useful for binding cytotoxic cells to target or drugs/toxins/radioisotopes to target
Drug conjugate	Drug delivery to the tumour. Internalization an advantage Disadvantage: only small numbers of chemotherapy molecules can be imported.
Radioisotope conjugate	Radiation with α or β particles at site of malignant cell focus
Toxin conjugate	Delivery of toxin into cell via internalized antibody.

Fig. 6.17 Antibody constructs with useful properties.

Improved cytotoxicity. Cytotoxicity of mouse monoclonals can be enhanced by coupling antibodies to potent toxins such as ricin or diphtheria toxin, radioactive compounds or cytotoxic drugs (Uhr, 1984). Cytotoxicity can also be enhanced by constructing biphenotypic antibodies linked by disulphide bonds at their Fc portions, each possessing different specificities. Despite the specificity of the antibody for the antigen on the tumour cell, the use of antibody toxins can bring problems of non-specific toxicity, in particular to the liver, due to clearance of toxin-rich immune complexes and cells by the reticuloendothelial system. Radiolabelled antibodies will cause cell damage to bystander cells in the immediate vicinity of the target. This will only be advantageous if the majority of the nearby cells are part of the malignancy.

Improving cooperation with the human immune system. Much imagination and ingenuity has gone into the construction of novel antibodies that confer human properties with the specificity of the mouse monoclonal. Chemically engineered constructs with human Fc fragments joined by disulphide links to the mouse variable portions have been made which allow human complement binding and ADCC cooperation (Baulianne *et al.*, 1984; Jones *et al.*, 1986). The *in vivo* survival of mouse monoclonals can be prolonged to that of human IgG by humanizing the Fc portion, or using mouse hybridoma–human myeloma fusion techniques, generating a hybrid antibody that has mouse light chains and human heavy chains. A sophisticated approach that has been successfully developed by Cobbold and Waldmann (1984) is to insert just the hypervariable portion of the mouse monoclonal DNA into the human DNA sequence of a secretory myeloma cell line. Such antibodies contain over 90% human material. They may, however, still induce anti-idiotypic antibodies against the mouse variable sequence.

Improving the antimalignant effect. The very specificity of monoclonals can be a disadvantage since it allows no latitude for binding if there are variations or mutations in the target antigen. This can be overcome by the use of cocktails of two or three antibodies. A relatively simple manoeuvre that avoids the problem of internalization and capping of the antitumour antibody is to use monovalent antibodies. Capping only occurs if the two arms of the antibody bind to separate surface antigen molecules. Univalent antibodies can be made by chemically dismantling the immunoglobulin molecule to leave only one light chain variable region or by recombining it with an irrelevant light chain by hybridoma fusion (Glennie and Stevenson, 1982; Hamblin, 1989). In this process the mouse monoclonal variable region is hybridized with a human invariable portion. These antibodies are far less capable of stimulating a neutralizing immune response, and have a prolonged half-life in the blood. The opportunity to use antibodies as 'magic bullets' has stimulated efforts to combine the antibody with drugs, radioactive compounds or toxins. Chlorambucil can be chemically linked to antibodies which then become a drug delivery system (Ghose et al., 1972). However, the cytotoxicity of drug bound to antibody is unlikely to be very powerful since only a few drug molecules can be carried on the antibody.

Radioactive compounds are more easily bound in useful therapeutic quantities, and several short-acting radionucleotides coupled to antibodies are finding increasing use in radioimaging. As a form of therapy radiolabelled antibodies are still being developed. The potential advantage of these compounds is the extension of the area of effective radiation to nearby tumour cells not bound by antibody (Larson, 1985). Plant and bacterial toxins which cause irreversible and lethal damage to RNA such as ricin, saporin and diphtheria toxin can be coupled to antibodies to render them highly toxic to the target cell (Vitetta et al., 1987). Such toxins are only effective if they enter the cell. Ricin has two chains: an A chain which is cytotoxic, and a B chain which binds to the cell and allows entry. By substituting the B chain with an antibody molecule with specificity for certain cells it is theoretically possible to generate the perfect magic bullet capable only of lethal damage to the target (Krolick et al., 1982). Ricin A chain antibody conjugates have been used in the treatment of GVHD and appear to be both safe and effective. Despite the promise of high specificity and therefore lack of systemic injury from these antibody conjugates there is still, however, a risk that the reticuloendothelial system will accumulate antibodies and sustain damage.

Improving access. The use of IgG or Fab fragments gives penetration to the tissues. Plasma exchange can temporarily reduce circulating tumour antigen and promote binding to the malignant cells but the process is cumbersome and relatively inefficient.

Clinical applications of monoclonals

The revolution in monoclonal antibody production and recombinant gene technology has opened up the prospect of designing and producing cells and antibodies with novel properties for use in the treatment of malignant blood disorders. This approach is in its infancy at present, but in the future may be revolutionary in the application of antibodies to treatment of malignant diseases in general (Hamblin, 1989).

Monoclonal antibodies and artificial constructs based on antigen-specific binding have begun to find a use in the *in vitro* treatment of autologous bone marrow to remove malignant cells, and in experimental use *in vivo* to treat lymphomas. Table 6.18 summarizes these preliminary experiences which are, as yet, disappointing. The inability of antibody treatments to eliminate bulk disease restricts their use at

Table 6.18 Clinical trials of antibody treatment for haematological malignancies (Janson et al., 1989)

Disease	Number of patients	Antigen	Antibody	Response
B lymphoma	37	Idiotype, CD20, lymphoma	Campath-1H, others	10% CR 40% PR
B-CLL	26	CD5, idiotype	T101	Minor and transient responses only
T lymphomas	45	CD5	T101, L17F12	<5% CR 35% PR or minor R
T-ALL	8	CD5, other T markers	Various	
B-ALL	4	CALLA	J-5	Transient fall in circulating blasts
AML	3	Myeloid antigens	Various	

CR, Complete remission; PR, partial remission; CLL, chronic lymphoblastic leukaemia; ALL, acute lymphoblastic leukaemia; AML, acute myeloid leukaemia.

present to treating minimal residual disease, and *in vitro* purging of bone marrow. It is likely that the improved constructs now being developed will widen the scope of these agents considerably in the future. For example, radiolabelled antibody with specificity for the reticuloendothelial system is being evaluated in dogs as a means of increasing the antileukaemic effect of preparative regimens for marrow transplants (Appelbaum, 1990).

Future developments

The present use of immunotherapeutic agents is at an early stage of development. We are only now beginning to find out the behaviour of recombinant factors in the complicated *in vivo* milieu. Schedules and doses for single-agent applications remain to be optimized. In future, the probable direction is likely to be the integration of treatment approaches with the prospect of obtaining better control and regulation of malignant cells.

Combination chemotherapy–cytokine treatment

Interferon α can synergize with chlorambucil in reducing tumour bulk in low-grade non-Hodgkin's lymphoma. A trial in multiple myeloma comparing IFN started during initial chemotherapy with IFN started during plateau phase is under way in the UK. Interleukin 2 has been used in conjunction with cyclophosphamide to treat melanoma, and there are ongoing studies evaluating chemotherapy–IL-2 combinations in other solid tumour trials. Since chemotherapy may damage the immune response, IFN and IL-2 may be beneficial in protecting against suppression of the immune response to the malignancy.

Combinations of cytokines

Animal experiments demonstrate that IL-2/IFN and IL-2/TNF combinations enhance the host response to syngeneic tumours. The interactions of cytokines active in the lymphoid system with haemopoietic growth factors have not been explored. Possible candidates are IL-1 and M-CSF. However some interactions may be unhelpful. For example, IFNα reduces tumour cell susceptibility to LAK cells (Gronberg et al., 1989).

Combinations with antibody treatments

Interleukin 2 can be used to enhance antibody-dependent cell cytotoxicity of NK cells by activating the cytotoxicity of the cell. *In vitro*, IL-2-mediated cytotoxicity is enhanced by anti-Fc antibodies. Antibodies could be used to deplete the recipient selectively of, for example, suppressor cells in order preferentially to amplify clones of cytotoxic helper cells and improve the antitumour response.

Artificially modified cytotoxic cells

The successful insertion of the neomycin resistance gene into cytotoxic TILs and their subsequent infusion and retrieval in the vicinity of the tumour marks a turning point in our ability to modify genetically cell function for specific purposes. The ability to insert novel cytokine genes into cells with no natural cytotoxic potential but the ability to bind to leukaemia targets could be used to enhance tumour cell killing to a much greater level than is possible now (Rosenberg et al., 1990; The TNF TIL Human Gene Therapy Clinical Protocol, 1990). Alternatively, improved cytotoxicity might be achieved by introducing appropriate recognition sites for malignant target cells into NK cells which otherwise express only non-MHC-restricted cytotoxicity. The construction of artificial binding sites between cytotoxic cells and ricin-conjugated antibodies could produce potent and specific killer cells with novel properties. Such developments may have far-reaching therapeutic possibilities with equal or superior efficacy to chemotherapy in the ability to eliminate overt disease as well as minimal residual disease.

Single-chain antigen-binding proteins linked to toxins have been genetically manufactured in *Escherichia coli*. Thus, Le Maistre *et al.* (1991) used a genetically engineered hybrid molecule composed of the binding site of IL-2 coupled to diphtheria toxin. This toxin was successfully used to reduce the lymphocyte count in pilot studies in patients with CLL.

The possibilities of manufacturing molecules which not only avoid the limitations of conventional monoclonals but combine the selectivity of antibodies with regulatory or cytotoxic functions are extensive (Uhr, 1984).

REFERENCES

Adler A, Chervenick PA, Whiteside TL et al. (1988) Interleukin-2 induction of lymphokine activated killer activity (LAK) in the peripheral blood and bone marrow of acute leukemia patients. I. Feasibility of LAK generation in adult patients with active disease and in remission. *Blood* 71, 709.

Allison MA, Jones S, McGuffey P (1989) Phase II trial of outpatient interkeukin-2 in malignant lymphoma, chronic lymphocytic leukaemia and selected solid tumours. *Journal of Clinical Oncology* 7, 75.

Allouche A, Sahraoui Y, Augery-Bourget Y et al. (1989) Presence of a p70 IL-2 binding peptide on leukemic cells from various hemopoietic lineages. *Journal of Immunology* 143, 2223.

Alter BP (1987) The bone marrow failure syndromes. In: Nathan DG, Oski FA (eds) *Hematology of Infancy and Childhood*. WB Saunders, Philadelphia, p. 159.

Anderson KC, Weinstein HJ (1990) Transfusion-associated graft-versus-host disease. *New England Journal of Medicine* 323, 315.

Anderson DC, Schmalstieg FC, Finegold MJ et al. (1985) The severe and moderate phenotypes of heritable Mac-1, LFA-1 deficiency: their quantitative definition and relation to leukocyte dysfunction and clinical features. *Journal of Infectious Disease* 152, 668.

Andreesen R, Gadd S, Brugger W et al. (1988) Activation of human monocyte-derived macrophages cultured on Teflon – response to interferon-gamma during terminal maturation in vitro. *Immunobiology* 177, 186.

Anichi A, Fossati G, Parmiani G et al. (1987) Clonal analysis of the cytolytic T cell response to human tumours. *Immunology Today* 8, 385.

Appelbaum FR (1990) Allogeneic marrow transplantation for myeloid leukaemias. *Journal of Cellular Biochemistry* 14A (suppl), 251.

Arkin S, Naprstek B, Guarini L et al. (1991) Expression of intercellular adhesion molecule-1 (CD54) on hematopoietic progenitors. *Blood* 77, 948.

Armitage RJ, Lai AP, Roberts PJ et al. (1986) Certain myeloid cells possess receptors for interleukin-2. *British Journal of Haematology* 64, 799.

Bagot M, Cordonnier C, Tilkin FF et al. (1986) A positive predictive test for graft versus-host disease in bone marow graft recipients. *Transplantation* 41, 316.

Bain B, Vas MR, Lowenstein L (1964) The development of large immature lymphocytes in mixed lymphocyte culture. *Blood* 23, 108.

Barnes DW, Loutit JH (1957) Treatment of murine leukaemia with X-rays and homologous bone marrow. *British Journal of Haematology* 3, 241.

Barnet D, Granger V, Reilly JT (1990) Expression of the p75 interleukin 2 receptor (beta subunit) in acute and chronic leukaemia. *British Journal of Haematology* 76, 314.

Baron S, Dianzani F, Stanton GJ (1982) General considerations of the interferon system. *Texas Report of Biological Medicine* 41, 1.

Barrett AJ, Jiang YZ (1992) The immunology of chronic myeloid leukaemia. *Bone Marrow Transplantation* 9, 305.

Barrett AJ, Staughton RCD, Bridgen D et al. (1976) Antilymphocyte globulin in the treatment of advanced Sezary syndrome. *Lancet* 1, 940.

Baulianne GL, Hozaumi N, Shulman MJ (1984) Production of mouse/human chimeric antibody. *Nature* 312, 643.

Bianchi A, Dodd L, Kornbluth J (1990) Selective deficiency in the ability of LAK cells from patients with multiple myeloma to lyse myeloma tumour cells. *Blood* 76, 201a.

Bierer BE, Peterson A, Barbosa J et al. (1988) Expression of the T-cell surface molecule CD2 and an epitope loss CD2 mutant to define the role of lymphocyte function associated antigen-3 (LFA-3) in T cell activation. *Proceedings of the National Academy of Sciences of the USA* 85, 1194.

Billaud M, Rousset F, Calender A et al. (1990) Low expression of lymphocyte function-associated antigen-1 and LFA-3 adhesion molecules is a common trait in Burkitt's lymphoma associated with and not associated with Epstein–Barr virus. *Blood* 75, 1827.

Blaise D, Olive D, Stoppa AM et al. (1990) Haematological and immunologic effects of the systemic administration of recombinant interleukin 2 after autologous bone marrow transplantation. *Blood* 76, 1092.

Blok WL, Lowenberg B, Sizoo W (1988) Disappearance of trisomy 8 after alpha-2 interferon in a patient with myelodysplastic syndrome. *New England Journal of Medicine* 318, 787.

Bluestone JA, Matis LA (1989) TCR γδ cells – minor redundant T cell subset or specialised immune system? *Journal of Immunology* 142, 1785.

Bonauida B, Wright SC (1986) Role of natural killer cytotoxic factors in the mechanism of target-cell killing by natural killer cells. *Journal of Clinical Immunology* 6, 1.

Borden EC, Ball LA (1981) Interferons: biochemical, cell growth, inhibitory and immunological effects. *Progress in Hematology* 12, 299.

Boughton BJ, O'Brien D, Simpson A (1991) Autologous IL-2/LAK cell therapy for AML in second complete remission. *Haematologica* 76 (suppl 4), 55.

Branca AA, Baglioni C (1981) Evidence that types I and II interferons have different receptors. *Nature* 294, 768.

Brandtzaeg P, Halstensen TS, Scott H et al. (1989) Epithelial homing of $\gamma\delta$ T-cells? *Nature* 341, 113.

Brenner MB, McLean J, Scheft H et al. (1987) Two forms of the T-cell receptor gamma protein found on peripheral blood cytotoxic T lymphocytes. *Nature* 325, 689.

Brenner MK (1988) Tumour necrosis factor. *British Journal of Haematology* 69, 149.

Brenner MK, Heslop HE (1991) Graft versus leukaemia effects after marrow transplantation in man. In: Proctor SJ (ed.) *Minimal Residual Disease in Leukaemia*, vol 4. Bailliere Tindall, London, p. 727.

Burdach SEG, Levitt LJ (1987) Receptor specific inhibition of bone marrow erythropoiesis by recombinant DNA-derived interleukin-2. *Blood* 69, 1368.

Burnet FM (1970) The concept of immunological surveillance. *Progress in Experimental Tumour Research* 13, 1.

Butturini A, Gale RP (1990) New strategies for T cell depletion. *Bone Marrow Transplantation* 6, 225.

Campana D, Sheridan B, Tidman N et al. (1986) Human leukocyte function associated antigens on lympho-haemopoietic precursor cells. *European Journal of Immunology* 16, 537.

Carron JA, Cawley JC (1989) IL-2 and myelopoiesis: IL-2 induces blast cell proliferation in some cases of acute myeloid leukaemia. *British Journal of Haematology* 73, 168.

Charak BS, Brynes RK, Groshen S et al. (1990) Bone marrow transplantation with interleukin-2 activated bone marrow followed by interleukin 2 therapy for acute myeloid leukaemia in mice. *Blood* 76, 2187.

Cobbold SP, Waldmann H (1984) Therapeutic potential of monovalent monoclonal antibodies. *Nature* 308, 460.

Collins T, Korman AJ, Wake CT et al. (1984) Immune interferon activates multiple class II major histocompatibility complex genes and the associated invariant chain gene in human endothelial cells and dermal fibroblasts. *Proceedings of the National Academy of Sciences of the USA* 81, 4917.

Cooper MR, Fefer A, Thompson J et al. (1986) Alpha-2-interferon/melphalan/prednisone in previously untreated patients with multiple myeloma — a phase I-II trial. *Cancer Treatment Report* 70, 473.

Cordingly FT, Bianchi A, Hoffbrand AV et al. (1988) Tumour necrosis factor as an autocrine tumour growth factor for chronic B cell malignancies. *Lancet* 1, 969.

Daley GQ, Van Etten RA, Baltimore D (1990) Induction of chronic myeloid leukemia in mice by the p210 *bcr/abl* gene of the Philadelphia chromosome. *Science* 247, 824.

Dearman RJ, Stevenson FK, Wrightham M et al. (1988) Lymphokine activated killer cells from normal and lymphoma subjects are cytotoxic for cells coated with antibody derivatives displaying human Fc. *Blood* 72, 1985.

Dowding C, Guo AP, Maisin D et al. (1991) The effects of interferon-α on the proliferation of CML progenitor cells in vitro are not related to the precise position of the M-BCR breakpoint. *British Journal of Haematology* 77, 165.

Dustin ML, Rothlein R, Bhan AK et al. (1986) A natural adhesion molecule (ICAM-1): induction by IL-1 and gamma-interferon, tissue distribution, biochemistry and function. *Journal of Immunology* 137, 245.

Dustin ML, Selvaraj P, Mattaliano RJ et al. (1987) Anchoring mechanisms for LFA-3 cell adhesion glycoprotein at membrane surfaces. *Nature* 329, 846.

Dustin ML, Singer KH, Tuck DT et al. (1988) Adhesion of T lymphoblasts to epidermal keratinocytes is regulated by interferon-gamma and is mediated by intracellular adhesion molecule-1 (ICAM-1). *Journal of Experimental Medicine* 167, 1323.

Editorial (1987) Treatment of myelodysplastic syndromes. *Lancet* 2, 717.

Ehrlich P (1906) *Collected Studies on Immunity*, vol II. John Wiley, New York, p. 442.

Enokihara H, Furusawa S, Nakakubo H et al. (1989) T cells from eosinophilic patients produce interleukin-5 with interleukin-2 stimulation. *Blood* 73, 1809.

Ettinghauser SE, Moore JG, White DE et al. (1987) Haematological effects of immunotherapy with lymphokine activated killer cells and recombinant interleukin-2 in cancer patients. *Blood* 69, 1654.

Everson TC (1964) Spontaneous regression of cancer. *Annals of the New York Academy of Sciences* 114, 721.

Falkenburg JHF, Goselingk HM, Van Der Harst D et al. (1990) Specific lysis of clonogenic leukaemic cells by cytotoxic T lymphocytes against minor histocompatibility antigens: an in vitro model for graft versus leukaemia. *Experimental Haematology* 18, 682.

Favrot MC, Floret D, Negrier S et al. (1989) Systemic interleukin-2 therapy in children with progressive neuroblastoma after high dose chemotherapy and bone marrow transplantation. *Bone Marrow Transplantation* 4, 499.

Fernandez-Botran R, Krammer PM, Diamantstein T et al. (1986) B cell stimulating factor 1 (BSF-1) promotes growth of helper T cell lines. *Journal of Experimental Medicine* 164, 580.

Fierro MY, Xin-Sheng L, Lusso P et al. (1988) In vitro and in vivo susceptibility of human leukaemia cells to lymphokine activated killer activity. *Leukaemia* 2, 50.

Figdor CG, Van Kooyk Y, Keizer GD (1990) Review: on the mode of action of LFA-1. *Immunology Today* 11, 277.

Fisch P, Malkovsky M, Braakman E et al. (1990a)

Gamma delta T cell clones and natural killer cells mediate distinct patterns of non-major histocompatibility complex-restricted cytolysis. *Journal of Experimental Medicine* 171, 1567.

Fisch P, Malkovsky M, Kovats S et al. (1990b) Recognition by human Vγ9/Vδ2 T-cells of a groEL homolog on Daudi Burkitt's lymphoma cells. *Science* 250, 1269.

Fischer A, Blanche S, Veber F et al. (1986) Correction of immune disorders by HLA matched and mismatched bone marrow transplantation. In: Gale RP, Champlin RE (eds) *Progress in Bone Marrow Transplantation*, Alan R Liss, New York, p. 911.

Fisher B, Packard BS, Read EJ (1989) Tumour localisation of adoptively transferred indium 111 labelled tumour infiltrating lymphocytes in patients with metastatic melanoma. *Journal of Clinical Oncology* 7, 250.

Fleischmann WR, Klimpel GR, Tyring SK et al. (1984) Interferon: antitumour actions. *Transplantation Proceedings* 16, 516.

Foa R, Melone G, Tosti S et al. (1989) Recombinant IL-2 in the treatment of acute leukaemia: a pilot study. *Blood* 74 (suppl.), 357a.

Foa R, Carretto P, Fierro MT et al. (1990a) Interleukin-2 does not promote the in-vitro and in-vivo proliferation and growth of human acute leukaemia cells of myeloid and lymphoid origin. *British Journal of Haematology* 75, 34.

Foa R, Fierro MT, Raspadori D et al. (1990b) Lymphokine activated killer (LAK) cell activity in B and T chronic lymphoid leukemia: defective LAK generation and reduced susceptibility of the leukemic cells to allogeneic and autologous LAK effectors. *Blood* 76, 1349.

Froom P, Aghai E, Dobinsky JB et al. (1987) Reduced natural killer activity in patients with Fanconi's anemia and in family members. *Leukemia Research* 11, 197.

Galvani DW (1989) The beneficial effects of alpha interferon in CGL are probably not mediated by NK cells. *British Journal of Haematology* 71, 233.

Galvani DW, Cawley JC (1989) Mechanism of action of alpha interferon in chronic granulocytic leukaemia: evidence for a preferential inhibition of late progenitors. *British Journal of Haematology* 73, 475.

Gatti RA, Good RA (1971) Occurrence of malignancy in immunodeficiency diseases: a literature review. *Cancer* 28, 89.

Gerlier D, Rabourdin-Combe C (1989) Antigen processing—from cell biology to molecular interactions. *Immunology Today* 10, 3.

Germain RN (1991) Antigen processing: the second class story. *Nature* 353, 605.

Germain RN, Hendrix LR (1991) MHC class II structure, occupancy and surface expression determined by post-endoplasmic reticulum antigen binding. *Nature* 353, 134.

Geser A, Lenoir GM, Anvret M et al. (1983) Epstein-Barr virus markers in a series of Burkitt's lymphomas from the west Nile district Uganda. *European Journal of Cancer and Clinical Oncology* 19, 1393.

Ghose T, Norwell ST, Guclin A et al. (1972) Immunotherapy of cancer with chlorambucil carrying antibody. *British Medical Journal* 3, 495.

Gibson FM, Malkovska V, Myint AA et al. (1991) Mechanism of suppression of normal hemopoietic activity by lymphokine activated killer cells and their products. *Experimental Hematology* 19, 659.

Gisslinger H, Ludwig H, Linkesch W et al. (1989) Long-term interferon therapy for thrombocytosis in myeloproliferative disease. *Lancet* 1, 634.

Gisslinger, H, Chott A, Linkesch W et al. (1990) Long term alpha interferon therapy in myelodysplastic syndromes. *Leukemia* 4, 91.

Glennie MJ, Stevenson GT (1982) Univalent antibodies kill tumour cells in vitro and in vivo. *Nature* 295, 712.

Gordon J, Abdul-Ahad AK, Hamblin TJ et al. (1984) Mechanisms of tumour cell escape encountered in treating lymphocytic leukaemia with anti-idiotypic antibody. *British Journal of Cancer* 49, 547.

Gottlieb D, Brenner MK, Heslop HE et al. (1989a) A phase I clinical trial of recombinant interleukin-2 following high dose chemo-radiotherapy for haematological malignancy: applicability to the elimination of minimal residual disease. *British Journal of Cancer* 60, 610.

Gottlieb DJ, Prentice HG, Heslop HE et al. (1989b) Effects of recombinant interleukin-2 administration on cytotoxic function following high dose chemo-radiotherapy for haematological malignancy. *Blood* 74, 2335.

Greaves MF, Paxton A, Janossy G et al. (1980) Acute lymphoblastic leukaemia associated antigen: III. Alterations in expression during treatment and in relapse. *Leukemia Research* 4, 1.

Green WR, Nowinski RC, Henney CS (1979) The generation and specificity of cytotoxic T cells raised against syngeneic tumor cells bearing AKR/Gross murine leukaemia virus antigens. *Journal of Experimental Medicine* 150, 51.

Greenberg PD (1986) Therapy of murine leukemia with cyclophosphamide and murine LYT-2 cells: cytotoxic T cells can mediate eradication of disseminated leukaemia. *Journal of Immunology* 136, 1917.

Greenberg PD (1991) Adoptive T cell therapy of tumors: mechanisms operative in the recognition and elimination of tumor cells. *Advances in Immunology* 49, 281.

Greenberg PD, Klarnet JP, Kern DE et al. (1989) Specific adoptive immunotherapy. In: *Immunity to Cancer II*. p. 349.

Gresser I (1991) Antitumour effects of interferons: past, present and future. *British Journal of Haematology* 79 (suppl 1): 1.

Grimm EA, Mazumder A, Zhang HZ et al. (1982) Lymphokine activated killer cell phenomenon. Lysis of natural killer-resistant fresh solid tumor cells by interleukin 2 activated autologous human peripheral blood lymphocytes. *Journal of Experimental Medicine* 155, 1823.

Grimm EA, Ramsey KM, Mazumder A (1983) Lymphokine activated killer cell phenomenon.

II. Precursor phenotype is serologically distinct from peripheral T lymphocytes, memory cytotoxic thymus derived lymphocytes and natural killer cells. *Journal of Experimental Medicine* 157, 884.

Gronberg A, Ferm M, Tsai L (1989) Interferon is able to reduce tumor cell susceptibility to human lymphokine activated killer (LAK) cells. *Cellular Immunology* I, 118, 10.

Gross L (1943) Intradermal immunisation of C3H mice against sarcomas that originate in animals of the same line. *Cancer Research* 3, 326.

Haddada H, De Vaux Saint Cyr C (1982) The role of natural killer cells in tumor rejection in hamsters. In: Serrou B, Rosenfeld C, Herberman, RB (eds) *Human Cancer Immunology*, vol 4: *Natural Killer Cells*. Elsevier Biomedical Press, Amsterdam, p. 231.

Hagenbeek A, Lu YL, Ger JA et al. (1991) Minimal residual disease in acute leukemia: preclinical studies. In: Champlin RE, Gale RP (eds) *New Strategies in Bone Marrow Transplantation*. Wiley-Liss, New York, p. 193.

Haller O, Hansson M, Kiessling R et al. (1977) Role of non-conventional natural killer cells in resistance against syngeneic tumor cells in vitro. *Nature* 270, 609.

Hamblin TJ (1989) Modifications of monoclonal antibodies for immunotherapy. In: Hamblin TJ (ed.) *Immunotherapy of Disease*. Kluwer, London, p. 143.

Hansson M, Beran M (1982) Inhibition of in-vitro granulopoiesis by autologous and allogeneic human NK cells. *Journal of Immunology* 129, 126.

Harada M, Nakao S, Kondo K (1986) Effect of activated lymphocytes on the regulation of haematopoiesis: enhancement and suppression of in vitro BFU-E growth by T cells stimulated by autologous non-T cells. *Blood* 67, 1143.

Harding CV, Levia-Cobian F, Unanue ER (1988) Mechanism of antigen processing. *Immunology Review* 10, 77.

Harley JB, Pajak ThF, McIntyre OR et al. (1979) Improved survival of increased-risk myeloma patients on combined triple alkylating agent therapy. *Blood* 54, 13.

Hauch M, Gazzola MV, Small T et al. (1990) Anti leukaemic potential of interleukin 2 activated natural killer cells after bone marrow transplantation for chronic myelogenous leukaemia. *Blood* 75, 2250.

Heisterkamp N, Jenster G, Hoeve J et al. (1990) Acute leukemia in bcr/abl transgenic mice. *Nature* 344, 251.

Herberman RB, Bellanti JA (1985) Immune defense mechanisms in tumor immunity. In: Bellanti JA (ed.) *Immunology III*. WB Saunders, London, p. 330.

Herberman RB, Ortaldo JR (1981) Natural killer cells: their role in defences against disease. *Science* 214, 24.

Herberman RB, Nunn ME, Holden HT et al. (1975) Natural cytotoxic reactivity of mouse lymphoid cells against syngeneic and allogeneic tumours: I: Distribution of reactivity and specificity. *International Journal of Cancer* 16, 216.

Hercend T, Takvorian T, Nowill A et al. (1986) Characterization of natural killer cells with anti-leukemia activity following allogeneic bone marrow transplantation. *Blood* 67, 722.

Herin M, Lemoine C, Weynants P et al. (1987) Production of stable cytolytic T-cell clones directed against autologous human melanoma. *Journal of International Cancer* 39, 390.

Hersey P, MacDonald M, Werkman H (1988) Western blot analysis of antigens on melanoma cells recognized by cytotoxic T cells. *Journal of the National Cancer Institute* 80, 826.

Heslop HE, Gottlieb DJ, Reittie JE et al. (1989a) Spontaneous and interleukin 2 induced secretion of tumour necrosis factor and gamma interferon following autologous marrow transplantation or chemotherapy. *British Journal of Haematology* 72, 122.

Heslop HE, Gottlieb DJ, Bianchi ASM et al. (1989b) In vivo induction of gamma interferon and tumour necrosis factor by interleukin 2 infusion following intensive chemotherapy or autologous marrow transplant. *Blood* 74, 1374.

Heslop HE, Duncombe AS, Reittie JE et al. (1991) Interleukin 2 infusion induces hemopoietic growth factors and modifies marrow regeneration. *British Journal of Haematology* 74, 2(a).

Higuchi CM, Thompson JA, Cox T et al. (1989) Lymphokine activated killer function following autologous bone marrow transplantation for refractory haematological malignancies. *Cancer Research* 49, 5509.

Hoshino S, Oshimi KK, Tsudo M et al. (1990) Flow cytometric analysis of expression of interleukin 2 receptor beta chain (p70–75) on various leukaemic cells. *Blood* 76, 767.

Howard FD, Ledbetter JA, Wong J et al. (1981) A human T-lymphocyte differentiation marker defined by monoclonal antibodies that block E-rosette formation. *Journal of Immunology* 126, 2117.

Hughes CC, Savage COS, Pober JS (1990) Endothelial cells augment T cell interleukin-2 production by a contact-dependent mechanism involving CD2/LFA-3 interaction. *Journal of Experimental Medicine* 171, 1453.

Hughes TP, Morgan GJ, Martiat P et al. (1991) Detection of residual leukaemia after bone marrow transplantation for chronic myeloid leukaemia: role of polymerase chain reaction in predicting relapse. *Blood* 77, 874.

Hunig T, Tiefenthaler G, Meyer Zum Buschenfelde KH et al. (1987) Alternative pathway activation of T cells by binding of CD2 to its cell surface ligand. *Nature* 326, 298.

Isaacs A, Lindenmann J (1957) Virus interference. *Proceedings of the Royal Society of London (Biology)* 147, 258.

Jablons DM, Mule JJ, McIntosh JK et al. (1989) IL-6/IFN-beta 2 as a circulating hormone. Induction by cytokine administration in humans. *Journal of Immunology* 142, 1542.

Janeway C (1991) MLs: makes a little sense. *Nature* 349, 459.

Janson CH, Tehrani M, Wigzell H et al. (1989) Rational

use of biological response modifiers in haematological malignancies – a review of treatment with interferon cytotoxic cells, and antibodies. *Leukemia Research* 13, 1039.

Jiang YZ, Borzy MS, Macdonald D et al. (1990) Defective natural immunity in patients with essential thrombocythaemia. *Experimental Haematology* 16, 644.

Jones PT, Dear PH, Foote J et al. (1986) Replacing the complementary-determining regions in a human antibody with those from a mouse. *Nature* 321, 522.

Jung S, Schluesener HJ (1991) Brief definitive report: human T lymphocytes recognize a peptide of single point-mutated, oncogenic ras proteins. *Journal of Experimental Medicine* 173, 273.

Jung LKL, Hara T, Fu SM (1984) Detection and functional studies of p60–65 (tac antigen) on activated human B cells. *Journal of Experimental Medicine* 160, 1597.

Kalter SP, Riggs SA, Cabanillas F et al. (1985) Aggressive non-Hodgkin's lymphomas in immunocompromised homosexual males. *Blood* 66, 655.

Kamel-Reid S, Letarte M, Sirard C et al. (1989) A model of human acute lymphoblastic leukemia in immune-deficient SCID mice. *Science* 246, 1597.

Kaufmann Y, Levanon M, Davidshon J (1987) Interleukin-2 induces human acute lymphocytic leukaemia cells to manifest lymphokine activated killer (LAK) cytotoxicity. *Journal of Immunology* 139, 977.

Kersey JH, Spector BD, Good R (1953) Primary immunodeficiency diseases and cancer: the Immunodeficiency Cancer Registry. *Journal of International Cancer* 12, 333.

Kiessling R, Klein E, Wizgzell H (1975) Natural killer cells in the mouse. I. Cytotoxic cells with specificity for mouse Moloney leukaemia cells. Specificity and distributions according to genotype. *European Journal of Immunology* 5, 112.

Kiessling IR, Hansson AM, Greenberg A (1984) Natural killer cells as regulators of malignant and normal cell growth. In: Yamamura Y, Tada T (eds) *Progress in Immunology*. Academic Press, Tokyo, p. 1181.

Kishimoto TK, O'Connor K, Lee A et al. (1987) Cloning of the beta subunit of the leukocyte adhesion proteins: homology to an extracellular matrix receptor defines a novel super-gene family. *Cell* 48, 681.

Klempner MS, Noring R, Mier JW et al. (1990) An acquired chemotactic defect in neutrophils from patients receiving interleukin-2 immunotherapy. *New England Journal of Medicine* 322, 959.

Kohl S, Springer TA, Schmalstieg FC et al. (1984) Defective natural killer cytotoxicity and polymorphonuclear leukocyte antibody dependent cellular cytotoxicity in patients with LFA-1/OKM-1 deficiency. *Journal of Immunology* 133, 2972.

Kohler G, Milstein C (1975) Continuous culture of fused cells secreting antibodies of predetermined specificity. *Nature* 256, 495.

Kolitz JE, Kempin SJ, Templeton MA et al. (1990) A pilot trial of rIL-2 and r-Interferon alpha 2a in low grade B cell malignancies. *Blood* 76, 357a.

Krensky AM, Samchez-Madrid F, Robbins E et al. (1983) The functional significance, distribution, and structure of LFA-1, LFA-2 and LFA-3: cell surface antigens associated with cytotoxic T lymphocyte-target interactions. *Journal of Immunology* 131, 611.

Krolick KA, Uhr JW, Slavin S et al. (1982) In vivo therapy of a murine B-cell tumour (BCL) using antibody-ricin A chain immunotoxins. *Journal of Experimental Medicine* 155, 1797.

Kurzinger K, Reynolds T, Germain RN et al. (1981) A novel lymphocyte function associated antigen (LFA-1): cellular distribution, quantitative expression and structure. *Journal of Immunology* 127, 596.

Larner AJ (1989) Monoclonal antibodies: a new class of reagents in cancer therapy. *Transfusion Science* 10, 15.

Larson SM (1985) Radiolabelled monoclonal antitumour antibodies in diagnosis and therapy. *Journal of Nuclear Medicine* 26, 538.

Lebleu B, Sen GC, Shaila S et al. (1976) Interferon, double-stranded RNA and protein phosphorylation. *Proceedings of the National Academy of Sciences of the USA* 73, 3107.

Le Maistre CF, Rosenblum MG, Reuben JM et al. (1991) Therapeutic effects of a genetically engineered toxin (DAB_{486} IL-2) in patients with chronic lymphocytic leukaemia. *Lancet* 337, 1124.

Lindenmann J, Burke D, Isaacs A (1957) Studies on the production, mode of action and properties of interferon. *British Journal of Experimental Pathology* 38, 551.

Lista P, Fierro MT, Xin-Sheng L et al. (1989) Lymphokine activated killer cells inhibit the clonogenic growth of leukemic stem cells. *European Journal of Haematology* 42, 425.

Litchfield MG, Hengartner H, Podack ER et al. (1988) Structure and function of human perforin. *Nature* 335, 448.

Long EO (1989) Intracellular traffic and antigen processing. *Immunology Today* 10, 232.

Lotteau V, Teyton L, Peleraux A et al. (1991) Intracellular transport of class II MHC molecules directed by invariant chain. *Nature* 348, 600.

Lotze MT, Matory YL, Ettinghausen SE et al. (1985) In vivo administration of purified human interleukin-2. II: Half life, immunologic effects and expansion of peripheral lymphoid cells in vivo with recombinant IL-2. *Journal of Immunology* 135, 2865.

Lotze MT, Roberts K, Custer MC et al. (1987) Specific binding and lysis of human melanoma by IL-2 activated cells coated with anti-T3 or anti-Fc receptor c•oss linked to anti-melanoma antibody. *Journal of Surgical Research* 42, 580.

Lotzova E, Savary CA, Herberman RB (1989) Induction of NK cell activity against fresh human leukemia cells in culture with interleukin 2. *Journal of Immunology* 138, 2718.

Lowrey DM, Hengartner H, Podack ER et al. (1989) Cloning analysis and expression of murine perforin I cDNA a component of cytolytic T-cell granules with homology to complement component C9. *Proceedings of the National Academy of Sciences of the USA* 86, 247.

McCune JM, Namikawa R, Kaneshima H et al. (1988) The SCID-hu mouse: murine model for the analysis of human hematolymphoid differentiation and function. Science 241, 1632.

Macdonald D, Gordon AA, Kajitani H et al. (1990a) Interleukin-2 treatment-associated eosinophilia is mediated by interleukin-5 production. British Journal of Haematology 76, 168.

Macdonald D, Adams JA, McCarthy DM et al. (1990b) Interleukin 2 inhibits the growth of human bone marrow derived fibroblasts. Acta Haematologica 83, 26.

Macdonald D, Jiang YZ, Gordon AA et al. (1990c) Recombinant interleukin-2 for acute myeloid leukaemia in first complete remission: a pilot study. Leukaemia Research 14, 967.

Macdonald D, Jiang YZ, Swirsky D et al. (1991) Acute myeloid leukaemia relapsing following interleukin-2 treatment expresses the alpha chain of the interleukin-2 receptor. British Journal of Haematology 77, 43.

McIntosh JK, Mule JJ, Merino MJ et al. (1988) Synergistic effects of immunotherapy with recombinant interleukin-2 and recombinant tumour necrosis factor-α. Cancer Research 48, 260.

Mackinnon S, Hows JM, Goldman JM (1990) Induction of in vitro graft versus leukaemia activity following bone marrow transplantation for chronic myeloid leukaemia. Blood 76, 2037.

Madden DR, Gorga JC, Strominger JL et al. (1991) The structure of HLA-B27 reveals nonamer self-peptides bound in an extended conformation. Nature 353, 321.

Maio M, Pinto A, Carbone A et al. (1990) Differential expression of CD54/intercellular adhesion molecule-1 in myeloid leukaemias and in lymphoproliferative disorders. Blood 76, 783.

Maiolo AT, Cortelezzi A, Calori R et al. (1990) Recombinant γ-interferon as first line therapy for high risk myelodysplastic syndromes. Leukemia 4, 480.

Makgoba MW, Sanders ME, Sha S (1989) The CD2-LFA-3 and LFA-1-ICAM-1 pathway: relevance to T cell recognition. Immunology Today 10, 417.

Male D, Champion B, Cooke A, Owen M (eds) (1991) Complement. In: Advanced Immunology, 2nd edn. Gower Medical, London, p. 152.

Malkovska V, Sondel PM (1990) Prospects for interleukin 2 therapy in hematologic malignant neoplasms. Journal of the National Cancer Institute Monographs 10, 69.

Malkovska V, Murphy J, Hudson L et al. (1987) Direct effect of interleukin-2 on chronic lymphocytic leukaemia B cell function and morphology. Clinical and Experimental Immunology 68, 677.

Malkovska V, Sondel PM, Malkovsky M (1989) Tumour immunotherapy. Cancer and Immunology 1, 883.

Malkovska V, Cigel F, Armstrong N et al. (1992) Anti-lymphoma activity of human γδ T cells in mice with severe combined immune deficiency. Cancer Research 52, 1.

Malkovsky M, Sondel PM (1987) Interleukin-2 and its receptor: structure, function and therapeutic potential. Blood Reviews 1, 254.

Malkovsky M, Brenner MK, Hunt R et al. (1986) T-cell depletion prevents potentiation of graft versus host disease by IL-2. Cellular Immunology 103, 476.

Malkovsky M, Loveland B, North M et al. (1987) Recombinant interleukin-2 directly augments the cytotoxicity of human monocytes. Nature 325, 262.

Mandelli F, Tribalto M, Avvisati G et al. (1988) Recombinant interferon alpha-2b (Intron A) as post-induction therapy for responding multiple myeloma patients. M84 protocol. Cancer Treatment Review 15 (suppl A), 43.

Mandelli F, Avvisati G, Amadori S et al. (1990) Maintenance treatment with recombinant interferon alfa-2b in patients with multiple myeloma responding to conventional induction chemotherapy. New England Journal of Medicine 322, 1430.

Manson LA (1991) Does antibody-dependent epitope masking permit progressive tumor growth in the face of cell-mediated cytotoxicity? Immunology Today 12, 352.

Marrack P, Kappler J (1988) T-cells can distinguish between allogeneic major histocompatibility complex products on different cell types. Nature 332, 840.

Masucci G, Poros A, Seeley JK et al. (1980) In vitro generation of K562 killers in human T-lymphocyte subsets. Cellular Immunology 52, 247.

Mathé G, Amiel JL, Schwartzenberg L (1965) Adoptive immunotherapy of acute leukaemia. Experimental and clinical results. Cancer Research 25, 1525.

Mathé G, Amiel JL, Schwarzenberg L (1969) Active immunotherapy for acute lymphoblastic leukaemia. Lancet 1, 697.

May D, Wandl UB, Niederle N (1989) Treatment of essential thrombocythaemia with interferon alpha-2b. Lancet 1, 96.

Meeker T, Lowder J, Cleroy M (1985) Emergence of idiotype variants during treatment of B-cell lymphoma with anti-idiotypic antibodies. New England Journal of Medicine 312, 1658.

Metchnikoff E (1899) Etudes sur la resorption des cellules. Annales de l'Institut Pasteur 13, 737.

Meuer SC, Roux MM, Schraven B (1989) The alternative pathway of T cell activation: biology, pathophysiology and perspectives for immunopharmacology. Clinical Immunology and Immunopathology 50, s133.

Michalevicz R, Campana D, Katz F et al. (1988) Recombinant interleukin 2 and anti-Tac influence the growth of enriched multipotent hemopoietic progenitors: proposed hypotheses for different responses in early and late progenitors. Leukemia Research 12, 113.

Miescher S, Whiteside TL, Moretta L et al. (1987) Clonal and frequency analysis of tumor infiltrating T lymphocytes from human solid tumors. Journal of Immunology 138, 4004.

Mitchell MS, Kempf RA, Harel W et al. (1988) Effectiveness and tolerability of low dose cyclophosphamide and low dose intravenous interleukin-

2 in disseminated melanoma. *Journal of Clinical Oncology* 6, 409.

Morhenn VB, Waster GJ, Cua AB et al. (1989) Effects of recombinant interleukin-1 and interleukin-2 on human keratinocytes. *Journal of Investigative Dermatology* 93, 121.

Mueller DL, Jenkins MK, Schwartz RH (1989) An accessory cell-derived co-stimulatory signal acts independently of protein kinase C activation to allow T cell proliferation and prevent the induction of unresponsiveness. *Journal of Immunology* 142, 2617.

Mukherji B, MacAlister TJ (1983) Brief definitive report: clonal analysis of cytotoxic T cell response against human melanoma. *Journal of Experimental Medicine* 158, 240.

Mukherji B, Guha A, Chakraborty NG et al. (1989) Clonal analysis of cytotoxic and regulatory T cell responses against human melanoma. *Journal of Experimental Medicine* 169, 1961.

Mule JJ, Smith CA, Rosenberg SA (1987) Interleukin 4 (B cell stimulating factor 1) can mediate the induction of lymphokine activated killer cell activity directed against fresh tumour cells. *Journal of Experimental Medicine* 166, 792.

Munker R, Koeffler P (1987) In vitro action of tumor necrosis factor on myeloid leukaemia cells. *Blood* 69, 1102.

Murphy M, Perussia B, Trinchieri G (1988) Effects of recombinant tumour necrosis factor, lymphotoxin, and immune interferon on proliferation and differentiation of enriched hematopoietic precursor cells. *Experimental Hematology* 16, 131.

Nagler A, Lanier LL, Phillips JH (1988) The effects of IL-4 on human natural killer cells. A potent regulator of IL-2 activation and proliferation. *Journal of Immunology* 1141, 2349.

Neimeyer CM, Sieff CA, Mathey-Prevot B et al. (1989) Expression of human interleukin 3 (multi-CSF) is restricted to human lymphocytes and T cell tumour lines. *Blood* 73, 945.

Newman RA, Warner JF, Dennert G (1984) NK recognition of target structures: is the transferrin receptor the NK target structure? *Journal of Immunology* 133, 1841.

Nickoloff BJ (1988) Review: role of interferon-gamma in cutaneous trafficking of lymphocytes with emphasis on molecular and cellular adhesion events. *Archive of Dermatology* 124, 1835.

Nickoloff BJ, Griffiths CEM (1989) T lymphocytes and monocytes bind to keratinocytes in frozen sections of biopsy specimens of normal skin treated with gamma interferon. *Journal of the American Academy of Dermatology* 20, 736.

Nunn ME, Herberman RB, Holden HT (1977) Natural killer cell mediated cytotoxicity in mice against nonlymphoid tumors and some normal cells. *International Journal of Cancer* 20, 231.

O'Brien TK, Stevens HAF, Knight RA et al. (1983) Recognition of marrow elements by natural killer cells: are NK cells involved in haemopoietic regulation? *British Journal of Haematology* 53, 161.

Okano A, Seruti C, Takasuki F et al. (1988) Effects of interleukin-6 on bone marrow in transplanted mice. *Transplantation* 47, 738.

Oshimi K, Atutusu M, Takei Y et al. (1986) Cytotoxicity of interleukin 2 activated lymphocytes for leukemia and lymphoma cells. *Blood* 68, 938.

Perrault C, Decary F, Brochu S et al. (1990) Minor histocompatibility antigens – a review. *Blood* 76, 1269.

Peters PM, Ortaldo JR, Shalaby MF et al. (1986) Natural killer sensitive targets stimulate production of alpha-TNF but not beta-TNF by highly purified human peripheral blood large granular lymphocytes. *Journal of Immunology* 137, 2592.

Phillips C, McMillan M, Flood PM et al. (1985) Identification of a unique tumor-specific antigen as a novel class I major histocompatibility molecule. *Proceedings of the National Academy of Sciences of the USA*, 82, 5140.

Phillips RA, Jewett MAS, Gallie BL (1989) Growth of human tumors in immune deficient scid-mice and nude mice. *Current Topics in Microbiology and Immunology* 152, 259.

Pierres M, Goridis C, Golstein P (1982) Inhibition of murine T cell mediated cytolysis and T cell proliferation by a rat monoclonal antibody immunoprecipitating two lymphoid cell surface polypeptides of 94 000 and 180 000 molecular weight. *European Journal of Immunology* 12, 60.

Purtillo DT, Sakamoto K, Barnabei V et al. (1982) Epstein–Barr virus induced diseases in boys with the X-linked lymphoproliferative syndrome (XLP). An update on the registry. *American Journal of Medicine* 73, 49.

Quesada JR, Reuben J, Manning JT et al. (1984) Alpha interferon for induction of remission in hairy cell leukemia. *New England Journal of Medicine* 310, 15.

Reem GH, Yeh NH (1984) Interleukin 2 regulates expression of its receptor and gamma interferon by T lymphocytes. *Science* 225, 429.

Rees ADM, Lombardi G, Scoging A (1989) Functional evidence for the recognition of endogenous peptides by autoreactive T cell clones. *International Immunology* 1, 624.

Reittie JE, Gottleib DJ, Heslop HE et al. (1989) Endogenously generated activated killer cells circulate after autologous and allogeneic marrow transplantation. *Blood* 73, 1351.

Riccardi C, Santoni A, Barlozzari T et al. (1982) In vitro role of NK cells against neoplastic or non-neoplastic cells. In: Herberman RB (ed.) *Natural Killer Cells*. Elsevier Biomedical Press, Amsterdam, p. 57.

Richards JM (1989) Therapeutic use of interleukin-2 and lymphokine activated killer (LAK) cells. *Blood Reviews* 3, 110.

Robertson M (1991) Proteasomes in the pathway. *Nature* 353, 300.

Robertson MJ, Ritz J (1990) Biology and clinical relevance of human natural killer cells. *Blood* 76, 2421.

Rosenberg SA, Lotze MT, Muul LM et al. (1985) Observations on the systemic administration of autologous lymphokine activated killer cells and recombinant interleukin-2 to patients with metastatic cancer. *New England Journal of Medicine* 313, 1485.

Rosenberg SA, Lotze MT, Muul LM et al. (1987) A progress report on the treatment of 157 patients with advanced cancer treated using lymphokine activated killer cells and interleukin-2 or high dose interleukin-2 alone. *New England Journal of Medicine* 319, 889.

Rosenberg SA, Packard BS, Aebersold PM et al. (1988a) Use of tumour infiltrating lymphocytes and interleukin-2 in the immunotherapy of patients with metastatic melanoma. *New England Journal of Medicine* 319, 1676.

Rosenberg SA, Schwarz SL, Spiess PJ (1988b) Combination immunotherapy for cancer: synergic antitumour interactions of interleukin-2, alpha interferon, and tumor infiltrating lymphocytes. *Journal of the National Cancer Institute* 80, 1393.

Rosenberg SA, Aebersold P, Cornetta K et al. (1990) Gene transfer into humans: immunotherapy of patients with advanced melanoma using tumour infiltrating lymphocytes modified by retroviral gene transduction. *New England Journal of Medicine* 323, 570.

Rosolen A, Nakanishi M, Poplack DG et al. (1989) Expression of interleukin-2 receptor beta subunit in hematopoietic malignancies. *Blood* 73, 1968.

Rudensky AY, Preston-Hurlburt P, Hong SC et al. (1991) Sequence analysis of peptides bound to MHC class II molecules. *Nature* 353, 622.

Sachs DH, Sharibi Y, Sykes M (1991) Chimerism and the induction of transplant tolerance. In: Gale RP, Champlin RK (eds) *New Strategies in Bone Marrow Transplantation.* Wiley-Liss, New York, p. 21.

Savary CA, Lotzova E (1990) Inhibition of human bone marrow and myeloid progenitors by interleukin 2 activated lymphocytes. *Experimental Hematology* 18, 1083.

Scala G, Allavena P, Djev JY et al. (1984) Human large granular lymphocytes are potent producers of interleukin-1. *Nature* 309, 56.

Schaafsma MR, Fibbe WE, Van Der Harst D et al. (1990) Increased numbers of circulating haematopoietic progenitor cells after treatment with high dose interleukin 2 in cancer patients. *British Journal of Haematology* 76, 180.

Schorle H, Holtschke T, Hünig T et al. (1991) Developmental function of T-cells in mice rendered interleukin-2 deficient by gene targeting. *Nature* 352, 621.

Schroff RW, Foon KA, Beatty SM (1985) Human antimurine immunoglobulin response in patients receiving monoclonal antibody therapy. *Cancer Research* 45, 879.

Schwartz RS (1975) Another look at immunologic surveillance. *New England Journal of Medicine* 293, 181.

Seewann HL, Gastl G, Lang A et al. (1988) Interferon-alpha in the treatment of idiopathic myelofibrosis. *Blut* 56, 161.

Selby P, Hobbs S, Viner C et al. (1987) Tumour necrosis factor in man: clinical and biological observations. *British Journal of Cancer* 56, 803.

Shabbad E, Cassel A, Froom P, Aghai E (1990) Effect of adherent cells on the regulation of BFU-E in patients with myeloproliferative disorders. *American Journal of Hematology* 33, 225.

Sharrock CEM, Kaminski E, Man S (1990) Limiting dilution analysis of human T cells: a useful clinical tool. *Immunology Today* 11, 281.

Shiloni I, Eisenthal A, Sachs D et al. (1987) Antibody-dependent cellular cytotoxicity mediated by murine lymphocytes activated in recombinant interleukin-2. *Journal of Immunology* 138, 1992.

Shinkai Y, Takio K, Okumura K (1988) Homology of perforin to the ninth component of complement. *Nature* 334, 525.

Shows TB, Sakaguchi AY, Naylor SL et al. (1982) Clustering of leucocyte and fibroblast interferon genes on human chromosome 9. *Science* 218, 373.

Shulman L, Revel M (1980) Interferon-dependent induction of mRNA activity for (2′−5′)-oligoisoadenylate synthetase. *Nature* 298, 98.

Sikora K, Lennox E (1982) Tumor antigens. In: Lachmann PJ, Peters DK (eds) *Clinical Aspects of Immunology.* Blackwell Scientific Publications, Oxford, p. 1249.

Silver RT (1990) A new treatment for polycythemia vera: recombinant interferon alfa. *Blood* 76, 664.

Slavin S, Ackerstein A, Naparstek E et al. (1990) The graft versus leukaemia (GVL) phenomenon: is GVL separable from GVHD? *Bone Marrow Transplantation* 6, 155.

Smith KA (1988) Interleukin-2 inception impact, and implications. *Science* 240, 1169.

Smythe MJ, Ortaldo JR, Bene W et al. (1990) IL-2 and IL-6 synergise to augment pore forming protein gene expression and cytotoxic potential of human peripheral blood T cells. *Journal of Immunology* 145, 1159.

Soiffer R, Murray C, Cochran K et al. (1990) Selective expansion of NK cells in patients given low dose recombinant IL-2 after BMT. *Blood* 76, 220a.

Sosman JA, Sondel PM (1987) The graft versus leukaemia effect following bone marrow transplantation: a review of laboratory and clinical data. *Hematology Review* 2, 77.

Sosman JA, Oettel KR, Hank JA et al. (1989) Specific recognition of human leukaemic cells by allogeneic T cell lines. *Transplantation* 48, 486.

Sosman JA, Oettel KR, Smith SD et al. (1990) Specific recognition of human leukaemic cells by allogeneic T cells. II. Evidence for HLA-D restricted determinants on leukaemic cells that are crossreactive with determinants present on unrelated non-leukaemic cells. *Blood* 75, 2005.

Spiegel RJ (1985) Phase I/II clinical trials. In: Kisner DL, Smyth JF (eds) *Interferon Alpha-2: Pre-clinical and Clinical Evaluation.* Martinus Nijhoff, Boston, p. 43.

Springer TA, Dustin ML, Kishimoto TK et al. (1987) The LFA1, CD2 and LFA3 molecules: cell adhesion receptors of the immune system. *Annual Review of Immunology* 5, 223.

Stein RC, Malkovska V, Morgan S et al. (1991) The

clinical effects of prolonged treatment of patients with advanced cancer with low-dose subcutaneous interleukin-2. *British Journal of Cancer* 63, 275.

Steis RG, Smith JW, Urbar WJ et al. (1988) Resistance to recombinant interferon alpha-2a in hairy cell leukaemia associated with neutralizing anti-interferon antibodies. *New England Journal of Medicine* 318, 1409.

Stevenson GT, Stevenson FK (1975) Antibody to a molecularly-defined antigen confined to a tumour cell surface. *Nature* 254, 714.

Stotter H, Weibke EA, Tomita S (1989) Cytokines alter target cell susceptibility to lysis. II: Evaluation of tumour infiltrating lymphocytes. *Journal of Immunology* 142, 1767.

Stutman O (1982) Natural cell-mediated cytotoxicity against tumors in mice. In: Serrou B, Rosenfeld C, Herberman RB (eds) *Human Cancer Immunology Vol. 4: Natural Killer Cells.* Elsevier Biomedical Press, Amsterdam, p. 205.

Stutman O, Paige CT, Figarella EF (1978) Natural cytotoxic cells against solid tumors in mice. I. Strain and age distribution and target cell susceptibility. *Journal of Immunology* 121, 1819.

Sullivan JL (1988) Epstein Barr virus and lymphoproliferative disorders. *Seminars in Hematology* 25, 269.

Swan F, Manning J, Ordonez N et al. (1991) The effect of MHC class 1 expression on survival in patients with large cell lymphoma (LCL). *Blood* 78 (suppl 1), 123a.

Takihara Y, Reimann J, Michalopoulos E et al. (1989) Diversity and structure of human T-cell receptor δ-chain genes in peripheral blood γ/δ-bearing T-lymphocytes. *Journal of Experimental Medicine* 169, 393.

Talmadge JE, Phillips H, Schindler J (1987) Systematic pre-clinical study on the therapeutic properties of recombinant human interleukin-2 for the treatment of metastatic disease. *Cancer Research* 47, 5725.

Talpaz AM, Kantarjian HM, Kurzrock R et al. (1988) Therapy of chronic myelogenous leukaemia: chemotherapy and interferons. *Seminars in Hematology* 25, 62.

The TNF/TIL Human Gene Therapy Clinical Protocol (1990) *Human Gene Therapy* 1, 441.

Thomas JA, Hotchin NA, Allday MJ et al. (1990) Immunohistology of Epstein–Barr virus-associated antigens in B cell disorders from immunocompromised individuals. *Transplantation* 49, 944.

Thompson JA, Peace DJ, Klarnet JP et al. (1986) Eradication of disseminated murine leukaemia by treatment with high dose interleukin-2. *Journal of Immunology* 137, 3675.

Tichelli A (1989) Treatment of thrombocytosis in myeloproliferative disorders with interferon-alpha. *Blut* 58, 15.

Topalian SL, Solomon D, Avis FP et al. (1988) Immunotherapy of patients with advanced cancer using tumour infiltrating lymphocytes and recombinant interleukin-2: a pilot study. *Journal of Clinical Oncology* 6, 839.

Tsudo M, Kitamura F, Miyasaka M (1989) Characterisation of the interleukin-2 receptor beta chain using three distinct monoclonal antibodies. *Proceedings of the National Academy of Sciences of the USA* 86, 1982.

Uhr JW (1984) Immunotoxins: harnessing nature's poisons. *Journal of Immunology* 133, i.

Van Kooyk Y, Van De Wiel-Van Kemenade P, Weder P et al. (1989) Enhancement of LFA-1 mediated cell adhesion by triggering through CD2 or CD3 on T lymphocytes. *Nature* 342, 811.

Veals SA, Kessler DS, Josiah S et al. (1991) Signal transduction pathway activating interferon-alpha-stimulated gene expression. *British Journal of Haematology* 79 (suppl 1), 9.

Vinci G, Vernant JP, Cordonnier C et al. (1987) In vitro inhibition of hematopoiesis by HNK 1, DR-positive T cells and monocytes after allogeneic bone marrow transplantation. *Experimental Hematology* 15, 54.

Vinci G, Vernant JP, Nakazawa M et al. (1988) In vitro inhibition of normal human hematopoiesis by marrow CD3+, CD8+, HLA-DR+, HNK1+ lymphocytes. *Blood* 72, 1616.

Visani G, Delwel R, Touw I et al. (1987) Membrane receptors for interleukin 2 on hematopoietic precursors in chronic myeloid leukaemia. *Blood* 68, 1182.

Vitetta ES, Fulton RJ, May RD et al. (1987) Redesigning nature's poisons to create anti-tumour reagents. *Science* 238, 1098.

Vogetseder W, Feichtinger H, Schulz TF et al. (1989) Expression of 7F7-antigen: a human adhesion molecule identical to ICAM-1 in human carcinomas and their stromal fibroblasts. *Journal of International Cancer* 43, 768.

Voogt PJ, Falkenburg JHF, Fibbe WE et al. (1989) Normal hematopoietic progenitor cells and malignant lymphohematopoietic cells show different susceptibility to direct cell-mediated MHC-nonrestricted lysis by T cells receptor-/CD3−, T cell receptor-δϑ+/CD3+ and T cell receptor-αβ+/CD3+ lymphocytes. *Journal of Immunology* 142, 1774.

Vose BM, Bonnard GD (1982) Human tumor antigens defined by cytotoxicity and proliferative response of cultured lymphoid cells. *Nature* 296, 359.

Walz G, Zanker B, Brand K et al. (1989) Sequential effects of interleukin 2-diphtheria toxin fusion protein on T-cell activation. *Proceedings of the National Academy of Sciences of the USA* 86, 9485.

Webb DSA, Gerrard TL (1990) IFN-alpha and IFN-gamma can affect both monocytes and tumor cells to modulate monocyte-mediated cytotoxicity. *Journal of Immunology* 144, 3643.

Weetman AP, Cohen S, Makgoba MW et al. (1989) Expression of an intercellular adhesion molecule, ICAM-1, by human thyroid cells. *Journal of Endocrinology* 122, 185.

West WH, Tauer KW, Yanelli JR et al. (1987) Constant infusion recombinant interleukin-2 in adoptive immunotherapy of advanced cancer. *New England Journal of Medicine* 316, 889.

Whitehead RP, Ward D, Hemingway L et al. (1990) Subcutaneous recombinant interleukin-2 in a dose escalating regimen in patients with metastatic renal

cell adenocarcinoma. *Cancer Research* 50, 6708.
Winkelhake JL, Stampfl S, Zimmerman RJ (1987) Synergistic effect of combination therapy with human recombinant interleukin 2 and tumor necrosis factor in murine tumor models. *Cancer Research* 47, 3948.
Wisniewski D, Strife A, Wachter M et al. (1985) Regulation of human peripheral blood erythroid burst-forming unit growth by T lymphocytes and T lymphocyte populations defined by OKT4 and OKT8 monoclonal antibodies. *Blood* 65, 456.
Wong GG, Clark SC (1988) Multiple actions of interleukin-6 within a cytokine network. *Immunology Today* 9, 137.
Zarling JM, Robins HI, Raich PC et al. (1978) Generation of cytotoxic T lymphocytes to autologous human leukemia cells by sensitization to pooled allogeneic normal cells. *Nature* 274, 269.
Ziegler JL (1991) Cancer in the immunocompromised host. In: Stites DP, Terr AL (eds) *Basic and Clinical Immunology*, 7th edn, Prentice Hall, London, p. 588.

Index

Page numbers in *italics* refer to figures and tables.

α₂-macroglobulin, 59, 60
α-fetoprotein, 325
α-helical cytokines, 20
ABC gene, 343
ABL gene, 158
ABMT *see* autologous bone marrow transplantation
acquired immune deficiency syndrome (AIDS), 282, 303, 309
acute lymphoblastic leukaemia (ALL), 2, 33, 75, 79, 88–90, 92, 93, 95, 96, 143–4, 156–78, 193, 229–36, 295
  adult, 96
  childhood, 141, 324
  stem cell derived, 78
  T cell, 81
  T-lineage, 295
  treatment problems, 97
  treatment schedule, 94
acute myeloid leukaemia (AML), 39, 76–88, 90, 97–107, 143–67, 179, 193, 204, 229, 282–327, 367
  clonality, 163
  diagnosis and prognosis, 165–6
  growth factors on, *294*
  hypoplastic, 307
  pathogenesis, 163–5
  treatment with HGF, 307–8
  treatment problems, 98
acute non-lymphoblastic leukaemia, 126
acute phase, protein, 87
acute promyelocytic leukaemia (APML), 39, 73, 82, 88, *101*, 152–3, 164, 181, 295
ADCC *see* antibody dependent cytotoxic cells
adenosine deaminase, 108
adenosine deaminase deficiency (ADA), 115–121, 180
adenosine triphosphate (ATP), 84, 150, 214, 343
adenovirus, 267
adenylate cyclase, 40, *41*, *42*
adhesion molecules, 177, 336, *337*, 337–9, 348
  cell adhesion, 54, 55, 336, 339, 348
    characteristics of, 338–9
  neural cell adhesion, 26, 350
  surface adhesion, 329
adult respiratory distress syndrome (ARDS), 288, 295, 307
agranulocytosis, 298
  idiosyncratic, 130
AIDS *see* acquired immune deficiency syndrome
ALL *see* acute lymphoblastic leukaemia
all-trans-retinoic acid (ATRA), 73, 82, *98*, 164
  and APML, 100–2
amidopyrine agranulocytosis, *131*, 132
AML *see* acute myeloid leukaemia
anaemia, 305, 309
  chemotherapy-induced, 303
  chronic, 303
  and cancer, *282*
  Diamond–Blackfan, 178
  post-chemotherapy, *282*
  renal disease, *282*
  Sl/SId, 289
  sickle cell, 181
  treatment with HGFs, 302–4
animal models,
  BMT, 195–200
  genetic disorders, *199*
  GvL, 227–8
  tumours, and IL-2, 370
antibody, 109, 287–8, 387
  anti-GM-CSF monoclonal, 21
  anti-IL-1 receptor, 287
  anti-IL-2 receptor, 287, 378
  antigens recognized by, 348
  artificial constructs, 389–90
  and leukaemia subgroups, *144*
  monoclonal, 4, 20, 30, 143, 326
    deficiencies in, 389
    modes of action of, 387–8
  polyclonal, 143
antibody dependent cytotoxic cells (ADCC), 331, 340–1, *349*, 357, 388, 391
antibody molecule, structure of, 172, *173*
antibody treatment,
  combinations, 394
  for haematological malignancies, *393*
  in vivo, 251
antibody-coated immunomagnetic beads, 52, 237
antigen, 74, 329
  carcinoembryonic, 325
  CD10, 77, 78
  CD13, 77, 78
  CD19, 77, 78
  CD33, 77, 78
  CD34, 4, 77, 78, 200, 201, 203, 204
  CD45 cell surface, 43
  CD5, 78
  CD7, 77, 78
  Class I, 83, 218, 219, *222*, 325
  DR, 246, 375
  endogenous, 344, 353
  exogenous, 353
  Hh, 216
  histocompatibility, 214
  human leukocyte (HLA), 169, 190, 191, 297, 335
  leukaemia and lymphoma cells, *346*
  MHC-restricted, 342
  minor, diversity of, 218
  minor histocompatibility, 214–17, 344, *345*, 345, 347
  oncofoetal, 342
  p24, 309
  retrovirally encoded, 345
  self-, 216, 342

Tac, 24, 59
transplantation, 211–12, 345
tumour, 216, 342
tumour specific (TSA), 342
Y chromosome determined (H–Y), 216, 217, 345
antigen presentation, 342–4, 344–7
antigen-presenting cells, 45
antigen-presenting groove, 217
antigen-processing,
  endogenous, 342, *343*
  exogenous, 342, *343*, 344
antilymphocyte globulin, 123, 125, 126, 251, 252, 255, 257
antimicrobial prophylaxis, 116
aplasia, 102
  chemotherapy-induced temporary, 89
  pure red cell, 115, 116
aplastic anaemia, *130–2*, 170, 178–9, 227, 203, 241, 246, 253, 257, *282*
  aetiology of, *123*
  diagnosis, 178
  and drug-induced cytopenias, 122–32
  with HGF, 297–9
  pathogenesis, 178–9
  pathophysiology of, 122–25
  severe (SAA), 190, 191, 206, 207, 253
  treatment, 125–7
APML *see* acute promyelocytic leukaemia
apoptosis, 46, 175, *351*, 353
ARDS *see* adult respiratory distress syndrome
arthritis, 49, 287, 288, 293, 295, 303
athymic (nu gene), 198
ATP *see* adenosine triphosphate
ATRA *see* all-trans-retinoic acid
autocrine stimulation, 163, 164, 175, 291
autoimmune disease, 9, *262*, 287
autoradiography, 30, 145

β₂-interferon (IL-4), *3*
β₂-microglobulin, 213
B cell, 4–7, *31*, 50, 77, 79, 215, 218, 219, 250, 298, 341, 354
  cyclic adenosine monophosphate on, *42*
  Epstein-Barr virus transformed, 34, 338
  pre-, 48, 76
  transmembrane signalling in, 41
B cell activation, 47
B cell ALL, 175
B cell CLL, 175
B cell clone, malignant, 90
B cell colony formation, IL-7-induced, 47
B cell diseases, 75
B cell growth factor, 351
B cell leukaemia, 289
B cell lymphoma, 176
B cell malignancy, *90*, *153*, *325*, *328*
B cell precursors, 15
B cell receptor gene rearrangement, 74
B lymphocytes *see* B cell
B lymphopoiesis, 7, 47
β-globin gene mutation, 180
β pleated sheet, 214, *216*

bacterial infection, 116, 259, 260, *265*, 298, 306–8, 340
bcl gene, 174, 175, 176, 177
BCR *see* break-point cluster region
beige mice, 326, *327*
BFU-E, 44–52, 115–16, 284, 301–3, 306, 312
biphenotypic leukaemia, 77–9
bladder cancer, 296
blast cell, 33, 45, 306, 307
blast colony, 5–7, 8, 54
Bloom's syndrome, *327*
Bone Marrow Transplant Registry (IBMTR), 191, 192
bone marrow transplantation (BMT), 85–115, 124–5, 147–52, 168–72, 190–270, 309, 324
  allogeneic *81*–100, *90*, 111, 190, 191, *196*, 207–81, 208, 224, 371, 376
    cure of leukaemia by, 225–33
  autologous, 73, 81, 92–100, 167, 177, 191, 208, 224, 258
    stem cell, 86
  changes in outcome, 193–4
  chimerism, 169–70
  complications, 171
  donor selection, 168–9
  graft failure, 170–1
  and HGFs, 311–14
  infections after, 258–66, 268–70
  marrow, 87, 89
  metabolic disturbance after, 242
  modification to, *195*
  non-haematological complications, 266–70
  purging, 171–2
  relapse, 171
  and second malignancies, *270*
  sources of stem cells for, 202
  syngeneic, 194
  timing of, 242
  viral infections after, 262–3
bone marrow transplantation (BMT) animal models of, 195–200
bone marrow transplantation (BMT) in aplastic anaemia, 126–7
bone marrow transplantation (BMT) conditions, 232–3
BPA *see* burst-promoting activity
break-point cluster region (BCR), 88, 90, 96, 103, 152–8, 175, 181, 346, 366
bronchiolitis, obstructive, 247
Bruton-type agammaglobulinaemia, 114
Burkitt-type lymphoma, 34, 81, 174, 175
burst-promoting activity (BPA), *3*, 12, 45, 51

c-fms (growth factor receptor gene), *153*, 164, 166, 168
c-fos gene, 168
c-kit, 2, 23
c-kit ligand (Steel factor), *3*
c-myc (nuclear proteins), *153*, 166, 168
c-sis (growth factor gene), 153
c-src (cytoplasmic protein tyrosine kinase), *153*
calcium pump, *42*, 151
Calmette–Guerin bacillus (BCG), 100, 324

CAM *see* cell adhesion molecule
cancer, 303
   bladder, 296
   breast, 296, 312
   and chronic anaemia, *282*
   gastrointestinal, 311
   lung, 296
   small cell, *31*
   treatment, 128–30
carcinoembryonic antigen, 325
Castleman's disease, 288
cDNA, 10–17, 25, 26, 28, 36, 220
   cloned, 37
   murine (IL-3), 13
cDNA clone, 12, 13
cell adhesion molecule (CAM), 54, *57*, 155, 293
cell death (apoptosis), 46, 175, 351, 353
central nervous system (CNS), 94
   relapse of, 95
CFU-E *see* erythroid colony forming cells
Chediak–Highashi disease, *114*, *119*, *327*, 352
chemotherapeutic agents, *237*
chemotherapeutic drug resistance, 73
chemotherapy 81–96, 102–30, 141, 166–8, 176, 295, 302–13, 353
   consolidation, 95
   and cure, 89
   cyclical, *85*
   cytotoxic, 308
   designing schedules, 90–3
   high-dose, 100, 190, 315
      and radiation, 253, 268
      and radiotherapy, 225
   high-intensity remission-induction, 83
   and IL-2, 378
   induction, 307
   intensive and unselective, 97
   low-dose cytotoxic, 306
   maintenance, 99
   MOPP, *112*
   post-remission, 99–100
   remission-induction, 307
   stem cell toxic, and radiotherapy, 234
   value of HGF in, 309–11
chemotherapy and radiation, *258*
chemotherapy-cytokine treatment, 393–4
chemotherapy-induced anaemia, 303
   aplasia, 89
chemotherapy-resistant relapse, 83
chimerism,
   and bone marrow transplantation (BMT), 169–70, 235
   and graft take, 256
   lineage-specific, 170
   split, 240
cholesterol, 284
   serum, 283
chondroitin sulphate, 28
chromium release assay, 223, 333
chromosome, 39, 77, 147, 165
   Philadelphia (Ph), 103, 142, *145*, 156, 157, 163
   translocations, 141, 142, 148

   Y, 39, 170
chromosome analysis, 74
chromosome translocation, 88
chronic granulomatous disease, *113*, *114*
chronic lymphocytic leukaemia (CLL), 80–5, *93*, 107, *153*, 287, 365
chronic myeloid leukaemia (CML) 28, 32, 76–93, 103–5, *142–62*, 171, 181, 192, 227–35, *327*, 342, 365–6
   BCR-ABL in, 74
   clonality of, 158
   detection and management of residual disease, 160–2
   pathogenicity of, 158–9
   Ph positive progenitor cells in, 79
   prognosis of, 159–60
   treatment strategies, *104*
chronic myelomonocytic leukaemia (CMML), *142*
cirrhosis, 247, *269*
cis-acting promotor elements, 155
cisplatin, 154, 311
class II, gene, 213
clone, GvL-reacting, 228
CML *see* chronic myeloid leukaemia
CMML *see* chronic myelomonocytic leukaemia
CMV *see* cytomegalovirus
co-trimoxazole, 116, 211, 252, 262
codon, 164
colitis, immune complex-induced, 287
compatibility testing, 220–24, *221*
complement fixation, 387–8
complementary DNA *see* cDNA
concanavalin A, 14, 48
conditioning regimens, 194, 240–2
congenital agranulocytosis *see* Kostmann's syndrome
congenital bone marrow disorders, 112–122
congenital disorders, *197*
congenital immune deficiency, 254
congenital neutropenia, *114*
   G-CSF in, 116
consolidation, of treatment, 99
Cos cell, 12, 15, 16, 23, 34, 26
cross-linking, chemical, 35
CTL *see* cytotoxic T lymphocyte
CTLp *see* cytotoxic T lymphocyte precursor
cure, *85*, 89–90
   definition of, 89
cyclosporin 84, 90, 100, 116, 123–5, 192, 235–57, 267, 270
cysteine residues (CCCC), 11, 21
cytogenetics blood and marrow cells, 87
cytokine synthesis inhibitory factor (CSIF), 3, 16
cytokines, 2, 16–19, 45, 58, 86, 112, 113–16, 117, *123*, 196, 211, 326–32, 348–9, 355
   α-helical, 20
   combinations, 394
   and interleukins, 355–8, 378
   regulation, 350
   in treatment, 357
cytomegalovirus (CMV), 169–71, 210, 259–65, 267
   immunoglobulin, 263

cytopenia, 130, 131, 305
    autoimmune, 247
    chemotherapy-induced, 314
    drug-induced, 127–32
        and aplastic anaemia, 122–32
        from idiosyncracy to drugs, 130
    immune, 131
    management of, 103
    post (BMT), 282
    post-chemotherapy, 282
cytotoxic chemotherapy, 197, 207
cytotoxic lymphocytes, 232, 255
cytotoxic T lymphocyte precursors (CTLp), 223, 224, 330, 331
cytotoxicity,
    antibody-dependent cellular, 305
    antitumour, 349
    binding sites for, 341
    improved, 390–1
cytotoxicity assay, 222, 331–3

Daudi lymphoma cell line, 331, 335, 347, 375
daunorubicin, 91, 94, 95, 98
deoxyhaemoglobin S, 303
deoxyribose-nucleic-acid see DNA
Dexter's long-term bone marrow culture system, 3
DIA see differentiation inhibiting activity
Diamond–Blackfan anaemia, 178
differentiation inhibiting activity (DIA), 3, 49
diphtheria toxin, 287, 392
disulphide bridge, 11, 19, 172
DNA, 9, 117, 146, 163, 219, 241
    binding protein, 4, 155
    fingerprinting method, 147
    human, 391
    insertion, 121
    methylation, 4
    packaging, 151
    probe, 170
    repair, 327
        genetical defects in, 180
    synthesis, 47
    transfected, 119, 151
    viral, 359
    viruses, 211, 262
    X-linked, 179
DNAse 1 hypersensitivity, 4
donor immune cells, 100
donor lymphocytes, 256–7
donor selection, and BMT, 168–9
donor T cell-mediated immune regulation, 104
donor T lymphocyte transfusion, 105
dot blot hybridization, 180
Down's syndrome, haemopoiesis in, 180
DRbl, gene, 220
drug-induced idiosyncratic cytopenia, 132
dyskeratosis, 178, 262

E2A, gene, 176
E-CFC see erythroid colony-forming cells

EBMT see European Cooperative Group for Bone Marrow Transplantation
EBV see Epstein-Barr virus
ECM see extracellular matrix
electron microscopy, 165
electroporation, 151, 152
ELISA see enzyme-linked immunosorbent assay
endonuclease, methylation-sensitive, 147
endoplasmic reticulum, 13, 213, 214
endothelial cells, 7
    human umbilical vein, 53
    retrovirus-immortalized, 53
    sinusoidal, 55
engraftment, 204–5
enzyme-linked immunosorbent assay (ELISA), 3
Eo-CSF see eosinophil colony-stimulating factor
eosinophil, 31–3, 45, 56, 156, 283–6, 290–2, 298, 300, 354
eosinophil colony-stimulating factor (Eo-CSF), 3, 46, 52
Epstein-Barr virus (EBV), 16, 226, 264, 325
    B cells, 34, 162, 328, 361
    related lymphoma, 270, 327
erythroid burst-promoting activity, 5, 311
erythroid cells, 4, 144
erythroid colony-forming cells (CFU-E), 29, 33, 105, 115, 306, 369
erythroid progenitors, 31, 77
erythroleukaemia, 105, 144, 163
erythropoiesis (BFU-E), 47, 77, 102, 115, 117, 205, 283, 304
erythropoietin 8–35, 46–51, 105, 116, 124, 206, 282–314, 316
    biotinylated, 36
    human, recombinant, 302
    receptor, 21, 24, 29, 33, 35, 40
essential thrombocythaemia (ET), 77, 105, 106, 162
exon, 9, 14, 213, 220
extracellular matrix (ECM), 57–8

FAB see French-American-British classification
FACs cell sorting, 235
factor-dependent myeloid cell lines, 291
Fanconi anaemia, 112–17, 125, 130–2, 178–80, 194, 204, 241–2, 327
Fc immunoglobulin region, 354
    receptor binding, 341
Felty's syndrome, 301
fetal liver, 203–4
fibroblast, 7, 24, 31, 50, 53, 58
fibroblast growth factor (bFGF), 58
fingerprinting method, DNA, 147
flow cytometry, 7, 87, 143
fluorescent in situ hybridization, 74
fluorescent-activated cell sorter (FACS), 88, 235
fms, gene, 167
French-American-British classification (FAB), of leukaemia, 144, 295
Friend erythroleukaemia virus, 105, 360
fungal infection, 116–17, 259, 260, 265, 282, 298, 308, 340

fusion protein, 176

G6PD *see* glucose-6-phosphate dehydrogenase
G protein-linked receptors, 28
G proteins, *42*
G-CSF *see* granulocyte colony-stimulating factor
GAG *see* glycosaminoglycan
Gaucher's disease, *114*
GC *see* guanosine-cytosine pairs
gel electrophoresis, 15, 149
GEMM-CFC, 44, 48, 52, 311
gene insertion, *120*
gene therapy, 117–22, 121–2
gene transfer, 152
genes, of special interest, 152–6
genetic markers, 152
genome libraries, 12
Glanzmann's disease, *113, 114, 180*
glucose-6-phosphate dehydrogenase (G6PD), 77, 103, 126, 149, 162, 179
glycogen storage disease, *282*, 300
glycoprotein, 21–2, 26
glycosaminoglycan (GAG), *54*, 57, 58
glycosylation, 11, 18–19, 35, 293
  N-linked, 12, 16, 17
  O-linked, 12, 15, 26
GM-CSF *see* granulocyte-macrophage colony-stimulating factor
Golgi, *13*, 343
graft failure, 169, 253–8
  and bone marrow transplantation (BMT), 170–1
  conditions predisposing to, 253–6
  risk factors for, *254*
graft rejection, 220, 340
  mechanisms of, *255*
  treatment of, 257–8
graft versus leukaemia (GvL), 195, 199, 212, 215, 225–7, 231–5, 325, 334, 345–7, 355, 370, 386
  and cure of malignant disease, 227–31
  in humans, 227
graft-versus-host disease (GVHD) 171, 190–233, 242–6, 266–87, 325, 340, 370
  acute, 198, 210, 243, 252, 259, *261*
    amplification, 245
    effector mechanisms, 245–6
    initiation, 245
    pathophysiology of, 245–8
  agents blocking, 251
  autologous, 234
  chronic, 198–9, 210, *243*, 247–8, 252, 259, 261
    immune deficiency and infection, *262*
  combination treatment for, 251
  cytokines in, 246–7
  and graft take, 256
  and haemopoietic recovery, *207*
  prevention and treatment, 195, 248–52
granulocyte function defects, *113*
granulocyte-macrophage colony-stimulating factor (GM-CSF), 1–19, 26–60, 98–132, 164, 262–351
  binding, protein, 36
  receptor, 39

granulocytosis, peripheral, 281
granulopoiesis, 77, 87, 101, 102, 105, 115, 132, 205
granzymes, *351*, 352
GroEl chaperonin, 60, *226*
growth factor, 115–16, 125, *197*
  and aplastic anaemia, 127
  binding,
    to receptors, kinetics of, 28–30
    to soluble protein, 41, 59
    to soluble receptors, 59–60
  on colony formation, in Ogawa's blast colony assay, *5*
  defects of, and microenvironment, 124
  genes, 9, 37–40, 56, 164
    chromosomal localization of, 37–40
  haemopoietic, 10
  independent colonies, 290
  interactions, 11
    complex, 57
  levels, regulation of, *59*
  membrane-bound, *57*, 58–9
  models for immobilization of, *57*
  modified, 286–7
  modulation, 58
  molecular biology of, and their receptors, 10–43
  production, 47
  receptors, 30–5, 57, 215
    factors affecting, *54*
  recombinant, 326
  response, 53–60
  soluble, 10, *59*
  target cell interactions, 43–60
  therapy, 288–9
guanine nucleotide regulatory proteins, *42*
guanosine triphosphate, 40, *42*
  dependent coupling, 40

H-*ras* gene, 165, 168
haematological malignancies, 142, 355
  antibody treatment for, *393*
  cure by autologous BMT, 233–8
  genes in, *153*
  immune responses against, 348–9
  mechanisms of cure, *90*
  with study of immune interactions, 329–36
haematological recovery,
  after BMT, 205–6
  factors affecting, 206–8
haematopoietin receptor superfamily, 21, 23, 24, 25, 26
haemoglobin F (HbF), 303
haemoglobinopathies, 112, *113*, 179–80
haemoietic growth factor/interleukin growth factors, 35
haemophilia, *180*
Haemophilus influenzae, 262
haemopoiesis, 3, 45–60, 86, 97, 128, 326
  clonal, 162, 179
  clonal pluripotent cell origin of, 77
  in Down's syndrome, *180*
  dysplastic, 78, 102
  growth factors in, *3*

and interleukin 2 (IL-2), 374–5
  monoclonal, 179
  normal, 73, 78, 80
  recovery after BMT, 204–6
  reinducing, 103
haemopoietic cell culture technology, 43
haemopoietic cells, 3, 30, 43
  adherent (cobblestone areas), 7–8
  malignant, 141
  non-adherent, 6
  signal transduction in, 42
haemopoietic colony formation, 3, 49–50
haemopoietic growth factor genes (HGF) 38
haemopoietic growth factor receptors (HGF), 11, 21–8, 30, 31
haemopoietic growth factors (HGF), 1, 10, 29, 41, 53, 73, 98–9, 281–8
  clinical application, 281–316
  experimental background, 288–292
  exposure to, 289–92
  human, and targets, 44–50
  molecular cloning of, and interleukins, 12–18
  and neutropenia, 299–301
  recombinant, 2
  therapy,
    clinical, 294–6, 296–314
    principles and practice of, 292–6
haemopoietic lineages, 112
haemopoietic microenvironment, 88, 123
haemopoietic precursors, 126
haemopoietic progenitor cells, 1, 6, 29, 40, 55, 119, 144
haemopoietic recovery, 258
  and cytotoxic drug dose, 129
  factors affecting pattern of, 207
  spontaneous recipient, 253
haemopoietic stem cells, 7, 54, 55, 86, 152
  measurement of, 4–9
haemopoietic system, 1
haemopoietic target cells, 40
hairy cell leukaemia (HCL), 73, 93, 108, 143, 156, 178, 208, 308, 361, 363–4
  interferon, in, 363–5, 384–5
haplotypes, 217
HbF see haemoglobin F
HCL see hairy cell leukaemia
helix, 20, 214, 216
heat shock proteins, 215
helix-loop-helix protein, 155
helix-turn-helix DNA-binding motif, 176
  protein, 155
helper T lymphocyte precursor (HTLp) assay, 330, 331
heparan sulphate, 28, 57
heparin, 59, 268
heparin-affinity chromatography, 58
hepatitis, 211, 258, 261, 265, 269
hepatocyte, 3, 31
herpes simplex virus (HSV), 210, 211, 253, 264, 265, 266
heterodimer, 17, 174, 338
  class 1, 343
HEV see high endothelial venule

HGF see haemopoietic growth factors
high endothelial venule (HEV), 155
HILDA see human interleukin for DA cells
histocompatibility, 197, 214, 345, 347
HIV see human immunodeficiency virus
HLA see human leukocyte antigen
Hodgkin's disease, 82, 83, 110–12, 142, 178
homeobox genes, 4, 155
homing receptor, 55, 155
homodimer, 17, 58
Hox gene, 2, 4
HPRT see hypoxanthine phosphoribosyl transferase
HTLp see helper T lymphocyte precursor
HTLV virus, 226
human β-globin gene, 119
human erythropoietin transgene, 291
human immune system, improving cooperation with, 391
human immuno-deficiency virus (HIV), 258, 261, 265, 303, 309, 327, 328
human interleukin for DA cells (HILDA), 3, 49
human leukocyte antigen (HLA), 115–16, 126, 190–1, 203, 212–13, 297, 335, 344
  antigen-antibody complexes, 220
  complex, 170
  disparity, donor-recipient, 195
  matched donor-recipient pairs, 194
  matched siblings, 245
  mismatched random pairing, 221
  restriction, 216
  serotyping, 219
  typing, 169, 217, 218
human urinary CSF, 311
Hurler's disease, 199, 239
hybrid receptor, 26
hybridoma fusion, 391
hypervariable region (HVR), 177
hypogammaglobulinaemia, 113, 262
hypoplastic myelodysplasia, 179
hyposplenism, 252, 261
hypoxanthine phosporibosyl transferase (HPRT), 119, 147, 167, 306

ICAM-1, 338, 339, 340, 348
idarubicin, 98, 98
idiopathic neutropenia, 282, 300–1
idiopathic pulmonary fibrosis, 49, 288
idiosyncratic marrow suppression, 130–2
IFNβ see interferon gene
IFNγ see interferon gene
IgA see immunoglobulin A
IgG see immunoglobulin G
IgM see immunoglobulin M
IL see interleukin
IL-7, 15–16, 19, 35, 42, 48, 58, 59
immune deficiency symdromes, severe, 217, 247
immune dysregulation, 209, 267
immune marrow suppression, 132
immune recovery,
  after BMT, 208–11
  factors affecting, 210–11
  treatment approaches to improve, 211
immune regulatory cells, autologous, 89

immune surveillance, 325
immune system, 88
  and haematological malignancies, 326-9
immune-mediated myelosuppression, 123-4
immunoglobulin A (IgA), 209, 261
  E (IgE), 47, 287
  G (IgG), 209, 391, 392
  G1 (IgG1), 47
  gene, 87, 153, 172, 175
  heavy chain, 75, 173, 177
  isotypes, 169
  M (IgM), 209, 388, 389
  superfamily, 22, 337
immunological recovery, 258
immunological techniques, 236-7
immunosuppressive agents, 125-6, 259, 261, 297
immunotherapy, 89, 92, 324-95, 355-93
  cellular and humeral approaches to, 349
infection,
  cytomegalovirus, 263-4
  from blood products, 258
  gram-negative, 259
  gram-positive, 259
  treatment with HGF, 308-9
infectious complications, 258-9
inherited deficiencies, 180-1
inositol lipids, hydrolysis of, 40
inositol phosphate metabolism, 42
integrins, 337, 338
intensity, of treatment, 95-6
interferon, 3, 10, 74-110, 104, 112, 160-2, 286, 304, 308, 326-67, 394
  in hairy cell leukaemia, 363-5
  IFNα, 10, 17, 49, 355
  IFNγ, 10-17, 35-7, 57, 102, 116-17, 210-19, 246, 336-8, 353, 358, 359
  and leukaemia cell lines, 82
  receptor, 26, 34
  stimulated genes (ISG), 358, 359
  stimulated response element (ISRE), 358, 360
interleukin 1 (IL-1), 1, 14-15, 22-58, 164-78, 257-94, 301, 336-73
interleukin 2 (IL-2), 6-47, 59, 93, 100-6, 156, 176, 210-51, 304-62, 350, 352, 353, 367-70, 368, 368-94, 393, 394
  in allogeneic BMT, 377
  and animal tumours, 370
  in autologous BMT, 377
  clinical trials of, 372-9
  intraperitoneal, 198, 199
  and its receptor, 369
  and subcutaneous low-dose, 378
  therapeutic index of, 378
interleukin 3 (IL-3), 3, 5-57, 102, 114-16, 121-7, 193, 211, 291, 298, 301-9, 369
interleukin 4 (IL-4), 3, 15, 21-35, 42, 47-8, 59, 206-91, 211, 382
interleukin 5 (IL-5), 24-41, 47-8, 369
interleukin 6 (IL-6), 5-51, 109, 164, 175, 269, 301-2, 382-3
interleukin-7 (IL-7), 15-19, 26, 35, 42, 58-9, 286
interleukin-8 (IL-8), 16, 34, 49, 288
interleukin 9 (IL-9), 3, 16, 37, 49

interleukin-10 (IL-10), 328
interleukin-11 (IL-11), 302
intermittent highdose treatment, 85
interstitial pneumonitis, 171, 191, 241, 263, 266, 267
intrathecal methotrexate (IT MTX), 94
intravenous immunoglobulin, 114
intron, 9, 10, 122
intron-exon organization, 15
iron chelation, 114, 117

K cells, 354
K-ras gene, 165
K-ras mutation, 163
Karnofsky performance score, 194
karyotype, 76, 144-5, 169
keratinocytes, 31, 223, 233, 246, 329
keratoconjunctivitis, 269
kinase C, 42
Kostmann's syndrome, 299
Krabbé disease, 200

LAD see leukocyte adhesion deficiency
LAK see lymphokine activated killer
Langerhans cell, 244, 262
LAP see leukocyte alkaline phosphatase
leucine zipper protein, 155
leukaemia, 9, 203, 237, 270, 307
  acute, 142, 160, 324, 352
    and, CML 371
    stem cell derived, 78
  biphenotypic, 77-9
  blast cells, 29, 33, 75, 371
  classification of, 143
  colony-forming cells, 79
  congenital and infant, 172, 176
  diversity of cell populations in, 79
  dysregulation, 79
  end-stage, 191
  French-American-British classification, 144
  promyelocytic see acute promyelocytic leukaemia
  stem cell, 8, 77-9, 81
  transgenic, in mice, 335
leukaemia inhibitory factor (LIF), 2, 3, 5, 17, 49, 56-7, 292
leukapheresis, 203, 314, 383
leukocyte adhesion deficiency (LAD), 180, 282, 300
leukocyte alkaline phosphatase (LAP), 156
leukocyte isoenzymes, 169
leukocytes, 239, 337
leukocytosis, 286, 289, 357
leukoencephalopathy, multifocal, 269
leukopenia, acute, 293
LFA-1, 338, 339, 340
LIF see leukaemia inhibitory factor
ligand, 21, 29, 354
  blotting technique, 36
  cognate, 21
  ECM cell adhesion, 57
  SCF/c/kit, 58
limiting dilution assay, 223
  technique, 227, 330

loop, immunoglobulin-like, 22
lung cancer, small cell, *31*
    adenocarcinoma, 296
lymphocyte, 29, *123*, 123, *222*, 233, 340
    accessory cell, 338
    activating factor (IL-1), *3*
    activation markers, 336
    allogeneic, 242
    alloreactive, 89, 325, 329, 386
    autologous, 329
    CD3 receptor, 249, 254
    depletion of, 249–50
    function, changes in, 375–6
    interaction with targets, 339–42
    ontogeny, 75
    retrovirus tagging of, *120*
    subset, 375–6
    T4, 340, 353
    T8, 340, 353
    target cell, 338
    tumour-specific, 384–5
lymphocytic lymphoma, small cell, 175
lymphocytotoxicity, 126
lymphoid atrophy, *262*
lymphoid chimerism, 198
lymphoid marker, 79
lymphoid neoplasia, 172–8, 175
    diagnosis/clonality, 172–4
    minimal residual disease, 177–8
    pathogenesis, 174–6
    prognosis, 176–7
lymphokine-activated killer cells (LAK), 9, 50, 100–10, 196, 228, 331–78
lymphoma, 75, 89, *90*, 236, 313
    B cell, 176, 371
    Burkitt-type, 81
    diffuse large cell, 91
    effect of IL-2 on, 370–2
    follicular, 178
    Hodgkin's, 82–3, 110–12, *142*, 178
    mantle zone, 175
    NHL, 93, 109–10, *111*, 154, 175, *270*, 313, 365, 376, 393
    ontogeny of, 74–5
    small cell lymphocytic, 175
    spontaneous, 352
    T cell, 371
    treatment by (IL-2), 376
lymphopenia, 126, 246, 374
lymphopoiesis, 7, 48, 50, 86
    regulation of, 52
lymphopoietic growth factors, 44
lymphoproliferative disorders, 365
lymphoreticular malignancy, 325
lymphotoxin, 18, 353, 379
Lyon hypothesis, 77

M-CSF *see* macrophage colony-stimulating factor
macrophage, 7, 14, *31*–2, 45–7, 56, *123*, 290, 341–54
    colony-stimulating factor (M-CSF), 2, 12–20, 39–58, *114*, *164*, 284–5, 308, 314, 382–4
        receptor, 167

magnetic resonance imaging (MRI), 151
maintenance, of treatment, 99
major break-point cluster region (M-BCR), 157, 159
major histocompatibility complex (MHC), 197–8, 212, 216–18, 253–4, 325–53, 361
    molecule, 218–19, 233, 341, 342, 346, 353
        structure, *215*
    molecule expression, failure of, 348
        function of, 214
        and minor histocompatibility antigens, 214–17
mantle zone lymphoma, 175
Maroteaux–Lamy disorder, *199*
marrow ablative treatment, 91
marrow aspiration, 141
marrow purging, 234, 236–8
marrow stromal cells, 52
mast cell growth factor (Steel factor), *3*
maturation-inducing agents, 89
MDR1 *see* multidrug-resistance gene
MDS *see* myelodysplastic syndrome
MECLR *see* mixed epidermal lymphocyte culture
megakaryoblastic cells, *144*
megakaryocyte (MK), *31*, 48, 76, 105, *106*, 124, 167, 200
    cell line, human, 16
    stimulating factors, 206
megakaryocytopoiesis (Mk-CFC), 48, 49, 77, 115, 283, 284, 302
melanoma, 296, 325, 345, 393
    malignant, 312
melphalan, 109, *128*, 267, 310, 311, 365
mesangial cells, *31*
messenger RNA *see* mRNA
metabolic disorders, *239*
MF *see* myelofibrosis
MHC *see* major histocompatibility complex
microglia, *239*
microinjection, *151*, 152
minimal residual disease (MRD), 90, 181
    and relapse, 87–8
Minor histocompatibility antigen system, 217, 218
mixed epidermal lymphocyte culture (MECLR), 223
mixed lymphocyte culture (MLC), 221
mixed lymphocyte reaction (MLR), 169
Mk-CFC *see* megakaryopoiesis
MLC *see* mixed lymphocyte reaction
MLR *see* mixed lymphocyte reaction
molecular mass (Mr), 35
monoclonal antibodies, 30, *248*, 250, 257, 326, 388, 389
    clinical applications of, 392–3
    therapeutic use of, 388–9
monocytes, *31*–3, 45, 52, 123, 167, 284, 293, 298, 340
monocytic leukaemia, 78
monocytosis, 86
monozygosity, in donor-recipient pairs, 169
MPD *see* myeloproliferative disorders
MRI *see* magnetic resonance imaging
mRNA, 7–17, 57, 157, 164, 175, 176
multi-colony-stimulating factor, *3*
multidrug resistance gene (MDR1), 3, 7, 84, *153*, 166, 168, 176

multiple drug-resistance gene (MDR), 76, 84–97,
    102–3, 123–6, 167–8, *282*, 304–5
myeloablative regimens, 191
myelodysplasia, 89, *123*, 124, 167–8, 304, 305
    clonality of, 167
    pathogenesis, 167–8
    prognosis, 168
    treatment with HGFs, 305–6
myelofibrosis (MF), 77, 85, 105, 206, 366
myeloid malignancies, 76–7
    phenotype and precursor origin, 76
myeloma, 75, *87*, *93*, 310
    multiple, 365
    treatment, *108*
myeloproliferative disorders (MPD), 76, 82, 158, 162–3,
    352, 366–7
    clonality, 162
    non-leukaemic, 105–7
    pathogenesis and prognosis, 163
    stem cell clone, *106*
    syndrome, 56, 291
    treatment, *106*
myelosuppression, 108, 128
    immune-mediated, 123–4

N-CAM *see* neuronal cell adhesion molecule
N-linked glycosylation, 16, 17
N-linked oligosaccharides, 19
N-*ras* gene, 165, 168
N-*ras* mutation, 163
NAP-1 *see* neutrophil activating protein
natural killer cell (NK), 9, *31*, 83, *90*, 105–6, 196,
    209–63, 298, 326–31, 349–58, 370
    ligand, *226*
    markers, 255
neo gene, 119
nerve growth factor receptor superfamily, 27
neural cell adhesion molecule, 26, 350
neuroblastoma, 236, 238
neuronal cell adhesion molecule, 26
neutropenia, 132, 259, 281, 289, 305–15, 357
    absolute, growth factors on, *312*
    amidopyrine-induced, *130*
    autoimmune, *128*
    congenital, 116, *282*, 299–300
    cyclic, *282*, 301
    growth factors and recovery from, *310*
    idiopathic, *282*, 300–1
    immune-mediated, 301
    treatment with HGFs, 299–301
neutrophil, 29–45, 53, 56, 101, 108, 116–17, 167, 208,
    284, 290–311, 354
    activating protein (NAP-1), 3
    chemotactic defect, 375
    CML 35, 29, *31*, 32, 45, 116, 290, 292, 293, 304
new typing technique, 219–20
NHL *see* non-Hodgkin's lymphoma
Niemann–Pick disorder, *199*
NK *see* natural killer cell
non-Hodgkin's lymphoma (NHL), 93, 109–11, 154, 175,
    270, 313, 365, 376, 393
non-immunological techniques, 237–8
non-malignant disorders,
    cure by BMT, 238–42
    with matched sibling donors, *196*
Northern analysis, 146–7, 175

nucleic acid hybridization technique, 164
nucleoside phosphorylase, 119
nude mice, athymic, 227, 228, *335*

O-linked glycosylation, 15, 26
objectives, of treatment, 84, *85*
Ogawa's blast colony assay, colony formation in, *5*
oligonucleotide probing, 219, *221*
oncogene, 154, 155
    recessive (tumour suppressor factor), 39
osteoclast, 3, 50
osteonecrosis, *269*
osteopetrosis, *113*, *114*, *199*, 200, 242

p53 gene, 165
pancreatitis, 56
pancytopenia, 85, 99, 126, *128*, 244, 253
    peripheral, 297
    progressive, 102
paracrine stimulation, 175
paraprotein analysis, 87
paroxysmal nocturnal haemoglobinuria (PNH), 126,
    179
PCR analysis, 230
PCR *see* polymerase chain reaction
PEG *see* polyethylene glycol
Pelger–Huet anomaly, 300
penicillin, 192, 252, 259, 262
peptide binding site, 215
peripheral blood, as sources of stem cells, 202
pertussis toxin, *42*, 42
PGK *see* phosphoglycerate kinase
PHA *see* phytohaemagglutinin
Philadelphia chromosome (Ph), 103, 142, *145*,
    150–9, 163, 175, 342
phorbol ester, 37, 82
phorbol myristate acetate, 116
phosphoglycerate kinase (PGK), 147, 167, 306
phosphorylation, tyrosine, 24, 43
phytohaemagglutinin (PHA), 209, 298
plasma cell dyscrasias, 175
plasma cell leukaemia, 288
platelet derived growth factor (PDGF), 7
platelet transfusion support, 206
PNH *see* paroxysmal nocturnal haemoglobinuria
polycythaemia vera (PV), 77, 105, 106, 162, 284, 285,
    291, 366
polymerase chain reaction (PCR), 87–8, 142–8,
    161–77, 180, 220, 230
PP *see* primary polycythaemia
prl gene, 176
probe,
    chromosome specific, 74
    minisatellite, 170
    oligonucleotide, 179, 180, 220
    recombinant DNA, 177
    synthetic oligonucleotide, 170
    synthetic primer, 220
prolactin receptor, 26
proliferative assays, 329–31
promyelocytic leukaemia *see* acute promyelocytic
    leukaemia

protein folding, 11, 19–20
protein G, 42
protein kinase (PK), 22, 42, 360
protein phosphorylation, *41*, *42*, 43, 150
protein tyrosine kinase (PTK), 22, 40, 41, 150, 175
protein tyrosine phosphatases, 40
proto-oncogenes, *153*, 166
PTK *see* protein tyrosine kinase
pulmonary fibrosis, idiopathic, 288
Purtillo's syndrome, *327*
PV *see* polycythaemia vera

radio-immunoassay (RIA), 3, 143, 149–50
radioreceptor-binding assays, 11
radiotherapy, 89, 91, 111
RAR chain, 164
RAR *see* retinoic acid receptor
RAR α/*myl* gene, 100, 152, 153, 181
ras gene, *153*, 160, 165, 346
ras gene family, 160
Rauscher virus leukaemia model, 227
RB gene, 169
RB *see* retinoblastoma gene
receptor,
　chain, 38
　colony-stimulating factor, 1, 21–3
　erythropoietin, 24, 29, 33, 35
　　human, 40
　GM-CSF down regulated, 36
　GM-CSF down regulated M-CSF, 36
　granulocyte colony-stimulating factor, 26, 32
　granulocyte macrophage colony-stimulating, 23–4, 32
　IL-1, 22–3, 33
　IL-2, 24–5, 33–4, 41
　IL-3, 24, 33, 41
　IL-4, 25, 34
　IL-5, 24, 25, 28, 34, 41
　IL-6, 26–7, 34
　IL-7, 34
　IL-8, 34
　immunoglobulin-like, 21–3
　interferon, 26, 34
　kinetics of growth factor binding to, 28–30
　M-CSF/CSF-1 (c-fms), 21–23, 32–33, 39, 40, 41
　PDGF, 39, 40
　SCF, 33
　SCF (c-kit), 41
　soluble, *59*
　　growth factor binding to, 59–60
　TGF, 28
　TNF, 27, 35
receptor binding, 20–1, 21
receptor characterization, 35–6
receptor genes,
　chromosomal localization of, 37–40
　human IFN, 40
receptor ligand studies, 11
receptor numbers and affinities, 32–5
receptor regulation, 36–7
receptor research, methods used in, 28–30
receptor TGF, 34–5
receptor-ligand complex, 29, 30

receptor-mediated protein tyrosine phosphorylation, 40
recombinant growth factors, 52
red cell aplasia, *114*, 128
refractory anaemia, 76
regulatory factors, and immune recovery, 206
relapse, 87–8, 161, 235
　and bone marrow transplantation (BMT), 171
　post-transplant cytogenetic, 105
remission,
　and all-trans-retinoic acid (ATRA), 101
　treatment after, 95
remission induction, 85, 85–7, 97–9, 102
　for acute myeloid leukaemia (AML), 91
　haematological changes during, 86
　marrow, 177
renal allograft rejection, 287
renal failure, *269*
　chronic, 303
residual disease detection technique, 87
restriction fragment length polymorphism (RFLP), 147, 152, 169, 179–80, 219–20, 306
reticular dysgenesis, *113*, 114
reticulocyte, 283, 284, 311
reticuloendothelial system, 83, 239
　cooperation with, 388
retinoblastoma gene (RB), 154, 175
retinoic acid receptor (RAR), 100, 102, 152, *153*, 181
retroviral ADA gene insertion, *114*
retroviral structure, 118, 291
retroviral vectors, *151*, 152
retrovirally encoded antigen, 345
retrovirus, 105, 118, 119, 172, 290
　modification, for gene transfer, 118
　structure of, *119*
　transforming, 106
reverse transcriptase, 105, 118
RFLP *see* restriction fragment length polymorphism
RIA *see* radio-immunoassay; radioimmunoassay
ribonucleic acid *see* RNA
ricin-conjugated antibodies, 250, 392
RNA, 119, 146, 163, 206
　viral, 118
RNA polymerase enzymes, 4
RNA tumour viruses, 154

SAA *see* severe aplastic anaemia
sarcoma, soft tissue, 310
Scatchard method, 29, 30, 34
SCF, 19, 20, 41, 49, 58
SCID mice, 196–8, 326, *327*, 335
SCID *see* severe combined immune deficiency; severe combined immunodeficiency syndromes
semisolid culture technology, 5
serine proteases and esterases, 351
serine/threonine phosphorylation, 42
serological typing methods, 219
serum-free culture conditions, influence of, 50–1
severe aplastic anaemia (SAA), 124, 126, 127, 298
severe combined immunodeficiency (SCID), 9, 114, 156, 191, 203, 240–1, 254, 326–7, 335, 340
sicca syndrome, 247, 262

sickle cell anaemia, *114*, 179, 181, 192, *282*, 303
  fetal haemoglobin production on, 117
sickle mice, *199*
signal sequence, *9*, 13
  hydrophobic, 11
signal transduction, *25*, 40–3
signal-transducing IL-1 receptor, 22
single high dose treatment, *85*
Southern analysis (blotting), *87*, 103, 145–7, 153, 158–9, 172, 177
spleen colony-forming cells (CFU-S), 6, 291
splenectomy, 108, 111, 242, 291, 364
Steel factor, 2, *3*, 14, 33, 46, 289
stem cell, 1, 6
  autologous, 233
  bone marrow,
    defects in, 191
    for bone marrow transplantation (BMT), 202
  defects, *113*, 124–5
  DNA, 124
  early haemopoietic, 5
  and engraftment, 200–4
  exhaustion, 315
  factor (SCF) (Steel factor), 2, *3*, 5, 14, 33, 46, 289, *294*
  haemopoietic, 7, 54, 152
  infection, 119–20, 121
  inhibitor, 58
  leukaemic, 77–9, *81*, 88
  normal, *81*, 86
  pluripotent, 78, *81*, 86, 118, 121, 122, 162
  retrovirus-infected, 291
  studies, and purging, *197*
  surface markers, 77
  transplantation, autologous, 86
stromal cell, 4, *6*, 6, 43, 55
stromal layers, colony formation on, 7–8
superantigen heat-shock protein, 347
surface marker studies, *87*, 165
SV-40 transfected epithelial cells, 53
Schwachmann–Diamond syndrome, 178

T cell, 4–6, 13, *31*–3, 48–50, 79, 118–20, 167, 192–3, 196, 216, *231*, 248–50, 298, 326–31, 336–8, 344, 353, 355, 370
  acute lymphoblastic leukaemia, 81
  clones, 233, 293
  colony formation, 47
  cytotoxic, 329
    suppressor, 336, 354
  depletion, 193, 249–50
  in facilitating graft take, 255–6
  functional defects, *113*
  growth factor, 14, 47
  helper cytotoxic, 336
  helper: suppressor, 309
  leukaemia/lymphoma, adult, 379
  lymphoma, 379
  malignancy, *153*
  non-alloreactive, 230
  phosphoinositide pathway in, *42*
  receptor (TCR), 75, *174*, 339
    gene, 87

  receptor (TCR) gene rearrangement, 74
T cytotoxic/suppressor cells, 375
T lymphocyte-depleted syngeneic marrow cells, 198
T lymphotropic virus, 1, 169
T suppressor cells,
  cytotoxic prethymic, 247
  donor, *262*
T-depleted syngeneic marrow, 199
Tac antigen, 24, 59
target cells, 1, 54, 60
TBI total body irradiation, fractionated, 226, 269
TCR *see* T cell receptor
TdT *see* terminal deoxyribosyltransferase
terminal deoxyribosyltransferase (TdT), 77, *78*
TGF *see* transforming growth factor
thalassaemia, *113*–14, 181, 192, 194, 238, 241, 269
thrombocythaemia (ET), 367
thrombocytopenia, *113*, *128*, 131, 305, *357*, 374
  treatment with HGFs, 301–2
thrombocytosis, *357*
thrombopoiesis, 87, 105, 117
thymidine uptake, tritiated, *222*
thymidine suicide technique, 302
thymus, atrophy of, 56
TIL *see* tumour-infiltrating lymphocyte
tissue antigens, diversity of, 217–18
tissue damage, after BMT, *269*
tissue typing and matching, 211–24
TNF *see* tumour necrosis factor
total body irradiation *see* TBI
toxicity, and HGF therapy, 293–4
transferrin receptor, 350
transforming growth factor (TGF), 2–3, 17, 28, 34–5, 45, 50, 58–9,355
transfusion, 102, *114*, 117
transgene,
  GM-CSF, 56
  HGF, 56
transgenic mice, 290, 315
translocation, 96, 174
transplantation antigens, 211–12, 345
tritiated thymidine, 329
  and autoradiography, 284
trophoblast, *31*, 32
TSA *see* tumour specific antigen
tumour,
  antigens, 216, 342
  bulk, 84
  cells, as targets for immune attack, 336–48, 389
  immunobiology, 326–55
    and clinical studies, 336
  markers, *153*
  regulation, role of NK cells in, 352–3
  solid, 9, *270*, 315
  suppressor gene, 39, *153*, 168
tumour necrosis factor (TNF), 17–18, 45–58, 110, *120*, 152, 210–304
  receptor, 27, 35
tumour-infiltrating lymphocyte (TIL), *120*, 150, *357*, 370, 386
tumour-specific antigens (TSAs), 342
tumour-specific immune cells, 383–6
tumour-specific lymphocytes, 384–5

twin, identical, as donor, 228
twitcher mouse, *199*
tyrosine kinase activity, 21, 22, 29, 41, *42*, 150, 157

umbilical cord blood, as sources of stem cells, 204
urokinase, inhibitor of, 156

veno-occlusive disease, 266, 268
viral infection, 209, *265*
  and haemopoietic recovery, *207*, 260
viral infections, after BMT, 262–3
viral neoantigens, 334
virus, 344
  DNA, GVHD and GVL, 264
  EBV, 16, *226*, 264, 270, 325, 329
  Friend erythroleukaemia, 105, 360
  GP55 glycoprotein, 105
  hepatitis, 261
  herpes group, infections with, 264
  HIV, *258*, 265, 303, 309
  HSV, 210, 211, 253, 264, 265, 266
  HTLV, *226*
  influenza, 358
  oncogenic, 344
  RNA tumour, 154
  T lymphotropic, 1, 169

VZV, 210, 252, 264, 265
vitamin D3, 82
volunteer donors, unrelated, 224
von Willebrand disease, *180*

W locus, 2
Waldenstrom's macroglobulinaemia, *75*, 175
western analysis, 149
Western blotting, 143, 175
Whitlock-Witte cultures, 50
Wiskott-Aldrich disease, 1, *114*, 254, *327*
Wolman's disease, 242

X chromosome, 39, 77
X-linked chronic granulomatous disease, *180*
X-linked lymphoproliferative syndrome, 328
xenograft resistance, 196
Xenopus oocytes, 11, 15
xeroderma pigmentosum, *180*
xid gene, 197

Y chromosome, 39, 170
Y chromosome determined antigens (H-Y), 216, 217, 345

zinc finger protein, 155